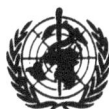

WORLD HEALTH ORGANIZATION

INTERNATIONAL AGENCY FOR RESEARCH ON CANCER

IARC MONOGRAPHS

ON THE

EVALUATION OF CARCINOGENIC

RISKS TO HUMANS

Hormonal Contraception and Post-menopausal Hormonal Therapy

VOLUME 72

This publication represents the views and expert opinions
of an IARC Working Group on the
Evaluation of Carcinogenic Risks to Humans,
which met in Lyon,

2–9 June 1998

1999

IARC MONOGRAPHS

In 1969, the International Agency for Research on Cancer (IARC) initiated a programme on the evaluation of the carcinogenic risk of chemicals to humans involving the production of critically evaluated monographs on individual chemicals. The programme was subsequently expanded to include evaluations of carcinogenic risks associated with exposures to complex mixtures, life-style factors and biological agents, as well as those in specific occupations.

The objective of the programme is to elaborate and publish in the form of monographs critical reviews of data on carcinogenicity for agents to which humans are known to be exposed and on specific exposure situations; to evaluate these data in terms of human risk with the help of international working groups of experts in chemical carcinogenesis and related fields; and to indicate where additional research efforts are needed.

The lists of IARC evaluations are regularly updated and are available on Internet: http://www.iarc.fr/.

This project was supported by Cooperative Agreement 5 UO1 CA33193 awarded by the United States National Cancer Institute, Department of Health and Human Services. Additional support has been provided since 1986 by the European Commission, since 1993 by the United States National Institute of Environmental Health Sciences and since 1995 by the United States Environmental Protection Agency through Cooperative Agreement Assistance CR 824264.

IARC Library Cataloguing in Publication Data

Hormonal contraception and post-menopausal hormonal therapy /
    IARC Working Group on the Evaluation of Carcinogenic
    Risks to Humans (1999 : Lyon, France).

    (IARC monographs on the evaluation of carcinogenic risks to humans ; 72)

    1. Carcinogens – congresses 2. Hormones – therapeutic use
    I. IARC Working Group on the Evaluation of Carcinogenic Risks to Humans
    II. Series

    ISBN 92 832 1272 X   (NLM Classification: W1)
    ISSN 1017-1606

PRINTED IN FRANCE

CONTENTS

NOTE TO THE READER

The term 'carcinogenic risk' in the *IARC Monographs* series is taken to mean the probability that exposure to an agent will lead to cancer in humans.

Inclusion of an agent in the *Monographs* does not imply that it is a carcinogen, only that the published data have been examined. Equally, the fact that an agent has not yet been evaluated in a monograph does not mean that it is not carcinogenic.

The evaluations of carcinogenic risk are made by international working groups of independent scientists and are qualitative in nature. No recommendation is given for regulation or legislation.

Anyone who is aware of published data that may alter the evaluation of the carcinogenic risk of an agent to humans is encouraged to make this information available to the Unit of Carcinogen Identification and Evaluation, International Agency for Research on Cancer, 150 cours Albert Thomas, 69372 Lyon Cedex 08, France, in order that the agent may be considered for re-evaluation by a future Working Group.

Although every effort is made to prepare the monographs as accurately as possible, mistakes may occur. Readers are requested to communicate any errors to the Unit of Carcinogen Identification and Evaluation, so that corrections can be reported in future volumes.

IARC WORKING GROUP ON HORMONAL CONTRACEPTION AND POST-MENOPAUSAL HORMONAL THERAPY

Lyon, 2–9 June 1998

LIST OF PARTICIPANTS

Members

R.A. Baan[1], Hammarskjoldlaan 47, 2286 GX Rijswijk, The Netherlands

E. Barrett-Connor, Division of Epidemiology, Department of Family and Preventive Medicine, University of California, 9500 Gilman Drive—Mail Code 0607, San Diego School of Medicine, La Jolla, CA 92093-0607, United States

V. Beral, Cancer Epidemiology Unit, Imperial Cancer Research Fund, University of Oxford, Gibson Building, The Radcliffe Infirmary, Oxford OX2 6HE, United Kingdom

M.C. Bosland, Nelson Institute of Environmental Medicine, NYU Medical Center, Long Meadow Road, Tuxedo, NY 10987, United States

L. Cook[2], Fred Hutchinson Cancer Research Center, 1124 Columbia Street, Seattle, WA 98104, United States

S. Franceschi, Epidemiology Unit, Aviano Cancer Centre, via Pedemontana Occidentale 12, 33081 Aviano PN, Italy

E. Hirvonen, Department of Obstetrics and Gynecology, Helsinki University Central Hospital, Annankatu 15 B 16, 00120 Helsinki, Finland

A. Jordan, Division of Reproductive and Urologic Drug Products, Center for Drug Evaluation and Research, Food and Drug Administration, HFD-580, 5600 Fishers Lane, Rockville, MD 20857, United States

D.G. Kaufman, Department of Pathology, University of North Carolina at Chapel Hill, School of Medicine, 515 Brinkhous-Bullitt Building, CB 7525, Chapel Hill, NC 27599-7525, United States

T. Key, Cancer Epidemiology Unit, Imperial Cancer Research Fund, University of Oxford, Gibson Building, The Radcliffe Infirmary, Oxford OX2 6HE, United Kingdom

R.J.B. King, School of Biological Sciences, University of Surrey, Guildford GU2 5XH, United Kingdom

---

[1] Present address: Unit of Carcinogen Identification and Evaluation, IARC

[2] Present address: Department of Community Health Sciences, The University of Calgary, 3330 Hospital Drive NW, Calgary, Alberta T2N 4N1, Canada

C. La Vecchia, Institute of Pharmacological Research 'Mario Negri', via Eritrea 62, 20157 Milan, Italy (*Chairperson*)

P. Lumbiganon, Department of Obstetrics and Gynecology, Faculty of Medicine, Khon Kaen University, Khon Kaen 40002, Thailand

R. Luoto, Department of Epidemiology and Health Promotion, National Public Health Institute, Mannerheimintie 166, 00300 Helsinki, Finland

O. Meirik, Unit for Epidemiological Research, United Nations Development Programme, United Nations Family Planning Agency, World Health Organization, World Bank Special Programme of Research, Development and Research Training in Human Reproduction, World Health Organization, 1211 Geneva 27, Switzerland

K. Mitsumori, Division of Pathology, National Institute of Health Sciences, 1-18-1 Kamiyoga, Setagaya-ku, Tokyo 158, Japan

A. Molinolo, Hormonal Carcinogenesis Laboratory, Institute of Experimental Biology and Medicine CONICET, Vuelta de Obligado 2490, 1428 Buenos Aires, Argentina

H. Olsson, Department of Oncology, University Hospital, 22185 Lund, Sweden

I.R. Persson, Department of Medical Epidemiology, Karolinska Institute, PO Box 281, 171 77 Stockholm, Sweden

L. Rosenberg, Slone Epidemiology Unit, Boston University School of Medicine, 1371 Beacon Street, Brookline, MA 02146, United States

D. Roy, Department of Environmental Health Sciences, University of Alabama, 1665 University Boulevard, Ryals Building No. 309E, Birmingham, AL 35294, United States

H. Seifried, Chemical and Physical Carcinogenesis Branch, National Cancer Institute, 6006 Executive Boulevard, Suite 220—MSC 7055, Bethesda, MD 20892-7055, United States (*and Representative of the National Cancer Institute*)

F. Sullivan, Harrington House, 8 Harrington Road, Brighton BN1 6RE, East Sussex, United Kingdom

D.B. Thomas, Program in Epidemiology, Fred Hutchinson Cancer Research Center, 1100 Fairview Avenue North, MP-474, Seattle, WA 98109, United States

J.D. Yager, Department of Environmental Health Sciences, School of Hygiene and Public Health, Johns Hopkins University, 615 North Wolfe Street, Baltimore, MD 21205-2179, United States

Secretariat

E. Banks, Cancer Epidemiology Unit, Imperial Cancer Research Fund, University of Oxford, Gibson Building, The Radcliffe Infirmary, Oxford OX2 6HE, United Kingdom

H. Jernström, Department of Family and Preventive Medicine, University of California, 9500 Gilman Drive—Mailcode 0607, San Diego, La Jolla, CA 92093-0607, United States

E. Heseltine, 24290 St Léon-sur-Vézère, France (*Editor*)

IARC

M. Blettner[1], Unit of Carcinogen Identification and Evaluation (*Responsible Officer*)

C. Genevois-Charmeau, Unit of Carcinogen Identification and Evaluation

Y. Grosse, Unit of Carcinogen Identification and Evaluation

S. Klug, Unit of Field and Intervention Studies

D. McGregor, Unit of Carcinogen Identification and Evaluation

N. Muñoz, Unit of Field and Intervention Studies

C. Partensky, Unit of Carcinogen Identification and Evaluation

I. Persson, Unit of Multistage Carcinogenesis

B. Rachet, Programme of Epidemiology for Cancer Prevention

J. Rice, Unit of Carcinogen Identification and Evaluation (*Head of Programme*)

A. Sasco, Programme of Epidemiology for Cancer Prevention

J. Smith, Unit of Field and Intervention Studies

J. Wilbourn, Unit of Carcinogen Identification and Evaluation

Technical assistance

M. Lézère

A. Meneghel

D. Mietton

J. Mitchell

S. Reynaud

S. Ruiz

J. Thévenoux

---

[1] Present address: Department of Epidemiology and Medical Statistics, School of Public Health, Postfach 100131, 33501 Bielefeld, Germany

PREAMBLE

IARC MONOGRAPHS PROGRAMME ON THE EVALUATION OF CARCINOGENIC RISKS TO HUMANS

PREAMBLE

1. BACKGROUND

In 1969, the International Agency for Research on Cancer (IARC) initiated a programme to evaluate the carcinogenic risk of chemicals to humans and to produce monographs on individual chemicals. The *Monographs* programme has since been expanded to include consideration of exposures to complex mixtures of chemicals (which occur, for example, in some occupations and as a result of human habits) and of exposures to other agents, such as radiation and viruses. With Supplement 6 (IARC, 1987a), the title of the series was modified from *IARC Monographs on the Evaluation of the Carcinogenic Risk of Chemicals to Humans* to *IARC Monographs on the Evaluation of Carcinogenic Risks to Humans*, in order to reflect the widened scope of the programme.

The criteria established in 1971 to evaluate carcinogenic risk to humans were adopted by the working groups whose deliberations resulted in the first 16 volumes of the *IARC Monographs series*. Those criteria were subsequently updated by further ad-hoc working groups (IARC, 1977, 1978, 1979, 1982, 1983, 1987b, 1988, 1991a; Vainio *et al.*, 1992).

2. OBJECTIVE AND SCOPE

The objective of the programme is to prepare, with the help of international working groups of experts, and to publish in the form of monographs, critical reviews and evaluations of evidence on the carcinogenicity of a wide range of human exposures. The *Monographs* may also indicate where additional research efforts are needed.

The *Monographs* represent the first step in carcinogenic risk assessment, which involves examination of all relevant information in order to assess the strength of the available evidence that certain exposures could alter the incidence of cancer in humans. The second step is quantitative risk estimation. Detailed, quantitative evaluations of epidemiological data may be made in the *Monographs*, but without extrapolation beyond the range of the data available. Quantitative extrapolation from experimental data to the human situation is not undertaken.

The term 'carcinogen' is used in these monographs to denote an exposure that is capable of increasing the incidence of malignant neoplasms; the induction of benign neoplasms may in some circumstances (see p. 19) contribute to the judgement that the exposure is carcinogenic. The terms 'neoplasm' and 'tumour' are used interchangeably.

Some epidemiological and experimental studies indicate that different agents may act at different stages in the carcinogenic process, and several mechanisms may be involved. The aim of the *Monographs* has been, from their inception, to evaluate evidence of carci- nogenicity at any stage in the carcinogenesis process, independently of the underlying mechanisms. Information on mechanisms may, however, be used in making the overall evaluation (IARC, 1991a; Vainio *et al.*, 1992; see also pp. 25–27).

The *Monographs* may assist national and international authorities in making risk assessments and in formulating decisions concerning any necessary preventive measures. The evaluations of IARC working groups are scientific, qualitative judgements about the evidence for or against carcinogenicity provided by the available data. These evaluations represent only one part of the body of information on which regulatory measures may be based. Other components of regulatory decisions vary from one situation to another and from country to country, responding to different socioeconomic and national priorities. **Therefore, no recommendation is given with regard to regulation or legislation, which are the responsibility of individual governments and/or other international organizations.**

The *IARC Monographs* are recognized as an authoritative source of information on the carcinogenicity of a wide range of human exposures. A survey of users in 1988 indi- cated that the *Monographs* are consulted by various agencies in 57 countries. About 4000 copies of each volume are printed, for distribution to governments, regulatory bodies and interested scientists. The Monographs are also available from IARC*Press* in Lyon and via the Distribution and Sales Service of the World Health Organization in Geneva.

3.   SELECTION OF TOPICS FOR MONOGRAPHS

Topics are selected on the basis of two main criteria: (a) there is evidence of human exposure, and (b) there is some evidence or suspicion of carcinogenicity. The term 'agent' is used to include individual chemical compounds, groups of related chemical compounds, physical agents (such as radiation) and biological factors (such as viruses). Exposures to mixtures of agents may occur in occupational exposures and as a result of personal and cultural habits (like smoking and dietary practices). Chemical analogues and compounds with biological or physical characteristics similar to those of suspected carcinogens may also be considered, even in the absence of data on a possible carcino- genic effect in humans or experimental animals.

The scientific literature is surveyed for published data relevant to an assessment of carcinogenicity. The IARC information bulletins on agents being tested for carcino- genicity (IARC, 1973–1996) and directories of on-going research in cancer epide- miology (IARC, 1976–1996) often indicate exposures that may be scheduled for future meetings. Ad-hoc working groups convened by IARC in 1984, 1989, 1991, 1993 and 1998 gave recommendations as to which agents should be evaluated in the IARC Mono- graphs series (IARC, 1984, 1989, 1991b, 1993, 1998a,b).

As significant new data on subjects on which monographs have already been prepared become available, re-evaluations are made at subsequent meetings, and revised monographs are published.

4. DATA FOR MONOGRAPHS

The *Monographs* do not necessarily cite all the literature concerning the subject of an evaluation. Only those data considered by the Working Group to be relevant to making the evaluation are included.

With regard to biological and epidemiological data, only reports that have been published or accepted for publication in the openly available scientific literature are reviewed by the working groups. In certain instances, government agency reports that have undergone peer review and are widely available are considered. Exceptions may be made on an ad-hoc basis to include unpublished reports that are in their final form and publicly available, if their inclusion is considered pertinent to making a final evaluation (see pp. 25–27). In the sections on chemical and physical properties, on analysis, on production and use and on occurrence, unpublished sources of information may be used.

5. THE WORKING GROUP

Reviews and evaluations are formulated by a working group of experts. The tasks of the group are: (i) to ascertain that all appropriate data have been collected; (ii) to select the data relevant for the evaluation on the basis of scientific merit; (iii) to prepare accurate summaries of the data to enable the reader to follow the reasoning of the Working Group; (iv) to evaluate the results of epidemiological and experimental studies on cancer; (v) to evaluate data relevant to the understanding of mechanism of action; and (vi) to make an overall evaluation of the carcinogenicity of the exposure to humans.

Working Group participants who contributed to the considerations and evaluations within a particular volume are listed, with their addresses, at the beginning of each publication. Each participant who is a member of a working group serves as an individual scientist and not as a representative of any organization, government or industry. In addition, nominees of national and international agencies and industrial associations may be invited as observers.

6. WORKING PROCEDURES

Approximately one year in advance of a meeting of a working group, the topics of the monographs are announced and participants are selected by IARC staff in consultation with other experts. Subsequently, relevant biological and epidemiological data are collected by the Carcinogen Identification and Evaluation Unit of IARC from recognized sources of information on carcinogenesis, including data storage and retrieval systems such as MEDLINE and TOXLINE.

For chemicals and some complex mixtures, the major collection of data and the preparation of first drafts of the sections on chemical and physical properties, on analysis, on production and use and on occurrence are carried out under a separate contract funded by the United States National Cancer Institute. Representatives from industrial associations may assist in the preparation of sections on production and use. Information on production and trade is obtained from governmental and trade publications and, in some cases, by direct contact with industries. Separate production data on some agents may not be available because their publication could disclose confidential information. Information on uses may be obtained from published sources but is often complemented by direct contact with manufacturers. Efforts are made to supplement this information with data from other national and international sources.

Six months before the meeting, the material obtained is sent to meeting participants, or is used by IARC staff, to prepare sections for the first drafts of monographs. The first drafts are compiled by IARC staff and sent before the meeting to all participants of the Working Group for review.

The Working Group meets in Lyon for seven to eight days to discuss and finalize the texts of the monographs and to formulate the evaluations. After the meeting, the master copy of each monograph is verified by consulting the original literature, edited and prepared for publication. The aim is to publish monographs within six months of the Working Group meeting.

The available studies are summarized by the Working Group, with particular regard to the qualitative aspects discussed below. In general, numerical findings are indicated as they appear in the original report; units are converted when necessary for easier comparison. The Working Group may conduct additional analyses of the published data and use them in their assessment of the evidence; the results of such supplementary analyses are given in square brackets. When an important aspect of a study, directly impinging on its interpretation, should be brought to the attention of the reader, a comment is given in square brackets.

7.   EXPOSURE DATA

Sections that indicate the extent of past and present human exposure, the sources of exposure, the people most likely to be exposed and the factors that contribute to the exposure are included at the beginning of each monograph.

Most monographs on individual chemicals, groups of chemicals or complex mixtures include sections on chemical and physical data, on analysis, on production and use and on occurrence. In monographs on, for example, physical agents, occupational exposures and cultural habits, other sections may be included, such as: historical perspectives, description of an industry or habit, chemistry of the complex mixture or taxonomy. Monographs on biological agents have sections on structure and biology, methods of detection, epidemiology of infection and clinical disease other than cancer.

For chemical exposures, the Chemical Abstracts Services Registry Number, the latest Chemical Abstracts Primary Name and the IUPAC Systematic Name are recorded; other synonyms are given, but the list is not necessarily comprehensive. For biological agents, taxonomy and structure are described, and the degree of variability is given, when applicable.

Information on chemical and physical properties and, in particular, data relevant to identification, occurrence and biological activity are included. For biological agents, mode of replication, life cycle, target cells, persistence and latency and host response are given. A description of technical products of chemicals includes trade names, relevant specifications and available information on composition and impurities. Some of the trade names given may be those of mixtures in which the agent being evaluated is only one of the ingredients.

The purpose of the section on analysis or detection is to give the reader an overview of current methods, with emphasis on those widely used for regulatory purposes. Methods for monitoring human exposure are also given, when available. No critical evaluation or recommendation of any of the methods is meant or implied. The IARC published a series of volumes, *Environmental Carcinogens: Methods of Analysis and Exposure Measurement* (IARC, 1978–93), that describe validated methods for analysing a wide variety of chemicals and mixtures. For biological agents, methods of detection and exposure assessment are described, including their sensitivity, specificity and reproducibility.

The dates of first synthesis and of first commercial production of a chemical or mixture are provided; for agents which do not occur naturally, this information may allow a reasonable estimate to be made of the date before which no human exposure to the agent could have occurred. The dates of first reported occurrence of an exposure are also provided. In addition, methods of synthesis used in past and present commercial production and different methods of production which may give rise to different impurities are described.

Data on production, international trade and uses are obtained for representative regions, which usually include Europe, Japan and the United States of America. It should not, however, be inferred that those areas or nations are necessarily the sole or major sources or users of the agent. Some identified uses may not be current or major applications, and the coverage is not necessarily comprehensive. In the case of drugs, mention of their therapeutic uses does not necessarily represent current practice, nor does it imply judgement as to their therapeutic efficacy.

Information on the occurrence of an agent or mixture in the environment is obtained from data derived from the monitoring and surveillance of levels in occupational environments, air, water, soil, foods and animal and human tissues. When available, data on the generation, persistence and bioaccumulation of the agent are also included. In the case of mixtures, industries, occupations or processes, information is given about all agents present. For processes, industries and occupations, a historical description is also given, noting variations in chemical composition, physical properties and levels of occupational exposure with time and place. For biological agents, the epidemiology of infection is described.

Statements concerning regulations and guidelines (e.g., pesticide registrations, maximal levels permitted in foods, occupational exposure limits) are included for some countries as indications of potential exposures, but they may not reflect the most recent situation, since such limits are continuously reviewed and modified. The absence of information on regulatory status for a country should not be taken to imply that that country does not have regulations with regard to the exposure. For biological agents, legislation and control, including vaccines and therapy, are described.

8.   STUDIES OF CANCER IN HUMANS

(a)   Types of studies considered

Three types of epidemiological studies of cancer contribute to the assessment of carcinogenicity in humans—cohort studies, case–control studies and correlation (or ecological) studies. Rarely, results from randomized trials may be available. Case series and case reports of cancer in humans may also be reviewed.

Cohort and case–control studies relate the exposures under study to the occurrence of cancer in individuals and provide an estimate of relative risk (ratio of incidence or mortality in those exposed to incidence or mortality in those not exposed) as the main measure of association.

In correlation studies, the units of investigation are usually whole populations (e.g. in particular geographical areas or at particular times), and cancer frequency is related to a summary measure of the exposure of the population to the agent, mixture or exposure circumstance under study. Because individual exposure is not documented, however, a causal relationship is less easy to infer from correlation studies than from cohort and case–control studies. Case reports generally arise from a suspicion, based on clinical experience, that the concurrence of two events—that is, a particular exposure and occurrence of a cancer—has happened rather more frequently than would be expected by chance. Case reports usually lack complete ascertainment of cases in any population, definition or enumeration of the population at risk and estimation of the expected number of cases in the absence of exposure. The uncertainties surrounding interpretation of case reports and correlation studies make them inadequate, except in rare instances, to form the sole basis for inferring a causal relationship. When taken together with case–control and cohort studies, however, relevant case reports or correlation studies may add materially to the judgement that a causal relationship is present.

Epidemiological studies of benign neoplasms, presumed preneoplastic lesions and other end-points thought to be relevant to cancer are also reviewed by working groups. They may, in some instances, strengthen inferences drawn from studies of cancer itself.

(b)   Quality of studies considered

The Monographs are not intended to summarize all published studies. Those that are judged to be inadequate or irrelevant to the evaluation are generally omitted. They may be mentioned briefly, particularly when the information is considered to be a useful supplement to that in other reports or when they provide the only data available. Their inclusion does not imply acceptance of the adequacy of the study design or of the analysis and interpretation of the results, and limitations are clearly outlined in square brackets at the end of the study description.

It is necessary to take into account the possible roles of bias, confounding and chance in the interpretation of epidemiological studies. By 'bias' is meant the operation of factors in study design or execution that lead erroneously to a stronger or weaker association than in fact exists between disease and an agent, mixture or exposure circumstance. By 'confounding' is meant a situation in which the relationship with disease is made to appear stronger or weaker than it truly is as a result of an association between the apparent causal factor and another factor that is associated with either an increase or decrease in the incidence of the disease. In evaluating the extent to which these factors have been minimized in an individual study, working groups consider a number of aspects of design and analysis as described in the report of the study. Most of these considerations apply equally to case–control, cohort and correlation studies. Lack of clarity of any of these aspects in the reporting of a study can decrease its credibility and the weight given to it in the final evaluation of the exposure.

Firstly, the study population, disease (or diseases) and exposure should have been well defined by the authors. Cases of disease in the study population should have been identified in a way that was independent of the exposure of interest, and exposure should have been assessed in a way that was not related to disease status.

Secondly, the authors should have taken account in the study design and analysis of other variables that can influence the risk of disease and may have been related to the exposure of interest. Potential confounding by such variables should have been dealt with either in the design of the study, such as by matching, or in the analysis, by statistical adjustment. In cohort studies, comparisons with local rates of disease may be more appropriate than those with national rates. Internal comparisons of disease frequency among individuals at different levels of exposure should also have been made in the study.

Thirdly, the authors should have reported the basic data on which the conclusions are founded, even if sophisticated statistical analyses were employed. At the very least, they should have given the numbers of exposed and unexposed cases and controls in a case–control study and the numbers of cases observed and expected in a cohort study. Further tabulations by time since exposure began and other temporal factors are also important. In a cohort study, data on all cancer sites and all causes of death should have been given, to reveal the possibility of reporting bias. In a case–control study, the effects of investigated factors other than the exposure of interest should have been reported.

Finally, the statistical methods used to obtain estimates of relative risk, absolute rates of cancer, confidence intervals and significance tests, and to adjust for confounding should have been clearly stated by the authors. The methods used should preferably have been the generally accepted techniques that have been refined since the mid-1970s. These methods have been reviewed for case–control studies (Breslow & Day, 1980) and for cohort studies (Breslow & Day, 1987).

(c)   *Inferences about mechanism of action*

Detailed analyses of both relative and absolute risks in relation to temporal variables, such as age at first exposure, time since first exposure, duration of exposure, cumulative exposure and time since exposure ceased, are reviewed and summarized when available. The analysis of temporal relationships can be useful in formulating models of carcinogenesis. In particular, such analyses may suggest whether a carcinogen acts early or late in the process of carcinogenesis, although at best they allow only indirect inferences about the mechanism of action. Special attention is given to measurements of biological markers of carcinogen exposure or action, such as DNA or protein adducts, as well as markers of early steps in the carcinogenic process, such as proto-oncogene mutation, when these are incorporated into epidemiological studies focused on cancer incidence or mortality. Such measurements may allow inferences to be made about putative mechanisms of action (IARC, 1991a; Vainio *et al.*, 1992).

(d)   *Criteria for causality*

After the individual epidemiological studies of cancer have been summarized and the quality assessed, a judgement is made concerning the strength of evidence that the agent, mixture or exposure circumstance in question is carcinogenic for humans. In making its judgement, the Working Group considers several criteria for causality. A strong association (a large relative risk) is more likely to indicate causality than a weak association, although it is recognized that relative risks of small magnitude do not imply lack of causality and may be important if the disease is common. Associations that are replicated in several studies of the same design or using different epidemiological approaches or under different circumstances of exposure are more likely to represent a causal relationship than isolated observations from single studies. If there are inconsistent results among investigations, possible reasons are sought (such as differences in amount of exposure), and results of studies judged to be of high quality are given more weight than those of studies judged to be methodologically less sound. When suspicion of carcinogenicity arises largely from a single study, these data are not combined with those from later studies in any subsequent reassessment of the strength of the evidence.

If the risk of the disease in question increases with the amount of exposure, this is considered to be a strong indication of causality, although absence of a graded response is not necessarily evidence against a causal relationship. Demonstration of a decline in risk after cessation of or reduction in exposure in individuals or in whole populations also supports a causal interpretation of the findings.

Although a carcinogen may act upon more than one target, the specificity of an association (an increased occurrence of cancer at one anatomical site or of one morphological type) adds plausibility to a causal relationship, particularly when excess cancer occurrence is limited to one morphological type within the same organ.

Although rarely available, results from randomized trials showing different rates among exposed and unexposed individuals provide particularly strong evidence for causality.

When several epidemiological studies show little or no indication of an association between an exposure and cancer, the judgement may be made that, in the aggregate, they show evidence of lack of carcinogenicity. Such a judgement requires first of all that the studies giving rise to it meet, to a sufficient degree, the standards of design and analysis described above. Specifically, the possibility that bias, confounding or misclassification of exposure or outcome could explain the observed results should be considered and excluded with reasonable certainty. In addition, all studies that are judged to be methodologically sound should be consistent with a relative risk of unity for any observed level of exposure and, when considered together, should provide a pooled estimate of relative risk which is at or near unity and has a narrow confidence interval, due to sufficient population size. Moreover, no individual study nor the pooled results of all the studies should show any consistent tendency for the relative risk of cancer to increase with increasing level of exposure. It is important to note that evidence of lack of carcinogenicity obtained in this way from several epidemiological studies can apply only to the type(s) of cancer studied and to dose levels and intervals between first exposure and observation of disease that are the same as or less than those observed in all the studies. Experience with human cancer indicates that, in some cases, the period from first exposure to the development of clinical cancer is seldom less than 20 years; latent periods substantially shorter than 30 years cannot provide evidence for lack of carcinogenicity.

9. STUDIES OF CANCER IN EXPERIMENTAL ANIMALS

All known human carcinogens that have been studied adequately in experimental animals have produced positive results in one or more animal species (Wilbourn *et al.*, 1986; Tomatis *et al.*, 1989). For several agents (aflatoxins, 4-aminobiphenyl, azathioprine, betel quid with tobacco, bischloromethyl ether and chloromethyl methyl ether (technical grade), chlorambucil, chlornaphazine, ciclosporin, coal-tar pitches, coal-tars, combined oral contraceptives, cyclophosphamide, diethylstilboestrol, melphalan, 8-methoxypsoralen plus ultraviolet A radiation, mustard gas, myleran, 2-naphthylamine, nonsteroidal oestrogens, oestrogen replacement therapy/steroidal oestrogens, solar radiation, thiotepa and vinyl chloride), carcinogenicity in experimental animals was established or highly suspected before epidemiological studies confirmed their carcinogenicity in humans (Vainio *et al.*, 1995). Although this association cannot establish that all agents and mixtures that cause cancer in experimental animals also cause cancer in humans, nevertheless, **in the absence of adequate data on humans, it is biologically plausible and prudent to regard agents and mixtures for which there is *sufficient evidence* (see p. 24) of carcinogenicity in experimental animals as if they presented a carcinogenic risk to humans**. The possibility that a given agent may cause cancer through a species-specific mechanism which does not operate in humans (see p. 27) should also be taken into consideration.

The nature and extent of impurities or contaminants present in the chemical or mixture being evaluated are given when available. Animal strain, sex, numbers per group, age at start of treatment and survival are reported.

Other types of studies summarized include: experiments in which the agent or mixture was administered in conjunction with known carcinogens or factors that modify carcinogenic effects; studies in which the end-point was not cancer but a defined precancerous lesion; and experiments on the carcinogenicity of known metabolites and derivatives.

For experimental studies of mixtures, consideration is given to the possibility of changes in the physicochemical properties of the test substance during collection, storage, extraction, concentration and delivery. Chemical and toxicological interactions of the components of mixtures may result in nonlinear dose–response relationships.

An assessment is made as to the relevance to human exposure of samples tested in experimental animals, which may involve consideration of: (i) physical and chemical characteristics, (ii) constituent substances that indicate the presence of a class of substances, (iii) the results of tests for genetic and related effects, including studies on DNA adduct formation, proto-oncogene mutation and expression and suppressor gene inactivation. The relevance of results obtained, for example, with animal viruses analogous to the virus being evaluated in the monograph must also be considered. They may provide biological and mechanistic information relevant to the understanding of the process of carcinogenesis in humans and may strengthen the plausibility of a conclusion that the biological agent under evaluation is carcinogenic in humans.

(a)   Qualitative aspects

An assessment of carcinogenicity involves several considerations of qualitative importance, including (i) the experimental conditions under which the test was per-formed, including route and schedule of exposure, species, strain, sex, age, duration of follow-up; (ii) the consistency of the results, for example, across species and target organ(s); (iii) the spectrum of neoplastic response, from preneoplastic lesions and benign tumours to malignant neoplasms; and (iv) the possible role of modifying factors.

As mentioned earlier (p. 11), the *Monographs* are not intended to summarize all published studies. Those studies in experimental animals that are inadequate (e.g., too short a duration, too few animals, poor survival; see below) or are judged irrelevant to the evaluation are generally omitted. Guidelines for conducting adequate long-term carcinogenicity experiments have been outlined (e.g. Montesano *et al.*, 1986).

Considerations of importance to the Working Group in the interpretation and eva-luation of a particular study include: (i) how clearly the agent was defined and, in the case of mixtures, how adequately the sample characterization was reported; (ii) whether the dose was adequately monitored, particularly in inhalation experiments; (iii) whether the doses and duration of treatment were appropriate and whether the survival of treated animals was similar to that of controls; (iv) whether there were adequate numbers of animals per group; (v) whether animals of each sex were used; (vi) whether animals were allocated randomly to groups; (vii) whether the duration of observation was adequate; and (viii) whether the data were adequately reported. If available, recent data on the incidence of specific tumours in historical controls, as well as in concurrent controls, should be taken into account in the evaluation of tumour response.

When benign tumours occur together with and originate from the same cell type in an organ or tissue as malignant tumours in a particular study and appear to represent a stage in the progression to malignancy, it may be valid to combine them in assessing tumour incidence (Huff *et al.*, 1989). The occurrence of lesions presumed to be pre-neoplastic may in certain instances aid in assessing the biological plausibility of any neo-plastic response observed. If an agent or mixture induces only benign neoplasms that appear to be end-points that do not readily progress to malignancy, it should nevertheless be suspected of being a carcinogen and requires further investigation.

(b)   Quantitative aspects

The probability that tumours will occur may depend on the species, sex, strain and age of the animal, the dose of the carcinogen and the route and length of exposure. Evidence of an increased incidence of neoplasms with increased level of exposure strengthens the inference of a causal association between the exposure and the develop-ment of neoplasms.

The form of the dose–response relationship can vary widely, depending on the particular agent under study and the target organ. Both DNA damage and increased cell division are important aspects of carcinogenesis, and cell proliferation is a strong deter-minant of dose–response relationships for some carcinogens (Cohen & Ellwein, 1990). Since many chemicals require metabolic activation before being converted into their reactive intermediates, both metabolic and pharmacokinetic aspects are important in determining the dose–response pattern. Saturation of steps such as absorption, activation, inactivation and elimination may produce nonlinearity in the dose–response relationship, as could saturation of processes such as DNA repair (Hoel *et al.*, 1983; Gart *et al.*, 1986).

(c)   Statistical analysis of long-term experiments in animals

Factors considered by the Working Group include the adequacy of the information given for each treatment group: (i) the number of animals studied and the number examined histologically, (ii) the number of animals with a given tumour type and (iii) length of survival. The statistical methods used should be clearly stated and should be the generally accepted techniques refined for this purpose (Peto *et al.*, 1980; Gart *et al.*, 1986). When there is no difference in survival between control and treatment groups, the Working Group usually compares the proportions of animals developing each tumour type in each of the groups. Otherwise, consideration is given as to whether or not appropriate adjustments have been made for differences in survival. These adjustments can include: comparisons of the proportions of tumour-bearing animals among the effective number of animals (alive at the time the first tumour is discovered), in the case where most differences in survival occur before tumours appear; life-table methods, when tumours are visible or when they may be considered 'fatal' because mortality rapidly follows tumour development; and the Mantel-Haenszel test or logistic regression, when occult tumours do not affect the animals' risk of dying but are 'incidental' findings at autopsy.

In practice, classifying tumours as fatal or incidental may be difficult. Several survival-adjusted methods have been developed that do not require this distinction (Gart *et al.*, 1986), although they have not been fully evaluated.

10. OTHER DATA RELEVANT TO AN EVALUATION OF CARCINOGENICITY AND ITS MECHANISMS

In coming to an overall evaluation of carcinogenicity in humans (see pp. 25–27), the Working Group also considers related data. The nature of the information selected for the summary depends on the agent being considered.

For chemicals and complex mixtures of chemicals such as those in some occupational situations or involving cultural habits (e.g. tobacco smoking), the other data considered to be relevant are divided into those on absorption, distribution, metabolism and excretion; toxic effects; reproductive and developmental effects; and genetic and related effects.

Concise information is given on absorption, distribution (including placental transfer) and excretion in both humans and experimental animals. Kinetic factors that may affect the dose–response relationship, such as saturation of uptake, protein binding, metabolic activation, detoxification and DNA repair processes, are mentioned. Studies that indicate the metabolic fate of the agent in humans and in experimental animals are summarized briefly, and comparisons of data on humans and on animals are made when possible. Comparative information on the relationship between exposure and the dose that reaches the target site may be of particular importance for extrapolation between species. Data are given on acute and chronic toxic effects (other than cancer), such as organ toxicity, increased cell proliferation, immunotoxicity and endocrine effects. The presence and toxicological significance of cellular receptors is described. Effects on reproduction, teratogenicity, fetotoxicity and embryotoxicity are also summarized briefly.

Tests of genetic and related effects are described in view of the relevance of gene mutation and chromosomal damage to carcinogenesis (Vainio *et al.*, 1992; McGregor *et al.*, 1999). The adequacy of the reporting of sample characterization is considered and, where necessary, commented upon; with regard to complex mixtures, such comments are similar to those described for animal carcinogenicity tests on p. 18. The available data are interpreted critically by phylogenetic group according to the end-points detected, which may include DNA damage, gene mutation, sister chromatid exchange, micronucleus formation, chromosomal aberrations, aneuploidy and cell transformation. The concentrations employed are given, and mention is made of whether use of an exogenous metabolic system *in vitro* affected the test result. These data are given as listings of test systems, data and references. The Genetic and Related Effects data presented in the *Monographs* are also available in the form of Graphic Activity Profiles (GAP) prepared in collaboration with the United States Environmental Protection Agency (EPA) (see also

Waters *et al.*, 1987) using software for personal computers that are Microsoft Windows®
compatible. The EPA/IARC GAP software and database may be downloaded free of
charge from *www.epa.gov/gapdb*.

Positive results in tests using prokaryotes, lower eukaryotes, plants, insects and
cultured mammalian cells suggest that genetic and related effects could occur in
mammals. Results from such tests may also give information about the types of genetic
effect produced and about the involvement of metabolic activation. Some end-points
described are clearly genetic in nature (e.g., gene mutations and chromosomal aberrations), while others are to a greater or lesser degree associated with genetic effects (e.g.
unscheduled DNA synthesis). In-vitro tests for tumour-promoting activity and for cell
transformation may be sensitive to changes that are not necessarily the result of genetic
alterations but that may have specific relevance to the process of carcinogenesis. A
critical appraisal of these tests has been published (Montesano *et al.*, 1986).

Genetic or other activity manifest in experimental mammals and humans is regarded
as being of greater relevance than that in other organisms. The demonstration that an
agent or mixture can induce gene and chromosomal mutations in whole mammals indicates that it may have carcinogenic activity, although this activity may not be detectably
expressed in any or all species. Relative potency in tests for mutagenicity and related
effects is not a reliable indicator of carcinogenic potency. Negative results in tests for
mutagenicity in selected tissues from animals treated *in vivo* provide less weight, partly
because they do not exclude the possibility of an effect in tissues other than those
examined. Moreover, negative results in short-term tests with genetic end-points cannot
be considered to provide evidence to rule out carcinogenicity of agents or mixtures that
act through other mechanisms (e.g. receptor-mediated effects, cellular toxicity with regenerative proliferation, peroxisome proliferation) (Vainio *et al.*, 1992). Factors that may
lead to misleading results in short-term tests have been discussed in detail elsewhere
(Montesano *et al.*, 1986).

When available, data relevant to mechanisms of carcinogenesis that do not involve
structural changes at the level of the gene are also described.

The adequacy of epidemiological studies of reproductive outcome and genetic and
related effects in humans is evaluated by the same criteria as are applied to epidemiological studies of cancer.

Structure–activity relationships that may be relevant to an evaluation of the carcinogenicity of an agent are also described.

For biological agents—viruses, bacteria and parasites—other data relevant to
carcinogenicity include descriptions of the pathology of infection, molecular biology
(integration and expression of viruses, and any genetic alterations seen in human
tumours) and other observations, which might include cellular and tissue responses to
infection, immune response and the presence of tumour markers.

11.   SUMMARY OF DATA REPORTED

In this section, the relevant epidemiological and experimental data are summarized. Only reports, other than in abstract form, that meet the criteria outlined on p. 11 are considered for evaluating carcinogenicity. Inadequate studies are generally not summarized: such studies are usually identified by a square-bracketed comment in the preceding text.

(a)   Exposure

Human exposure to chemicals and complex mixtures is summarized on the basis of elements such as production, use, occurrence in the environment and determinations in human tissues and body fluids. Quantitative data are given when available. Exposure to biological agents is described in terms of transmission and prevalence of infection.

(b)   Carcinogenicity in humans

Results of epidemiological studies that are considered to be pertinent to an assessment of human carcinogenicity are summarized. When relevant, case reports and correlation studies are also summarized.

(c)   Carcinogenicity in experimental animals

Data relevant to an evaluation of carcinogenicity in animals are summarized. For each animal species and route of administration, it is stated whether an increased incidence of neoplasms or preneoplastic lesions was observed, and the tumour sites are indicated. If the agent or mixture produced tumours after prenatal exposure or in single-dose experiments, this is also indicated. Negative findings are also summarized. Dose–response and other quantitative data may be given when available.

(d)   Other data relevant to an evaluation of carcinogenicity and its mechanisms

Data on biological effects in humans that are of particular relevance are summarized. These may include toxicological, kinetic and metabolic considerations and evidence of DNA binding, persistence of DNA lesions or genetic damage in exposed humans. Toxicological information, such as that on cytotoxicity and regeneration, receptor binding and hormonal and immunological effects, and data on kinetics and metabolism in experimental animals are given when considered relevant to the possible mechanism of the carcinogenic action of the agent. The results of tests for genetic and related effects are summarized for whole mammals, cultured mammalian cells and nonmammalian systems.

When available, comparisons of such data for humans and for animals, and particularly animals that have developed cancer, are described.

Structure–activity relationships are mentioned when relevant.

For the agent, mixture or exposure circumstance being evaluated, the available data on end-points or other phenomena relevant to mechanisms of carcinogenesis from studies in humans, experimental animals and tissue and cell test systems are summarized within one or more of the following descriptive dimensions:

(i) Evidence of genotoxicity (structural changes at the level of the gene): for example, structure–activity considerations, adduct formation, mutagenicity (effect on specific genes), chromosomal mutation/aneuploidy

(ii) Evidence of effects on the expression of relevant genes (functional changes at the intracellular level): for example, alterations to the structure or quantity of the product of a proto-oncogene or tumour-suppressor gene, alterations to metabolic activation/inactivation/DNA repair

(iii) Evidence of relevant effects on cell behaviour (morphological or behavioural changes at the cellular or tissue level): for example, induction of mitogenesis, compensatory cell proliferation, preneoplasia and hyperplasia, survival of premalignant or malignant cells (immortalization, immunosuppression), effects on metastatic potential

(iv) Evidence from dose and time relationships of carcinogenic effects and interactions between agents: for example, early/late stage, as inferred from epidemiological studies; initiation/promotion/progression/malignant conversion, as defined in animal carcinogenicity experiments; toxicokinetics

These dimensions are not mutually exclusive, and an agent may fall within more than one of them. Thus, for example, the action of an agent on the expression of relevant genes could be summarized under both the first and second dimensions, even if it were known with reasonable certainty that those effects resulted from genotoxicity.

12.   EVALUATION

Evaluations of the strength of the evidence for carcinogenicity arising from human and experimental animal data are made, using standard terms.

It is recognized that the criteria for these evaluations, described below, cannot encompass all of the factors that may be relevant to an evaluation of carcinogenicity. In considering all of the relevant scientific data, the Working Group may assign the agent, mixture or exposure circumstance to a higher or lower category than a strict interpretation of these criteria would indicate.

(a)   Degrees of evidence for carcinogenicity in humans and in experimental animals and supporting evidence

These categories refer only to the strength of the evidence that an exposure is carcinogenic and not to the extent of its carcinogenic activity (potency) nor to the mechanisms involved. A classification may change as new information becomes available.

An evaluation of degree of evidence, whether for a single agent or a mixture, is limited to the materials tested, as defined physically, chemically or biologically. When the agents evaluated are considered by the Working Group to be sufficiently closely related, they may be grouped together for the purpose of a single evaluation of degree of evidence.

(i)   Carcinogenicity in humans

The applicability of an evaluation of the carcinogenicity of a mixture, process, occupation or industry on the basis of evidence from epidemiological studies depends on the variability over time and place of the mixtures, processes, occupations and industries. The Working Group seeks to identify the specific exposure, process or activity which is considered most likely to be responsible for any excess risk. The evaluation is focused as narrowly as the available data on exposure and other aspects permit.

The evidence relevant to carcinogenicity from studies in humans is classified into one of the following categories:

Sufficient evidence of carcinogenicity: The Working Group considers that a causal relationship has been established between exposure to the agent, mixture or exposure circumstance and human cancer. That is, a positive relationship has been observed between the exposure and cancer in studies in which chance, bias and confounding could be ruled out with reasonable confidence.

Limited evidence of carcinogenicity: A positive association has been observed between exposure to the agent, mixture or exposure circumstance and cancer for which a causal interpretation is considered by the Working Group to be credible, but chance, bias or confounding could not be ruled out with reasonable confidence.

Inadequate evidence of carcinogenicity: The available studies are of insufficient quality, consistency or statistical power to permit a conclusion regarding the presence or absence of a causal association between exposure and cancer, or no data on cancer in humans are available.

Evidence suggesting lack of carcinogenicity: There are several adequate studies covering the full range of levels of exposure that human beings are known to encounter, which are mutually consistent in not showing a positive association between exposure to the agent, mixture or exposure circumstance and any studied cancer at any observed level of exposure. A conclusion of 'evidence suggesting lack of carcinogenicity' is inevitably limited to the cancer sites, conditions and levels of exposure and length of observation covered by the available studies. In addition, the possibility of a very small risk at the levels of exposure studied can never be excluded.

In some instances, the above categories may be used to classify the degree of evidence related to carcinogenicity in specific organs or tissues.

(ii)   *Carcinogenicity in experimental animals*

The evidence relevant to carcinogenicity in experimental animals is classified into one of the following categories:

Sufficient evidence of carcinogenicity: The Working Group considers that a causal relationship has been established between the agent or mixture and an increased incidence of malignant neoplasms or of an appropriate combination of benign and malignant neoplasms in (a) two or more species of animals or (b) in two or more independent studies in one species carried out at different times or in different laboratories or under different protocols.

Exceptionally, a single study in one species might be considered to provide sufficient evidence of carcinogenicity when malignant neoplasms occur to an unusual degree with regard to incidence, site, type of tumour or age at onset.

Limited evidence of carcinogenicity: The data suggest a carcinogenic effect but are limited for making a definitive evaluation because, e.g. (a) the evidence of carcinogenicity is restricted to a single experiment; or (b) there are unresolved questions regarding the adequacy of the design, conduct or interpretation of the study; or (c) the agent or mixture increases the incidence only of benign neoplasms or lesions of uncertain neoplastic potential, or of certain neoplasms which may occur spontaneously in high incidences in certain strains.

Inadequate evidence of carcinogenicity: The studies cannot be interpreted as showing either the presence or absence of a carcinogenic effect because of major qualitative or quantitative limitations, or no data on cancer in experimental animals are available.

Evidence suggesting lack of carcinogenicity: Adequate studies involving at least two species are available which show that, within the limits of the tests used, the agent or mixture is not carcinogenic. A conclusion of evidence suggesting lack of carcinogenicity is inevitably limited to the species, tumour sites and levels of exposure studied.

(b)   Other data relevant to the evaluation of carcinogenicity and its mechanisms

Other evidence judged to be relevant to an evaluation of carcinogenicity and of sufficient importance to affect the overall evaluation is then described. This may include data on preneoplastic lesions, tumour pathology, genetic and related effects, structure–activity relationships, metabolism and pharmacokinetics, physicochemical parameters and analogous biological agents.

Data relevant to mechanisms of the carcinogenic action are also evaluated. The strength of the evidence that any carcinogenic effect observed is due to a particular mechanism is assessed, using terms such as weak, moderate or strong. Then, the Working Group assesses if that particular mechanism is likely to be operative in humans. The strongest indications that a particular mechanism operates in humans come from data on humans or biological specimens obtained from exposed humans. The data may be considered to be especially relevant if they show that the agent in question has caused changes in exposed humans that are on the causal pathway to carcinogenesis. Such data may, however, never become available, because it is at least conceivable that certain compounds may be kept from human use solely on the basis of evidence of their toxicity and/or carcinogenicity in experimental systems.

For complex exposures, including occupational and industrial exposures, the chemical composition and the potential contribution of carcinogens known to be present are considered by the Working Group in its overall evaluation of human carcinogenicity. The Working Group also determines the extent to which the materials tested in experimental systems are related to those to which humans are exposed.

(c)   Overall evaluation

Finally, the body of evidence is considered as a whole, in order to reach an overall evaluation of the carcinogenicity to humans of an agent, mixture or circumstance of exposure.

An evaluation may be made for a group of chemical compounds that have been eva-luated by the Working Group. In addition, when supporting data indicate that other, related compounds for which there is no direct evidence of capacity to induce cancer in humans or in animals may also be carcinogenic, a statement describing the rationale for this conclusion is added to the evaluation narrative; an additional evaluation may be made for this broader group of compounds if the strength of the evidence warrants it.

The agent, mixture or exposure circumstance is described according to the wording of one of the following categories, and the designated group is given. The categorization of an agent, mixture or exposure circumstance is a matter of scientific judgement, reflec-ting the strength of the evidence derived from studies in humans and in experimental animals and from other relevant data.

Group 1 —The agent (mixture) is carcinogenic to humans.
The exposure circumstance entails exposures that are carcinogenic to humans.

This category is used when there is *sufficient evidence* of carcinogenicity in humans. Exceptionally, an agent (mixture) may be placed in this category when evidence of carci-nogenicity in humans is less than sufficient but there is *sufficient evidence* of carcino-genicity in experimental animals and strong evidence in exposed humans that the agent (mixture) acts through a relevant mechanism of carcinogenicity.

Group 2

This category includes agents, mixtures and exposure circumstances for which, at one extreme, the degree of evidence of carcinogenicity in humans is almost sufficient, as well as those for which, at the other extreme, there are no human data but for which there is evidence of carcinogenicity in experimental animals. Agents, mixtures and exposure circumstances are assigned to either group 2A (probably carcinogenic to humans) or group 2B (possibly carcinogenic to humans) on the basis of epidemiological and experi-mental evidence of carcinogenicity and other relevant data.

Group 2A—The agent (mixture) is probably carcinogenic to humans.
The exposure circumstance entails exposures that are probably carcinogenic to humans.

This category is used when there is *limited evidence* of carcinogenicity in humans and *sufficient evidence* of carcinogenicity in experimental animals. In some cases, an agent (mixture) may be classified in this category when there is *inadequate evidence* of carcinogenicity in humans, *sufficient evidence* of carcinogenicity in experimental animals and strong evidence that the carcinogenesis is mediated by a mechanism that also operates in humans. Exceptionally, an agent, mixture or exposure circumstance may be classified in this category solely on the basis of *limited evidence* of carcinogenicity in humans.

Group 2B—The agent (mixture) is possibly carcinogenic to humans.
The exposure circumstance entails exposures that are possibly carcinogenic to
humans.

This category is used for agents, mixtures and exposure circumstances for which there is *limited evidence* of carcinogenicity in humans and less than *sufficient evidence* of carcinogenicity in experimental animals. It may also be used when there is *inadequate evidence* of carcinogenicity in humans but there is *sufficient evidence* of carcinogenicity in experimental animals. In some instances, an agent, mixture or exposure circumstance for which there is *inadequate evidence* of carcinogenicity in humans but *limited evidence* of carcinogenicity in experimental animals together with supporting evidence from other relevant data may be placed in this group.

Group 3—The agent (mixture or exposure circumstance) is not classifiable as to its carcinogenicity to humans.

This category is used most commonly for agents, mixtures and exposure circumstances for which the *evidence of carcinogenicity* is *inadequate* in humans and *inadequate* or *limited* in experimental animals.

Exceptionally, agents (mixtures) for which the *evidence of carcinogenicity* is *inadequate* in humans but *sufficient* in experimental animals may be placed in this category when there is strong evidence that the mechanism of carcinogenicity in experimental animals does not operate in humans.

Agents, mixtures and exposure circumstances that do not fall into any other group are also placed in this category.

Group 4—The agent (mixture) is probably not carcinogenic to humans.

This category is used for agents or mixtures for which there is *evidence suggesting lack of carcinogenicity* in humans and in experimental animals. In some instances, agents or mixtures for which there is *inadequate evidence* of carcinogenicity in humans but *evidence suggesting lack of carcinogenicity* in experimental animals, consistently and strongly supported by a broad range of other relevant data, may be classified in this group.

References
Breslow, N.E. & Day, N.E. (1980) *Statistical Methods in Cancer Research*, Vol. 1, *The Analysis of Case–Control Studies* (IARC Scientific Publications No. 32), Lyon, IARC

Breslow, N.E. & Day, N.E. (1987) *Statistical Methods in Cancer Research*, Vol. 2, *The Design and Analysis of Cohort Studies* (IARC Scientific Publications No. 82), Lyon, IARC

Cohen, S.M. & Ellwein, L.B. (1990) Cell proliferation in carcinogenesis. *Science*, **249**, 1007–1011

Gart, J.J., Krewski, D., Lee, P.N., Tarone, R.E. & Wahrendorf, J. (1986) *Statistical Methods in Cancer Research*, Vol. 3, *The Design and Analysis of Long-term Animal Experiments* (IARC Scientific Publications No. 79), Lyon, IARC

Hoel, D.G., Kaplan, N.L. & Anderson, M.W. (1983) Implication of nonlinear kinetics on risk estimation in carcinogenesis. *Science*, **219**, 1032–1037

Huff, J.E., Eustis, S.L. & Haseman, J.K. (1989) Occurrence and relevance of chemically induced benign neoplasms in long-term carcinogenicity studies. *Cancer Metastasis Rev.*, **8**, 1–21

IARC (1973–1996) *Information Bulletin on the Survey of Chemicals Being Tested for Carcinogenicity/Directory of Agents Being Tested for Carcinogenicity*, Numbers 1–17, Lyon

IARC (1976–1996)

    Directory of On-going Research in Cancer Epidemiology 1976. Edited by C.S. Muir & G. Wagner, Lyon

    Directory of On-going Research in Cancer Epidemiology 1977 (IARC Scientific Publications No. 17). Edited by C.S. Muir & G. Wagner, Lyon

    Directory of On-going Research in Cancer Epidemiology 1978 (IARC Scientific Publications No. 26). Edited by C.S. Muir & G. Wagner, Lyon

    Directory of On-going Research in Cancer Epidemiology 1979 (IARC Scientific Publications No. 28). Edited by C.S. Muir & G. Wagner, Lyon

    Directory of On-going Research in Cancer Epidemiology 1980 (IARC Scientific Publications No. 35). Edited by C.S. Muir & G. Wagner, Lyon

    Directory of On-going Research in Cancer Epidemiology 1981 (IARC Scientific Publications No. 38). Edited by C.S. Muir & G. Wagner, Lyon

    Directory of On-going Research in Cancer Epidemiology 1982 (IARC Scientific Publications No. 46). Edited by C.S. Muir & G. Wagner, Lyon

    Directory of On-going Research in Cancer Epidemiology 1983 (IARC Scientific Publications No. 50). Edited by C.S. Muir & G. Wagner, Lyon

    Directory of On-going Research in Cancer Epidemiology 1984 (IARC Scientific Publications No. 62). Edited by C.S. Muir & G. Wagner, Lyon

    Directory of On-going Research in Cancer Epidemiology 1985 (IARC Scientific Publications No. 69). Edited by C.S. Muir & G. Wagner, Lyon

    Directory of On-going Research in Cancer Epidemiology 1986 (IARC Scientific Publications No. 80). Edited by C.S. Muir & G. Wagner, Lyon

    Directory of On-going Research in Cancer Epidemiology 1987 (IARC Scientific Publications No. 86). Edited by D.M. Parkin & J. Wahrendorf, Lyon

    Directory of On-going Research in Cancer Epidemiology 1988 (IARC Scientific Publications No. 93). Edited by M. Coleman & J. Wahrendorf, Lyon

    Directory of On-going Research in Cancer Epidemiology 1989/90 (IARC Scientific Publications No. 101). Edited by M. Coleman & J. Wahrendorf, Lyon

    Directory of On-going Research in Cancer Epidemiology 1991 (IARC Scientific Publications No.110). Edited by M. Coleman & J. Wahrendorf, Lyon

    Directory of On-going Research in Cancer Epidemiology 1992 (IARC Scientific Publications No. 117). Edited by M. Coleman, J. Wahrendorf & E. Démaret, Lyon

    Directory of On-going Research in Cancer Epidemiology 1994 (IARC Scientific Publications No. 130). Edited by R. Sankaranarayanan, J. Wahrendorf & E. Démaret, Lyon

Directory of On-going Research in Cancer Epidemiology 1996 (IARC Scientific Publications No. 137). Edited by R. Sankaranarayanan, J. Wahrendorf & E. Démaret, Lyon

IARC (1977) *IARC Monographs Programme on the Evaluation of the Carcinogenic Risk of Chemicals to Humans*. Preamble (IARC intern. tech. Rep. No. 77/002), Lyon

IARC (1978) *Chemicals with* Sufficient Evidence *of Carcinogenicity in Experimental Animals—* IARC Monographs *Volumes 1–17* (IARC intern. tech. Rep. No. 78/003), Lyon

IARC (1978–1993) *Environmental Carcinogens. Methods of Analysis and Exposure Measurement*:

Vol. 1. *Analysis of Volatile Nitrosamines in Food* (IARC Scientific Publications No. 18). Edited by R. Preussmann, M. Castegnaro, E.A. Walker & A.E. Wasserman (1978)

Vol. 2. *Methods for the Measurement of Vinyl Chloride in Poly(vinyl chloride), Air, Water and Foodstuffs* (IARC Scientific Publications No. 22). Edited by D.C.M. Squirrell & W. Thain (1978)

Vol. 3. *Analysis of Polycyclic Aromatic Hydrocarbons in Environmental Samples* (IARC Scientific Publications No. 29). Edited by M. Castegnaro, P. Bogovski, H. Kunte & E.A. Walker (1979)

Vol. 4. *Some Aromatic Amines and Azo Dyes in the General and Industrial Environment* (IARC Scientific Publications No. 40). Edited by L. Fishbein, M. Castegnaro, I.K. O'Neill & H. Bartsch (1981)

Vol. 5. *Some Mycotoxins (IARC Scientific Publications No. 44)*. Edited by L. Stoloff, M. Castegnaro, P. Scott, I.K. O'Neill & H. Bartsch (1983)

Vol. 6. *N-Nitroso Compounds (IARC Scientific Publications No. 45)*. Edited by R. Preussmann, I.K. O'Neill, G. Eisenbrand, B. Spiegelhalder & H. Bartsch (1983)

Vol. 7. *Some Volatile Halogenated Hydrocarbons* (IARC Scientific Publications No. 68). Edited by L. Fishbein & I.K. O'Neill (1985)

Vol. 8. *Some Metals: As, Be, Cd, Cr, Ni, Pb, Se, Zn* (IARC Scientific Publications No. 71). Edited by I.K. O'Neill, P. Schuller & L. Fishbein (1986)

Vol. 9. *Passive Smoking (IARC Scientific Publications No. 81)*. Edited by I.K. O'Neill, K.D. Brunnemann, B. Dodet & D. Hoffmann (1987)

Vol. 10. *Benzene and Alkylated Benzenes (IARC Scientific Publications No. 85)*. Edited by L. Fishbein & I.K. O'Neill (1988)

Vol. 11. *Polychlorinated Dioxins and Dibenzofurans* (IARC Scientific Publications No. 108). Edited by C. Rappe, H.R. Buser, B. Dodet & I.K. O'Neill (1991)

Vol. 12. *Indoor Air* (IARC Scientific Publications No. 109). Edited by B. Seifert, H. van de Wiel, B. Dodet & I.K. O'Neill (1993)

IARC (1979) *Criteria to Select Chemicals for* IARC Monographs (IARC intern. tech. Rep. No. 79/003), Lyon

IARC (1982) *IARC Monographs on the Evaluation of the Carcinogenic Risk of Chemicals to Humans*, Supplement 4, *Chemicals, Industrial Processes and Industries Associated with Cancer in Humans* (IARC Monographs, Volumes 1 to 29), Lyon

IARC (1983) *Approaches to Classifying Chemical Carcinogens According to Mechanism of Action* (IARC intern. tech. Rep. No. 83/001), Lyon

IARC (1984) *Chemicals and Exposures to Complex Mixtures Recommended for Evaluation in IARC Monographs and Chemicals and Complex Mixtures Recommended for Long-term Carcinogenicity Testing* (IARC intern. tech. Rep. No. 84/002), Lyon

IARC (1987a) *IARC Monographs on the Evaluation of Carcinogenic Risks to Humans*, Supplement 6, *Genetic and Related Effects: An Updating of Selected* IARC Monographs *from Volumes 1 to 42*, Lyon

IARC (1987b) *IARC Monographs on the Evaluation of Carcinogenic Risks to Humans*, Supplement 7, *Overall Evaluations of Carcinogenicity: An Updating of* IARC Monographs *Volumes 1 to 42*, Lyon

IARC (1988) *Report of an IARC Working Group to Review the Approaches and Processes Used to Evaluate the Carcinogenicity of Mixtures and Groups of Chemicals* (IARC intern. tech. Rep. No. 88/002), Lyon

IARC (1989) *Chemicals, Groups of Chemicals, Mixtures and Exposure Circumstances to be Evaluated in Future IARC Monographs, Report of an ad hoc Working Group* (IARC intern. tech. Rep. No. 89/004), Lyon

IARC (1991a) *A Consensus Report of an IARC Monographs Working Group on the Use of Mechanisms of Carcinogenesis in Risk Identification* (IARC intern. tech. Rep. No. 91/002), Lyon

IARC (1991b) *Report of an ad-hoc* IARC Monographs *Advisory Group on Viruses and Other Biological Agents Such as Parasites* (IARC intern. tech. Rep. No. 91/001), Lyon

IARC (1993) *Chemicals, Groups of Chemicals, Complex Mixtures, Physical and Biological Agents and Exposure Circumstances to be Evaluated in Future* IARC Monographs, *Report of an ad-hoc Working Group* (IARC intern. Rep. No. 93/005), Lyon

IARC (1998a) *Report of an ad-hoc* IARC Monographs *Advisory Group on Physical Agents* (IARC Internal Report No. 98/002), Lyon

IARC (1998b) *Report of an ad-hoc* IARC Monographs *Advisory Group on Priorities for Future Evaluations* (IARC Internal Report No. 98/004), Lyon

McGregor, D.B., Rice, J.M. & Venitt, S., eds (1999) *The Use of Short and Medium-term Tests for Carcinogens and Data on Genetic Effects in Carcinogenic Hazard Evaluation* (IARC Scientific Publications No. 146), Lyon, IARC

Montesano, R., Bartsch, H., Vainio, H., Wilbourn, J. & Yamasaki, H., eds (1986) *Long-term and Short-term Assays for Carcinogenesis—A Critical Appraisal* (IARC Scientific Publications No. 83), Lyon, IARC

Peto, R., Pike, M.C., Day, N.E., Gray, R.G., Lee, P.N., Parish, S., Peto, J., Richards, S. & Wahrendorf, J. (1980) Guidelines for simple, sensitive significance tests for carcinogenic effects in long-term animal experiments. In: *IARC Monographs on the Evaluation of the Carcinogenic Risk of Chemicals to Humans*, Supplement 2, *Long-term and Short-term Screening Assays for Carcinogens: A Critical Appraisal*, Lyon, pp. 311–426

Tomatis, L., Aitio, A., Wilbourn, J. & Shuker, L. (1989) Human carcinogens so far identified. *Jpn. J. Cancer Res.*, **80**, 795–807

Vainio, H., Magee, P.N., McGregor, D.B. & McMichael, A.J., eds (1992) *Mechanisms of Carcinogenesis in Risk Identification* (IARC Scientific Publications No. 116), Lyon, IARC

Vainio, H., Wilbourn, J.D., Sasco, A.J., Partensky, C., Gaudin, N., Heseltine, E. & Eragne, I. (1995) *Identification of human carcinogenic risk in* IARC Monographs. *Bull. Cancer,* **82,** 339–348 (in French)

Waters, M.D., Stack, H.F., Brady, A.L., Lohman, P.H.M., Haroun, L. & Vainio, H. (1987) Appendix 1. Activity profiles for genetic and related tests. In: *IARC Monographs on the Evaluation of Carcinogenic Risks to Humans*, Suppl. 6, *Genetic and Related Effects: An Updating of Selected IARC Monographs from Volumes 1 to 42*, Lyon, IARC, pp. 687–696

Wilbourn, J., Haroun, L., Heseltine, E., Kaldor, J., Partensky, C. & Vainio, H. (1986) Response of experimental animals to human carcinogens: an analysis based upon the IARC Monographs Programme. *Carcinogenesis*, **7**, 1853–1863

GENERAL REMARKS

Oestrogens and progestogens (progestins) and their medical uses for contraception and for post-menopausal hormonal therapy were considered by previous working groups, in 1974 (IARC, 1974), 1978 (IARC, 1979) and 1987 (IARC, 1987). The monographs included in this volume incorporate new data that have become available. They also reflect modifications to the Preamble to the *IARC Monographs* (IARC, 1991), which permit more explicit inclusion of information on mechanisms of carcinogenesis (Vainio *et al.*, 1992) and of data on effects other than cancer in the evaluation process.

IARC Monographs Volume 21 (IARC, 1979) gives a general discussion of sex hormones and cancer, and the principles described in that volume remain applicable, especially in the section 'General Conclusions on Sex Hormones': 'Steroid hormones are essential for the growth, differentiation and function of many tissues in both animals and humans. It has been established by animal experimentation that modification of the hormonal environment by surgical removal of endocrine glands, by pregnancy or by exogenous administration of steroids can increase or decrease the spontaneous occurrence of tumours or the induction of tumours by applied carcinogenic agents .... The incidence of tumours in humans could be altered by exposure to various exogenous hormones, singly or in combination.' These statements underline the facts that oestrogens and progestogens occur naturally and that the hormonal milieu and dose are generally inextricably involved in the carcinogenic effects of oestrogens and progestogens.

Naturally occurring and synthetic oestrogens and progestogens are among the most widely used drugs in medicine; however, the use of specific agents, combinations and regimens for contraception and for post-menopausal hormonal therapy varies from one geographic region to another and among countries, and the use of oestrogens and progestogens in medical practice continues to evolve rapidly. Moreover, the doses prescribed have changed significantly since previous evaluations in the *IARC Monographs*. The drugs themselves are complex and often cannot be classified simply as oestrogens or progestogens; some have multiple endocrine actions that may vary from one tissue to another. Accordingly, the substances evaluated in these monographs may differ from those evaluated under the same names by previous working groups.

Hormonal contraceptives

Oral contraceptives allow effective, convenient family planning for women and couples worldwide, and they have revolutionized the reproductive lives of millions of women since their introduction in the 1960s. When combined oral contraceptives are used correctly, the pregnancy rate is 0.1 per 100 woman–years, while the pregnancy rate with use of progestogen-only pills is somewhat higher (0.5 per 100 woman–years). Combined oral contraceptives prevent pregnancy primarily by inhibiting ovulation, while progestogen-only pills act mainly by altering the cervical mucus. Use of combined oral contraceptives leads to regular monthly bleeding in most women. Most of the studies of side-effects of hormonal contraceptives have been conducted with combined oral contraceptives; limited data are available for progestogen-only contraceptives, but they are generally regarded as safe.

In the 1960s, combined oral contraceptive preparations contained 100–150 μg ethinyloestradiol[1] and about 1–5 mg of a progestogen. The doses of both ethinyloestradiol and progestogens were successively lowered, and today preparations containing less than 50 μg ethinyloestradiol are generally used. The 'pill' most commonly used worldwide today contains 30 μg ethinyloestradiol and 150 μg levonorgestrel. New synthetic progestogens, i.e. desogestrel, gestodene and norgestimate, have been introduced. Combined oestrogen plus progestogen preparations are also available in injectable form, and progestogen-only preparations are available as tablets, injections, implants and intrauterine devices. Combined and progestogen-only tablets are used not only prophylactically but also as emergency contraceptives up to 72 h after intercourse.

The hormones that make up the various oral contraceptives affect not only the reproductive system but other bodily systems as well, and their effects on the prevalence and incidence of various diseases have been the subject of numerous studies over the past decades. Shortly after the introduction of combined oral contraceptives in about 1960, case reports were published of venous thrombolic disease, stroke and myocardial infarct in women using them. These reports spurred a large number of epidemiological studies of the cardiovascular effects of combined oral contraceptives. The relationship between use of combined oral contraceptives and acute myocardial infarct, stroke and venous thromboembolism has been reviewed (Chasan-Taber & Stampfer, 1998; WHO Scientific Group on Cardiovascular Disease and Steroid Hormone Contraception, 1998) and is summarized below.

The review of Chasan-Taber and Stampfer (1998) of 374 epidemiological studies led them to conclude that non-smoking women under 40 years of age who use oral contraceptives have little or no increase in their risk for myocardial infarct when compared with women who do not use these preparations. The WHO Scientific Group on Cardiovascular Disease and Steroid Hormone Contraception (1998) concluded that the risk for myocardial infarct is not increased by use of combined oral contraceptive by women who do not smoke, whose blood pressure is checked regularly and who do not have hypertension or diabetes, regardless of age; however, use of combined oral contraceptives increases the already elevated risk for myocardial infarct among women with cardiovascular risk factors, such as smoking and hypertension.

The risk for ischaemic stroke among women who do not smoke, have their blood pressure checked regularly and do not have hypertension is 1.5-fold higher for those who

---

[1] Throughout this volume, the term ethinyloestradiol is used for 17α-ethinyloestradiol.

currently use low-dose combined oral contraceptives than for those who do not (WHO Scientific Group on Cardiovascular Disease and Steroid Hormone Contraception, 1998). Combined oral contraceptives cause a small increase in blood pressure, even at low doses. A study in China showed an increase of 1.8–2.3 mm Hg (0.24–0.30 kPa) in diastolic pressure (Shen *et al.*, 1994). Among women who use combined oral contraceptives, the risk for haemorrhagic stroke is not increased in those who do not smoke, are not hypertensive and are under the age of 35 years, but may be increased by twofold in women aged 35 years or older. In general, use of combined oral contraceptives by women with risk factors for stroke adversely modifies their already elevated baseline risk (WHO Scientific Group on Cardiovascular Disease and Steroid Hormone Contraception, 1998).

The WHO Scientific Group on Cardiovascular Disease and Steroid Hormone Contraception (1998) concluded that current users of combined oral contraceptives have a three- to sixfold increase in the risk for venous thromboembolism in comparison with non-users; the excess risk is probably highest during the first year of use and declines thereafter, but it persists until discontinuation. Combined oral contraceptives containing desogestrel or gestodene have been associated in some studies with a greater increase in risk for venous thromboembolic disease than that reported with combined oral contraceptives containing levonorgestrel, but other studies have not come to the same conclusion. Smoking and hypertension do not appear to elevate the risk for venous thromboembolism.

The risk for gall-bladder disease, including gallstones, has been associated with current use of combined oral contraceptives, which may enhance the development of symptoms of already existing gallstones, with or without enhancement of gallstone formation (Thijs & Knipschild, 1993). Low-dose oral contraceptives appear to confer a lower risk for gall-bladder disease than high-dose oral contraceptives (Strom *et al.*, 1986; Vessey & Painter, 1994).

Use of combined oral contraceptives confers several benefits other than contraception. Their use has been associated with a reduced risk for benign breast disease, although it is not yet clear whether low-dose oral contraceptives have the same protective effect as high-dose preparations (McGonigle & Huggins, 1991). It has been reported that oral contraceptive users have a reduced risk for uterine myomas and for undergoing surgery for uterine myomas (Lumbagnon *et al.*, 1996). Other non-contraceptive benefits of combined oral contraceptive use include a reduced risk for iron deficiency anaemia, because of decreased menstrual blood loss, and lower frequencies of dysmenorrhoea and functional ovarian cysts (Mehta, 1993; Mishell, 1993). Two reviews also indicate a lower risk for uterine salpingitis in women who have contracted a sexually transmitted disease (Mishell, 1993; Burkman, 1994).

The newer progestogens used in low-dose combined oral contraceptives, desogestrel and gestodene, have fewer androgenic effects than those used earlier. Patients with acne have shown improvement after treatment with pills containing desogestrel, gestodene or norgestimate in randomized controlled trials (Mango *et al.*, 1996; Redmond *et al.*, 1997).

Post-menopausal hormonal therapy

With improvements in health and longevity, an increasing proportion of women's lives is lived after the menopause. In developed countries, life expectancy is such that, on average, women are expected to live half of their adult lives after the menopause, with the associated reductions in the concentrations of endogenous oestrogen and progestogen.

Post-menopausal oestrogen therapy, introduced more than 50 years ago, was originally prescribed for the short-term relief of menopausal symptoms; interest in the risks and benefits of long-term therapy is relatively recent (see review by Ettinger, 1998). Studies of the health outcomes of oestrogen use after the menopause are heavily weighted by studies of oestrogens and of combined oestrogen and progestogen from the United States, where the oestrogens used are conjugated equine oestrogens and the progestogen is medroxyprogesterone acetate. The use of transdermal oestradiol[1] is relatively new, and few data on disease outcomes are available.

Post-menopausal oestrogen therapy is the most commonly prescribed medication in the United States. Nevertheless, even there, most post-menopausal women are not treated, and most of those who are prescribed oestrogen therapy discontinue it within a few years because of its side-effects or fear of cancer. Evidence of an increased risk for cancer is reviewed in this volume. The carcinogenic risks must be placed in the perspective of potential benefits (Grady *et al.*, 1992). The best-established benefit is the prevention of osteoporotic fractures (Lufkin *et al.*, 1992). Because coronary heart disease is the most common fatal disease among women in most developed countries, any significant reduction in risk for that outcome is important. As recently reviewed (Barrett-Connor & Grady, 1998), a meta-analysis of 25 studies of oestrogen therapy showed an overall relative risk for coronary heart disease of 0.70 (95% confidence interval [CI], 0.65–0.75), most of the use being of conjugated equine oestrogens alone, and seven studies of oestrogen plus a progestogen showed an overall relative risk of 0.66 (95% CI, 0.53–0.84). At present, the evidence that oestrogen prevents heart disease is consistent but circumstantial. The other most important postulated benefit of post-menopausal oestrogen therapy is the prevention of memory loss or dementia. As reviewed by Yaffe *et al.* (1998), a meta-analysis of 10 published studies showed a summary odds ratio of 0.71 (95% CI, 0.53–0.96) for the risk of developing dementia. The major well-documented non-cancer risks associated with post-menopausal oestrogen use are gall-bladder disease and deep-vein thrombosis or pulmonary embolism. In a large cohort study (Grodstein *et al.*, 1994), a twofold increase in the risk for cholecystectomy (relative risk [RR], 2.1; 95% CI, 1.9–2.4) was seen among post-menopausal women using hormones. The first published data showing a two- to fourfold increase in the risk for venous thromboembolic disease was published in 1996 (Daly *et al.*, 1996; Grodstein *et al.*, 1996; Jick *et al.*, 1996), and the results were confirmed in a randomized clinical trial (Grady *et al.*, 1997).

---

[1] Throughout this volume, the term oestradiol is used for oestradiol-17β.

The favourable health profiles of women who use oestrogens undoubtedly have contributed to the apparent protective effect of these drugs against cardiovascular disease and memory loss or dementia.

Methodological considerations in the interpretation of epidemiological studies

All possible reasons for discrepancies in the results of epidemiological studies must be considered critically. Broadly, the roles of chance, bias, confounding and biological susceptibility should be weighed before a final interpretation is made.

Chance: Many of the studies summarized clearly suffer from small numbers, particularly in relevant potential high-risk strata, e.g., with long-term exposure. All of the studies include associations with 'ever-use', but such analyses are rather uninformative and probably misleading, since the results become incomparable due to variations in exposure. Only a minority of the studies were large enough and had meaningfully large numbers of subjects in the long-duration sub-categories (e.g., Brinton *et al.*, 1986; Ewertz, 1988; Bergkvist *et al.*, 1989; Colditz *et al.*, 1995; Newcomb *et al.*, 1995; Persson *et al.*, 1997).

Five meta-analyses of the combined results from several (but different) sets of studies were conducted to improve the statistical power of subgroup analyses (Armstrong, 1988; Dupont & Page, 1991; Steinberg *et al.*, 1991; Sillero-Arenas *et al.*, 1992; Colditz *et al.*, 1993). Even these analyses arrived at different results: two failed to demonstrate an association between increased risk for breast cancer and long-term exposure. A collaborative re-analysis of most of the epidemiological evidence (Collaborative Group on Hormonal Factors in Breast Cancer, 1997), which included more studies with greater statistical power, showed a slight but significant relation between current long-term pre-menopausal use of oestrogens and breast cancer risk. Nevertheless, there was insufficient power to examine the association for users of regimens with progestogens only and for women with long duration of treatment in the distant past.

Biases: Non-differential measurement errors, e.g. imprecise classification of exposure to hormones, would be expected to attenuate (bias towards the null) any true association with the risk for breast cancer. For instance, in the collaborative re-analysis (Collaborative Group on Hormonal Factors in Breast Cancer, 1997), information on the hormonal constituents of the consumed drugs was available for only 40% of the subjects, indicating that there may be important heterogeneity with regard to compound types, regimens and schedules of exposure. Studies that provide precise measurements of the particular post-menopausal hormonal therapy used should, if there is a true link, achieve the most valid estimates.

More serious are biases that could systematically distort the results. In cohort studies, there is a possibility of surveillance bias, e.g. that subjects prescribed post-menopausal hormonal therapy more often undergo mammography (Barrett-Connor, 1991). Differential use of mammography was addressed in previous studies (Colditz *et al.*, 1995; Persson *et al.*, 1997) and studies performed within breast screening programmes (Brinton *et al.*, 1988; Schairer *et al.*, 1994; Persson *et al.*, 1997), and a positive risk relationship was seen. An additional complexity with regard to detection is the possibility that post-menopausal hormonal regimens enhance the density of the mammogram, depending on the treatment regimen (Persson *et al.*, 1997), and reduce the sensitivity of mammography to detect small tumours (Laya *et al.*, 1996).

In case–control studies, a general concern is recall bias, meaning that affected women report exposure more accurately than do controls; however, there is some empirical evidence that differential misclassification by case–control status is not a problem (Goodman *et al.*, 1990). Bias in the selection of controls is another possibility in many of the cited studies. Hospital-based studies (e.g. Harris *et al.*, 1992; La Vecchia *et al.*, 1995; Levi *et al.*, 1996; Tavani *et al.*, 1997) may be inherently biased, since hospitalized control subjects may have conditions related to exposure to hormones (e.g. fracture cases would be expected to have less exposure to hormones). Valid selection of controls should follow the study base principle, i.e. that controls are randomly sampled from the population and time that generated the cases. Even when population-based controls are used, as in the random-digit dialling procedure (Wingo *et al.*, 1987; Stanford *et al.*, 1995), there may be selection of subjects with regard to exposure variables (Olson *et al.*, 1992).

Confounding: It is clear that women taking post-menopausal hormonal therapy have anamnestic or behavioural features that may correlate with the risk for breast cancer (Barrett-Connor, 1991). Ethnicity and socioeconomic status are possible confounders. Obesity, linked to less use of hormones and to increased risk for post-menopausal breast cancer, and alcohol consumption (Rosenberg *et al.*, 1993) are examples of life-style factors that could be confounders. Time of natural or surgical menopause (oophorectomy) is a particularly important determinant of breast cancer risk and also of use of post-menopausal hormonal therapy (Colditz, 1996). The type and time of menopause and reproductive factors are crucial possible confounders.

The approaches used to deal with confounding have varied, particularly with regard to the variables of menopause (Pike *et al.*, 1998). One difficulty is classification of the menopausal status and age of women who have had a hysterectomy (without oophorectomy) or who started hormone use before the cessation of natural menses. In the collaborative analysis (Collaborative Group on Hormonal Factors in Breast Cancer, 1997), women of unknown age at menopause were excluded (18% of all subjects), implying that a substantial number of women who used bleeding-provoking oestrogen–progestogen regimens were not included in the analyses. Confounding by indication—the reason for treatment—is difficult to rule out; however, it is reasonable to believe that menopausal symptoms or osteoporosis would be associated with low levels of endogenous oestrogens.

All of these issues relate to the validity of the results of the individual studies. The approaches used to deal with aspects of validity vary among the studies, and this heterogeneity may be an important explanation for the inconsistencies among studies. A critical evaluation of validity is therefore basic to an interpretation of the results of any study.

Biological interpretation: As mentioned above, one reason for differences among the results may be the lack of sufficiently large numbers of women exposed for long enough sufficiently long ago, i.e. effects of both duration and latency. Even the collaborative analysis (Collaborative Group on Hormonal Factors in Breast Cancer, 1997) suggests that the number of women with such exposure is insufficient.

Even if issues of validity are properly addressed and the risk relationships are analysed in comparable ways, there may still be true differences in the effects of hormones on breast cancer development, due to differences in susceptibility factors. A number of such factors are considered in the monographs, e.g. obesity, ovarian status, age at diagnosis, use of combined oral contraceptives, reproductive factors, alcohol consumption, cigarette smoking, benign breast disease and family history. The only factor shown in several studies to modify the effects of hormones on the risk for breast and endometrial cancer is body mass (Brinton, 1997; Collaborative Group on Hormonal Factors in Breast Cancer, 1997). Hypothetically, differences in the degree of obesity in some study populations in the United States (Colditz *et al.*, 1995; Newcomb *et al.*, 1995; Stanford *et al.*, 1995), as compared with those in European studies (Ewertz, 1988; Bergkvist *et al.*, 1989; Persson *et al.*, 1997), could explain the inconsistent results. A definite difficulty in most studies of interactive effects is lack of power due to small numbers within subgroups.

New, very large, rigorously designed studies are needed. The underlying hypothesis should be supported by the results of clinical or basic research on hormonal pathways and mechanisms.

Studies in experimental animals

The results of studies in experimental animals (mice, rats, dogs and monkeys) are a fundamental component of the evaluation of agents for carcinogenicity. The results of whole-animal bioassays ideally provide data on tumour incidence, type and multiplicity in relevant tissues and organs and potential mechanisms of carcinogenesis. The use of rodents (rats and mice) allows the formation of test groups comprised of sufficient numbers of animals to provide statistically meaningful comparisons among groups, multiple groups exposed to agents at different doses and testing of both males and females. A major additional advantage of animal bioassays is that individual compounds or combinations of specific compounds can be tested for carcinogenicity, which is not possible in most epidemiological studies.

In practice, however, for several reasons, there are limitations to the data. Thus, while experimental animals provide the advantages mentioned above, depending on the agents being tested, they may not be an appropriate surrogate for human exposure because of fundamental pharmacokinetic and/or toxicokinetic differences. In addition, there are no appropriate animal models of menopause; the only approach available, ovariectomized animals, is likely to be biologically different from spontaneous menopause. The manner in which humans and test animals are exposed could lead to significant differences in carcinogenic effects. For example, test animals are generally exposed in the diet at constant doses. With sex hormones in particular, humans may be exposed to oestrogen–progestogen combinations in ratios that vary at different times during the month. Such a pattern of exposure is not generally used in bioassays. In addition, the doses used are generally high, and non-physiological metabolism of such high doses raises concern about potential toxicity that may compromise the responses.

In these monographs, only results available in the public domain, principally the peer-reviewed literature, are used in the evaluations. Published studies were not necessarily designed for the purpose of providing a comprehensive bioassay: frequently dose-response data were not obtained, the group sizes were not optimal and not all tissues were evaluated for the presence of tumours, thus reducing the sensitivity of the study. Further-more, the final evaluations and classifications of carcinogenicity require that such agents produce malignant tumours in at least two species and/or each sex and/or more than one tissue/organ system. Because of these considerations, the Working Group tried to be as selective as practical in choosing studies for evaluating the carcinogenicity of oestrogens and progestogens.

Hormonal activitivy in relation to human carcinogenesis

The two main categories of compounds in oral contraceptives and post-menopausal hormonal therapy have either oestrogenic or progestogenic effects: in some cases, overlap of biological activities occurs. The relevance of the effects of oestrogens and progestogens to carcinogenic effects in humans varies with the target tissue. The main human tissues affected are breast, endometrium, cervix and ovary, with minor effects on the liver and colon. Only in the endometrium is there a clear-cut hypothesis about the molecular events that cause oestrogens to increase cancer risk and progestogens to antagonize the effects of oestrogens. These changes can be modelled in terms of receptor-mediated hormone effects on cell proliferation (King, 1997), but the genotoxic effects of oestrogen metabolites may also be important (Yager & Liehr, 1996). In the breast, it is clear that exposure to oestrogens increases cancer incidence, but whether progestogens have a stimulatory, inhibitory or benign role is unclear (Key & Pike, 1988; King, 1993). In the ovary, some of the effects may be indirect, acting by altering ovulation rates. In the cervix, the mechanisms are more obscure: human papillomavirus (see IARC, 1995), an important contributory agent to cervical cancer, has a weak glucocorticoid or progestogen response element in its DNA which indicates a possible stimulatory mechanism (Villa, 1997). In the liver, the relation with infection by hepatitis viruses B and C (see IARC, 1994) has been little studied.

The majority of the above responses can be explained by oestrogen and progestogen receptor mechanisms (King, 1991), but non-receptor processes may also exist (Duval *et al.*, 1983; Yager & Liehr, 1996). Cell proliferation may be the most important receptor-mediated mechanism by which hormonally active compounds act in carcinogenesis at hormone-sensitive target tissues. Cell proliferation is fundamental to the process of carcino-genesis; it is an essential (co)factor and enhances cancer incidence (i.e. tumour promoting) by preferentially stimulating the growth of genetically altered and preneoplastic cells (Preston-Martin *et al.*, 1990). Most if not all steroid hormonal stimulation of cell prolife-ration involves autocrine and paracrine events secondary to the steroid–hormone receptor complex interaction with hormone-response elements in the promoter region of relevant genes; this has been shown for breast and endometrial epithelium (Boyd, 1996; Snedeker

& Diaugustine, 1996). Exposure to certain hormones can result in the production of reactive intermediates which, either *per se* or via secondary generation of reactive oxygen species, can cause genetic damage in some tissues under certain conditions (Yager & Liehr, 1996). The significance of this property is not clear. The following approximations indicate how the doses of hormones used in experimental studies relate both to receptor and non-receptor mechanisms and to the doses achieved *in vivo* with oral contraceptives or post-menopausal hormonal therapy. In humans, the doses of hormones in oral contraceptives and post-menopausal hormonal therapy are usually in the low range of micro-grams per kilogram body weight per day, which generate plasma hormone levels of nano-grams (progestogens) or picograms (oestrogens) per litre (Orme *et al.*, 1983; Barnes & Lobo, 1987). These are the concentrations at which receptor-mediated events can be satu-rated *in vitro*. At appreciably higher concentrations, non-receptor mechanisms, such as induction of genetic damage, become detectable. It should be borne in mind that at concen-trations of micrograms per millilitre, these compounds can have surfactant effects (Duval *et al.*, 1983). As stated earlier, the significance of these non-receptor-mediated mechanisms is not clear; however, genetic and related effects in experimental systems have been reported by Vickers *et al.* (1989) (ethinyloestradiol plus a potent carcinogen) and Topinka *et al.* (1993) (cyproterone acetate) with doses relevant to use of oral contraceptives or post-menopausal hormonal therapy. In addition, Ghosh and Ghosh (1988), Pinto (1986) and Olsson *et al.* (1991a,b) observed genetic damage in women taking contraceptives or post-menopausal oestrogen therapy. Other factors involved in the carcinogenic process may also be involved in carcinogenic responses to hormones (Barrett & Tsutsui, 1996).

The changes made in the composition and mode of delivery of contraceptives were driven primarily by requirements for adequate contraception and minimization of side-effects, including those involving cardiovascular function. Effects on cancer development have not been a major consideration, especially as observations of effects may require extended use. For this reason, it is unclear how recent modifications in the composition and mode of use of contraceptives will affect cancer incidence. It is reasonable to expect that, because of these changes, the effects of contraceptives and post-menopausal hormonal therapy will have to be reviewed again in the future.

References

Armstrong, B.K. (1988) Oestrogen therapy after the menopause—boon or bane? *Med. J. Aust.*, **148**, 213–214

Barnes, R.B. & Lobo, R.A. (1987) Pharmacology of estrogens. In: Mishell, D.R., Jr, ed., *Menopause: Physiology and Pharmacology*, Chicago, IL, Year Book Medical, pp. 301–315

Barrett-Connor, E. (1991) Postmenopausal estrogen and prevention bias. *Ann. intern. Med.*, **115**, 455–456

Barrett-Connor, E. & Grady, D. (1998) Hormone replacement therapy, heart disease and other considerations. *Ann. Rev. public Health*, **19**, 55–72

Barrett, J.C. & Tsutsui, T. (1996) Mechanisms of estrogen-associated carcinogenesis. *Prog. clin. biol. Res.*, **394**, 105–111

Bergkvist, L., Adami, H.-O., Persson, I., Hoover, R. & Schairer, C. (1989) The risk of breast cancer after estrogen and estrogen-progestin replacement. *New Engl. J. Med.*, **321**, 293–297

Boyd, J. (1996) Estrogen as a carcinogen: The genetics and molecular biology of human endometrial carcinoma. In: Huff, J., Boyd, J. & Barrett, J.C., eds, *Cellular and Molecular Mechanisms of Hormonal Carcinogenesis: Environmental Influences*, New York, Wiley-Liss, pp. 151–173

Brinton, L.A. (1997) Hormone replacement therapy and risk for breast cancer. *Endocrinol. Metab. Clin. N. Am.*, **26**, 361–378

Brinton, L.A., Hoover, R. & Fraumeni, J.F., Jr (1986) Menopausal oestrogens and breast cancer risk: An expanded case–control study. *Br. J. Cancer*, **54**, 825–832

Brinton, L.A., Schairer, C., Hoover, R.N. & Fraumeni, J.F., Jr (1988) Menstrual factors and risk of breast cancer. *Cancer Invest.*, **6**, 245–254

Burkman, R.T., Jr (1994) Noncontraceptive effects of hormonal contraceptives: Bone mass, sexually transmitted disease and pelvic inflammatory disease, cardiovascular disease, menstrual function, and future fertility. *Am. J. Obstet. Gynecol.*, **170**, 1569–1575

Chasan-Taber, L. & Stampfer, M.J. (1998) Epidemiology of oral contraceptives and cardiovascular disease. *Ann. intern. Med.*, **128**, 467–477

Colditz, G.A. (1996) Postmenopausal estrogens and breast cancer. *J. Soc. gynecol. Invest.*, **3**, 50–56

Colditz, G.A., Egan, K.M. & Stampfer, M.J. (1993) Hormone replacement therapy and risk of breast cancer: Results from epidemiologic studies. *Am. J. Obstet. Gynecol.*, **168**, 1473–1480

Colditz, G.A., Hankinson, S.E., Hunter, D.J., Willett, W.C., Manson, J.E., Stampfer, M.J., Hennekens, C., Rosner, B. & Speizer, F.E. (1995) The use of estrogens and progestins and the risk of breast cancer in postmenopausal women. *New Engl. J. Med.*, **332**, 1589–1593

Collaborative Group on Hormonal Factors in Breast Cancer (1997) Breast cancer and hormone replacement therapy: Collaborative reanalysis of data from 51 epidemiological studies of 52 705 women with breast cancer and 108 411 women without breast cancer. *Lancet*, **350**, 1047–1059

Daly, E., Vessey, M.P., Hawkins, M.M., Carson, J.L., Gough, P. & Marsh, S. (1996) Risk of venous thromboembolism in users of hormone replacement therapy. *Lancet*, **348**, 977–980

Dupont, W.D. & Page, D.L. (1991) Menopausal estrogen replacement therapy and breast cancer. *Arch. intern. Med.*, **151**, 67–72

Duval, D., Durant, S. & Homo-Delarche, F. (1983) Non-genomic effects of steroids: Interactions of steroid molecules with membrane structures and functions. *Biochim. biophys. Acta*, **737**, 409–442

Ettinger, B. (1998) Overview of estrogen replacement therapy: A historical perspective. *Proc. Soc. exp. Biol. Med.*, **217**, 2–5

Ewertz, M. (1988) Influence of non-contraceptive exogenous and endogenous sex hormones on breast cancer risk in Denmark. *Int. J. Cancer*, **42**, 832–838

Ghosh, R. & Ghosh, P.K. (1988) Sister chromatid exchanges in the lymphocytes of control women, pregnant women, and women taking oral contraceptives: Effects of cell culture temperature. *Environ. mol. Mutag.*, **12**, 179–183

Goodman, M.T., Nomura, A.M., Wilkens, L.R. & Kolonel, L.N. (1990) Agreement between interview information and physician records on history of menopausal estrogen use. *Am. J. Epidemiol.*, **131**, 815–825

Grady, D., Rubin, S.M., Petitti, D.B., Fox, C.S., Black, D., Ettinger, B., Ernster, V.L. & Cummings, S.R. (1992) Hormone therapy to prevent disease and prolong life in postmenopausal women. *Ann. intern. Med.*, **117**, 1016–1037

Grady, D., Hulley, S.B. & Furberg, C. (1997) Venous thromboembolic events associated with hormone replacement therapy (Letter to the Editor). *J. Am. med. Assoc.*, **278**, 477

Grodstein, F., Colditz, G.A. & Stampfer, M.J. (1994) Postmenopausal hormone use and cholecystectomy in a large prospective study. *Obstet. Gynecol.*, **83**, 5–11

Grodstein, F., Stampfer, M.J., Goldhaber, S.Z., Manson, J.E., Colditz, G.A., Speizer, F.E., Willett, W.C. & Hennekens, C.H. (1996) Prospective study of exogenous hormones after risk of pulmonary embolism in women. *Lancet*, **348**, 983–987

Harris, R., Whittemore, A.S., Itnyre, J. & the Collaborative Ovarian Cancer Group (1992) Characteristics relating to ovarian cancer risk: Collaborative analysis of 12 US case–control studies. III. Epithelial tumors of low malignant potential in white women. *Am. J. Epidemiol.*, **136**, 1204–1211

IARC (1974) *IARC Monographs on the Evaluation of Carcinogenic Risk of Chemicals to Man*, Vol. 6, *Sex Hormones*, Lyon

IARC (1979) *IARC Monographs on the Evaluation of the Carcinogenic Risk of Chemicals to Humans*, Vol. 21, *Sex Hormones (II)*, Lyon

IARC (1987) *IARC Monographs on the Evaluation of Carcinogenic Risks to Humans*, Suppl. 7, *Overall Evaluations of Carcinogenicity: An Updating of* IARC Monographs *Volumes 1 to 42*, Lyon, pp. 272–310

IARC (1991) *A Consensus Report of an IARC Monographs Working Group on the Use of Mechanisms of Carcinogenesis in Risk Identification* (IARC intern. tech. Rep. No. 91/002), Lyon

IARC (1994) *IARC Monographs on the Evaluation of Carcinogenic Risks to Humans*, Vol. 59, *Hepatitis Viruses*, Lyon

IARC (1995) *IARC Monographs on the Evaluation of Carcinogenic Risks to Humans*, Vol. 64, *Human Papillomaviruses*, Lyon

Jick, H., Derby, L.E., Myers, M.W., Vasilakis, C. & Newton, K.M. (1996) Risk of hospital admission for idiopathic venous thromboembolism among users of postmenopausal oestrogens. *Lancet*, **348**, 981–983

Key, T.J.A & Pike, M.C. (1988) The role of oestrogens and progestagens in the epidemiology and prevention of breast cancer. *Eur. J. Cancer clin. Oncol.*, **24**, 29–43

King, R.J.B. (1991) A discussion of the roles of oestrogen and progestin in human mammary carcinogenesis. *J. Steroid Biochem. mol. Biol.*, **39**, 811–118

King, R.J.B. (1993) William L. McGuire Memorial Symposium. Estrogen and progestin effects in human breast carcinogenesis. *Breast Cancer Res. Treat.*, **27**, 3–15

King, R.J.B. (1997) Endometrial cancer: An introduction. In: Langdon, S.P., Miller, W.R. & Berchuck, A., eds, *Biology of Female Cancers*, Boca Raton, CRC Press, pp. 183–192

La Vecchia, C., Negri, E., Franceschi, S., Favero, A., Nanni, O., Filiberti, R., Conti, E., Montella, M., Veronesi, A., Ferraroni, M. & Decarli, A. (1995) Hormone replacement treatment and breast cancer risk: A cooperative Italian study. *Br. J. Cancer*, **72**, 244–248

Laya, M.B., Larson, E.B., Taplin, S.H. & White, E. (1996) Effect of estrogen replacement therapy on the specificity and sensitivity of screening mammography. *J. natl Cancer Inst.*, **88**, 643–649

Levi, F., Lucchini, F., Pasche, C. & La Vecchia, C. (1996) Oral contraceptives, menopausal hormone replacement treatment and breast cancer risk. *Eur. J. Cancer Prev.*, **5**, 259–266

Lufkin, E.G., Wahner, H.W., O'Fallon, W.M., Hodgson, S.F., Kotowicz, M.A., Lane, A.W., Judd, H.L., Caplan, R.H. & Riggs, B.L. (1992) Treatment of postmenopausal osteoporosis with transdermal estrogen. *Ann. intern. Med.*, **117**, 1–9

Lumbagnon, P., Rugpao, S., Phandhu-fung, S., Paopaiboon, M., Vudhikamraksa, N. & Werawatkul, Y. (1996) Protective effect of depot-medroxyprogesterone acetate on surgically treated uterine leiomyomas: A multicentre case–control study. *Br. J. Obstet. Gynaecol.*, **103**, 909–914

Mango, D., Ricci, S., Manna, P., Miggiano, G.A. & Serra, G.B. (1996) Clinical and hormonal effects of ethinylestradiol combined with gestodene and desogestrel in young women with acne vulgaris. *Contraception*, **53**, 163–170

McGonigle, K.F. & Huggins, G.R. (1991) Oral contraceptives and breast disease. *Fertil. Steril.*, **56**, 799–819

Mehta, S. (1993) Oral contraception—benefits and risks. In: Senanayake, P. & Kleinman, R.L., eds, *Family Planning. Meeting Challenges: Promoting Choices*, Carnforth, Parthenon Publishing Group, pp. 463–476

Mishell, D.R., Jr (1993) Noncontraceptive benefits of oral contraceptives. *J. reprod. Med.*, **38** (Suppl. 12), 1021–1029

Newcomb, P.A., Longnecker, M.P., Storer, B.E., Mittendorf, R., Baron, J., Clapp, R.W., Bogdan, G. & Willett, W.C. (1995) Long-term hormone replacement therapy and risk of breast cancer in postmenopausal women. *Am. J. Epidemiol.*, **142**, 788–795

Olson, S.H., Kelsey, J.L., Pearson, T.A. & Levin, B. (1992) Evaluation of random digit dialing as a method of control selection in case-control studies. *Am J. Epidemiol.*, **135**, 210-222

Olsson, H., Borg, A., Fernö, M., Ranstam, J. & Sigurdsson, H. (1991a) Her-2/neu and INT2 proto-oncogene amplification in malignant breast tumors in relation to reproductive factors and exposure to exogenous hormones. *J. natl Cancer Inst.*, **83**, 1483–1487

Olsson, H., Ranstam, J., Baldetorp, B., Ewers, S.-B., Fernö, M., Killander, D. & Sigurdsson, H. (1991b) Proliferation and DNA ploidy in malignant breast tumors in relation to early oral contraceptive use and early abortions. *Cancer*, **67**, 1285–1290

Orme, M.L.E., Back, D.J. & Breckenridge, A.M. (1983) Clinical pharmacokinetics of oral contraceptive steroids. *Clin. Pharmacokinet.*, **8**, 95–136

Persson, I., Thurfjell, E., Bergström, R. & Holmberg, L. (1997) Hormone replacement therapy and the risk of breast cancer. Nested case–control study in a cohort of Swedish women attending mammography screening. *Int. J. Cancer*, **72**, 758–761

Pike, M.C., Ross, R.K. & Spicer, D.V. (1998) Problems involved in including women with simple hysterectomy in epidemiologic studies measuring the effects of hormone replacement therapy in breast cancer risk. *Am. J. Epidemiol.*, **147**, 718–721

Pinto, M.R. (1986) Possible effects of hormonal contraceptives on human mitotic chromosomes. *Mutat. Res.*, **169**, 149–157

Preston-Martin, S., Pike, M.C., Ross, R.K., Jones, P.A. & Henderson, B.E. (1990) Increased cell division as a cause of human cancer. *Cancer Res.*, **50**, 7415–7421

Redmond, G.P., Olson, W.H., Lippman, J.S., Kafrissen, M.E., Jones, T.M. & Jorizzo, J.L. (1997) Norgestimate and ethinyl estradiol in the treatment of acne vulgaris: A randomized, placebo-controlled trial. *Obstet. Gynecol.*, **89**, 615–622

Rosenberg, L., Metzger, L.S. & Palmer, J.R. (1993) Alcohol consumption and risk of breast cancer: A review of the epidemiologic evidence. *Epidemiol. Rev.*, **15**, 133–144

Schairer, C., Byrne, C., Keyl, P.M., Brinton, L.A., Sturgeon, S.R. & Hoover, R.N. (1994) Menopausal estrogen and estrogen–progestin replacement therapy and risk of breast cancer (United States). *Cancer Causes Control*, **5**, 491–500

Shen, Q., Lin, D., Jiang, X., Li, H. & Zhang, Z. (1994) Blood pressure changes and hormonal contraceptives. *Contraception*, **50**, 131–141

Sillero-Arenas, M., Delgado-Rodriguez, M., Rodigues-Canteras, R., Bueno-Cavanillas, A. & Galvez-Vargas, R. (1992) Menopausal hormone replacement therapy and breast cancer: A meta-analysis. *Obstet. Gynecol.*, **79**, 286–294

Snedeker, S.M. & Diaugustine, R.P. (1996) Hormonal and environmental factors affecting cell proliferation and neoplasia in the mammary gland. *Prog. clin. biol. Res.*, **394,** 211–253

Stanford, J.L., Weiss, N.S., Voigt, L.F., Daling, J.R., Habel, L.A. & Rossing, M.A. (1995) Combined estrogen and progestin hormone replacement therapy in relation to risk of breast cancer in middle-aged women. *J. Am. med. Assoc.*, **274**, 137–142

Steinberg, K.K., Thacker, S.B., Smith, S.J., Stroup, D.F., Zack, M.M., Flanders, W.D. & Berkelman, R.L. (1991) A meta-analysis of the effect of estrogen replacement therapy on the risk of breast cancer. *J. Am. med. Assoc.*, **265**, 1985–1990

Strom, B.L., Tamragouri, R.N., Morse, M.L., Lazar, E.L., West, S.L., Stolley, P.D. & Jones, J.K. (1986) Oral contraceptives and other risk factors for gallbladder disease. *Clin. Pharmacol. Ther.*, **39**, 335–341

Tavani, A., Braga, C., La Vecchia, C., Negri, E. & Franceschi, S. (1997) Hormone replacement treatment and breast cancer risk: An age-specific analysis. *Cancer Epidemiol. Biomarkers Prev.*, **6**, 11-14

Thijs, C. & Knipschild, P. (1993) Oral contraceptives and the risk of gallbladder disease: A meta-analysis. *Am. J. public Health*, **83**, 1113–1120

Topinka, J., Andrae, U., Schwartz, L.R. & Wolff, T. (1993) Cyproterone acetate generates DNA adducts in rat liver and in primary rat hepatocyte cultures. *Carcinogenesis,* **14**, 423–427

Vainio, H., Magee, P.N., McGregor, D.B. & McMichael, A.J., eds (1992) *Mechanisms of Carcinogenesis in Risk Identification* (IARC Scientific Publications No. 116), Lyon, IARC

Vessey, M. & Painter, R. (1994) Oral contraceptive use and benign gallbladder disease; revisited. *Contraception*, **50**, 167–173

Vickers, A.E.M., Nelson, K., McCoy, Z. & Lucier, G.W. (1989) Changes in estrogen receptor, DNA ploidy, and estrogen metabolism in rat hepatocytes during a two-stage model for hepatocarcinogenesis using 17 alpha-ethinylestradiol as the promoting agent. *Cancer Res.*, **49**, 6512–6520

Villa, L.L. (1997) Human papillomaviruses and cervical cancer. *Adv. Cancer Res.*, **71**, 321–341

WHO Scientific Group on Cardiovascular Disease and Steroid Hormone Contraception (1998) *Cardiovascular Disease and Steroid Hormone Contraception* (WHO Technical Report Series 877), Geneva

Wingo, P.A., Layde, P.M., Lee, N.C., Rubin, G. & Ory, H.W. (1987) The risk of breast cancer in postmenopausal women who have used estrogen replacement therapy. *J. Am. med. Assoc.*, **257**, 209–215

Yaffe, K., Sawaya, G., Lieberburg, I. & Grady, D. (1998) Estrogen therapy in postmenopausal women. Effects on cognitive function and dementia. *J. Am. med. Assoc.*, **279**, 688–695

Yager, J.D. & Liehr, J.G. (1996) Molecular mechanisms of estrogen carcinogenesis. *Ann. Rev. Pharmacol. Toxicol.*, **36**, 203–232

THE MONOGRAPHS

ORAL CONTRACEPTIVES, COMBINED

1. Exposure

Combined oral contraceptives consist of the steroid hormone oestrogen in combination with a progestogen, taken primarily to prevent pregnancy. The same hormones can also be used in other forms for contraception. Combined oral contraceptive pills generally refer to pills in which an oestrogen and a progestogen are given concurrently in a monthly cycle. In contrast, a cycle of sequential oral contraceptive pills includes oestrogen-only pills followed by five to seven days of oestrogen plus progestogen pills. Sequential oral contraceptive pills were removed from the consumer market in the late 1970s; they are covered in an IARC monograph (IARC, 1979, 1987). Combined oral contraceptives are thus usually administered as a pill containing oestrogen and progestogen, which is taken daily for 20–22 days, followed by a seven-day pill-free interval (or seven days of placebo), during which time a withdrawal bleed is expected to occur. The most commonly used oestrogen is ethinyloestradiol, although mestranol is used in some formulations. The progestogens most commonly used in combined oral contraceptives are derived from 19-nortestosterone and include norethisterone, norgestrel and levonorgestrel, although many others are available (Kleinman, 1990) (see Annex 2, Table 1).

Chemical and physical data and information on the synthesis, production, use and regulations and guidelines for hormones used in combined oral contraceptives are given in Annex 1. Annex 2 (Table 1) lists the trade names of many contemporary combined oral contraceptives with their formulations.

Combined oral contraceptives are currently available in monophasic, biphasic and triphasic preparations, the terms referring to the number of different doses of progestogen they contain. Monophasic pills maintain a constant dose of oestrogen and progestogen, while multiphasic pills allow a lower total dose of progestogen to be given by reducing the amount of progestogen early in the 20–22-day period of exposure. Biphasic pills contain a lower dose of progestogen early in the cycle followed by a higher dose in the last 11 days. Triphasic pills consist of three doses of progestogen, increasing through the cycle, which may or may not be accompanied by variations in the dose of oestrogen (Kleinman, 1990).

Sequential pills contain only oestrogen during the first part of the cycle and an oestrogen and progestogen thereafter. In older regimens, oestrogen was given alone for the first 16 days of the cycle, followed by five days of combined oestrogen and progestogen. These preparations were withdrawn from use in many countries in the 1970s after concern about their association with endometrial cancer (IARC, 1974, 1979). The sequential combined oral contraceptive regimens available currently include oestrogen alone for a shorter interval, usually one week, followed by combined oestrogen and progestogen (Wharton & Blackburn, 1988; Kleinman, 1990).

Combined oral contraceptives act primarily by preventing ovulation, by inhibiting pituitary follicle-stimulating hormone and luteinizing hormone and by abolishing the pre-ovulatory surge in luteinizing hormone. The progestogen component renders the cervical mucus relatively impenetrable to sperm and may also reduce the receptivity of the endometrium to implantation (Williams & Stancel, 1996). Together, these actions make combined oral contraceptives very effective in preventing pregnancy, with fewer than one pregnancy per 100 users in the first year of use, when used correctly.

1.1   Historical overview

In the late nineteenth century, researchers noted that follicular development and ovulation were suppressed during pregnancy and that extracts of the corpus luteum inhibited ovulation in laboratory animals. In 1921, Ludwig Haberlandt proposed that extracts of the ovary itself could act as a contraceptive (Kleinman, 1990).

Three oestrogens were identified in 1929 and 1930, and progesterone was identified in 1934; however, there were no readily available oral equivalents until 1941, when Russell Marker synthesized diosgenin from extracts of the Mexican yam. Further experimentation yielded the synthesis of norethisterone (norethindrone in the United States) by Carl Djerassi in 1950 and norethynodrel by Frank B. Colton in 1952. These compounds were named progestogens (or progestins) due to their progesterone-like actions (Kleinman, 1990).

In the early 1950s, John Rock investigated the combination of oestrogen and progestogen for the treatment of infertility and found that women who were taking this compound did not ovulate. During 1956, Gregory Pincus, Celso-Ramon Garcia, John Rock and Edris Rice-Wray initiated clinical trials in Puerto Rico of the use of oral norethynodrel as a contraceptive. It was noted that the preparations containing the oestrogen mestranol as a contaminant were more effective in suppressing ovulation than those containing pure norethynodrel. In 1957, the combination of mestranol and norethynodrel was made available in the United States for regulation of menstruation, and in May 1960 it was approved as an oral contraceptive (McLaughlin, 1982; Kleinman, 1990). It was marketed as Enovid® and contained 150 µg mestranol and 9.35 mg norethynodrel (Thorogood & Villard-Mackintosh, 1993). Oral norethisterone (Norlutin®) was approved for menstrual regulation, but was not approved as an oral contraceptive until 1962, when it was combined with mestranol, as Ortho-Novum® (Drill, 1966). Interestingly, in 1959, about 500 000 women in the United States were taking Enovid® or Norlutin® for the treatment of 'menstrual disorders' (McLaughlin, 1982). Enovid® became available in the United Kingdom in 1960 (Thorogood & Villard-Mackintosh, 1993). Combined oral contraceptives were introduced throughout Europe and Latin America in the mid- to late 1960s, while use in many countries of Asia, Africa and the Middle East began in the 1970s and early 1980s (Wharton & Blackburn, 1988).

Figure 1 shows sales data for 1964–87 which have been converted into estimates of the percentages of women aged 15–44 buying the combined oral contraceptive pill from

Figure 1. Estimated percentages of women aged 15–44 buying oral contraceptives from pharmacies

(a) English-speaking countries, 1964 – 87

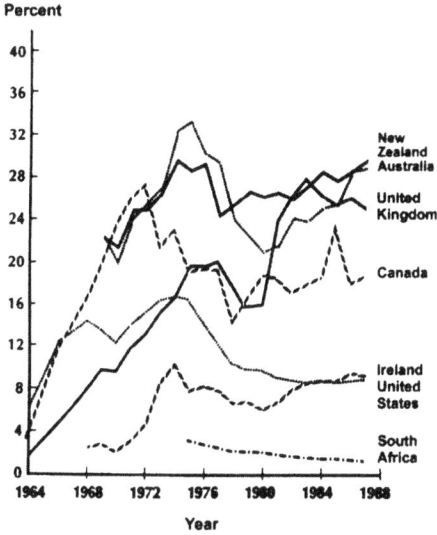

Percent

New Zealand
Australia
United Kingdom
Canada
Ireland
United States
South Africa

(b) Continental Europe, 1964 – 87

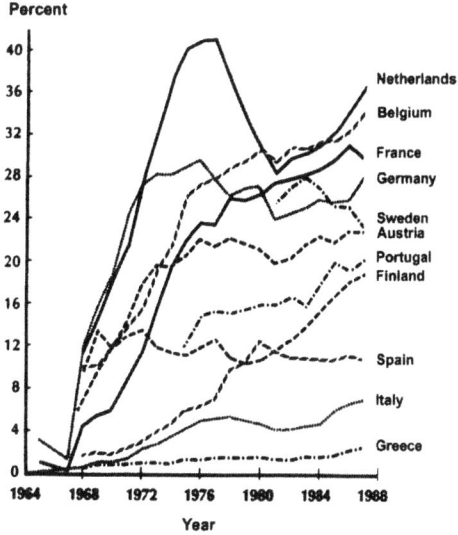

Percent

Netherlands
Belgium
France
Germany
Sweden
Austria
Portugal
Finland
Spain
Italy
Greece

(c) Latin America, 1968 – 87

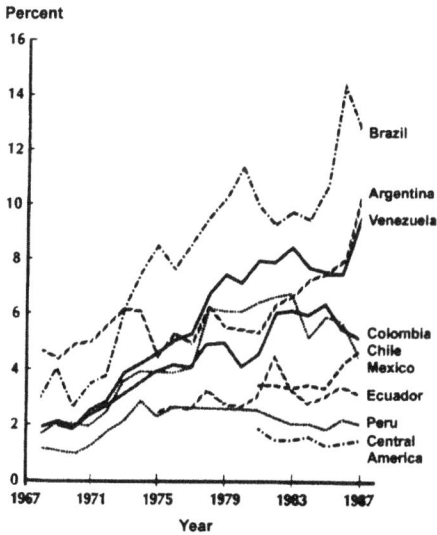

Percent

Brazil
Argentina
Venezuela
Colombia
Chile
Mexico
Ecuador
Peru
Central America

(d) Asia, Africa and the Near East, 1968 – 87

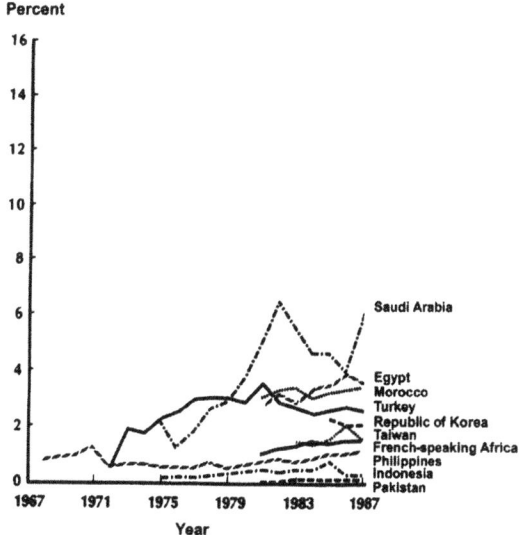

Percent

Saudi Arabia
Egypt
Morocco
Turkey
Republic of Korea
Taiwan
French-speaking Africa
Philippines
Indonesia
Pakistan

Adapted from Wharton and Blackburn (1988)

pharmacies. It shows the rapid increase in the use of the combined oral contraceptive pill in North America, Australia, New Zealand and many European countries in the late 1960s and early 1970s, as well as the decline in use in some countries in the late 1970s, corresponding to the period when the adverse cardiovascular effects of the combined oral contraceptive pill were becoming apparent. They also show the lower but generally increasing rates of combined oral contraceptive use over that time in Latin America, Asia and Africa, although it is important to bear in mind that these figures do not include combined oral contraceptives donated by aid agencies, which constitute up to a third of use in these places (Wharton & Blackburn, 1988).

From the first combined oral contraceptive pill to those available at the time of writing, the doses of oestrogen and progestogen have decreased by at least threefold, and the compositions of treatments have changed, as has the timing of administration of the various component hormones (Piper & Kennedy, 1987). As noted above, the first combined oral contraceptive contained 150 µg mestranol (oestrogen) and 9.35 mg norethynodrel (progestogen); in 1963, just under 50% of combined oral contraceptive pills used by a sample of British women contained 100 µg oestrogen and the remainder contained at least 50 µg oestrogen (Thorogood & Villard-Mackintosh, 1993). Nausea, headaches, vomiting and other side-effects were already thought to be related to high oestrogen levels when research in Britain in the late 1960s linked high oestrogen doses to thromboembolic disease. This finding resulted in the development and prescription of lower-dose pills in the 1970s and 1980s, with the eventual phasing out of those containing more than 50 µg of oestrogen. These lower-dose combined oral contraceptives were found to be just as effective in preventing pregnancy as the high-dose pills, but with fewer side-effects (Wharton & Blackburn, 1988). Most of the combined oral contraceptives prescribed now contain less than 50 µg oestrogen (Wharton & Blackburn, 1988), a dose of 30–35 µg being standard and doses of 20 µg being available (Kleinman, 1990).

The dose of progestogen has also decreased over time, and many different types have been developed (see Annex 2, Table 1). Use of combined oral contraceptives containing a high dose of progestogen peaked in 1972 in the United States, with gradual decreases since, facilitated by the introduction of biphasic and triphasic pills in the 1980s, which allowed the use of even lower doses of progestogen (Piper & Kennedy, 1987; Wharton & Blackburn, 1988). The so-called 'new-generation' progestogens (desogestrel, gestodene and norgestimate) were introduced in the mid-1980s, promising lower doses with equivalent efficacy. Studies published around 1995 showed these compounds to be associated with higher rates of venous thromboembolism than those seen with other progestogens (Jick et al., 1995; Farley et al., 1996), resulting in a decrease in the number of prescriptions of combined oral contraceptives containing new-generation progestogens.

1.2   Patterns of use of combined oral contraceptives

Over 200 million women worldwide have used combined oral contraceptives since 1960 (Kleinman, 1990), and over 60 million are using them currently (Wharton & Blackburn, 1988). The prevalence of combined oral contraceptive use varies enormously by country and region. Table 1 shows the percentage of married women or women in union aged 15–49 using any form of contraception (including traditional methods) and the percentage taking oral contraceptives. Although progestogen-only oral contraceptives are generally included in this figure, they constitute a relatively small proportion of use, even in the countries where they are most commonly used (see the monograph on 'Hormonal contraceptives, progestogens only'). The percentages are derived mainly from the Demographic and Health Surveys conducted by the United States Aid to International Development.

In 1988, the highest rates of combined oral contraceptive use were found in Europe, with over 40% of women in union of reproductive age using combined oral contraceptives in Belgium, Germany, Hungary and the Netherlands; in most other western European countries and in Australia and New Zealand, current use was 20–40%. Lower rates of use were found in Mediterranean Europe, including Spain, Italy and Greece. Use in the Americas and South-East Asia was generally intermediate, representing around 10–20% of eligible women, while countries in North Africa and the Middle East showed considerable variation in rates of use. The low rates of use of combined oral contraceptives in many countries of sub-Saharan Africa probably reflect low rates of contraceptive use overall and are in keeping with the large 'ideal family size' reported in those countries (Wharton & Blackburn, 1988). The low use in many eastern European and former Soviet Union countries probably reflects reliance on other methods of birth control, including abortion, and use of intrauterine devices (Popov *et al.*, 1993). Use of combined oral contraceptives is also uncommon in the Indian sub-continent. They are not licenced for contraceptive use in Japan, although high-dose preparations are available for the treatment of menstrual problems (Kleinman, 1996).

Patterns of use also vary from country to country. Table 2 shows the percentages of women who have ever used combined oral contraceptives by year of birth. The figures are those for the controls of population-based studies of use of combined oral contraceptives and breast cancer. Clearly, in the birth cohorts examined, any use of the pill depends on the age of the woman at the time combined oral contraceptives were introduced into a country as well as the overall prevalence and pattern of use. It is also clear that, in many countries in Europe and in Australia, New Zealand and North America, the vast majority of women born more recently will have taken combined oral contraceptives at some stage. In 1981, 81% of Swedish women aged 25–30 had ever used combined oral contraceptive pills, whereas in 1990–91, 88% of women born in 1960–65 had ever used them; 77% had begun use before the age of 20 (Ranstam & Olsson, 1993). In a United States survey conducted between 1976 and 1980, 15% of 15–19-year-olds and 34% of 20–24-year-olds were currently using combined oral contraceptives (Russell-Briefel *et al.*, 1985). In this context, it is important to note that women in high-prevalence countries who have never taken combined oral contraceptives may have particular characteristics, such as psychiatric illness. Indeed, in Sweden, women who have taken combined oral contraceptives are more likely to smoke, drink alcohol, be cohabiting, be older at their first full-term pregnancy and younger at menarche than women who have never taken them (Ranstam & Olsson, 1993).

Table 1. Contraceptive use among married women or women in union, aged 15–49, by country

Country or region	Year of survey	Any method (%)	Oral contra-ceptives (%)	No. of women (in thousands, 1990)	Calculated no. of oral contra-ceptive users (thousands)
Africa					
Algeria	1986–87	36	27		
	1992	51	39	3 300	1 287
Benin	1982	27	0		
	1996	16	1	800	8
Botswana	1984	28	10		
	1988	33	15	100	15
Burkina Faso	1993	8	2	1 600	32
Burundi	1987	9	0.25	800	2
Cameroon	1978	3	0		
	1991	16	1	1 600	19
Central African Republic	1994	15	1	500	5
Comoros	1996	21	3	75	2.2
Côte d'Ivoire	1980–81	4	1		
	1994	11	2	1 900	42
Egypt	1980	24	16		
	1984	30	17		
	1988	38	15		
	1991	48	16		
	1992	47	13		
	1995	48	10	8 300	863
Eritrea	1995	8	2		
Ethiopia	1990	4	2	8 300	158
Gambia	1990	12	3	100	3
Ghana	1979–80	12	3		
	1988	13	2		
	1993	20	3		
	1995	28	7	2 300	161
Kenya	1977–78	7	2		
	1984	17	3		
	1989	27	5		
	1993	33	10	3 100	298
Lesotho	1977	7	2		
	1991–92	23	7	200	14
Liberia	1986	6	3	400	13
Madagascar	1992	17	2	1 700	26
Malawi	1984	7	1		
	1992	13	2	1 400	31
Mali	1987	5	1		
	1995–96	7	3	1 900	59

Table 1 (contd)

Country or region	Year of survey	Any method (%)	Oral contra- ceptives (%)	No. of women (in thousands, 1990)	Calculated no. of oral contra- ceptive users (thousands)
Africa (contd)					
Mauritania	1981	1	0		
	1990	4	1	300	3
Mauritius	1975	46	21		
	1985	75	21		
	1991	75	21	200	42
Morocco	1970	1	1		
	1971	3	2		
	1972	4	3		
	1973	6	5		
	1974	7	6		
	1979	16	13		
	1979–80	19	13		
	1983–84	26	16		
	1987	36	23		
	1992	42	28		
	1995	50	32	3 300	1 063
Namibia	1989	26	7		
	1992	29	8	100	8.3
Niger	1992	4	2	1 300	20
Nigeria	1981–82	6	0		
	1990	6	1	18 100	217
Réunion	1990	73	40	100	40
Rwanda	1983	10	0		
	1992	21	3	900	27
Senegal	1978	4	0		
	1986	11	1		
	1992	7	2	1 200	26
South Africa	1975–76	50	14		
	1981–82	48	14		
	1988	50	13	4 300	568
Sudan	1979	5	3		
	1989–90	9	4		
	1992–93	10	5	3 700	185
Swaziland	1988	20	5	100	5.5
Togo	1988	34	0	600	2.4
Tunisia	1978	31	7		
	1983	41	5		
	1988	50	9		
	1994–95	60	7	1 100	80

Table 1 (contd)

Country or region	Year of survey	Any method (%)	Oral contra-ceptives (%)	No. of women (in thousands, 1990)	Calculated no. of oral contra-ceptive users (thousands)
Africa (contd)					
Uganda	1988–89	5	1		
	1995	15	3	2 600	68
Zambia	1992	15	4	1 200	52
Zimbabwe	1979	14	5		
	1984	38	23		
	1988	43	31		
	1994	48	33	1 400	463
Europe					
Austria	1981–82	71	40	1 200	480
Belgium	1966	72	5		
	1975	87	30		
	1982	81	32		
	1991	80	47	1 700	792
Bulgaria	1976	76	2	1 600	32
Czech Republic	1993	69	8	1 700	138
Denmark	1970	67	25		
	1975	63	22		
	1988	78	26	700	182
Finland	1971	77	20		
	1977	80	11		
	1989	70	15		
	1994	79	31	700	214
France	1972	64	11		
	1978	79	27		
	1988	80	27		
	1994	75	37	8 500	3 137
Germany	1985	78	34		
	1992	75	59	12 000	7 080
Hungary	1966	67	0		
	1974	74	27		
	1977	73	36		
	1986	73	39		
	1993	84	41	1 800	742
Italy	1979	78	14	9 600	1 344
Lithuania	1994–95	66	5	600	28

Table 1 (contd)

Country or region	Year of survey	Any method (%)	Oral contraceptives (%)	No. of women (in thousands, 1990)	Calculated no. of oral contraceptive users (thousands)
Europe (contd)					
Netherlands	1969	59	27		
	1975	75	50		
	1977	73	40		
	1982	69	39		
	1985	72	40		
	1988	70	43		
	1993	74	47	2 200	1 034
Norway	1977	71	13		
	1988	76	18	500	89
Poland	1972	60	2		
	1977	75	7	6 400	448
Portugal	1979–80	66	19	1 800	344
Romania	1978	58	1		
	1993	57	3	3 800	122
Slovakia	1991	74	5	1 000	50
Slovenia	1989	92	25		
Spain	1977	50	12		
	1985	59	16	6 400	992
Sweden	1981	78	23	1 200	276
Switzerland	1980	71	28		
	1994	82	34	1 000	341
United Kingdom	1970	75	19		
	1975	76	30		
	1976	77	32		
	1983	83	24		
	1986	81	19		
	1989	72	25	9 300	2 325
North America					
Canada	1984	73.1	11	4 200	462
United States	1965	63	15		
	1973	70	25		
	1976	68	23		
	1982	70	13		
	1988	74	15		
	1990	71	15	35 800	5 191
Latin America and the Caribbean					
Bolivia	1983	24	3		
	1989	30	2		
	1994	45	3	1 000	28

Table 1 (contd)

Country or region	Year of survey	Any method (%)	Oral contra- ceptives (%)	No. of women (in thousands, 1990)	Calculated no. of oral contra- ceptive users (thousands)
Latin America and the Caribbean (contd)					
Brazil	1986	66	25		
	1996	77	21	23 700	4 906
Colombia	1969	28	5		
	1976	43	14		
	1978	46	17		
	1980	49	17		
	1984	55	21		
	1986	65	16		
	1990	66	14		
	1995	72	13	4 700	606
Costa Rica	1976	68	23		
	1978	64	25		
	1981	65	21		
	1984	65	23		
	1986	68	19		
	1992–93	75	18	400	72
Cuba	1987	70	10	1 900	190
Dominican Republic	1975	32	8		
	1977	31	8		
	1980	42	9		
	1983	28	5		
	1986	50	9		
	1991	56	10		
	1996	64	13	1 000	129
Ecuador	1979	35	10		
	1982	40	10		
	1987	44	9		
	1989	53	9		
	1994	57	10	1 700	173
El Salvador	1975	22	7		
	1976	20	6		
	1978	34	9		
	1985	47	7		
	1988	47	8		
	1993	53	9	700	61
Guadeloupe	1976	44	10	100	10
Guatemala	1978	19	6		
	1983	25	5		
	1987	23	4		
	1995	31	4	1 300	49

Table 1 (contd)

Country or region	Year of survey	Any method (%)	Oral contra-ceptives (%)	No. of women (in thousands, 1990)	Calculated no. of oral contra-ceptive users (thousands)
Latin America and the Caribbean (contd)					
Guyana	1975	32	10	200	20
Haiti	1977	19	3		
	1983	7	2		
	1987	8	3		
	1989	10	4		
	1994	18	3	1000	31
Honduras	1981	27	12		
	1984	35	13		
	1987	41	13	700	94
Jamaica	1975–76	41	13		
	1979	55	24		
	1983	51	27		
	1989	55	20		
	1993	62	22	400	86
Martinique	1976	51	17	100	17
Mexico	1973	13	11		
	1976	29	12		
	1978	26	9		
	1979	38	15		
	1982	50	14		
	1987	53	10	13 000	1 261
Nicaragua	1981	27	11		
	1992–93	49	13	500	65
Panama	1976	57	19		
	1979	61	19		
	1984	58	12	300	35
Paraguay	1977	29	12		
	1979	32	10		
	1987	45	13		
	1990	48	14		
	1995–96	56	14	600	81
Peru	1969–70	26	3		
	1977–78	41	5		
	1981	41	5		
	1986	46	7		
	1991–92	59	6		
	1996	64	6	300	19

Table 1 (contd)

Country or region	Year of survey	Any method (%)	Oral contra- ceptives (%)	No. of women (in thousands, 1990)	Calculated no. of oral contra- ceptive users (thousands)
Latin America and the Caribbean (contd)					
Puerto Rico	1968	60	11		
	1974	62	20		
	1976	65	13		
	1982	70	9		
	1995–96	78	10	500	49
Trinidad and Tobago	1970–71	44	17		
	1977	54	19		
	1987	53	14	200	28
Venezuela	1977	60	19	2 700	506
Asia					
Bahrain	1989	53	13	100	13
Bangladesh	1975	8	3		
	1977	9	2		
	1979	13	4		
	1980	12	4		
	1981	20	4		
	1983	19	3		
	1985	25	5		
	1989	31	9		
	1991	40	14		
	1993	45	17	21 400	3 724
Burma	1991	17	4		
China	1982	70	6		
	1988	71	4		
	1992	77	3	222 700	5 968
Hong Kong	1969	42	16		
	1972	54	20		
	1977	77	28		
	1982	77	21		
	1984	72	22		
	1987	81	16	900	148
India	1980	32	1		
	1988	43	1		
	1992–93	41	1	159 000	1 908
Indonesia	1973	9	3		
	1976	26	15		
	1979	21	11		
	1980	26	14		
	1985	39	15		

Table 1 (contd)

Country or region	Year of survey	Any method (%)	Oral contra-ceptives (%)	No. of women (in thousands, 1990)	Calculated no. of oral contra-ceptive users (thousands)
Asia (contd)					
Indonesia (contd)	1987	51	18		
	1991	50	15		
	1994	55	17	31 400	5 369
Iran	1978	23	20		
	1992	65	23	9 200	2 116
Iraq	1974	14	8		
	1989	14	5	2 500	117.5
Japan	1969	52	1		
	1971	53	1		
	1973	59	1		
	1975	61	2		
	1977	60	2		
	1979	62	2		
	1984	57	1		
	1986	64	1		
	1988	56	1	18 600	186
Jordan	1972	21	13		
	1976	25	12		
	1983	26	8		
	1985	27	6		
	1990	35	5	500	23
Kuwait	1987	35	24	300	72
Malaysia	1966–67	9	4		
	1970	16	12		
	1974	36	18		
	1979	36	25		
	1981	42	17		
	1984	51	12		
	1988	48	15	2 600	390
Nepal	1976	3	1		
	1981	7	1		
	1986	15	1		
	1991	25	1		
	1996	29	1	3 500	49
Oman	1988	9	2	200	4.8
Pakistan	1975	4	1		
	1980	6	1		
	1984–85	9	1		
	1990–91	12	1	18 100	127

Table 1 (contd)

Country or region	Year of survey	Any method (%)	Oral contra-ceptives (%)	No. of women (in thousands, 1990)	Calculated no. of oral contra-ceptive users (thousands)
Asia (contd)					
Philippines	1968	15	1		
	1972	8	5		
	1973	18	7		
	1976	22	11		
	1977	22	11		
	1978	37	5		
	1979	37	6		
	1980	45	5		
	1981	48	16		
	1983	33	6		
	1988	36	7		
	1993	40	9		
	1995	53	11		
	1996	48	12	9 700	1 125
Quatar	1987	32	13	100	13
Republic of Korea	1991	79	3	7 600	228
Singapore	1970	45	38		
	1973	60	22		
	1977	71	17		
	1978	71	17		
	1982	74	12	500	57.9
Sri Lanka	1975	32	2		
	1982	55	3		
	1987	62	4	2 700	110.7
Thailand	1970	14	4		
	1973	26	11		
	1975	33	14		
	1978	53	22		
	1981	59	20		
	1984	65	20		
	1985	59	21		
	1987	66	19	9 000	1 674
Turkey	1963	22	1		
	1968	32	2		
	1973	38	4		
	1978	50	8		
	1983	51	8		
	1988	63	6		
	1993	63	5	9 400	461

Table 1 (contd)

Country or region	Year of survey	Any method (%)	Oral contra-ceptives (%)	No. of women (in thousands, 1990)	Calculated no. of oral contra-ceptive users (thousands)
Asia (contd)					
Viet Nam	1988	53	0		
	1994	65	2	10 000	210
Yemen	1979	1	1		
	1991–92	7	3	1 700	54
Oceania					
Australia	1986	76	24	2 600	624
New Zealand	1976	70	29	400	114

From Population Council (1994, 1995); Phai *et al.* (1996); Population Council (1996a,b); United Nations (1996); Population Council (1997a,b,c,d,e,f; 1998a,b); United States Census Bureau (1998)

Sales figures for 1987 show that more than 40% of oral contraceptives purchased by pharmacies in most 'developed' countries were monophasic preparations, containing less than 50 μg oestrogen; approximately 35% were triphasic preparations, 10% were mono-phasic preparations containing 50 μg oestrogen, about 8% were biphasic preparations containing less than 50 μg oestrogen, about 3% were sequential combined preparations, and around 2% contained progestogen alone. In 'developing' countries, just under 50% of preparations bought by pharmacies were monophasic preparations containing less than 50 μg oestrogen, approximately 10% were triphasic preparations and around 42% were monophasic preparations containing 50 μg oestrogen (Wharton & Blackburn, 1988). Most of the oral contraceptives provided by major aid organizations (United States Aid to International Development, United Nations Family Planning Agency, International Planned Parenthood Federation) contain 30 μg ethinyloestradiol and 150 μg levonorgestrel.

1.3   Exposure to other combinations of oestrogen and progestogen

Injectable combined hormonal contraceptives were first developed in the late 1960s and consist of a depot progestogen and oestrogen administered monthly. Formulations and brands of such preparations are listed in Table 3, with a list of some of the countries in which they are available. They are used in parts of Latin America, China, Spain, Portugal, Thailand, Indonesia and Singapore, although, as can be seen from Table 1 in the monograph on 'Hormonal contraceptives, progestogens only', they are unlikely to constitute a large proportion of the contraceptive use in these countries.

In Latin America, at least 1 million women use dihydroxyprogesterone acetophenide and oestradiol oenanthate, and the combination of dihydroxyprogesterone acetophenide

Table 2. Percentages of women who have ever used oral contraceptives, by year of birth

Country	Year of birth								
	< 1915	1915–19	1920–24	1925–29	1930–34	1935–39	1940–44	1945–49
Australia	0	3	18	36	55	69	80	85
Canada	1	6	26	42	53	67	79	84
China	–	–	1	2	19	36	39	39
Denmark	–	0	4	21	35	46	66	75
France	–	–	–	7	16	38	61	69
Germany	–	–	–	–	40	58	75	86
Italy	0	0.4	0.2	2	3	8	15	25
Netherlands	–	5	16	35	49	69	84	90
New Zealand	–	–	–	50	61	75	84	91
Norway	–	–	–	–	–	–	–	45
Sweden	–	–	–	–	–	–	65	82
United Kingdom	–	3	15	27	41	51	68	83
United States	1	4	14	28	43	60	75	85

From Collaborative Group on Hormonal Factors in Breast Cancer (1996a) Appendix 5

Table 3. Injectable contraceptives containing oestrogen and progesterone given monthly

Brand name	Composition	Dose (mg)	Availability
Anafertin, Yectames	Oestradiol oenanthate Dihydroxyprogesterone acetophenide	5 75	Many Latin American countries and Spain
Chinese injectable No. 1	Oestradiol valerate 17α-Hydroxyprogesterone caproate	5 250	China
Chinese injectable No. 2	Oestradiol Megestrol acetate	3.5 25	China
Cicnor, Damix, Progesterol, Segutalmes	Oestradiol oenanthate Medroxyprogesterone acetate	10 150	Portugal
Ciclofem, Ciclofemina, Cyclofem, Cyclo Geston	Oestradiol cypionate Medroxyprogesterone acetate	5 25	Registered in Guatamala, Indonesia, Mexico, Peru and Thailand
Chinese injectable No. 3, Mesigyna, Norigynon	Oestradiol valerate Norethisterone oenanthate	5 50	Argentina, Brazil and Mexico
Agurin, Ciclovar, Deproxone, Exuna, Horprotal, Neolutin, Normagest, Novular, Perlutal, Perlutale, Perlutan, Proter, Topasel, Uno Ciclo	Oestradiol oenanthate Dihydroxyprogesterone acetophenide	10 150	Many Latin American countries and Spain
Redimen, Soluna, Unijab	Oestradiol benzoate Dihydroxyprogesterone acetophenide	10 150	Peru and Singapore
Unalmes	Oestradiol oenanthate Alfasona acetophenide	10 120	Chile and Paraguay

From Kleinman (1990); Lande (1995)

and hydroxyprogesterone caproate (Chinese injectable No. 1) has been used by about 1 million women in China (Lande, 1995).

A relatively high dose of oestrogen and progestogen can be administered up to 72 h after unprotected intercourse as 'emergency contraception'. It is often given as 100 µg ethinyl-oestradiol and 0.5 mg levonorgestrel (or 1 mg norgestrel), as two tablets, immediately and a further equal dose 12 h later (Kleinman, 1990). A progestogen-only regimen is also available (see the monograph on 'Hormonal contraceptives, progestogens only').

2.   Studies of Cancer in Humans

2.1   Breast cancer

The relationship between the use of combined oral contraceptives and the risk for breast cancer was reviewed by a working group convened by IARC in 1979 (IARC, 1979). At the time, the results from several follow-up (Royal College of General Practitioners, 1974; Ory et al., 1976; Vessey et al., 1976) and case–control studies (Vessey et al., 1972, 1975; Paffenbarger et al., 1977; Sartwell et al., 1977; Kelsey et al., 1978; Lees et al., 1978) had been published. The data were sparse even for the analysis of use. The Group concluded that there was no clear evidence that use of combined oral contraceptives influences the risk for breast cancer.

In the two decades since the 1979 report, oral contraceptive formulations have been changed: The doses of oestrogen and progestogen have been lowered, the components used have changed, cyclic preparations with different doses at different times during the menstrual cycle have been introduced, and progestogen-only formulations have become available.

Various aspects of the use of combined oral contraceptives in relation to the incidence of breast cancer have been assessed in numerous epidemiological studies conducted since 1979. Several detailed reviews of the epidemiological evidence have been published (Prentice & Thomas, 1987; Olsson, 1989; Romieu et al., 1990; Malone, 1991; Thomas, 1991a; WHO, 1992; Malone et al., 1993; Schlesselman, 1995). In addition, a pooled analysis of the individual data from 54 studies was reported (Collaborative Group on Hormonal Factors in Breast Cancer, 1996a,b); the analyses covered an estimated 90% of the data available at that time.

Studies in which cases of breast cancer occurring before 1980 were analysed provide limited information on many aspects of the use of combined oral contraceptives that are of interest, notably use at a young age, long duration of use, recent use and use followed by a long latent period (Ravnihar et al., 1979; Jick et al., 1980; Brinton et al., 1982; Harris et al., 1982; Vessey et al., 1982; Janerich et al., 1983; Hennekens et al., 1984; Schildkraut et al., 1990; Morabia et al., 1993). The early studies have been reviewed in detail (Thomas, 1991a). The studies considered here are based on data collected since 1979 and are limited to those reported in English.

The follow-up studies are summarized in Table 4, the case–control studies in which hospitalized controls were used are summarized in Table 5 and the case–control studies in which controls from other sources were used are summarized in Table 6. When several reports are available on the same study, all are listed; however, the data shown are taken from the report (marked with an asterisk) that was based on the largest numbers. The studies are listed in order of the year of the first publication of results. Thus, follow-up data have been published from the Nurses' Health Study (Colditz *et al.*, 1994), in which data on the use of combined oral contraceptives and risk factors were collected by postal questionnaire and the diagnoses were verified from hospital records.

A variety of methods was used in the case–control studies. The data on use of combined oral contraceptives and other risk factors for breast cancer were obtained almost exclusively by personal interview; the diagnoses of breast cancer were generally verified from hospital or cancer registry records. In virtually all of the studies, relative risks were estimated after control for important potential confounding factors, such as reproductive variables and socioeconomic status. The Collaborative Group on Hormonal Factors in Breast Cancer (1996a,b) analysed all of the published and unpublished studies available to them, for a combined total of some 53 000 cases and 100 000 controls. Individual data from each of the studies were analysed centrally; combined relative risk estimates were obtained by a modification of the Mantel-Haenszel procedure, with stratification on study, age at diagnosis, parity and age at the birth of the first child.

Comparisons of any use of combined oral contraceptives ('ever use') with no use ('never use') yielded overall relative risk estimates close to 1.0 in most studies. In the analysis of the Collaborative Group on Hormonal Factors in Breast Cancer (1996a,b), the relative risk estimate was 1.17 [95% confidence interval [CI], 1.1–1.24] on the basis of data from hospital-based case–control studies, 1.0 [95% CI, 0.97–1.1] from case–control studies with population controls and 1.07 [95% CI, 1.00–1.14] from follow-up studies. These estimates were not significantly different. The characteristics of women who had ever used oral contraceptives varied, however, from study to study and changed over time: there was a tendency to use combined oral contraceptives at younger ages and for longer.

In the early and mid-1980s, a number of associations between the use of combined oral contraceptives and an increased risk for breast cancer were observed in subgroups of some epidemiological studies, and hypotheses were raised (and later refuted) to explain those observations. In 1981, Pike *et al.* observed that the risk for breast cancer more strongly tended to increase with increasing duration of use of combined oral contraceptives before the first full-term pregnancy than after, raising the hypothesis that use of these contraceptives before the first full-term pregnancy is more harmful. A few subsequent studies provided some support for this hypothesis (McPherson *et al.*, 1987; Rohan & McMichael, 1988; Olsson *et al.*, 1989, 1991a), but most studies did not (Meirik *et al.*, 1986, 1989; Romieu *et al.*, 1989; Stanford *et al.*, 1989; UK National Case–Control Study Group, 1989; Paul *et al.*, 1990; WHO Collaborative Study of Neoplasia and Steroid Contraceptives, 1990; Weinstein *et al.*, 1991; Wingo *et al.*, 1991; Ewertz, 1992;

Table 4. Follow-up studies of breast cancer associated with use of combined oral contraceptives

Reference	Country	Age at recruitment (years)	Size of cohort	Period of follow-up	No. of cases	Loss to follow-up (%)	Any use (%)	RR (95% CI), any versus none	RR (95% CI) for longest duration
Lipnick et al. (1986); Romieu et al. (1989); Colditz et al. (1994)* (Nurses' Health Study)	United States	30–55	118 273	1976–86	1 799	5	48	1.1 (0.97–1.2)	Not reported
Kay & Hannaford (1988)[a] (incidence)	United Kingdom	Not reported	47 000	1968–85	239	[61]	Not reported	Former use (99 cases in 134 079 person–years), 1.2 (0.9–1.6) Current use (44 cases in 104 505 person–years), 1.2 (0.84–1.9)	≥ 10 years, 1.4 (0.91–2.3)
Mills et al. (1989)	United States	≥ 25	20 341	1976–82	215	1	27	1.5 (0.94–2.5) based on 29 cases in 31 188 person–years among women ≤ 45 years of age in 1960	≥ 10 years, 1.4 (0.34–6.0) based on 2 cases in 1660 person–years among women ≤ 45 years of age in 1960
Vessey et al. (1989a)	United Kingdom	25–39	17 032	1968–87	189	0.3 per year	Not reported	Not reported	Ages 25–44, ≥ 10 years, 0.65/1000 person–years (14 cases) versus 0.62/1000 person–years for no use (49 cases) [RR, 1.0] Ages ≥ 45, ≥ 10 years, 1/1000 person–years versus (8 cases) 2.2/1000 person–years for no use (50 cases) [RR, 0.48]

Table 4 (contd)

Reference	Country	Age at recruitment (years)	Size of cohort	Period of follow-up	No. of cases	Loss to follow-up (%)	Any use (%)	RR (95% CI), any versus none	RR (95% CI) for longest duration
Beral et al. (1999)[a]	United Kingdom	Not reported	46 000	1968–93	259 (deaths[b])	25	63	1.1 (0.82–1.4)	≥ 10 years, 1.4 (0.86–2.1) (26 deaths)
Collaborative Group (1996b)	–	–	–	–	6 806	–	[38]	1.07 [1.00–1.14]	≥ 15 years, 1.1 [0.96–1.2]

RR, relative risk; CI, confidence interval

* Report from which data are taken

[a] Data from Royal College of General Pracitioners (1974)

[b] 154 deaths for any use, 105 deaths for no use

Table 5. Case–control studies of use of combined oral contraceptives and breast cancer with hospital controls

Reference	Country	Years of case diagnosis	Age (years)	No. of cases	No. of controls	Participation rate (%) Cases/Controls	Any use (%) Cases/Controls	RR (95% CI), ever versus never	RR (95% CI), longest duration
Vessey et al. (1983)	United Kingdom	1968–80	16–50	1 176	1 176	Not reported	46/47	0.98 (0.81–1.2)	≥ 97 months versus never 0.99 (0.67–1.4)
Rosenberg et al. (1984); Miller et al. (1986, 1989); Rosenberg et al. (1996)* (surveillance study)	United States	1977–92	25–59	3 540 (white women)	4 488	95	≥ 1 year of use [29/30]	≥ 1 year versus < 1 year 1.1 (1.0–1.3)	≥ 10 years versus < 1 year 0.9 (0.7–1.1)
Talamini et al. (1985)	Italy	1980–83	26–79	368	373	99	4/6	0.7 (0.4–1.4)	Not reported
Ellery et al. (1986)	Australia	1980–82	25–64	141	279	Not reported	[48/42]	0.9 (0.6–1.5)	≥ 6 years 1.3 (0.7–2.7)
La Vecchia et al. (1986, 1989); Tavani et al. (1993a)*	Italy	1983–91	<60	2 309	1 928	98/97	16/14	1.2 (1.0–1.4)	≥ 60 months versus never 0.8 (0.5–1.0)
McPherson et al. (1987)	United Kingdom	1980–84	16–44	351	351	Not reported	68/65	Not reported	≥ 12 years versus never 1.8 (0.82–3.9)
			≥ 45	774	774	Not reported	24/27	Not reported	≥ 12 years versus never 0.84 (0.39–1.8)
Ravnihar et al. (1988)	Slovenia	1980–83	25–54	534	1 989	Not reported	30/24	1.6 (1.3–2.1)	> 7 years versus never 2.4 (1.5–3.8)
Harris et al. (1990)	United States	1979–81	All	401	519	Not reported	19/23	0.8 (0.6–1.2)	≥ 5 years (age <50) 0.4 (0.2–0.8)

Table 5 (contd)

Reference	Country	Years of case diagnosis	Age (years)	No. of cases	No. of controls	Participation rate (%) Cases/Controls	Any use (%) Cases/Controls	RR (95% CI), ever versus never	RR (95% CI), longest duration
WHO Collaborative Study (1990)*; Ebeling et al. (1991); Thomas (1991b); Thomas et al. (1991, 1992, 1994)	10 countries: 3 developed, 7 developing	1979–86	<62	2 116	13 072	Not reported	34/34	1.2 (1.0–1.3)	>8 years 1.6 (1.2–2.0)
Clavel et al. (1991)	France	1983–87	25–56	464	542	99/99	[51/44]	1.5 (1.1–2.1)	≥21 years versus never 1.2 (0.4–3.9)
Bustan et al. (1993)	Indonesia	1990–91	25–55	119	258	90	32/21	1.8 (1.1–3.0)	>5 years 1.1 (0.6–2.1)
Gomes et al. (1995)	Brazil	1978–87	25–75	300	600	Not reported	21/15	1.8 (1.2–2.9)	Not reported
La Vecchia et al. (1995)	Italy	1991–94	<65	1 991	1 899	96/96	18/14	1.1 (0.9–1.4)	>8 years versus never 1.2 (0.7–1.9)
Lipworth et al. (1995)	Greece	1989–91	All	820	795	95/93	4/4	≤45 years of age 1.1 (0.60–2.0) >45 years of age 1.6 (0.82–3.3)	≤45 years of age, ≥3 years 0.47 (0.13–1.70) 45 years of age, ≥3 years 1.2 (0.32–4.2)
Palmer et al. (1995) (surveillance)	United States	1977–92	25–59	524 (black women)	1 021	95	[31/27]	≥1 year versus <1 year 1.6 (1.2–2.1)	≥10 years versus <1 year 1.1 (0.6–2.0)
Levi et al. (1996)	Switzerland	1990–95	<70	206	424	85	37/32	1.5 (1.1–2.3)	≥10 years versus never 2.4 (1.4–4.2)

Table 5 (contd)

Reference	Country	Years of case diagnosis	Age (years)	No. of cases	No. of controls	Participation rate (%) Cases/Controls	Any use (%) Cases/Controls	RR (95% CI), ever versus never	RR (95% CI), longest duration
Tomasson & Tomasson (1996)	Iceland	1965–89	25–69	1 062	5 622 (cancer detection clinic)	Not reported	Not reported	Not reported	> 8 years 0.96 (0.69–1.3)
Tryggvadóttir et al. (1997)	Iceland	1975–95	18–43	204	1 183 (cancer detection clinic)	Not reported	79/81	Not reported	> 8 years 1.3 (p = 0.55)
Collaborative Group (1996a)[a]	–	–	–	15 030	34 565	–	26/31	1.17 [1.1–1.24]	≥ 15 years versus never 1.1 [0.96–1.2]

RR, relative risk; CI, confidence interval
* Report from which data are taken
[a] Includes all studies mentioned above

Table 6. Case–control studies of use of combined oral contraceptives and breast cancer with controls other than hospitalized patients

Reference	Country	Years of case diagnosis	Age (years)	No. of cases	No. of controls	Participation rate (%) Cases/Controls	Any use (%) Cases/Controls	RR (95% CI), ever versus never	RR (95% CI), longest duration
Pike et al. (1981, 1983); Bernstein et al. (1990)*	United States	1972–83	< 37	439 (population-based)	439 (neighbours)	68/not reported	85/85	Not reported	> 8 years versus never 1.7 ($p_{trend} < 0.01$)
Centers for Disease Control Cancer and Steroid Hormone Study (1983a); Stadel et al. (1985); Cancer and Steroid Study (1986)*; Schlesselmann et al. (1987, 1988); Stadel et al. (1988); Wingo et al. (1991); Mayberry & Stoddard-Wright (1992) (CASH Study)	United States	1980–82	20–54	4 711 (population-based)	4 676 (random-digit dialling)	80/83	[63/64]	1.0 (0.9–1.1)	≥ 15 years versus never 0.9 (0.8–1.1)
Meirik et al. (1986)*; Lund et al. (1989); Meirik et al. (1989); Holmberg et al. (1994) (Sweden–Norway Joint National Study)	Sweden, Norway	1984–85	< 45	422 (population-based)	722 (population-based)	89/81	77/78	Not reported	≥ 12 years versus never 2.2 (1.2–4.0)
Paul et al. (1986, 1990*, 1995) (New Zealand National Study)	New Zealand	1983–87	25–54	891 (population-based)	1 864 (electoral rolls)	95/90	77/83	1.0 (0.82–1.3)	≥ 14 years versus never 1.1 (0.78–1.7)

Table 6 (contd)

Reference	Country	Years of case diagnosis	Age (years)	No. of cases	No. of controls	Participation rate (%) Cases/Controls	Any use (%) Cases/Controls	RR (95% CI), ever versus never	RR (95% CI), longest duration
Rohan & McMichael (1988)	Australia	1982–84	20–69	395 (population-based)	386 (electoral rolls)	[81/72]	49/49	1.1 (0.70–1.6)	> 7 years versus never 0.67 (0.38–1.2)
Yuan et al. (1988)	China	1984–85	20–69	534 (population-based)	534 (population-based)	94/99	[19/18]	1.1 (0.74–1.5)	≥ 10 years versus never 1.4 (0.62–3.2)
Jick et al. (1989)	United States	1975–83	< 43	127 (health plan)	174 (health plan)	Not reported	61/71	0.9 (0.4–1.9)	≥ 10 years 1.4 (0.4–4.6)
Olsson et al. (1989*, 1991a)	Sweden	1979–80 1982–85	≤ 46	174 (hospital)	459 (population-based)	100/92	82/72	[1.8]	Not reported
Stanford et al. (1989)	United States	1973–80	All	2 022	2 183 (screening programme)	78/83	24/24	1.0 (0.9–1.2)	≥ 15 years versus never 0.65 (0.3–1.6)
UK National Case–Control Study Group (1989*, 1990); Chilvers et al. (1994) (United Kingdom National Study)	United Kingdom	1980–85	< 36	755 (population-based)	755 (general practice)	72/89	[91/89]	Not reported	> 8 years versus never 1.7 ($p_{trend} < 0.001$)
Weinstein et al. (1991)	United States	1984–86	20–70	1 067 (population-based)	1 066 (drivers' license files)	66/41	26/23	1.2 (0.98–1.5)	≥ 4 years versus never 1.2 (0.82–1.6)

Table 6 (contd)

Reference	Country	Years of case diagnosis	Age (years)	No. of cases	No. of controls	Participation rate (%) Cases/Controls	Any use (%) Cases/Controls	RR (95% CI), ever versus never	RR (95% CI), longest duration
Ewertz (1992)	Denmark	1983–84	< 40	203	212	90/88	[81/79]	1.2 (0.73–1.9)	≥ 12 years versus
			40–59	856 (population-based)	778 (population-based)	89/80	36/37	Not reported	< 4 years 1.3 (0.82–2.0)
Rosenberg et al. (1992)	Canada	1982–86	< 70	607 (cancer hospital)	1 214 (neigh-bour-hood)	79/65	43/45	Not reported	≥ 15 years versus never 0.9 (0.4–1.7)
Ursin et al. (1992)	United States and Canada	1935–89	< 50	149 (2 regis-tries)	243 (sisters)	Not reported	[42/30]	1.7 (1.0–2.9)	≥ 7 years 2.0 (0.93–4.2)
Rookus et al. (1994)	Nether-lands	1986–89	20–54	918 (population-based)	918 (population-based)	60/72	85/85	1.1 (0.8–1.4)	≥ 12 years versus never 1.3 (0.9–1.9)
White et al. (1994)	United States	1983–90	21–45	747 (popu-lation-based)	961 (random-digit dialling)	83/78	78 (≥ 1 year)/ 76 (≥ 1 year)	1.0 (0.71–1.5)	≥ 10 years versus never 1.3 (0.92–1.9)
Brinton et al. (1995)	United States	1990–92	20–45	1 648 (popu-lation-based)	1 505 (random-digit dialling)	86/78	76/71 (≥ 6 months)	Not reported ≥ 6 months to < 5 years versus < 6 months 1.3 (1.1–1.5)	≥ 10 years versus < 6 months 1.3 (1.0–1.6)

Table 6 (contd)

Reference	Country	Years of case diagnosis	Age (years)	No. of cases	No. of controls	Participation rate (%) Cases/Controls	Any use (%) Cases/Controls	RR (95% CI), ever versus never	RR (95% CI), longest duration
Primic-Žakelj et al. (1995)	Slovenia	1988–90	25–54	624 (hospital)	624 (population-based)	94/83	48/48	1.1 (0.85–1.4)	> 8 years versus never 1.2 (0.76–1.7)
Newcomb et al. (1996)	United States	1988–91	<75	6 751 (population-based)	9 311 (drivers' licenses or Medicare)	81/84	38/39	1.1 (1.0–1.2)	≥ 15 years versus never 1.0 (0.8–1.4)
Rossing et al. (1996)	United States	1988–90	50–64	537 (population-based)	545 (random-digit dialling)	81/73	[47/41]	1.1 (0.8–1.4)	> 10 years versus never 0.8 (0.5–1.3)
Collaborative Group (1996b)[a]	–	–	–	31 089	37 676	–	[48/49]	1.0 [0.97–1.1]	≥ 15 years 1.1 (0.96–1.2)

RR, relative risk; CI, confidence interval
* Reports from which data are taken
[a] Includes all studies

Tavani *et al.*, 1993a; White *et al.*, 1994; Brinton *et al.*, 1995; Palmer *et al.*, 1995; Primic-Žakelj *et al.*, 1995; Collaborative Group on Hormonal Factors in Breast Cancer, 1996b; Levi *et al.*, 1996; Newcomb *et al.*, 1996; Rosenberg *et al.*, 1996). When the study from which the hypothesis arose was completed, with larger numbers, the effect was no longer seen (Bernstein *et al.*, 1990). Rather, the data now suggested that the increase in risk was related to use before the age of 25. Some subsequent evidence has suggested that the risk is greater the younger the woman is when she first uses combined oral contraceptives (White *et al.*, 1994), but most studies have not supported this idea (Meirik *et al.*, 1986; Ravnihar *et al.*, 1988; Rohan & McMichael, 1988; Stanford *et al.*, 1989; UK National Case–Control Study Group, 1989; Paul *et al.*, 1990; WHO Collaborative Study of Neoplasia and Steroid Contraceptives, 1990; Clavel *et al.*, 1991; Weinstein *et al.*, 1991; Wingo *et al.*, 1991; Ewertz, 1992; Rosenberg *et al.*, 1992; Tavani *et al.*, 1993a; Brinton *et al.*, 1995; Palmer *et al.*, 1995; Primic-Žakelj *et al.*, 1995; Levi *et al.*, 1996; Newcomb *et al.*, 1996; Rosenberg *et al.*, 1996; Rossing *et al.*, 1996). The study of Rookus *et al.* (1994) suggested an increased risk for breast cancer before the age of 35 for women who started to use combined oral contraceptives at an early age but no increased risk between the ages of 36 and 45. The Collaborative Group on Hormonal Factors in Breast Cancer (1996a,b) provided little support for the idea that the effect of combined oral contraceptives is modified by the timing in relation to the first pregnancy (Figure 2) or the age at first use, except perhaps that the relative risks were somewhat higher in current or recent users who began use before the age of 20 (Figure 3). There is, however, no evidence of any persistent excess risk many years after use has ceased for women who began use before the age of 20.

Data on the use of combined oral contraceptives in relation to age at the time of diagnosis of breast cancer are shown in Table 7. As evidence has accumulated, a relatively consistent finding has been an increased risk for breast cancer occurring before the age of 45, and particularly before 35, among users of combined oral contraceptives (Meirik *et al.*, 1986; McPherson *et al.*, 1987; Stanford *et al.*, 1989; UK National Case–Control Study Group, 1989; Bernstein *et al.*, 1990; Paul *et al.*, 1990; WHO Collaborative Study of Neoplasia and Steroid Contraceptives, 1990; Weinstein *et al.*, 1991; Wingo *et al.*, 1991; Rookus *et al.*, 1994; Brinton *et al.*, 1995; Palmer *et al.*, 1995; La Vecchia *et al.*, 1995; Newcomb *et al.*, 1996; Rosenberg *et al.*, 1996). Some studies have not shown such an increase, however (Vessey *et al.*, 1983; Ravnihar *et al.*, 1988; Ewertz, 1992; Rosenberg *et al.*, 1992; Tavani *et al.*, 1993a; White *et al.*, 1994; Primic-Žakelj *et al.*, 1995). Most of the studies show no overall increase in risk for older women, although the relative risk estimates were increased for older women in some studies (Vessey *et al.*, 1983; Ravnihar *et al.*, 1988; Rookus *et al.*, 1994). The Collaborative Group on Hormonal Factors in Breast Cancer (1996a,b) found little difference in risk according to the age at diagnosis of breast cancer once recency of use had been taken into account (Figure 4).

Data on the recency of use of combined oral contraceptives are shown in Table 8. A relatively consistent finding is that the risk for breast cancer is increased among women who have used these oral contraceptives recently, within the previous five to 10 years

Figure 2. Relative risk for breast cancer by time since last use of combined oral contraceptives and in relation to childbearing

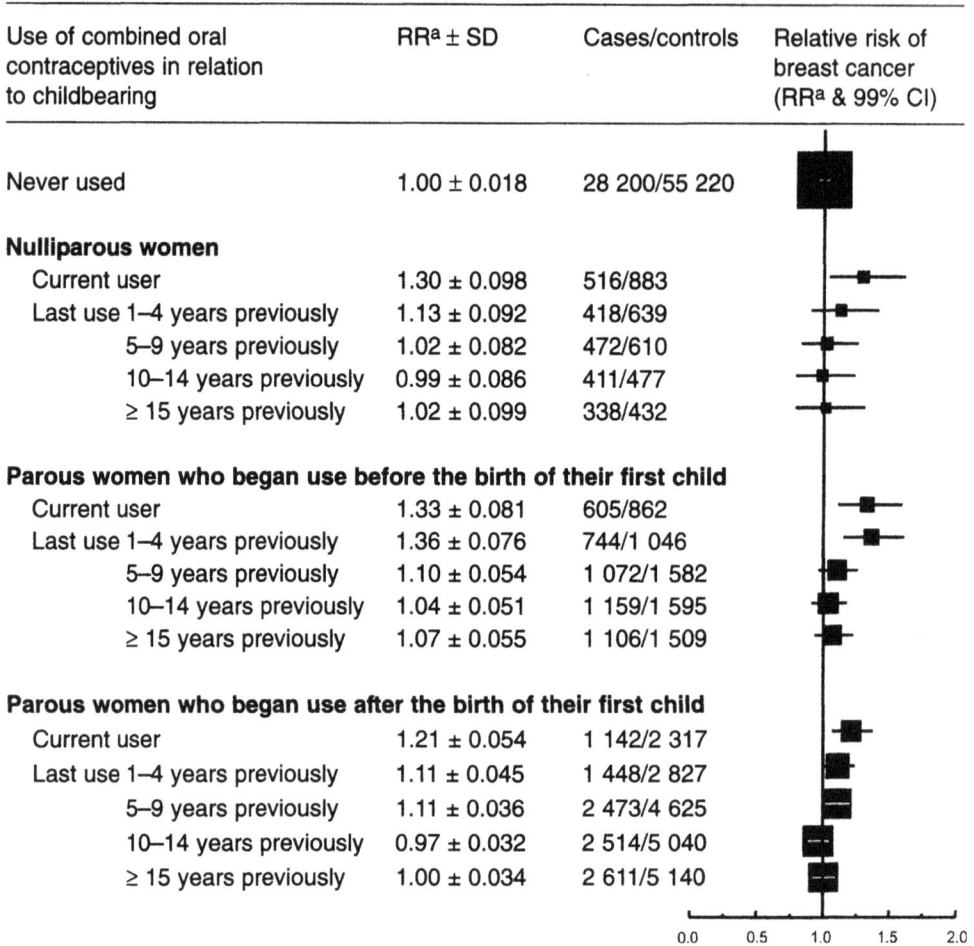

Use of combined oral contraceptives in relation to childbearing	RR[a] ± SD	Cases/controls	Relative risk of breast cancer (RR[a] & 99% CI)
Never used	1.00 ± 0.018	28 200/55 220	
Nulliparous women			
Current user	1.30 ± 0.098	516/883	
Last use 1–4 years previously	1.13 ± 0.092	418/639	
5–9 years previously	1.02 ± 0.082	472/610	
10–14 years previously	0.99 ± 0.086	411/477	
≥ 15 years previously	1.02 ± 0.099	338/432	
Parous women who began use before the birth of their first child			
Current user	1.33 ± 0.081	605/862	
Last use 1–4 years previously	1.36 ± 0.076	744/1 046	
5–9 years previously	1.10 ± 0.054	1 072/1 582	
10–14 years previously	1.04 ± 0.051	1 159/1 595	
≥ 15 years previously	1.07 ± 0.055	1 106/1 509	
Parous women who began use after the birth of their first child			
Current user	1.21 ± 0.054	1 142/2 317	
Last use 1–4 years previously	1.11 ± 0.045	1 448/2 827	
5–9 years previously	1.11 ± 0.036	2 473/4 625	
10–14 years previously	0.97 ± 0.032	2 514/5 040	
≥ 15 years previously	1.00 ± 0.034	2 611/5 140	

0.0   0.5   1.0   1.5   2.0

Adapted from Collaborative Group on Hormonal Factors in Breast Cancer (1996a,b)

[a] Relative risk (RR) given with 99% confidence interval (CI) relative to no use, stratified by study, age at diagnosis, parity and, where appropriate, age when first child was born and age when the risk for conceiving ceased

Size of square indicates the number of cases

Figure 3. Relative risk for breast cancer for various indices of the timing of combined oral contraceptive use within categories of time since last use

(a) Relative risk for breast cancer by duration of use and time since last use of combined oral contraceptives

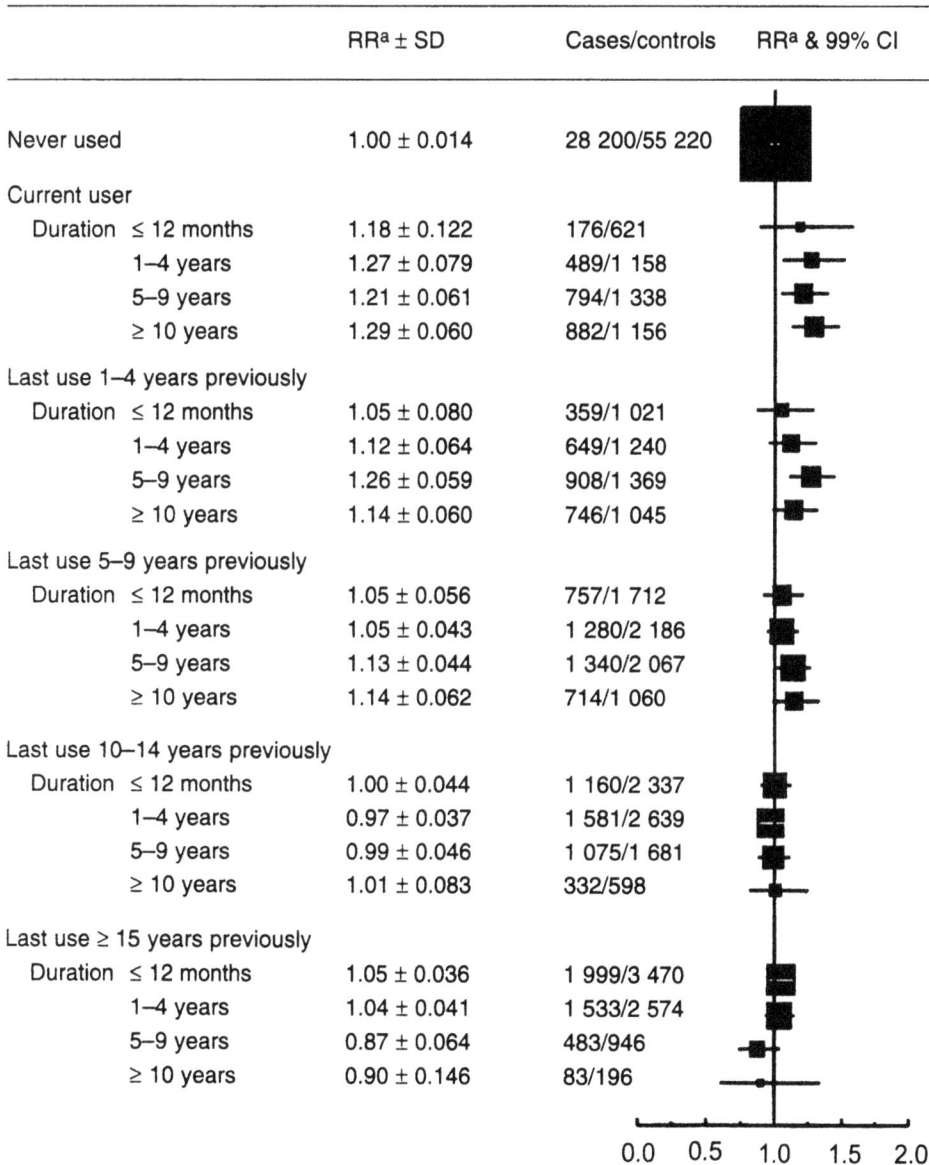

	RRa ± SD	Cases/controls	RRa & 99% CI
Never used	1.00 ± 0.014	28 200/55 220	
Current user			
Duration ≤ 12 months	1.18 ± 0.122	176/621	
1–4 years	1.27 ± 0.079	489/1 158	
5–9 years	1.21 ± 0.061	794/1 338	
≥ 10 years	1.29 ± 0.060	882/1 156	
Last use 1–4 years previously			
Duration ≤ 12 months	1.05 ± 0.080	359/1 021	
1–4 years	1.12 ± 0.064	649/1 240	
5–9 years	1.26 ± 0.059	908/1 369	
≥ 10 years	1.14 ± 0.060	746/1 045	
Last use 5–9 years previously			
Duration ≤ 12 months	1.05 ± 0.056	757/1 712	
1–4 years	1.05 ± 0.043	1 280/2 186	
5–9 years	1.13 ± 0.044	1 340/2 067	
≥ 10 years	1.14 ± 0.062	714/1 060	
Last use 10–14 years previously			
Duration ≤ 12 months	1.00 ± 0.044	1 160/2 337	
1–4 years	0.97 ± 0.037	1 581/2 639	
5–9 years	0.99 ± 0.046	1 075/1 681	
≥ 10 years	1.01 ± 0.083	332/598	
Last use ≥ 15 years previously			
Duration ≤ 12 months	1.05 ± 0.036	1 999/3 470	
1–4 years	1.04 ± 0.041	1 533/2 574	
5–9 years	0.87 ± 0.064	483/946	
≥ 10 years	0.90 ± 0.146	83/196	

```
        0.0   0.5   1.0   1.5   2.0
```

Figure 3 (contd)

(b) Relative risk for breast cancer by age at first use and time since last use of combined oral contraceptives

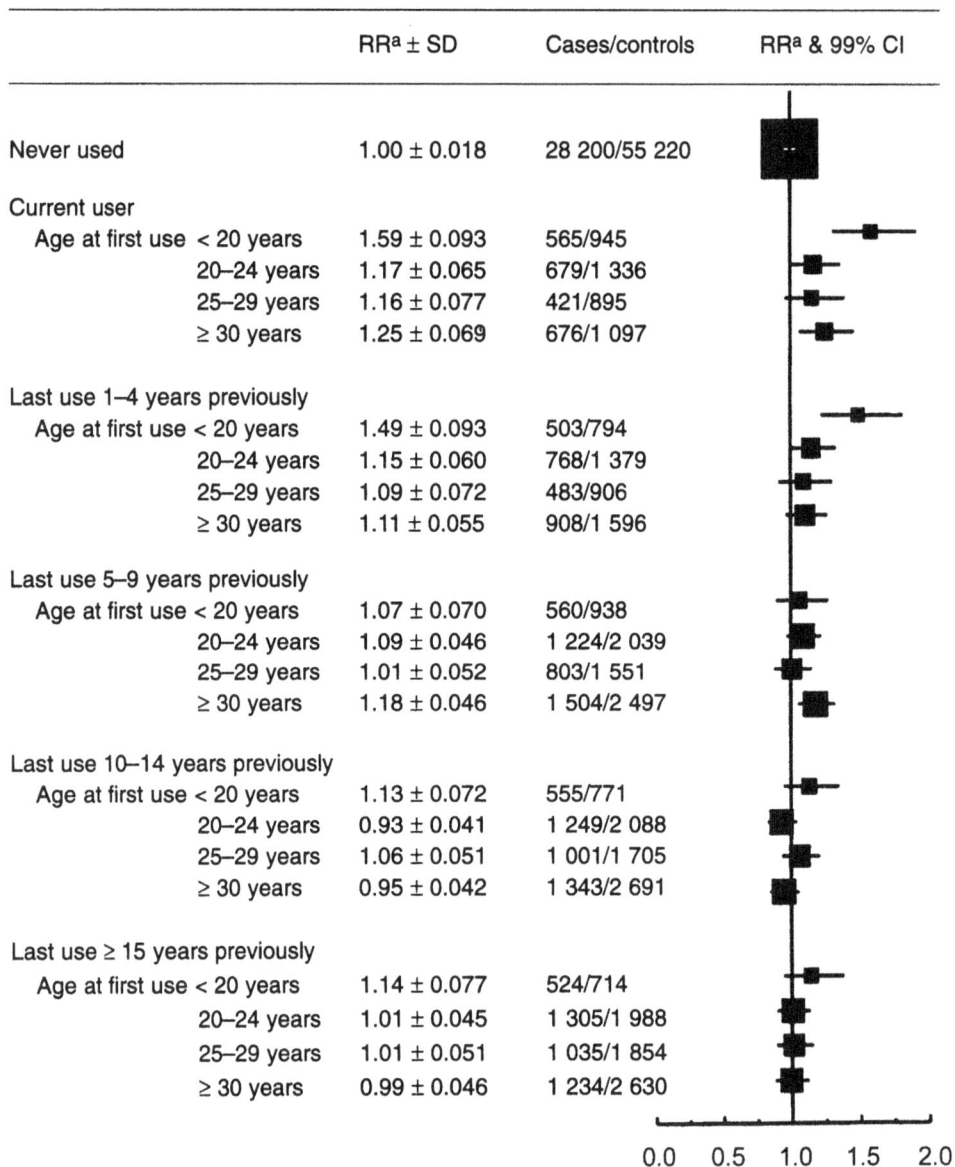

	RRa ± SD	Cases/controls	RRa & 99% CI
Never used	1.00 ± 0.018	28 200/55 220	
Current user			
Age at first use < 20 years	1.59 ± 0.093	565/945	
20–24 years	1.17 ± 0.065	679/1 336	
25–29 years	1.16 ± 0.077	421/895	
≥ 30 years	1.25 ± 0.069	676/1 097	
Last use 1–4 years previously			
Age at first use < 20 years	1.49 ± 0.093	503/794	
20–24 years	1.15 ± 0.060	768/1 379	
25–29 years	1.09 ± 0.072	483/906	
≥ 30 years	1.11 ± 0.055	908/1 596	
Last use 5–9 years previously			
Age at first use < 20 years	1.07 ± 0.070	560/938	
20–24 years	1.09 ± 0.046	1 224/2 039	
25–29 years	1.01 ± 0.052	803/1 551	
≥ 30 years	1.18 ± 0.046	1 504/2 497	
Last use 10–14 years previously			
Age at first use < 20 years	1.13 ± 0.072	555/771	
20–24 years	0.93 ± 0.041	1 249/2 088	
25–29 years	1.06 ± 0.051	1 001/1 705	
≥ 30 years	0.95 ± 0.042	1 343/2 691	
Last use ≥ 15 years previously			
Age at first use < 20 years	1.14 ± 0.077	524/714	
20–24 years	1.01 ± 0.045	1 305/1 988	
25–29 years	1.01 ± 0.051	1 035/1 854	
≥ 30 years	0.99 ± 0.046	1 234/2 630	

0.0   0.5   1.0   1.5   2.0

Figure 3 (contd)

**(c) Relative risk for breast cancer by time since first use and time
since last use of combined oral contraceptives**

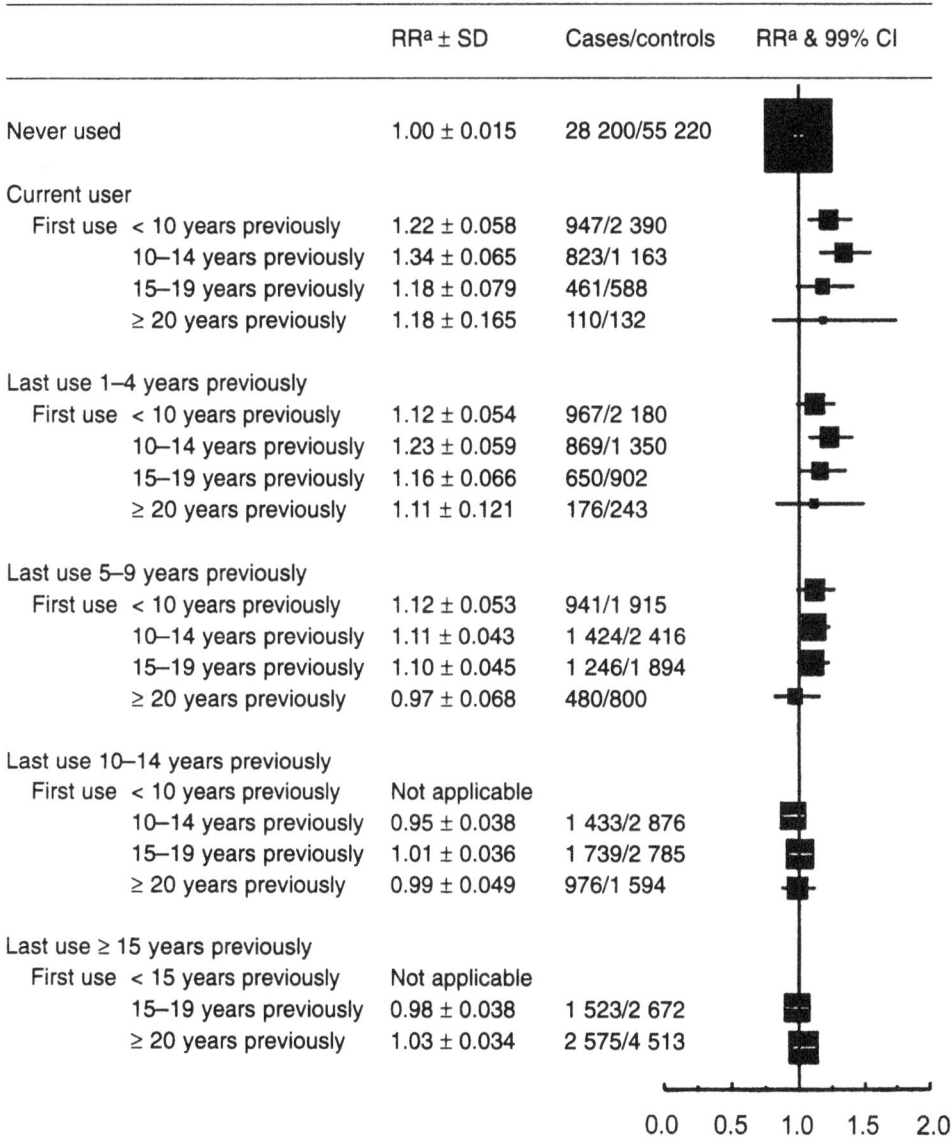

	RR^a ± SD	Cases/controls	RR^a & 99% CI
Never used	1.00 ± 0.015	28 200/55 220	
Current user			
First use < 10 years previously	1.22 ± 0.058	947/2 390	
10–14 years previously	1.34 ± 0.065	823/1 163	
15–19 years previously	1.18 ± 0.079	461/588	
≥ 20 years previously	1.18 ± 0.165	110/132	
Last use 1–4 years previously			
First use < 10 years previously	1.12 ± 0.054	967/2 180	
10–14 years previously	1.23 ± 0.059	869/1 350	
15–19 years previously	1.16 ± 0.066	650/902	
≥ 20 years previously	1.11 ± 0.121	176/243	
Last use 5–9 years previously			
First use < 10 years previously	1.12 ± 0.053	941/1 915	
10–14 years previously	1.11 ± 0.043	1 424/2 416	
15–19 years previously	1.10 ± 0.045	1 246/1 894	
≥ 20 years previously	0.97 ± 0.068	480/800	
Last use 10–14 years previously			
First use < 10 years previously	Not applicable		
10–14 years previously	0.95 ± 0.038	1 433/2 876	
15–19 years previously	1.01 ± 0.036	1 739/2 785	
≥ 20 years previously	0.99 ± 0.049	976/1 594	
Last use ≥ 15 years previously			
First use < 15 years previously	Not applicable		
15–19 years previously	0.98 ± 0.038	1 523/2 672	
≥ 20 years previously	1.03 ± 0.034	2 575/4 513	

0.0 0.5 1.0 1.5 2.0

Adapted from Collaborative Group on Hormonal Factors in Breast Cancer (1996a,b)

Of 15 tests for heterogeneity, one within each time since last use category, two are statistically significant: age at first use in current users (χ^2 = 12.7, degrees of freedom (d.f.) = 3, p = 0.005) and age at first use by women whose last use was 1–4 years previously (χ^2 = 12.6, d.f. = 3, p = 0.006).

^{a} Relative risk (given with 99% confidence interval) relative to no use, stratified by study, age at diagnosis, parity, and, where appropriate, the age when first child was born and age when risk for conceiving ceased.

Table 7. Use of combined oral contraceptives and risk for breast cancer risk according to age at diagnosis

Reference	Years of diagnosis	Comparison	Age at diagnosis (years)	Users No. of cases	No. of controls or person–years	RR	95% CI
Vessey et al. (1983)	1968–80	Ever versus never	<36	210	210	0.94	0.57–1.5
			36–40	257	257	0.86	0.56–1.3
			41–45	388	388	0.72	0.51–1.0
			46–50	321	321	1.5	1.0–2.2
Meirik et al. (1986)	1984–85	≥ 12 years versus never	<45	39	23	2.2	1.2–4.0
McPherson et al. (1987)	1980–84	≥ 12 years versus never	<45	21	20	1.8	0.82–3.9
			≥45	13	23	0.84	0.39–1.8
Ravnihar et al. (1988)	1980–83	Ever versus never	<35	31	96	1.5	0.68–3.4
			35–44	84	249	1.7	1.2–2.4
			45–54	57	122	1.5	1.0–2.3
Romieu et al. (1989)	1976–86	Current versus never	30–34	3	8 090[a]	0.71	0.19–2.6
		Past versus never		18	51 417[a]	0.67	0.3–1.4
		Current versus never	35–39	6	6 674[a]	1.0	0.43–2.4
		Past versus never		100	114 278[a]	1.0	0.74–1.5
		Current versus never	40–44	13	4 369[a]	2.7	1.5–4.6
		Past versus never		153	119 882[a]	1.1	0.89–1.5
		Current versus never	45–49	8	2 635[a]	1.6	0.81–3.3
		Past versus never		196	91 394[a]	1.2	0.95–1.4
		Current versus never	50–54	2	777[a]	1.1	0.28–4.4
		Past versus never		133	61 657[a]	1.1	0.90–1.4
		Current versus never	55–59	0	72[a]	–	
		Past versus never		69	29 144[a]	1.0	0.80–1.4
		Current versus never	60–64	0	5[a]	–	
		Past versus never		16	5 056[a]	1.2	0.72–2.1

Table 7 (contd)

Reference	Years of diagnosis	Comparison	Age at diagnosis (years)	Users No. of cases	No. of controls or person-years	RR	95% CI
Stanford et al. (1989)	1973–80	Ever versus never	<40	76	92	1.0	0.5–1.9
			40–44	208	235	1.4	0.9–1.9
			45–49	385	377	1.1	0.8–1.4
			50–54	425	448	0.8	0.6–1.1
			55–59	331	366	0.99	0.6–1.5
			≥60	597	665	1.0	0.5–2.2
UK National Case–Control Study (1989)	1982–85	> 8 years versus never	<35	198	143	1.74	p_{trend} < 0.001
Bernstein et al. (1990)	1972–83	Ever versus never	<37			RR, 1.0 per year of use	
Paul et al. (1990)	1983–87	Ever versus never	25–34	59	370	1.2	0.44–3.4
			35–44	286	711	1.2	0.78–1.8
			45–54	340	455	1.0	0.77–1.3
WHO Collaborative Study (1990)	1979–86	Ever versus never	<35	160	1 613	1.3	0.95–1.7
			≥35	560	2 814	1.1	0.98–1.3
Weinstein et al. (1991)	1984–86	Ever versus never	20–49	175	145	1.4	1.0–2.0
			50–70	101	95	1.1	0.79–1.5
Wingo et al. (1991)	1980–82	Ever versus never	20–34	425	547	1.4	1.0–2.1
			35–44	1 190	1 031	1.1	0.9–1.3
			45–54	888	991	0.9	0.8–1.0

Table 7 (contd)

Reference	Years of diagnosis	Comparison	Age at diagnosis (years)	Users No. of cases	No. of controls or person–years	RR	95% CI
Ewertz (1992)	1983–84	≥ 12 years versus never	< 40	20	22	1.1	0.5–2.2
			40–59	83	67	1.3	0.82–2.0
Rosenberg et al. (1992)	1982–86	≥ 10 years versus never	< 40	13	27	0.8	0.3–2.5
			40–69	46	95	0.9	0.6–1.3
Tavani et al. (1993a)	1983–91	Ever versus never	< 60	371	265	1.2	1.0–1.4
			< 40	130	151	0.9	0.6–1.2
Rookus et al. (1994)	1986–89	≥ 12 years versus never	< 35	20	8	2.9	
			36–45	75	79	1.1	
			46–54	41	21	2.3	
White et al. (1994)	1983–90	≥ 1 year versus < 1 year	< 46	583	733	1.0	0.81–1.3
Brinton et al. (1995)	1990–92	≥ 6 months versus < 6 months or never	< 35	206	193	1.7	1.2–2.6
			35–39	379	336	1.4	1.0–1.8
			40–44	674	545	1.1	0.9–1.4
			45–49	203	184	1.2	0.8–1.8
			50–54	138	142	0.94	0.6–1.4
Palmer et al. (1995)	1977–92	≥ 3 years versus < 1 year	< 45	87	142	2.2	1.5–3.2
			45–59	27	31	1.3	0.7–2.4
Primic-Žakelj et al. (1995)	1988–90	Ever versus never	Pre-menopausal	250	249	1.0	0.80–1.4
			Post-menopausal	48	50	1.4	0.82–2.4

Table 7 (contd)

Reference	Years of diagnosis	Comparison	Age at diagnosis (years)	Users		RR	95% CI
				No. of cases	No. of controls or person–years		
Newcomb et al. (1996)	1988–91	Ever versus never	< 35	139	400	1.4	0.8–2.3
			35–44	723	1 155	1.0	0.8–1.3
			45–54	809	1 112	1.1	0.9–1.3
			≥ 55	591	780	1.0	0.9–1.2
Rosenberg et al. (1996)	1977–92	≥ 1 year versus < 1 year	25–34	184	422	1.7	1.3–2.3
			35–44	455	606	0.9	0.7–1.0
			45–59	389	333	1.2	1.0–1.4
Rossing et al. (1996)	1988–90	Ever versus never	50–64	253	226	1.1	0.8–1.4

RR, relative risk; CI, confidence interval
[a] Person–years

Figure 4. Age-specific relative risk for breast cancer by time since last use of combined oral contraceptives

Age at diagnosis of breast cancer and duration of use of combined oral contraceptives	RR[a] ± SD	Cases/ controls	Age-specific relative risk of breast cancer (RR[a] & 99% CI)
Age < 30 at diagnosis			
never user	1.00 ± 0.118	290/2 995	
< 5 years since last use; < 20 at first use	1.95 ± 0.134	348/916	
< 5 years since last use; ≥ 20 at first use	1.14 ± 0.098	254/1 075	
5–9 years since last use	1.16 ± 0.143	134/412	
≥ 10 years since last use	insufficient data	18/48	
Age 30–34 at diagnosis			
never user	1.00 ± 0.067	690/2 093	
< 5 years since last use; < 20 at first use	1.54 ± 0.101	437/498	
< 5 years since last use; ≥ 20 at first use	1.13 ± 0.058	745/1 454	
5–9 years since last use	1.08 ± 0.060	629/1 163	
≥ 10 years since last use	0.96 ± 0.085	293/586	
Age 35–39 at diagnosis			
never user	1.00 ± 0.047	1 459/3 322	
< 5 years since last use; < 20 at first use	1.27 ± 0.116	237/278	
< 5 years since last use; ≥ 20 at first use	1.16 ± 0.055	965/1 660	
5–9 years since last use	1.00 ± 0.049	899/1 582	
≥ 10 years since last use	1.03 ± 0.044	1 286/2 081	
Age 40–44 at diagnosis			
never user	1.00 ± 0.035	2 958/5 392	
< 5 years since last use; < 20 at first use	insufficient data	45/43	
< 5 years since last use; ≥ 20 at first use	1.22 ± 0.057	942/1 443	
5–9 years since last use	1.13 ± 0.051	1 024/1 528	
≥ 10 years since last use	1.01 ± 0.034	2 222/3 258	
Age > 45 at diagnosis			
never user	1.00 ± 0.017	22 803/41 418	
< 5 years since last use; < 20 at first use	insufficient data	1/4	
< 5 years since last use; ≥ 20 at first use	1.11 ± 0.053	1 029/1 577	
5–9 years since last use	1.15 ± 0.043	1 405/2 340	
≥ 10 years since last use	0.99 ± 0.021	4 427/8 468	

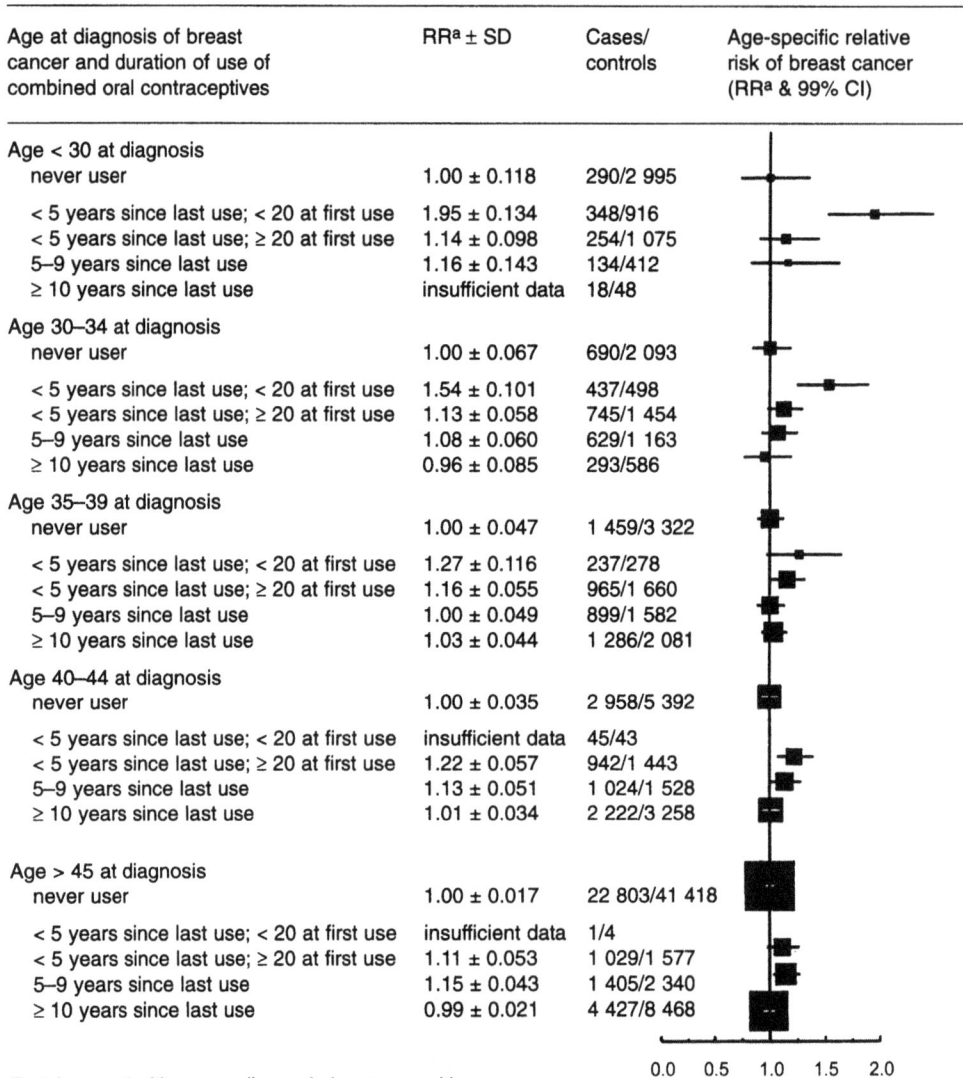

0.0 0.5 1.0 1.5 2.0

Test for trend with age at diagnosis in women with:
last use < 5 years ago, age at first use < 20: χ^2 (1 d.f.) = 5.2; p = 0.02
last use < 5 years ago, age at first use ≥ 20: χ^2 (1 d.f.) = 0.0; NS
last use 5–9 years ago: χ^2 (1 d.f.) = 1.2; NS
last use ≥ 10 years ago: χ^2 (1 d.f.) = 0.1; NS

Adapted from Collaborative Group on Hormonal Factors in Breast Cancer (1996a,b)
d.f., degree of freedom
[a] Relative risk (given with 99% confidence interval) relative to no use, stratified by study, age at diagnosis, parity and, where appropriate, the age when her first child was born and the age when her risk for conceiving ceased.

Table 8. Risk for breast cancer in relation to time since last use (recency of use) of combined oral contraceptives

Reference	Years of case diagnosis	Time since last use (years)	Age (years)	Users (cases/ controls)	RR (95% CI)
Vessey et al. (1983)	1968–80	≤ 1	16–50	58/69	0.99 (0.76–1.3)
		> 1–≤ 4		122/119	0.95 (0.7–1.3)
		> 4–≤ 8		125/101	1.3 (0.98–1.8)
		> 8		90/136	0.67 (0.48–0.94)
Meirik et al. (1986)	1984–85	Current use	< 45	80/80	1.5 (0.8–2.8)
		1–2		30/25	1.8 (0.9–3.7)
		3–5		45/35	1.9 (1.0–3.3)
		6–8		45/49	1.4 (0.8–2.4)
		9–11		36/55	1.0 (0.6–1.7)
		≥ 12		90/127	0.9 (0.6–1.4)
Rohan & McMichael (1988)	1982–84	≤ 8	20–69	81/71	1.2 (0.7–2.2)
		9–14		51/62	0.87 (0.50–1.5)
		≥ 15		55/52	1.1 (0.62–1.9)
Stanford et al. (1989)	1973–80	Current use	All	47/57	0.81 (0.5–1.2)
		1–3		93/96	1.0 (0.7–1.4)
		4–6		102/109	1.0 (0.8–1.4)
		≥ 7		221/251	0.96 (0.8–1.2)
Romieu et al. (1989)	1976–86	Current use	30–64	32/22 622[a]	1.6 (1.1–2.2)
		< 1		205/129 638[a]	1.1 (0.97–1.3)
		1–2		156/123 636[a]	1.1 (0.89–1.3)
		3–4		86/72 837[a]	0.97 (0.78–1.2)
		5–9		159/104 277[a]	1.1 (0.96–1.4)
		10–14		57/33 206[a]	1.1 (0.83–1.4)
		≥ 15		6/3 195[a]	1.1 (0.47–2.4)
WHO Collaborative Study (1990)	1979–86	Current use	< 62	127/747	1.7 (1.3–2.1)
		4–35 months		120/751	1.4 (1.1–1.8)
		3–9		234/1 374	1.2 (0.98–1.4)
		> 9		213/1 388	0.91 (0.77–1.1)
Clavel et al. (1991)	1983–87	Current use	20–55	41/45	1.4 (0.9–2.4)
		< 5		75/80	1.6 (1.0–2.5)
		5–9		66/56	1.6 (1.0–2.4)
		≥ 10		55/55	1.5 (0.9–2.3)

Table 8 (contd)

Reference	Years of case diagnosis	Time since last use (years)	Age (years)	Users (cases/ controls)	RR (95% CI)
Wingo *et al.* (1991)	1980–82	< 1	20–34	Not given	1.7 (1.1–2.6)
		1–< 2			1.1 (0.6–2.1)
		2–3			1.2 (0.7–1.9)
		4–5			1.8 (1.1–3.0)
		6–7			1.5 (0.9–2.5)
		8–9			1.5 (0.9–2.6)
		10–11			1.3 (0.7–2.4)
		12–13			1.0 (0.5–1.8)
		14–15			$p_{trend} = 0.5$
		16–17			
		18–19			
		≥ 20			
			35–44	Not given	1.2 (0.8–1.8)
					1.2 (0.7–2.3)
					1.5 (1.0–2.2)
					1.2 (0.9–1.6)
					1.1 (0.8–1.5)
					1.0 (0.7–1.3)
					1.0 (0.7–1.3)
					0.9 (0.7–1.2)
					1.0 (0.7–1.3)
					1.2 (0.8–1.7)
					0.9 (0.5–1.5)
					0.6 (0.3–1.5)
					$p_{trend} < 0.01$
			45–54	Not given	0.8 (0.4–1.5)
					0.8 (0.3–2.2)
					1.0 (0.7–1.5)
					1.1 (0.8–1.4)
					1.0 (0.8–1.3)
					1.3 (0.9–1.7)
					0.9 (0.7–1.2)
					0.8 (0.6–1.1)
					0.8 (0.6–1.1)
					0.6 (0.5–0.8)
					1.0 (0.7–1.5)
					0.6 (0.4–0.8)
					$p_{trend} < 0.01$

Table 8 (contd)

Reference	Years of case diagnosis	Time since last use (years)	Age (years)	Users (cases/ controls)	RR (95% CI)
Ewertz (1992)	1983–84	< 5 5–9 ≥ 10	< 40	56/65 46/37 59/58	1.0 (0.59–1.8) 1.5 (0.81–2.8) 1.2 (0.68–2.1)
			40–59	118/92 87/70 90/121	Reference 0.97 (0.64–1.5) 0.58 (0.39–0.85)
Tavani et al. (1993a)	1983–91	<5 5–9 ≥ 10	< 60	97/82 105/75 166/103	1.3 (1.0–1.9) 1.1 (0.8–1.6) 1.2 (0.9–1.5)
Rookus et al. (1994)	1986–89	< 3	46–54	Not given	1.9 (0.9–4.1)
White et al. (1994)	1983–90	Current use < 5 5–9 10–14 ≥ 15	21–45	59/88 102/131 135/171 171/226 116/111	1.3 (0.83–1.9) 1.3 (0.91–1.8) 1.0 (0.75–1.4) 0.88 (0.65–1.2) 0.96 (0.67–1.4)
Brinton et al. (1995)	1990–92	< 5 5–9 ≥ 10	20–34	135/Not given 40/Not given 31/Not given	2.0 (1.3–3.1) 1.5 (0.8–2.6) 1.2 (0.6–2.2)
			35–39	106/Not given 72/Not given 201/Not given	1.5 (0.9–2.2) 1.3 (0.9–2.0) 1.3 (0.9–1.9)
			40–44	57/Not given 91/Not given 526/Not given	1.2 (0.8–2.0) 1.2 (0.8–1.7) 1.1 (0.9–1.4)
La Vecchia et al. (1995)	1991–94	< 10 ≥ 10	< 35	Not given Not given	1.4 (0.7–2.7) 1.6 (0.4–6.0)
			35–44	Not given Not given	1.9 (1.2–2.9) 1.3 (0.9–2.0)
			45–64	Not given Not given	1.3 (0.8–2.3) 1.1 (0.8–1.4)

Table 8 (contd)

Reference	Years of case diagnosis	Time since last use (years)	Age (years)	Users (cases/ controls)	RR (95% CI)
Palmer *et al.* (1995)	1977–92	< 2 2–4 5–9 10–14 ≥ 15	25–59 (women with ≥ 3 years of use)	19/29 6/28 26/37 14/35 14/7	3.1 (1.5–6.3) 0.9 (0.3–2.4) 2.5 (1.4–4.5) 1.0 (0.5–2.1) 4.7 (1.7–13)
Paul *et al.* (1995)	1983–87	< 1 1–4 5–9 ≥ 10	25–34	18/147 17/85 20/96 4/42	1.3 (0.42–4.1) 1.9 (0.61–6.1) 1.4 (0.46–4.3) 0.36 (0.08–1.6)
			35–44	31/76 40/93 65/188 150/354	1.2 (0.65–2.1) 1.4 (0.82–2.5) 1.1 (0.65–1.7) 1.2 (0.78–1.9)
			45–54	21/20 30/43 63/78 226/314	1.5 (0.78–2.9) 0.90 (0.53–1.5) 1.0 (0.69–1.6) 0.99 (0.74–1.3)
Primic-Žakelj *et al.* (1995)	1988–90	< 6 months 7 months–5 years 6–10 11–15 > 15	25–54	32/16 43/38 54/68 94/102 75/75	2.3 (1.2–4.5) 1.3 (0.78–2.1) 0.89 (0.57–1.4) 1.0 (0.71–1.4) 1.1 (0.76–1.7)
Levi *et al.* (1996)	1990–95	< 5 5–14 ≥ 15	< 70	22/40 33/40 22/54	1.9 (0.9–3.6) 2.4 (1.4–4.4) 1.0 (0.6–1.8)
Newcomb *et al.* (1996)	1988–91	< 2 2–4 5–9 ≥ 10	< 35	30/109 25/64 47/127 37/100	1.3 (0.6–2.6) 1.9 (0.9–3.8) 1.5 (0.8–2.7) 1.1 (0.6–2.2)
			35–44	26/21 19/40 108/164 570/930	2.0 (1.1–3.9) 0.7 (0.4–1.3) 1.1 (0.8–1.5) 1.0 (0.8–2.1)

Table 8 (contd)

Reference	Years of case diagnosis	Time since last use (years)	Age (years)	Users (cases/ controls)	RR (95% CI)
Newcomb et al. (1996) (contd)			45–54	8/8	1.4 (0.5–4.0)
				10/12	1.3 (0.5–3.1)
				45/66	0.9 (0.6–1.4)
				746/1 026	1.1 (0.9–1.3)
		< 5	55–74	11/7	2.2 (0.8–5.7)
		5–9		24/41	0.8 (0.5–1.4)
		≥ 10		556/732	1.0 (0.9–1.2)
Rosenberg et al. (1996)	1977–92	< 3	25–34	80/184	1.9 (1.3–2.8)
		3–4		18/57	1.8 (0.9–3.3)
		5–9		53/112	1.6 (1.0–2.4)
		10–14		22/48	1.3 (0.7–2.3)
		≥ 15		0/3	–
			35–44	36/94	0.7 (0.5–1.2)
				25/50	0.8 (0.4–1.4)
				92/176	0.8 (0.5–1.0)
				157/159	1.1 (0.8–1.5)
				124/99	0.8 (0.6–1.2)
			45–54	16/29	0.9 (0.5–1.9)
				15/17	1.7 (0.8–3.8)
				70/80	1.0 (0.7–1.5)
				110/79	1.4 (1.0–1.9)
				159/106	1.2 (0.9–1.6)
Rossing et al. (1996)	1988–90	≤ 10	50–64	29/24	1.1 (0.6–2.0)
		11–15		57/43	1.4 (0.9–2.1)
		16–20		65/57	1.1 (0.7–1.7)
		21–25		57/59	0.9 (0.6–1.4)
		≥ 26		43/42	0.9 (0.6–1.5)

RR, relative risk; CI, confidence interval
[a] Person–years

(Meirik *et al.*, 1986; Rohan & McMichael, 1988; Romieu *et al.*, 1990; WHO Colla-borative Study of Neoplasia and Steroid Contraceptives, 1990; Wingo *et al.*, 1991; White *et al.*, 1994; Brinton *et al.*, 1995; Paul *et al.*, 1995; Primic-Žakelj *et al.*, 1995; La Vecchia *et al.*, 1995; Levi *et al.*, 1996; Newcomb *et al.*, 1996; Rosenberg *et al.*, 1996). In the study of La Vecchia *et al.* (1995), the increase was greater for women with longer use. Another consistent finding is that there is little or no increase in risk, or possibly even a decrease, among women who last used combined oral contraceptives at least 10 years previously (Meirik *et al.*, 1986; Rohan & McMichael, 1988; Romieu *et al.*, 1989; Stanford *et al.*, 1989; WHO Collaborative Study of Neoplasia and Steroid Contraceptives, 1990; Wingo *et al.*, 1991; White *et al.*, 1994; Brinton *et al.*, 1995; Paul *et al.*, 1995; Primic-Žakelj *et al.*, 1995; Levi *et al.*, 1996; Newcomb *et al.*, 1996; Rosenberg *et al.*, 1996; Rossing *et al.*, 1996); however, there was little or no variation in risk with recency of use in the studies of Vessey *et al.* (1983), Stanford *et al.* (1989), Ewertz (1992), Tavani *et al.* (1993a) or Rossing *et al.* (1996). The studies of Clavel *et al.* (1991) and Palmer *et al.* (1995) showed increased risks for users of these oral contraceptives that appeared to be unrelated to the recency of use. The estimated relative risk for breast cancer overall in the collaborative reanalysis was 1.24 (95% CI, 1.17–1.3) for current users, 1.16 (95% CI, 1.1–1.22) for users 1–4 years after stopping, 1.07 (95% CI, 1.0–1.12) for users 5–9 years after stopping and 1.0 (95% CI, 0.96–1.1) for users 10 or more years after stopping (Collaborative Group on Hormonal Factors in Breast Cancer, 1996b; Figure 5).

The relationship between recency of use and the risk for breast cancer at different ages was not assessed in many studies. Among those in which it was, that of Rookus *et al.* (1994) showed an increased risk associated with recent use for older but not younger women. In the studies of Wingo *et al.* (1991), Brinton *et al.* (1995), Paul *et al.* (1995) and Rosenberg *et al.* (1996), the increase in risk for recent users was most apparent in women under 35 years of age; in the study of La Vecchia *et al.* (1995), the increase for recent users was greatest among women aged 35–44; in the Nurses' Health Study (Romieu *et al.*, 1989), the point estimates of relative risk were increased for current users aged 40–45 and 45–49 and not younger users, but there were very few current users in any age group. In the study of Newcomb *et al.* (1996), the point estimates of relative risk were elevated for recent users in every age group, from < 35 through 55 and older (see Figure 4).

Data on the duration of use have been inconsistent, some studies suggesting increasing risk with increasing duration of use overall, before a first pregnancy or after starting at a young age. Long use is highly correlated with recent use, and it has been difficult to disentangle their effects. In studies in which recency of use was taken into account, there has been no clear trend for an increased risk with increasing duration (Romieu *et al.*, 1989; Paul *et al.*, 1990; WHO Collaborative Study of Neoplasia and Steroid Contraceptives, 1990; Wingo *et al.*, 1991; Palmer *et al.*, 1995; Primic-Žakelj *et al.*, 1995; Newcomb *et al.*, 1996; Rosenberg *et al.*, 1996). It is too early, however, to rule out a greater increase in risk for recent users who have used combined oral contraceptives for a very long time beginning at young ages, because the data on this issue are sparse (Collaborative Group on Hormonal Factors in Breast Cancer, 1996a,b; Figure 3).

Figure 5. Relative risk for breast cancer by time since last use of combined oral contraceptives

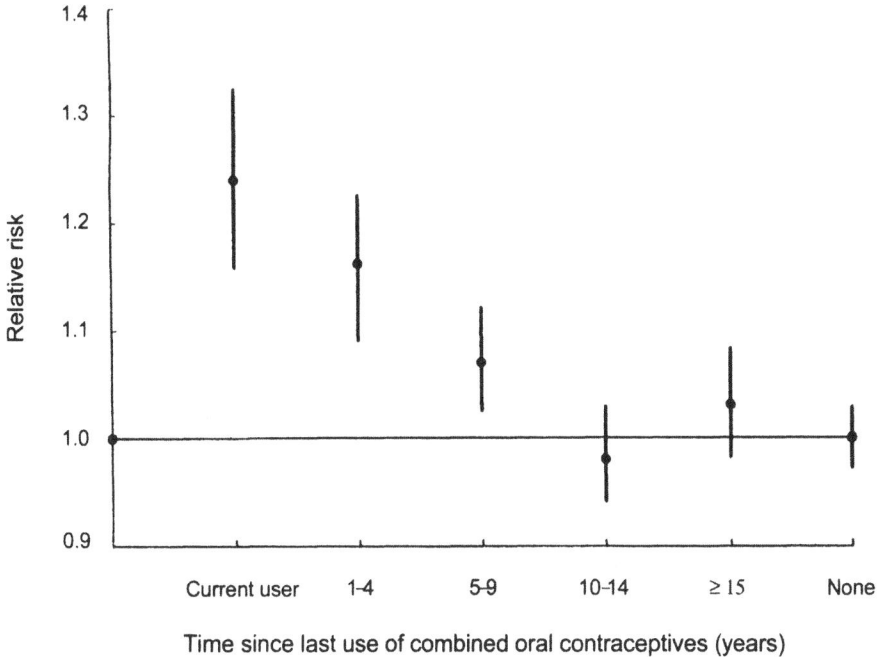

Time since last use of combined oral contraceptives (years)

From Collaborative Group on Hormonal Factors in Breast Cancer (1996b)
Relative risk (given with 95% confidence interval (CI)) relative to no use, stratified by study, age at diagnosis, parity, age at first birth and age at which risk for conceiving ceased

It has also been suggested that the risk for breast cancer associated with use of combined oral contraceptives varies according to the constituents of the formulation, e.g. that preparations with 'high potency' progestogens (as defined by their effect on the uterus) are the most harmful (Pike *et al.*, 1983). It has been difficult to study individual formulations because there are many of them, there are relatively few users of any particular one, and women tend to use several over the course of their reproductive lives. Little support for a differential effect according to the type of oestrogen or progestogen or the dose is provided in most studies (Vessey *et al.*, 1983; Cancer and Steroid Hormone Study of the Centers for Disease Control and the National Institute of Child Health and Human Development, 1986; Ravnihar *et al.*, 1988; UK National Case–Control Study Group, 1989; Clavel *et al.*, 1991; Ebeling *et al.*, 1991; Thomas *et al.*, 1992; Rookus *et al.*, 1994; Collaborative Group on Hormonal Factors in Breast Cancer, 1996a; Rosenberg *et al.*, 1996), although others indicate an effect (McPherson *et al.*, 1987; Ewertz, 1992; White *et al.*, 1994). Data from the Collaborative Group on Hormonal Factors in Breast Cancer (1996a,b) (Figures 6–10) show that there is little variation according to type or dose of oral contraceptive.

Figure 6. Relative risk (RR) for breast cancer by time since last use and oestrogen and progestogen type and dose of combined oral contraceptives last used

(a) Oestrogen type and dose

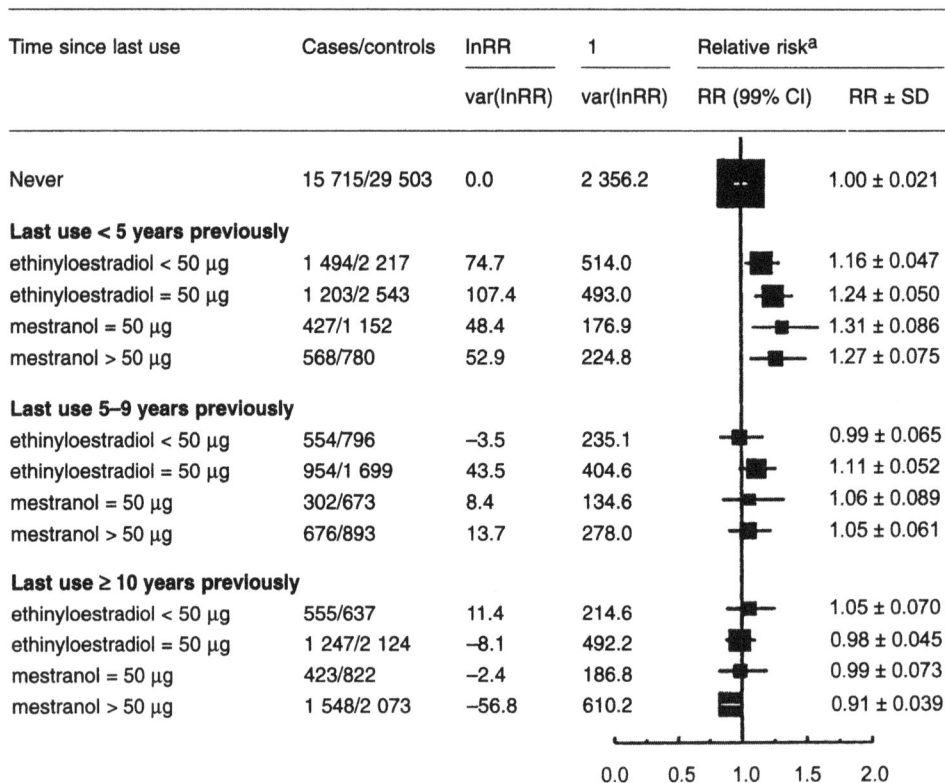

Time since last use	Cases/controls	lnRR $\frac{}{}$ var(lnRR)	1 $\frac{}{}$ var(lnRR)	Relative risk[a] RR (99% CI)	RR ± SD
Never	15 715/29 503	0.0	2 356.2	■	1.00 ± 0.021
Last use < 5 years previously					
ethinyloestradiol < 50 µg	1 494/2 217	74.7	514.0	■	1.16 ± 0.047
ethinyloestradiol = 50 µg	1 203/2 543	107.4	493.0	■	1.24 ± 0.050
mestranol = 50 µg	427/1 152	48.4	176.9	■	1.31 ± 0.086
mestranol > 50 µg	568/780	52.9	224.8	■	1.27 ± 0.075
Last use 5–9 years previously					
ethinyloestradiol < 50 µg	554/796	–3.5	235.1	■	0.99 ± 0.065
ethinyloestradiol = 50 µg	954/1 699	43.5	404.6	■	1.11 ± 0.052
mestranol = 50 µg	302/673	8.4	134.6	■	1.06 ± 0.089
mestranol > 50 µg	676/893	13.7	278.0	■	1.05 ± 0.061
Last use ≥ 10 years previously					
ethinyloestradiol < 50 µg	555/637	11.4	214.6	■	1.05 ± 0.070
ethinyloestradiol = 50 µg	1 247/2 124	–8.1	492.2	■	0.98 ± 0.045
mestranol = 50 µg	423/822	–2.4	186.8	■	0.99 ± 0.073
mestranol > 50 µg	1 548/2 073	–56.8	610.2	■	0.91 ± 0.039

0.0   0.5   1.0   1.5   2.0

Trend for heterogeneity by type and dose of oestrogen in women with:
Last use < 5 years previously: χ^2 (3 d.f.) = 2.9; NS
Last use 5–9 years previously: χ^2 (3 d.f.) = 2.3; NS
Last use ≥ 10 years previously: χ^2 (3 d.f.) = 4.0; NS

Figure 6 (contd)

(b) Progestogen type and dose

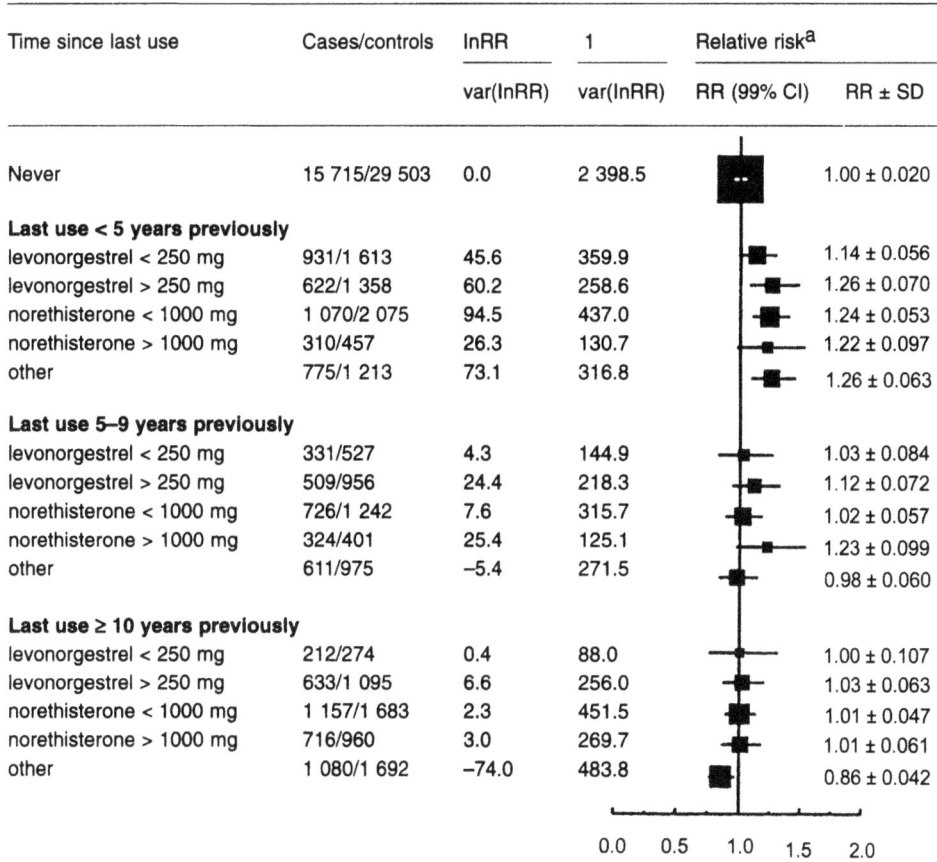

Time since last use	Cases/controls	lnRR var(lnRR)	1 var(lnRR)	Relative risk[a] RR (99% CI)	RR ± SD
Never	15 715/29 503	0.0	2 398.5		1.00 ± 0.020
Last use < 5 years previously					
levonorgestrel < 250 mg	931/1 613	45.6	359.9		1.14 ± 0.056
levonorgestrel > 250 mg	622/1 358	60.2	258.6		1.26 ± 0.070
norethisterone < 1000 mg	1 070/2 075	94.5	437.0		1.24 ± 0.053
norethisterone > 1000 mg	310/457	26.3	130.7		1.22 ± 0.097
other	775/1 213	73.1	316.8		1.26 ± 0.063
Last use 5–9 years previously					
levonorgestrel < 250 mg	331/527	4.3	144.9		1.03 ± 0.084
levonorgestrel > 250 mg	509/956	24.4	218.3		1.12 ± 0.072
norethisterone < 1000 mg	726/1 242	7.6	315.7		1.02 ± 0.057
norethisterone > 1000 mg	324/401	25.4	125.1		1.23 ± 0.099
other	611/975	−5.4	271.5		0.98 ± 0.060
Last use ≥ 10 years previously					
levonorgestrel < 250 mg	212/274	0.4	88.0		1.00 ± 0.107
levonorgestrel > 250 mg	633/1 095	6.6	256.0		1.03 ± 0.063
norethisterone < 1000 mg	1 157/1 683	2.3	451.5		1.01 ± 0.047
norethisterone > 1000 mg	716/960	3.0	269.7		1.01 ± 0.061
other	1 080/1 692	−74.0	483.8		0.86 ± 0.042

0.0   0.5   1.0   1.5   2.0

Trend for heterogeneity by type and dose of progestogen in women with:
Last use < 5 years previously: χ^2 (4 d.f.) = 2.6; NS
Last use 5–9 years previously: χ^2 (4 d.f.) = 5.4; NS
Last use ≥ 10 years previously: χ^2 (4 d.f.) = 9.1; $p = 0.003$

Adapted from Collaborative Group on Hormonal Factors in Breast Cancer (1996a,b)
d.f., degrees of freedom; NS, not significant; CI, confidence interval; SD, standard deviation
[a] Relative to no use, stratified by study, age at diagnosis, parity, age at first birth and age at which risk for conceiving ceased

Figure 7. Relative risk (RR) for breast cancer by time since last use and type of oestrogen and progestogen in the oral contraceptive

(a) First used

Oestrogen and progestogen	Cases/controls	Relative risk[a] RR & 99% CI	RR ± SD
Never	15 715/29 503		1.00 ± 0.020
Last use < 5 years previously			
ethinyloestradiol and norgestrel	882/2 089		1.14 ± 0.058
ethinyloestradiol and norethisterone	782/1 185		1.17 ± 0.061
mestranol and norethisterone	839/1 610		1.30 ± 0.064
ethinyloestradiol and lynoestrenol	112/234		1.03 ± 0.141
mestranol and lynoestrenol	171/274		1.42 ± 0.146
ethinyloestradiol and ethynodiol	109/125		1.64 ± 0.202
mestranol and ethynodiol	280/409		1.20 ± 0.101
mestranol and chlormadinone or norethynodrel	308/501		1.14 ± 0.095
ethinyloestradiol and desogestrel or gestodene	32/50		0.82 ± 0.234
other	117/177		1.11 ± 0.147
Last use 5–9 years previously			
ethinyloestradiol and norgestrel	540/1 065		1.14 ± 0.070
ethinyloestradiol and norethisterone	499/688		1.08 ± 0.072
mestranol and norethisterone	697/1 120		1.08 ± 0.062
ethinyloestradiol and lynoestrenol	64/118		0.92 ± 0.178
mestranol and lynoestrenol	125/232		0.98 ± 0.136
ethinyloestradiol and ethynodiol	49/84		1.02 ± 0.209
mestranol and ethynodiol	245/353		1.06 ± 0.099
mestranol and chlormadinone acetate	76/173		0.86 ± 0.145
mestranol and norethynodrel	212/224		1.14 ± 0.116
other	90/175		0.89 ± 0.145
Last use ≥ 10 years previously			
ethinyloestradiol and norgestrel	658/1 176		1.02 ± 0.062
ethinyloestradiol and norethisterone	745/1 031		0.99 ± 0.057
mestranol and norethisterone	1 372/1 908		0.99 ± 0.045
ethinyloestradiol and lynoestrenol	55/114		1.10 ± 0.213
mestranol and lynoestrenol	210/308		1.10 ± 0.121
ethinyloestradiol and ethynodiol	69/124		0.81 ± 0.154
mestranol and ethynodiol	338/480		0.91 ± 0.077
mestranol and chlormadinone acetate	128/238		0.81 ± 0.111
mestranol and norethynodrel	430/569		0.84 ± 0.067
other	123/193		0.92 ± 0.132

0.0   0.5   1.0   1.5   2.0

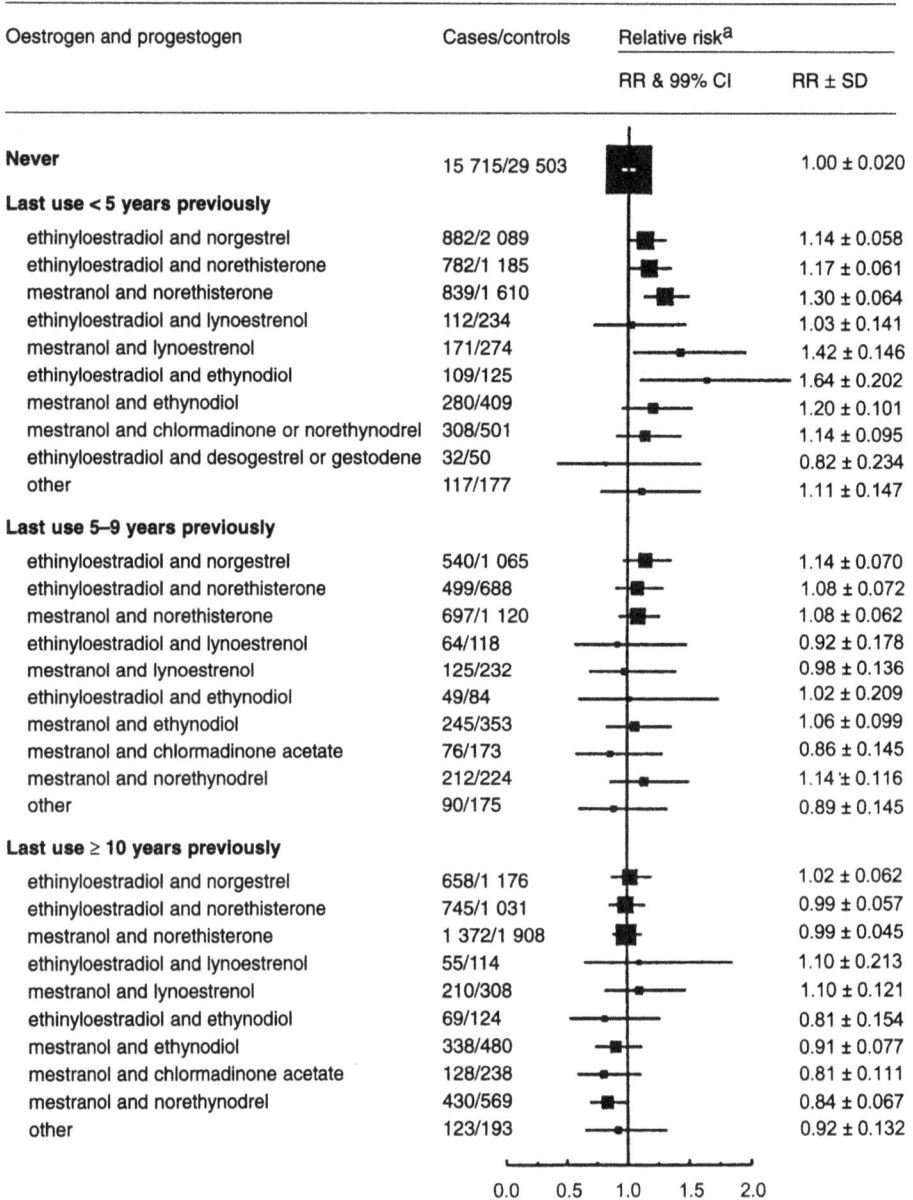

Test for heterogeneity by type of oral contraceptive in women with:
Last use < 5 years previously: χ^2 (9 d.f.) = 13.3; NS
Last use 5–9 years previously: χ^2 (9 d.f.) = 6.0; NS
Last use ≥ 10 years previously: χ^2 (9 d.f.) = 10.8; NS

Figure 7 (contd)

(b) Most used

Oestrogen and progestogen	Cases/controls	RR ± SD
Never	15 715/29 503	1.00 ± 0.021
Last use < 5 years previously		
ethinyloestradiol and norgestrel	1 168/2 513	1.16 ± 0.051
ethinyloestradiol and norethisterone	835/1 307	1.16 ± 0.058
mestranol and norethisterone	807/1 644	1.24 ± 0.063
ethinyloestradiol and lynoestrenol	163/332	1.12 ± 0.122
mestranol and lynoestrenol	149/217	1.45 ± 0.168
ethinyloestradiol and ethynodiol	137/161	1.49 ± 0.169
mestranol and ethynodiol	241/320	1.19 ± 0.110
mestranol and chlormadinone or norethynodrel	181/305	1.10 ± 0.115
ethinyloestradiol and desogestrel or gestodene	30/22	
other	101/147	1.28 ± 0.175
Last use 5–9 years previously		
ethinyloestradiol and norgestrel	631/1 226	1.12 ± 0.064
ethinyloestradiol and norethisterone	506/723	1.04 ± 0.070
mestranol and norethisterone	729/1 176	1.07 ± 0.060
ethinyloestradiol and lynoestrenol	108/172	1.13 ± 0.159
mestranol and lynoestrenol	123/217	0.93 ± 0.134
ethinyloestradiol and ethynodiol	67/118	1.05 ± 0.183
mestranol and ethynodiol	224/307	1.00 ± 0.102
mestranol and chlormadinone acetate	66/137	0.91 ± 0.165
mestranol and norethynodrel	168/170	1.21 ± 0.133
other	85/162	1.00 ± 0.160
Last use ≥ 10 years previously		
ethinyloestradiol and norgestrel	553/1 089	1.03 ± 0.066
ethinyloestradiol and norethisterone	764/1 054	1.00 ± 0.057
mestranol and norethisterone	1 425/1 963	0.99 ± 0.044
ethinyloestradiol and lynoestrenol	83/148	1.12 ± 0.174
mestranol and lynoestrenol	335/443	1.05 ± 0.097
ethinyloestradiol and ethynodiol	82/153	0.78 ± 0.136
mestranol and ethynodiol	316/460	0.89 ± 0.078
mestranol and chlormadinone acetate	126/235	0.75 ± 0.107
mestranol and norethynodrel	398/527	0.83 ± 0.069
other	120/190	0.94 ± 0.134

Relative risk[a] — RR & 99% CI. Scale: 0.0 0.5 1.0 1.5 2.0

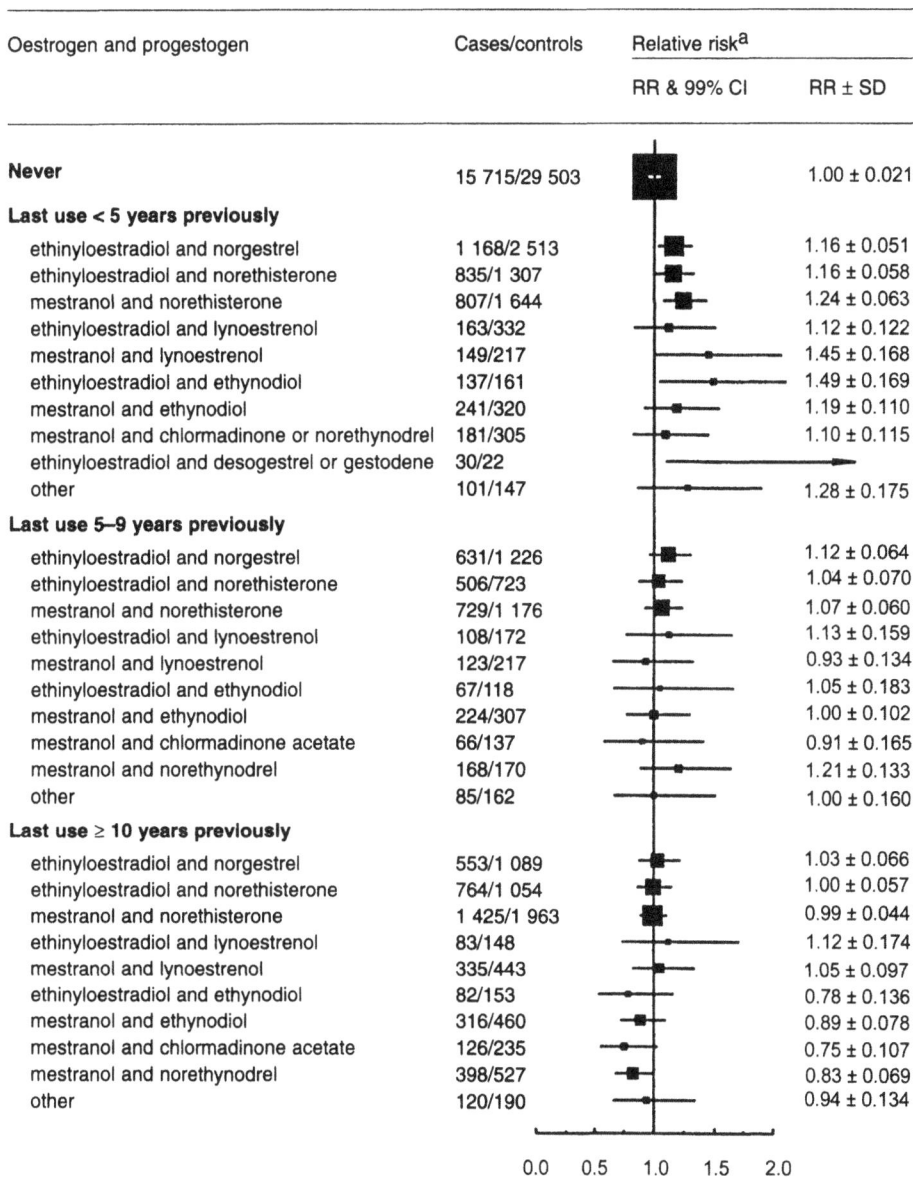

Test for heterogeneity by type of oral contraceptive in women with:
Last use < 5 years previously: χ^2 (9 d.f.) = 12.0; NS
Last use 5–9 years previously: χ^2 (9 d.f.) = 4.4; NS
Last use ≥ 10 years previously: χ^2 (9 d.f.) = 14.4; NS

Figure 7 (contd)

(c) Last used

Oestrogen and progestogen	Cases/controls	Relative risk[a]	
		RR & 99% CI	RR ± SD
Never	15 715/29 503		1.00 ± 0.019
Last use < 5 years previously			
ethinyloestradiol and norgestrel	1 564/3 003		1.17 ± 0.045
ethinyloestradiol and norethisterone	744/1 172		1.15 ± 0.060
mestranol and norethisterone	705/1 455		1.30 ± 0.069
ethinyloestradiol and lynoestrenol	129/319		1.05 ± 0.129
mestranol and lynoestrenol	40/107		
ethinyloestradiol and ethynodiol	132/160		1.46 ± 0.168
mestranol and ethynodiol	196/242		1.33 ± 0.133
mestranol and chlormadinone or norethynodrel	117/216		0.96 ± 0.129
ethinyloestradiol and desogestrel or gestodene	109/118		1.26 ± 0.180
other	75/98		1.37 ± 0.212
Last use 5–9 years previously			
ethinyloestradiol and norgestrel	848/1 504		1.07 ± 0.055
ethinyloestradiol and norethisterone	481/677		1.08 ± 0.073
mestranol and norethisterone	685/1 099		1.12 ± 0.063
ethinyloestradiol and lynoestrenol	104/188		0.93 ± 0.142
mestranol and lynoestrenol	31/99		
ethinyloestradiol and ethynodiol	61/116		0.94 ± 0.178
mestranol and ethynodiol	199/265		0.98 ± 0.107
mestranol and chlormadinone acetate	44/82		0.95 ± 0.207
mestranol and norethynodrel	134/147		1.09 ± 0.137
other	74/126		0.97 ± 0.172
Last use ≥ 10 years previously			
ethinyloestradiol and norgestrel	856/1 388		1.02 ± 0.055
ethinyloestradiol and norethisterone	749/1 026		1.03 ± 0.059
mestranol and norethisterone	1 360/1 930		0.98 ± 0.044
ethinyloestradiol and lynoestrenol	101/183		0.93 ± 0.145
mestranol and lynoestrenol	113/217		0.95 ± 0.142
ethinyloestradiol and ethynodiol	90/143		0.93 ± 0.150
mestranol and ethynodiol	275/410		0.86 ± 0.081
mestranol and chlormadinone acetate	117/204		0.79 ± 0.115
mestranol and norethynodrel	358/474		0.81 ± 0.072
other	113/177		0.94 ± 0.139

0.0   0.5   1.0   1.5   2.0

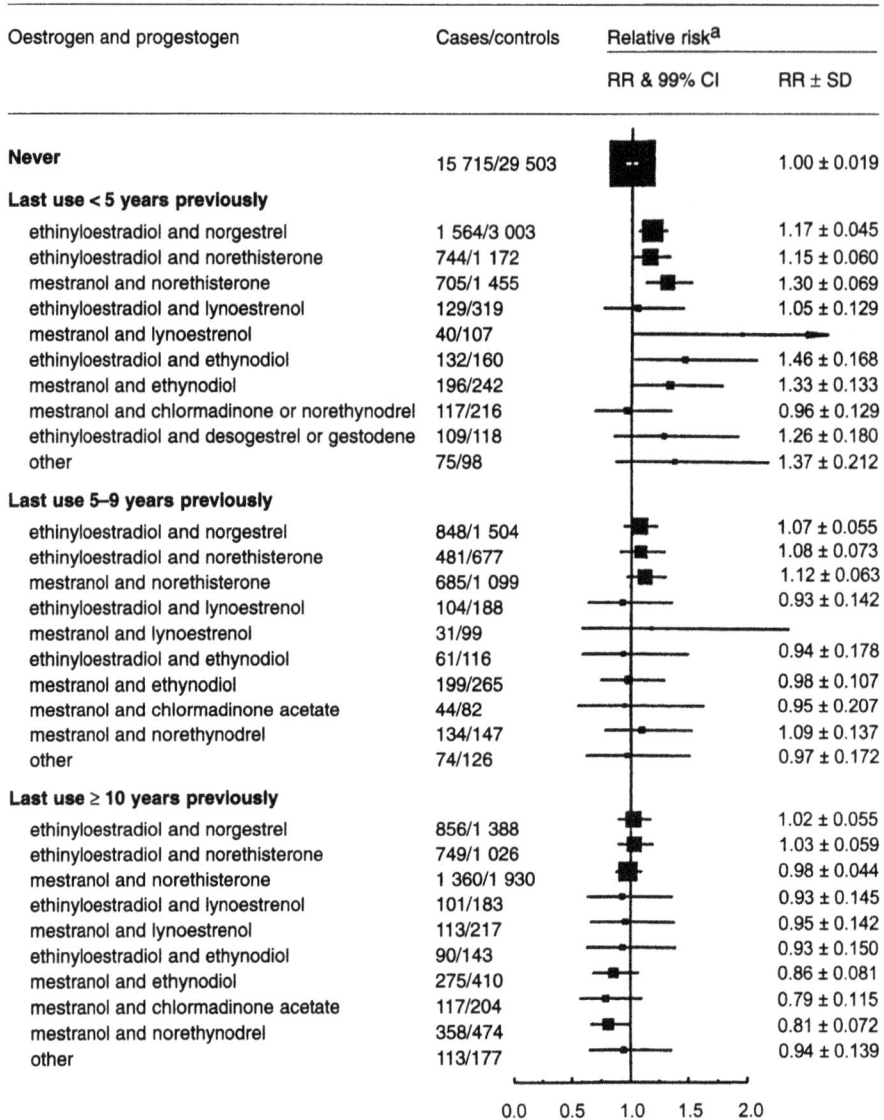

Test for heterogeneity by type of oral contraceptive in women with:
Last use < 5 years previously: χ^2 (9 d.f.) = 13.6; NS
Last use 5–9 years previously: χ^2 (9 d.f.) = 3.4; NS
Last use ≥ 10 years previously: χ^2 (9 d.f.) = 11.5; NS

Adapted from Collaborative Group on Hormonal Factors in Breast Cancer (1996a,b)
CI, confidence interval; SD, standard deviation; d.f., degrees of freedom; NS, not significant
[a] Relative to no use, stratified by study, age at diagnosis, parity, age at first birth and age at which risk for conceiving ceased

Figure 8. Relative risk (RR) for breast cancer by type and dose of progestogen in the oral contraceptive last used, grouped according to type and dose of oestrogen

(a) Last use < 5 years previously

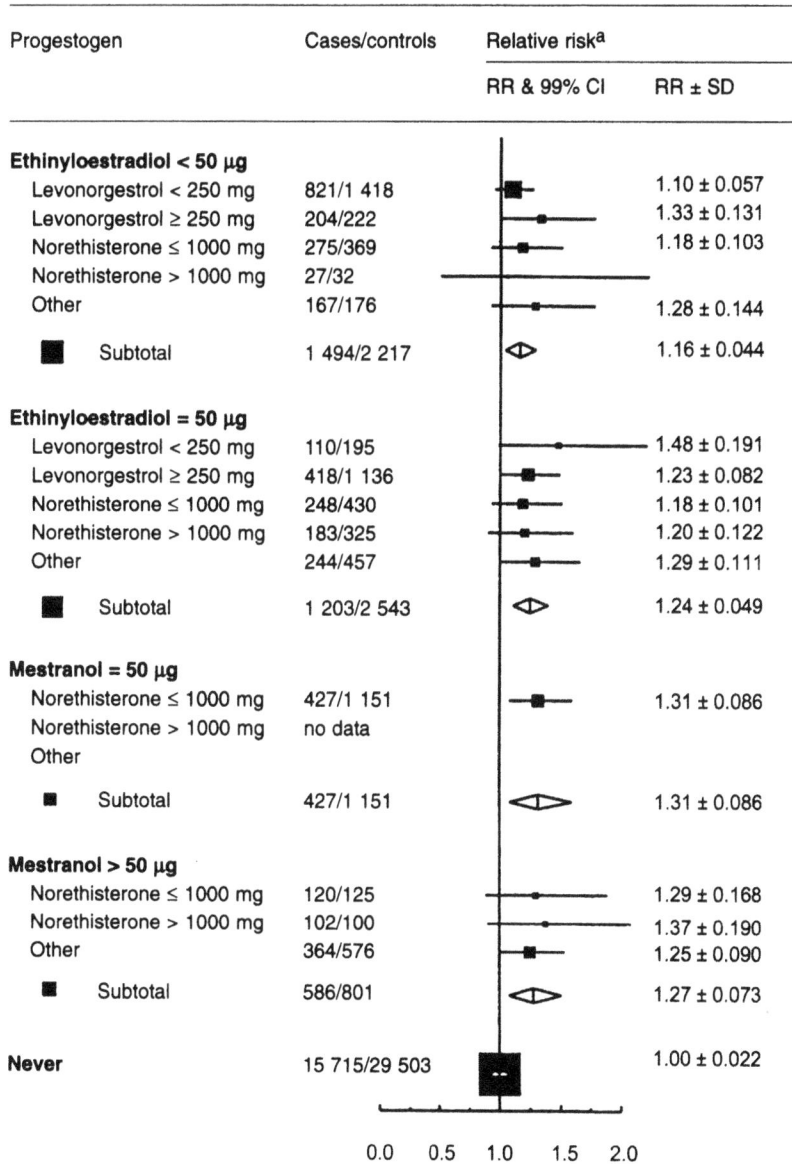

Progestogen	Cases/controls	Relative risk[a]	
		RR & 99% CI	RR ± SD
Ethinyloestradiol < 50 µg			
Levonorgestrol < 250 mg	821/1 418		1.10 ± 0.057
Levonorgestrol ≥ 250 mg	204/222		1.33 ± 0.131
Norethisterone ≤ 1000 mg	275/369		1.18 ± 0.103
Norethisterone > 1000 mg	27/32		
Other	167/176		1.28 ± 0.144
■ Subtotal	1 494/2 217		1.16 ± 0.044
Ethinyloestradiol = 50 µg			
Levonorgestrol < 250 mg	110/195		1.48 ± 0.191
Levonorgestrol ≥ 250 mg	418/1 136		1.23 ± 0.082
Norethisterone ≤ 1000 mg	248/430		1.18 ± 0.101
Norethisterone > 1000 mg	183/325		1.20 ± 0.122
Other	244/457		1.29 ± 0.111
■ Subtotal	1 203/2 543		1.24 ± 0.049
Mestranol = 50 µg			
Norethisterone ≤ 1000 mg	427/1 151		1.31 ± 0.086
Norethisterone > 1000 mg	no data		
Other			
■ Subtotal	427/1 151		1.31 ± 0.086
Mestranol > 50 µg			
Norethisterone ≤ 1000 mg	120/125		1.29 ± 0.168
Norethisterone > 1000 mg	102/100		1.37 ± 0.190
Other	364/576		1.25 ± 0.090
■ Subtotal	586/801		1.27 ± 0.073
Never	15 715/29 503		1.00 ± 0.022

0.0 0.5 1.0 1.5 2.0

Test for heterogeneity by type and dose of progestogen within oral contraceptives containing:
Ethinyloestradiol < 50 µg : χ^2 (4 d.f.) = 3.2; NS
Ethinyloestradiol = 50 µg : χ^2 (4 d.f.) = 1.7; NS
Mestranol > 50 µg : χ^2 (2 d.f.) = 0.3; NS

Figure 8 (contd)

(b) Last use 5–9 years previously

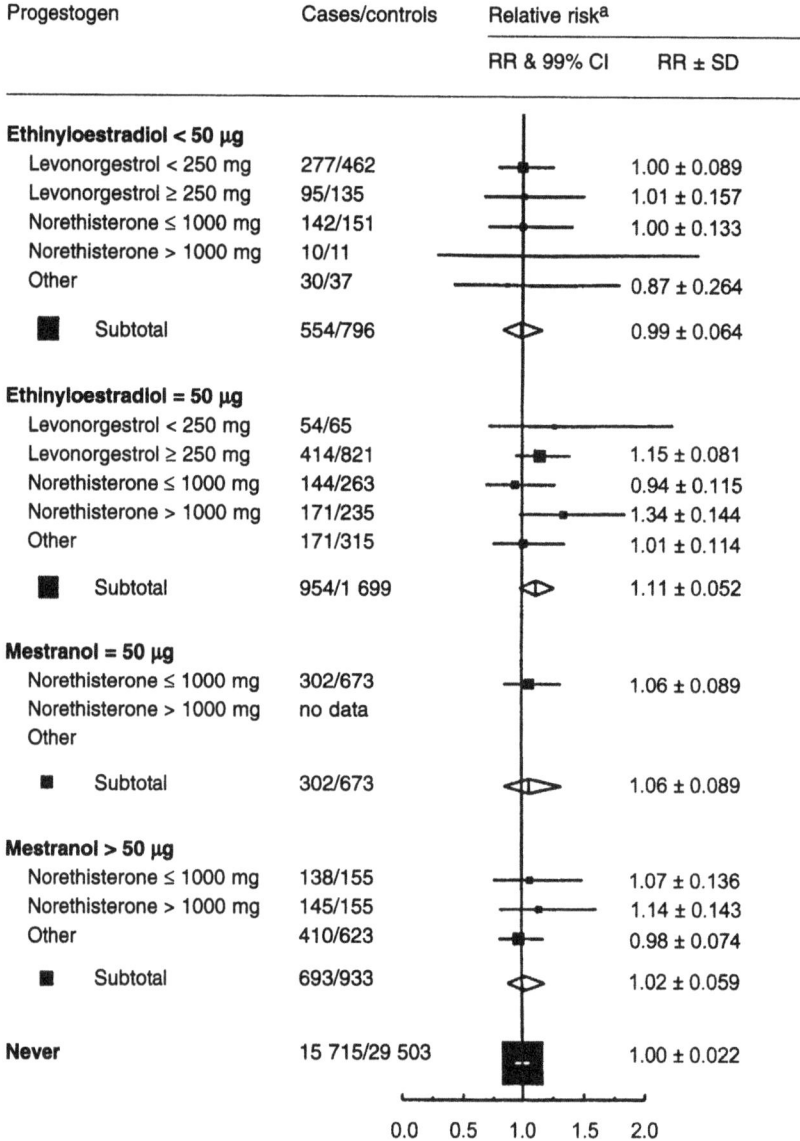

Progestogen	Cases/controls	Relative risk[a]	
		RR & 99% CI	RR ± SD

Ethinyloestradiol < 50 µg

Levonorgestrol < 250 mg	277/462		1.00 ± 0.089
Levonorgestrol ≥ 250 mg	95/135		1.01 ± 0.157
Norethisterone ≤ 1000 mg	142/151		1.00 ± 0.133
Norethisterone > 1000 mg	10/11		
Other	30/37		0.87 ± 0.264
Subtotal	554/796		0.99 ± 0.064

Ethinyloestradiol = 50 µg

Levonorgestrol < 250 mg	54/65		
Levonorgestrol ≥ 250 mg	414/821		1.15 ± 0.081
Norethisterone ≤ 1000 mg	144/263		0.94 ± 0.115
Norethisterone > 1000 mg	171/235		1.34 ± 0.144
Other	171/315		1.01 ± 0.114
Subtotal	954/1 699		1.11 ± 0.052

Mestranol = 50 µg

Norethisterone ≤ 1000 mg	302/673		1.06 ± 0.089
Norethisterone > 1000 mg	no data		
Other			
Subtotal	302/673		1.06 ± 0.089

Mestranol > 50 µg

Norethisterone ≤ 1000 mg	138/155		1.07 ± 0.136
Norethisterone > 1000 mg	145/155		1.14 ± 0.143
Other	410/623		0.98 ± 0.074
Subtotal	693/933		1.02 ± 0.059

Never	15 715/29 503		1.00 ± 0.022

```
        0.0   0.5   1.0   1.5   2.0
```

Test for heterogeneity by type and dose of progestogen within oral contraceptives containing:
Ethinyloestradiol < 50 µg   : χ^2 (4 d.f.) = 0.9; NS
Ethinyloestradiol = 50 µg   : χ^2 (4 d.f.) = 5.6; NS
Mestranol > 50 µg   : χ^2 (2 d.f.) = 1.2; NS

Figure 8 (contd)

(c) Last use ≥ 10 years previously

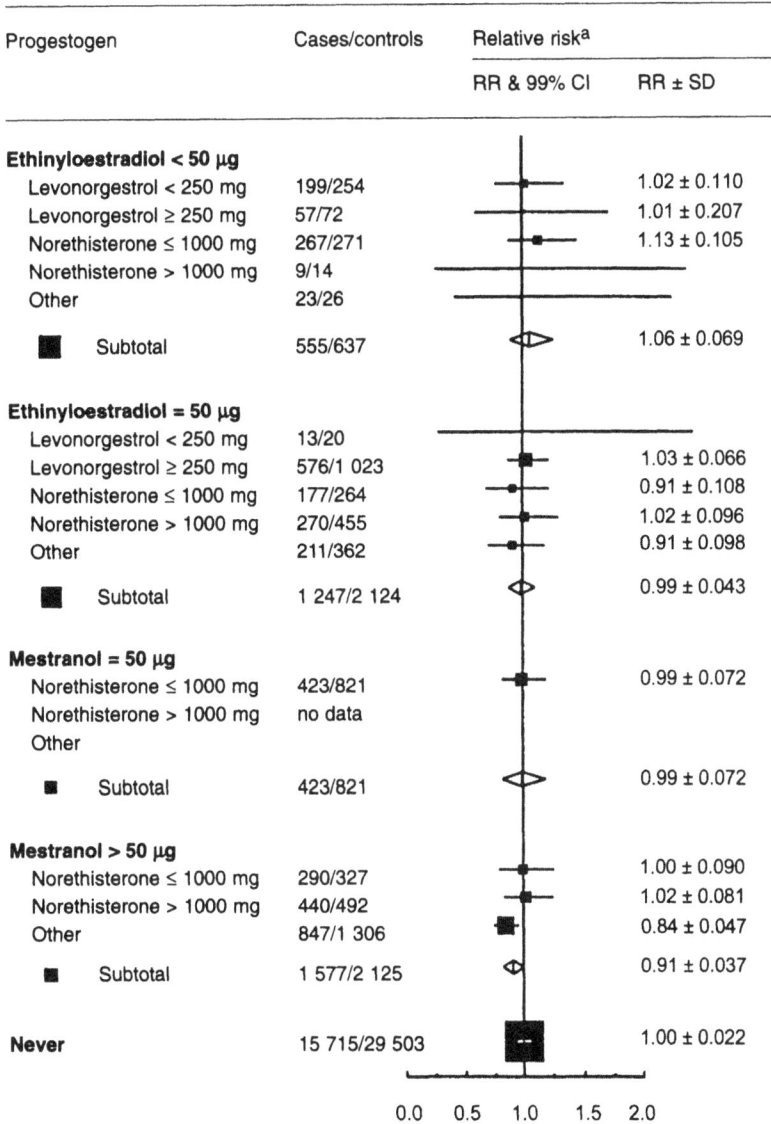

Progestogen	Cases/controls	Relative risk[a]	
		RR & 99% CI	RR ± SD

Ethinyloestradiol < 50 μg

Levonorgestrol < 250 mg	199/254		1.02 ± 0.110
Levonorgestrol ≥ 250 mg	57/72		1.01 ± 0.207
Norethisterone ≤ 1000 mg	267/271		1.13 ± 0.105
Norethisterone > 1000 mg	9/14		
Other	23/26		
■ Subtotal	555/637		1.06 ± 0.069

Ethinyloestradiol = 50 μg

Levonorgestrol < 250 mg	13/20		1.03 ± 0.066
Levonorgestrol ≥ 250 mg	576/1 023		0.91 ± 0.108
Norethisterone ≤ 1000 mg	177/264		1.02 ± 0.096
Norethisterone > 1000 mg	270/455		0.91 ± 0.098
Other	211/362		
■ Subtotal	1 247/2 124		0.99 ± 0.043

Mestranol = 50 μg

Norethisterone ≤ 1000 mg	423/821		0.99 ± 0.072
Norethisterone > 1000 mg	no data		
Other			
■ Subtotal	423/821		0.99 ± 0.072

Mestranol > 50 μg

Norethisterone ≤ 1000 mg	290/327		1.00 ± 0.090
Norethisterone > 1000 mg	440/492		1.02 ± 0.081
Other	847/1 306		0.84 ± 0.047
■ Subtotal	1 577/2 125		0.91 ± 0.037

| **Never** | 15 715/29 503 | | 1.00 ± 0.022 |

```
0.0   0.5   1.0   1.5   2.0
```

Test for heterogeneity by type and dose of progestogen within oral contraceptives containing:
Ethinyloestradiol < 50 μg : χ^2 (4 d.f.) = 1.2; NS
Ethinyloestradiol = 50 μg : χ^2 (4 d.f.) = 1.8; NS
Mestranol > 50 μg : χ^2 (2 d.f.) = 5.2; NS

Adapted from Collaborative Group on Hormonal Factors in Breast Cancer (1996a,b)
CI, confidence interval; SD, standard deviation; d.f., degrees of freedom; NS, not significant
[a] Relative to no use, stratified by study, age at diagnosis, parity, age at first birth and age at which risk for conceiving ceased

Figure 9. Relative risk (RR) for breast cancer by type and dose of oestrogen in the oral contraceptive last used, grouped according to type and dose of

(a) Last use < 5 years previously

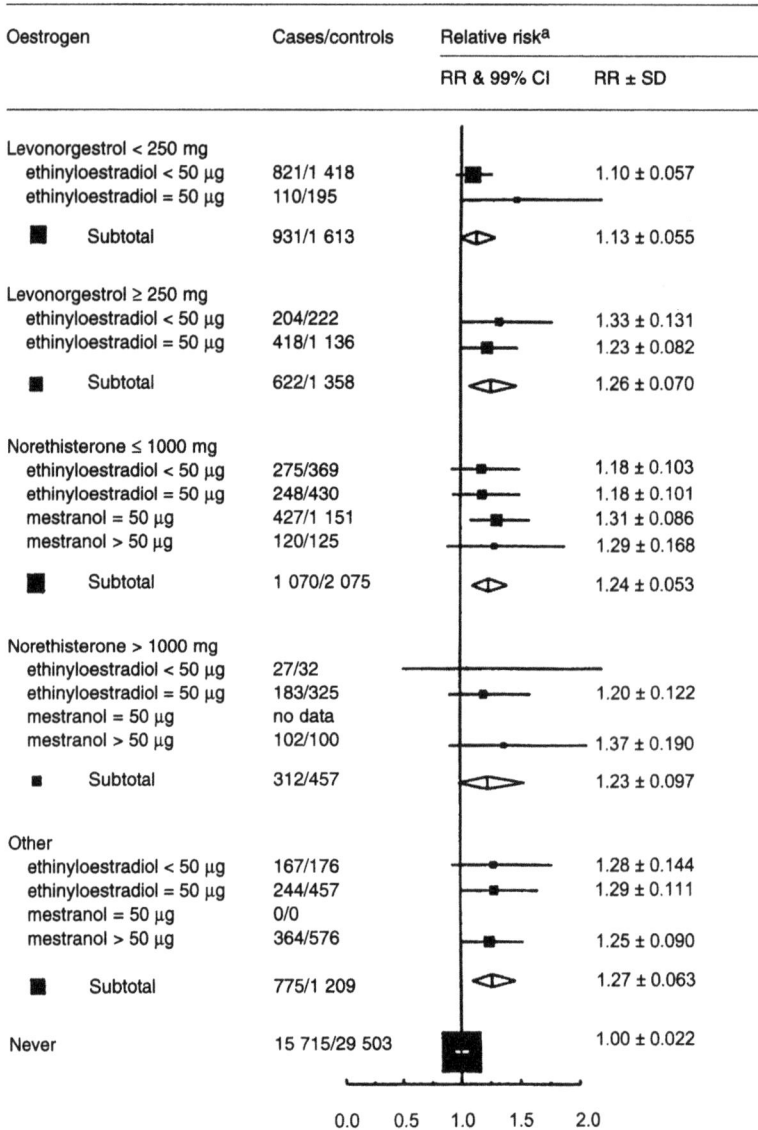

Oestrogen	Cases/controls	Relative risk[a]	
		RR & 99% CI	RR ± SD
Levonorgestrol < 250 mg			
ethinyloestradiol < 50 μg	821/1 418		1.10 ± 0.057
ethinyloestradiol = 50 μg	110/195		
Subtotal	931/1 613		1.13 ± 0.055
Levonorgestrol ≥ 250 mg			
ethinyloestradiol < 50 μg	204/222		1.33 ± 0.131
ethinyloestradiol = 50 μg	418/1 136		1.23 ± 0.082
Subtotal	622/1 358		1.26 ± 0.070
Norethisterone ≤ 1000 mg			
ethinyloestradiol < 50 μg	275/369		1.18 ± 0.103
ethinyloestradiol = 50 μg	248/430		1.18 ± 0.101
mestranol = 50 μg	427/1 151		1.31 ± 0.086
mestranol > 50 μg	120/125		1.29 ± 0.168
Subtotal	1 070/2 075		1.24 ± 0.053
Norethisterone > 1000 mg			
ethinyloestradiol < 50 μg	27/32		
ethinyloestradiol = 50 μg	183/325		1.20 ± 0.122
mestranol = 50 μg	no data		
mestranol > 50 μg	102/100		1.37 ± 0.190
Subtotal	312/457		1.23 ± 0.097
Other			
ethinyloestradiol < 50 μg	167/176		1.28 ± 0.144
ethinyloestradiol = 50 μg	244/457		1.29 ± 0.111
mestranol = 50 μg	0/0		
mestranol > 50 μg	364/576		1.25 ± 0.090
Subtotal	775/1 209		1.27 ± 0.063
Never	15 715/29 503		1.00 ± 0.022

0.0   0.5   1.0   1.5   2.0

Test for heterogeneity by type and dose of oestrogen within oral contraceptives containing:
Levonorgestrol < 250 mg   : χ^2 (1 d.f.) = 3.2; NS
Levonorgestrol > 250 mg   : χ^2 (1 d.f.) = 0.3; NS
Norethisterone < 1000 mg   : χ^2 (3 d.f.) = 1.2; NS
Norethisterone > 1000 mg   : χ^2 (2 d.f.) = 0.8; NS
Other   : χ^2 (2 d.f.) = 0.1; NS

Figure 9 (contd)

(b) Last use 5–9 years previously

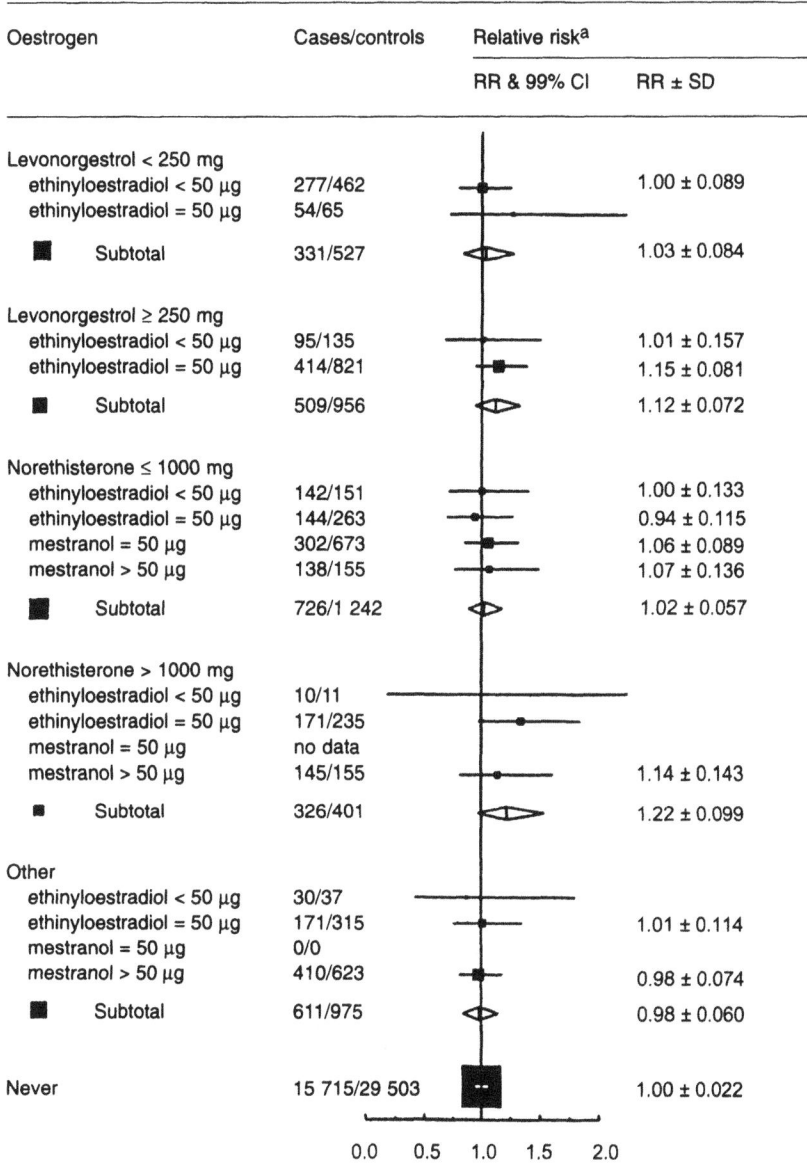

Oestrogen	Cases/controls	Relative risk[a]	
		RR & 99% CI	RR ± SD
Levonorgestrol < 250 mg			
ethinyloestradiol < 50 μg	277/462		1.00 ± 0.089
ethinyloestradiol = 50 μg	54/65		
Subtotal	331/527		1.03 ± 0.084
Levonorgestrol ≥ 250 mg			
ethinyloestradiol < 50 μg	95/135		1.01 ± 0.157
ethinyloestradiol = 50 μg	414/821		1.15 ± 0.081
Subtotal	509/956		1.12 ± 0.072
Norethisterone ≤ 1000 mg			
ethinyloestradiol < 50 μg	142/151		1.00 ± 0.133
ethinyloestradiol = 50 μg	144/263		0.94 ± 0.115
mestranol = 50 μg	302/673		1.06 ± 0.089
mestranol > 50 μg	138/155		1.07 ± 0.136
Subtotal	726/1 242		1.02 ± 0.057
Norethisterone > 1000 mg			
ethinyloestradiol < 50 μg	10/11		
ethinyloestradiol = 50 μg	171/235		
mestranol = 50 μg	no data		
mestranol > 50 μg	145/155		1.14 ± 0.143
Subtotal	326/401		1.22 ± 0.099
Other			
ethinyloestradiol < 50 μg	30/37		
ethinyloestradiol = 50 μg	171/315		1.01 ± 0.114
mestranol = 50 μg	0/0		
mestranol > 50 μg	410/623		0.98 ± 0.074
Subtotal	611/975		0.98 ± 0.060
Never	15 715/29 503		1.00 ± 0.022

0.0 0.5 1.0 1.5 2.0

Test for heterogeneity by type and dose of oestrogen within oral contraceptives containing:
Levonorgestrol < 250 mg   : χ^2 (1 d.f.) = 1.0; NS
Levonorgestrol > 250 mg   : χ^2 (1 d.f.) = 0.5; NS
Norethisterone < 1000 mg   : χ^2 (3 d.f.) = 0.8; NS
Norethisterone > 1000 mg   : χ^2 (2 d.f.) = 2.3; NS
Other   : χ^2 (2 d.f.) = 0.2; NS

Figure 9 (contd)

(c) Last use ≥ 10 years previously

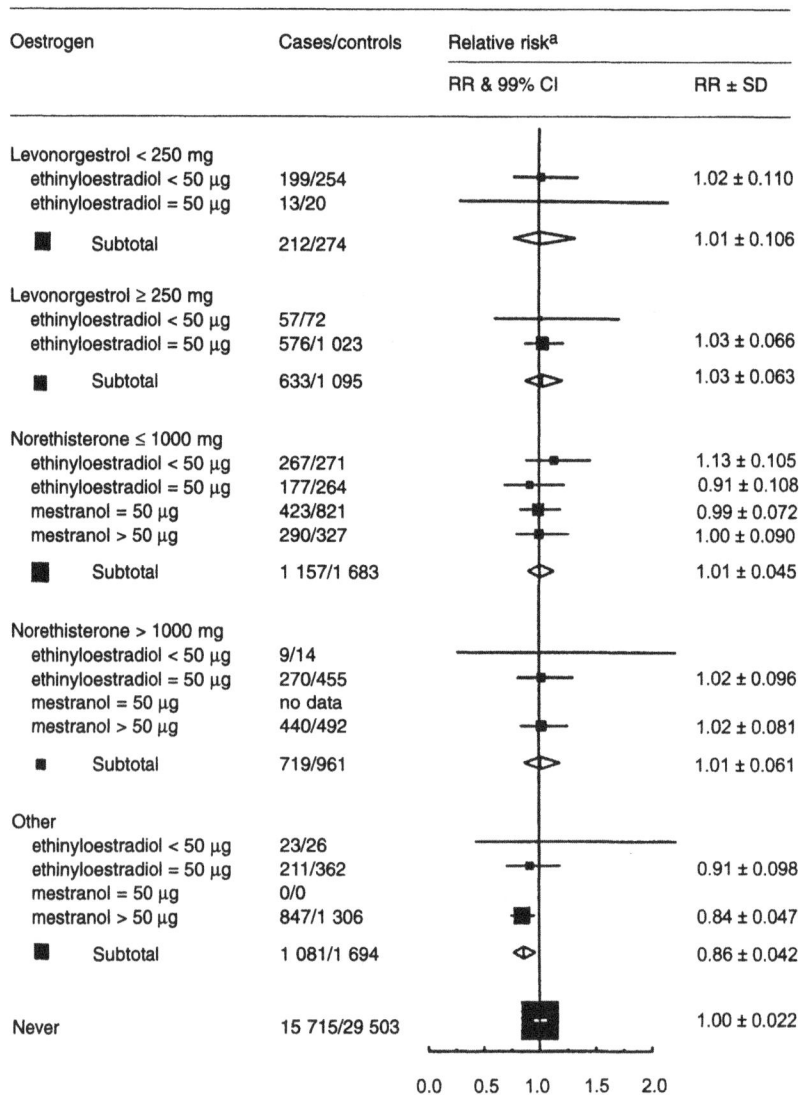

Oestrogen	Cases/controls	Relative risk[a]	
		RR & 99% CI	RR ± SD

Levonorgestrol < 250 mg			
ethinyloestradiol < 50 μg	199/254		1.02 ± 0.110
ethinyloestradiol = 50 μg	13/20		
■ Subtotal	212/274		1.01 ± 0.106
Levonorgestrol ≥ 250 mg			
ethinyloestradiol < 50 μg	57/72		
ethinyloestradiol = 50 μg	576/1 023		1.03 ± 0.066
■ Subtotal	633/1 095		1.03 ± 0.063
Norethisterone ≤ 1000 mg			
ethinyloestradiol < 50 μg	267/271		1.13 ± 0.105
ethinyloestradiol = 50 μg	177/264		0.91 ± 0.108
mestranol = 50 μg	423/821		0.99 ± 0.072
mestranol > 50 μg	290/327		1.00 ± 0.090
■ Subtotal	1 157/1 683		1.01 ± 0.045
Norethisterone > 1000 mg			
ethinyloestradiol < 50 μg	9/14		
ethinyloestradiol = 50 μg	270/455		1.02 ± 0.096
mestranol = 50 μg	no data		
mestranol > 50 μg	440/492		1.02 ± 0.081
■ Subtotal	719/961		1.01 ± 0.061
Other			
ethinyloestradiol < 50 μg	23/26		
ethinyloestradiol = 50 μg	211/362		0.91 ± 0.098
mestranol = 50 μg	0/0		
mestranol > 50 μg	847/1 306		0.84 ± 0.047
■ Subtotal	1 081/1 694		0.86 ± 0.042
Never	15 715/29 503		1.00 ± 0.022

```
           0.0   0.5   1.0   1.5   2.0
```

Test for heterogeneity by type and dose of oestrogen within oral contraceptives containing:
Levonorgestrol < 250 mg   : χ^2 (1 d.f.) = 0.2; NS
Levonorgestrol > 250 mg   : χ^2 (1 d.f.) = 0.0; NS
Norethisterone < 1000 mg   : χ^2 (3 d.f.) = 2.2; NS
Norethisterone > 1000 mg   : χ^2 (2 d.f.) = 0.4; NS
Other   : χ^2 (2 d.f.) = 0.6; NS

Adapted from Collaborative Group on Hormonal Factors in Breast Cancer (1996a,b)

CI, confidence interval; SD, standard deviation; d.f., degrees of freedom; NS, not significant

[a] Relative to no use, stratifed by study, age at diagnosis, parity, age at first birth and age at which risk for conceiving ceased

Figure 10. Relative risk (RR) for breast cancer by time since last use and type of combined oral contraceptive last used

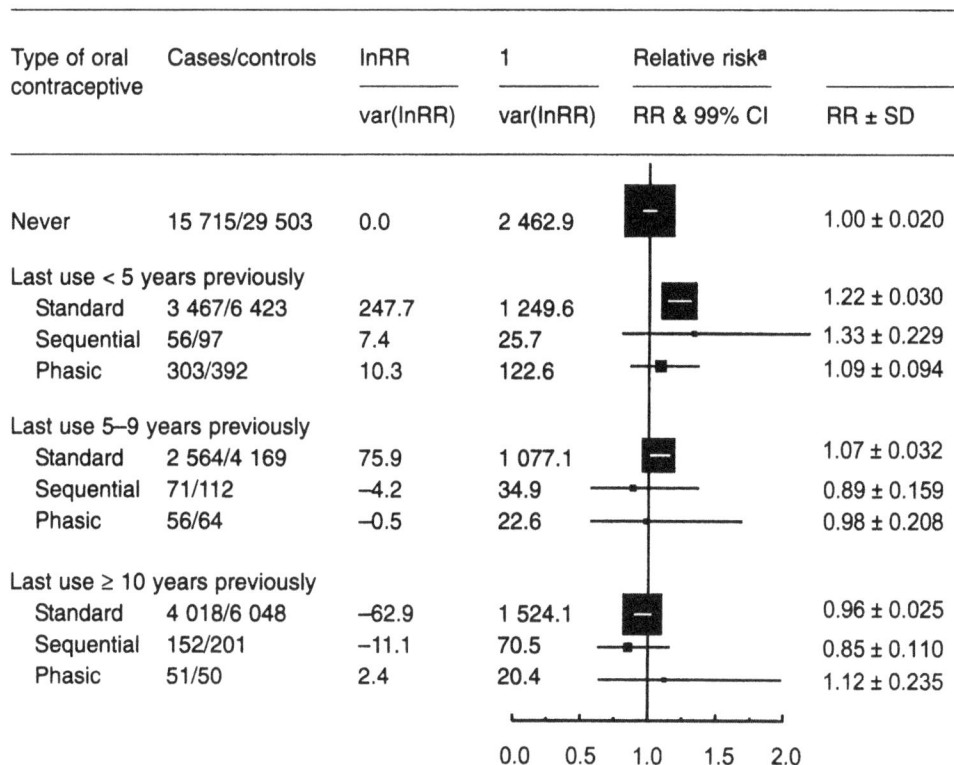

Type of oral contraceptive	Cases/controls	lnRR var(lnRR)	1 var(lnRR)	Relative risk[a] RR & 99% CI	RR ± SD
Never	15 715/29 503	0.0	2 462.9		1.00 ± 0.020
Last use < 5 years previously					
Standard	3 467/6 423	247.7	1 249.6		1.22 ± 0.030
Sequential	56/97	7.4	25.7		1.33 ± 0.229
Phasic	303/392	10.3	122.6		1.09 ± 0.094
Last use 5–9 years previously					
Standard	2 564/4 169	75.9	1 077.1		1.07 ± 0.032
Sequential	71/112	−4.2	34.9		0.89 ± 0.159
Phasic	56/64	−0.5	22.6		0.98 ± 0.208
Last use ≥ 10 years previously					
Standard	4 018/6 048	−62.9	1 524.1		0.96 ± 0.025
Sequential	152/201	−11.1	70.5		0.85 ± 0.110
Phasic	51/50	2.4	20.4		1.12 ± 0.235

0.0   0.5   1.0   1.5   2.0

Test for heterogeneity by type of oral contraceptives in women with:
Last use < 5 years previously : χ^2 (2 d.f.) = 1.7; NS
Last use 5–9 years previously: χ^2 (2 d.f.) = 1.4; NS
Last use ≥ 10 years previously: χ^2 (3 d.f.) = 1.5; NS

Adapted from Collaborative Group on Hormonal Factors in Breast Cancer (1996a,b)
CI, confidence interval; SD, standard deviation; d.f., degrees of freedom; NS, not significant
[a] Relative to no use, stratified by study, age at diagnosis, parity, age at first birth and age at which risk for conceiving ceased

A few studies indicate that the effect of use of combined oral contraceptives on the risk for breast cancer might be greater among women who have another risk factor than among those without the factor; however, there is no consistent evidence to suggest that the effect of combined oral contraceptives is modified by important risk factors such as benign breast disease, parity and menopausal status. There has been particular concern that a family history of breast cancer might modify an effect of the use of these contraceptives on the risk for breast cancer, but the results to date suggest that the risk is similar among users of these contraceptives with and without a family history of breast cancer (see Figure 11).

Information on the relation of use of oral contraceptives to breast cancer risk among women with mutations in the *BrCA1* or *BrCA2* gene is available from one small study in which 14 such women were compared with 36 women with breast cancer who did not have the mutations (Ursin *et al.*, 1997). A statistically significantly increased relative risk was observed among women who had used oral contraceptives for more than two years before their first full-term pregnancy.

Information on the relationship between use of combined oral contraceptives and the spread of the breast cancer at the time of diagnosis is much sparser than information on overall incidence. The collaborative reanalysis found that the relative risk was greater for localized tumours than for those that had spread beyond the breast (Collaborative Group on Hormonal Factors in Breast Cancer, 1996b). The estimated relative risk for disease localized to the breast was significantly increased for women who had used combined oral contraceptives in the previous five years (1.2), but declined to 1.1 five to nine years after they had stopped use and to 1.0, 10 or more years after stopping. For cancer that had spread beyond the breast, the relative risks were 1.1 for women who had used combined oral contraceptives in the previous five years, 0.96 five to nine years after stopping and 0.93 (significant) 10 or more years after stopping; all of these estimates were compatible with 1.0.

The most consistent findings to date are: a small increase in the risk for breast cancer among current and recent users of combined oral contraceptives; a decline in the risk relative to that of women who have never used them some 10 years after stopping; and little or no increase in risk with increasing duration of use after recency has been taken into account.

The possibility that biased recall might explain the observed increases was assessed in detail by the UK National Case–Control Study Group (1989) and Rookus *et al.* (1994). On the basis of reported use and records of use of combined oral contraceptives, they concluded that only a small part of the observed increase in risk could be explained by reporting bias. Data from follow-up studies are sparser than those from case–control studies. Greater assurance that reporting bias can be ruled out entirely, or that it plays only a small role, will be supplied if positive associations based on larger numbers are produced by the studies now in progress. The important known risk factors for breast cancer, such as age at first birth, parity and age at menopause, were controlled for and they seem unlikely to account for the observed increases. The increases have been observed across

Figure 11. Relative risk (RR) for breast cancer by time since last use of combined oral contraceptives and various characteristics of women

(a) Last use < 5 years previously

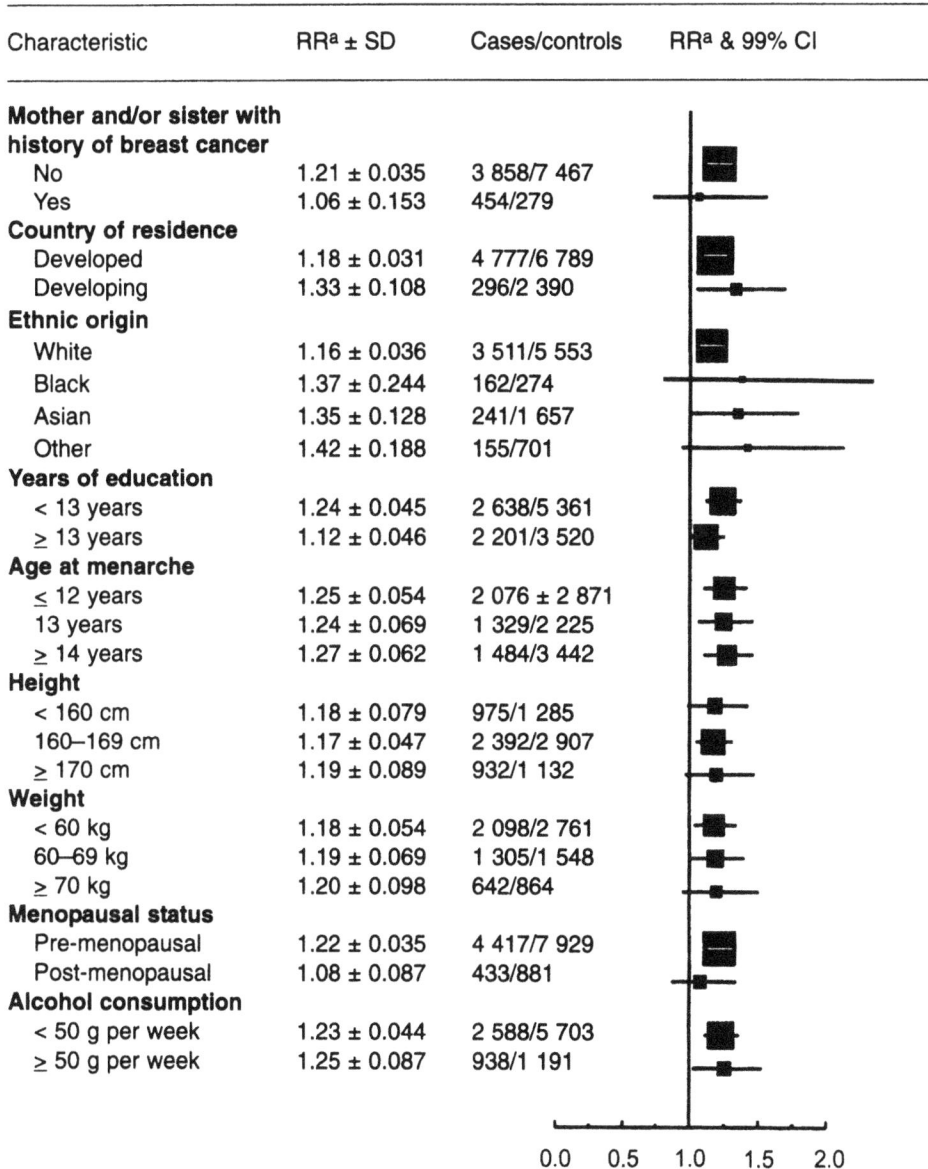

Characteristic	RR^a ± SD	Cases/controls	RR^a & 99% CI
Mother and/or sister with history of breast cancer			
No	1.21 ± 0.035	3 858/7 467	
Yes	1.06 ± 0.153	454/279	
Country of residence			
Developed	1.18 ± 0.031	4 777/6 789	
Developing	1.33 ± 0.108	296/2 390	
Ethnic origin			
White	1.16 ± 0.036	3 511/5 553	
Black	1.37 ± 0.244	162/274	
Asian	1.35 ± 0.128	241/1 657	
Other	1.42 ± 0.188	155/701	
Years of education			
< 13 years	1.24 ± 0.045	2 638/5 361	
≥ 13 years	1.12 ± 0.046	2 201/3 520	
Age at menarche			
≤ 12 years	1.25 ± 0.054	2 076 ± 2 871	
13 years	1.24 ± 0.069	1 329/2 225	
≥ 14 years	1.27 ± 0.062	1 484/3 442	
Height			
< 160 cm	1.18 ± 0.079	975/1 285	
160–169 cm	1.17 ± 0.047	2 392/2 907	
≥ 170 cm	1.19 ± 0.089	932/1 132	
Weight			
< 60 kg	1.18 ± 0.054	2 098/2 761	
60–69 kg	1.19 ± 0.069	1 305/1 548	
≥ 70 kg	1.20 ± 0.098	642/864	
Menopausal status			
Pre-menopausal	1.22 ± 0.035	4 417/7 929	
Post-menopausal	1.08 ± 0.087	433/881	
Alcohol consumption			
< 50 g per week	1.23 ± 0.044	2 588/5 703	
≥ 50 g per week	1.25 ± 0.087	938/1 191	

0.0   0.5   1.0   1.5   2.0

Global test for heterogeneity: χ^2 (14 d.f.) = 11.0; NS

Figure 11 (contd)

(b) Last use 5–9 years previously

Characteristic	RR[a] ± SD	Cases/controls	RR[a] & 99% CI
Mother and/or sister with history of breast cancer			
No	1.07 ± 0.031	3 270/6 377	
Yes	1.03 ± 0.128	468/367	
Country of residence			
Developed	1.06 ± 0.028	4 036/6 354	
Developing	1.31 ± 0.121	203/1 334	
Ethnic origin			
White	1.04 ± 0.033	2 974/5 023	
Black	1.26 ± 0.237	159/229	
Asian	1.19 ± 0.140	165/954	
Other	1.18 ± 0.168	135/503	
Years of education			
< 13 years	1.04 ± 0.041	2 014/4 106	
≥ 13 years	1.08 ± 0.042	2 090/3 421	
Age at menarche			
≤ 12 years	1.13 ± 0.048	1 825/2 651	
13 years	1.18 ± 0.065	1 136/1 894	
≥ 14 years	1.03 ± 0.054	1 179/2 780	
Height			
< 160 cm	1.17 ± 0.076	862/1 183	
160–169 cm	1.03 ± 0.042	1 991/2 822	
≥ 170 cm	1.13 ± 0.082	845/1 089	
Weight			
< 60 kg	1.07 ± 0.051	1 643/2 274	
60–69 kg	0.99 ± 0.059	1 088/1 575	
≥ 70 kg	1.12 ± 0.081	713/1 036	
Menopausal status			
Pre-menopausal	1.07 ± 0.035	2 987/5 175	
Post-menopausal	1.05 ± 0.057	903/1 836	
Alcohol consumption			
< 50 g per week	1.07 ± 0.039	2 121/4 354	
≥ 50 g per week	1.08 ± 0.074	870/1 118	

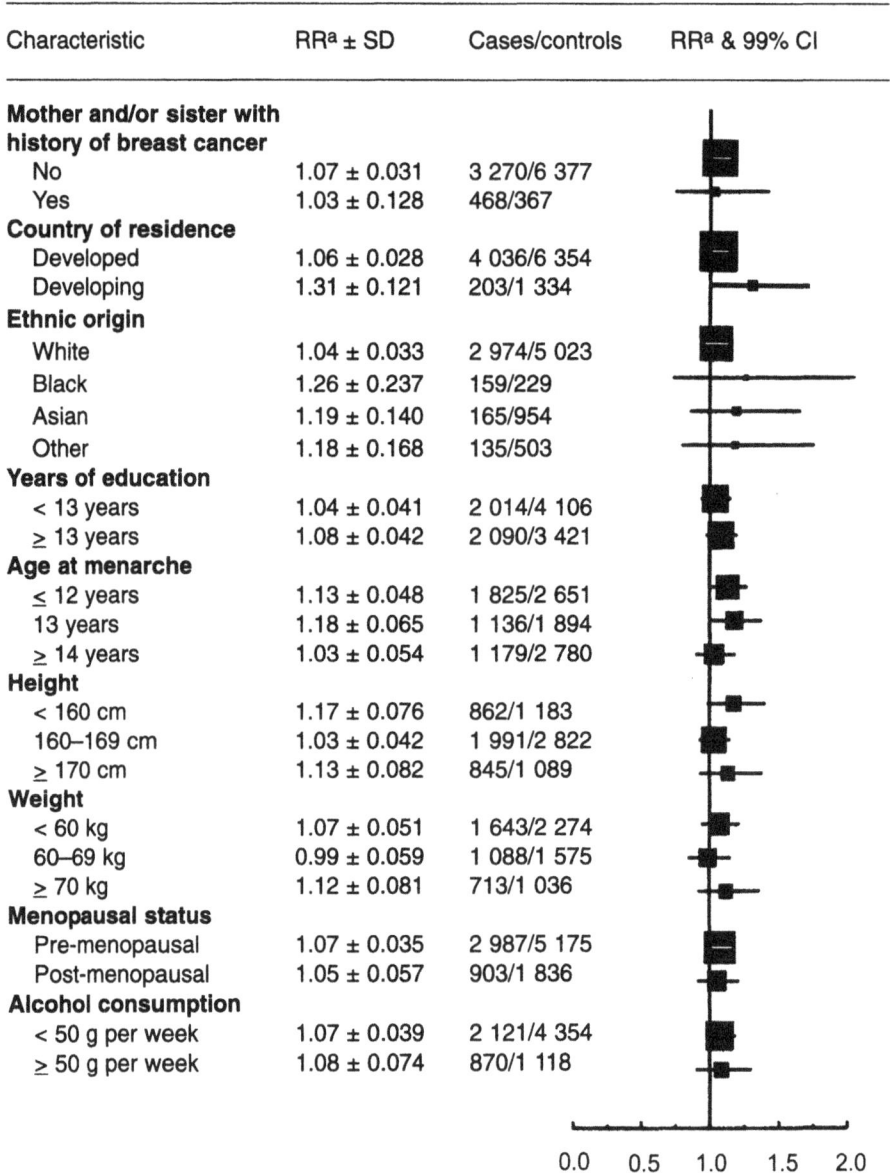

0.0　0.5　1.0　1.5　2.0

Global test for heterogeneity: χ^2 (14 d.f.) = 14.5; NS

Figure 11 (contd)

(c) Last use ≥ 10 years previously

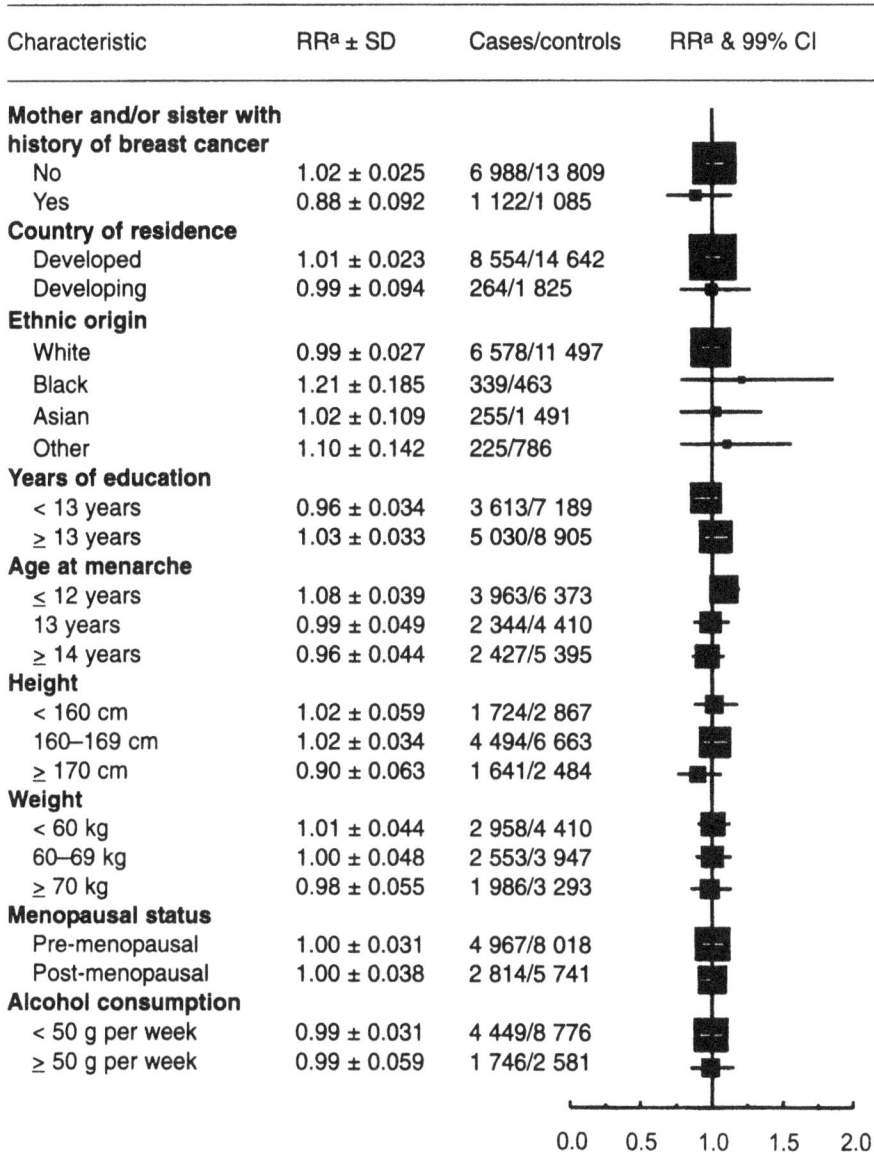

Characteristic	RR^a ± SD	Cases/controls	RR^a & 99% CI
Mother and/or sister with history of breast cancer			
No	1.02 ± 0.025	6 988/13 809	
Yes	0.88 ± 0.092	1 122/1 085	
Country of residence			
Developed	1.01 ± 0.023	8 554/14 642	
Developing	0.99 ± 0.094	264/1 825	
Ethnic origin			
White	0.99 ± 0.027	6 578/11 497	
Black	1.21 ± 0.185	339/463	
Asian	1.02 ± 0.109	255/1 491	
Other	1.10 ± 0.142	225/786	
Years of education			
< 13 years	0.96 ± 0.034	3 613/7 189	
≥ 13 years	1.03 ± 0.033	5 030/8 905	
Age at menarche			
≤ 12 years	1.08 ± 0.039	3 963/6 373	
13 years	0.99 ± 0.049	2 344/4 410	
≥ 14 years	0.96 ± 0.044	2 427/5 395	
Height			
< 160 cm	1.02 ± 0.059	1 724/2 867	
160–169 cm	1.02 ± 0.034	4 494/6 663	
≥ 170 cm	0.90 ± 0.063	1 641/2 484	
Weight			
< 60 kg	1.01 ± 0.044	2 958/4 410	
60–69 kg	1.00 ± 0.048	2 553/3 947	
≥ 70 kg	0.98 ± 0.055	1 986/3 293	
Menopausal status			
Pre-menopausal	1.00 ± 0.031	4 967/8 018	
Post-menopausal	1.00 ± 0.038	2 814/5 741	
Alcohol consumption			
< 50 g per week	0.99 ± 0.031	4 449/8 776	
≥ 50 g per week	0.99 ± 0.059	1 746/2 581	

0.0   0.5   1.0   1.5   2.0

Global test for heterogeneity: χ^2 (14 d.f.) = 13.5; NS

Adapted from Collaborative Group on Hormonal Factors in Breast Cancer (1996a,b)

SD, standard deviation; CI, confidence interval; d.f., degrees of freedom; NS, not significant

^{a} Relative risk relative to no use, stratified by study, age at diagnosis, parity and, where appropriate, age when first child was born and age when risk for conceiving ceased

case–control studies of various designs, both population- and hospital-based, suggesting that selection bias in the enrolment of cases or controls is not the explanation for the observed increases. The associations have also been observed across different populations. If biased recall, selection bias and confounding are unlikely explanations of the findings, the remaining explanations are that the associations are real (i.e. combined oral contraceptives act as a tumour promoter), that they are due to detection bias (i.e. breast cancer is diagnosed earlier in women who have used combined oral contraceptives) or both. There are few data on the mortality rates of users of these contraceptives, although two studies reported estimates close to 1.0 (Colditz *et al.*, 1994; Beral *et al.*, 1999).

2.2   Endometrial cancer

Combined and sequential oral contraceptives are discussed separately in relation to the risk for endometrial cancer, as use of these two preparations may have different impacts. Most of the information on the risk for endometrial cancer in relation to use of combined oral contraceptives concerns monophasic pills, i.e. with fixed doses of an oestrogen and a progestogen during a cycle. There is no information about the specific, long-term risk for endometrial cancer associated with use of the multiphasic oral contraceptives available since the early 1980s, in which varying doses of oestrogen and progestogen are given concurrently over one cycle.

2.2.1   *Combined oral contraceptives*

The cohort studies in which use of combined oral contraceptives and the risk for endometrial cancer have been investigated are summarized in Table 9 and the case–control studies in Table 10, with the risk associated with the duration and recency of use when available. Risk estimates by weight, parity (or gravidity) or use of post-menopausal oestrogen therapy are given in the text.

(a)   *Descriptive studies*

Several analyses have suggested that increased use of combined oral contraceptives can partially explain the decreasing rates of mortality from uterine corpus cancer (i.e. excluding those from cervical cancer) seen between 1960 and the 1980s (Beral *et al.*, 1988; Persson *et al.*, 1990; dos Santos Silva & Swerdlow, 1995). The decrease is particularly notable among women aged 55 or younger, who are most likely to have used combination oral contraceptives. Interpretation of these trends is complicated by improvements in cancer treatment over time and by lack of correction for the proportion of women who have had their uterus removed and are no longer at risk for developing (or dying from) endometrial cancer. Furthermore, the rate of death from uterine corpus cancer has generally been decreasing since the early 1950s, a decade before oral contraceptives were available. Thus, while it is plausible that increased use of combined oral contraceptives could have preceded and then paralleled the decrease in mortality from endometrial cancer, the magnitude of any decrease in the rate of death from uterine corpus cancer related to increased use of oral contraceptives remains unclear.

Table 9. Cohort studies of use of oral contraceptive pills[a] (not otherwise specified) and risk for endometrial cancer (by duration and recency of use when available)

Reference	Cohort enrolment		End of follow-up	Type/measure of therapy	No. of cases	No. of person-years	RR (95% CI)
	Year/age	Source population/ response/follow-up					
Trapido (1983)	1970/25–57 years	97 300 residents of Boston, USA, and 14 contiguous towns/70%	Dec. 1976	No use	75	296 501	Referent
				Any use	18	124 851	1.4 (NR)
				Duration (months)			
				1–11	6	33 997	1.7 (NR)
				12–23	4	21 978	1.9 (NR)
				24–35	3	21 437	1.6 (NR)
				36–59	2	28 705	0.6 (NR)
				≥ 60	3	18 734	1.5 (NR)
Beral *et al.* (1988, 1999)	May 1968– June 1969	46 000 British women identified by general practitioners/NA	April 1987 (incidence) Dec. 1993 (mortality)	No use	16	182 866	Referent
				Any use	2	257 028	0.2 (0.0–0.7)
				No use	6	335 998	Referent
				Any use	2	517 519	0.3 (0.1–1.4)
Vessey & Painter (1995)	1968–74/ 25–39 years	17 032 patients at 17 family planning clinics, UK/NA	Oct. 1993	No use	14	NR	Referent
				Any use	1	NR	0.1 (0.0–0.7)

RR, relative risk; CI, confidence interval; NR, not reported; NA, not applicable
[a] May be use of either combined or sequential oral contraceptive pills, but the majority of women used combined

Table 10. Case–control studies of use of oral contraceptive pills and risk for endometrial cancer (by duration and recency of use when available)

Reference	Location/period/age	Source of controls	Ascertainment of use	Participation (%) Cases	Participation (%) Controls	Type/measure of therapy	No. of subjects Cases	No. of subjects Controls	OR (95% CI)
Weiss & Sayvetz (1980)	Washington State, USA/ Jan. 1975–Dec. 1977/36–55 years	General population	Personal interviews	83	96	*Combined* No use, < 1 year's use ≥ 1 year's use	93 17	173 76	Referent 0.5 (0.1–1.0)
Kaufman et al. (1980)	USA and Canada/ July 1976–Dec. 1979/ < 60 years	Hospital patients	Personal interviews	96[a]	96[a]	*Combined* No use Any use *Duration (years)* < 1 1–2 ≥ 3 Unknown *Recency (years)* ≥ 5 With duration ≥ 1 year	136 16 5 6 5 0 12 8	411 99 14 32 53 6 60 52	Referent [0.4 (0.2–0.8)[b]] 0.8 (NR) 0.5 (NR) 0.3 (NR) 0.6 (0.3–1.2) 0.5 (0.2–1.0)
Kelsey et al. (1982)	Connecticut, USA/ July 1977–Mar. 1979/ 45–74 years	Hospital patients	Personal interviews	67	72	*Sequential/combined* No use For each + 5 years of use *Age 45–55 years* No use *Duration (years)* ≤ 2.5 > 2.5	NR NA 31 4 2	NR NA 256 42 44	Referent 0.6 (0.3–1.5) Referent 0.9 (NR) 0.5 (NR)
Hulka et al. (1982)	North Carolina, USA/ Jan. 1970–Dec. 1976/ < 60 years	General population	Personal interviews and medical record reviews	90[a]	90[a]	*Combined* No use, < 6 months' use ≥ 6 months' use *Recency (years)* < 1 ≥ 1 *Duration (years)* < 5 ≥ 5	74 5 0 5 3 2	172 31 13 14 14 17	Referent 0.4 (NR) 0 0.9 (NR) 0.6 (NR) 0.3 (NR)

Table 10 (contd)

Reference	Location/period/age	Source of controls	Ascertainment of use	Participation (%) Cases	Participation (%) Controls	Type/measure of therapy	No. of subjects Cases	No. of subjects Controls	OR (95% CI)
Henderson et al. (1983a)	Los Angeles county, USA/Jan. 1972–Dec. 1979/≤ 45 years	Residents in neighbourhood of cases	Telephone interviews	81	NR	*Combined* No use	67	50	Referent
						Duration (years)			
						<2	23	22	0.8 (NR)
						2–3	12	11	0.8 (NR)
						4–5	4	9	0.3 (NR)
						≥6	4	18	0.1 (NR)
Cancer and Steroid Hormone Study (1987)	Eight US areas/Dec 1980–Dec 1982/20–54 years	General population	Personal interviews	73	84	*Combined* No use	250	1 147	Referent
						Combined only	NR	NR	0.5 (0.4–0.6)
						Duration (months)			
						3–6	24	186	0.9 (0.5–1.5)
						–11	13	80	1.3 (0.6–2.6)
						12–23	20	266	0.7 (0.4–1.2)
						24–71	26	576	0.4 (0.3–0.7)
						72–119	12	317	0.4 (0.2–0.8)
						≥ 120	15	241	0.4 (0.2–0.8)
						Recency (years)			
						<5	12	471	0.3 (0.1–0.5)
						5–9	22	417	0.4 (0.2–0.6)
						10–14	30	368	0.5 (0.3–0.8)
						≥15	9	144	0.3 (0.2–0.6)
La Vecchia et al. (1986)	Greater Milan, Italy/Jan. 1979–Nov. 1985/<60 years	Hospital patients	Personal interviews	98c	98c	*Combined* Non-user	163	1 104	Referent
						Any use	7	178	0.5 (0.2–1.1)
Pettersson et al. (1986)	Uppsala, Sweden/Jan. 1980–Dec. 1981/<60 years	General population	Personal interviews	93	80	*Not specified* No use	96	91	Referent
						Any use	12	22	0.5 (0.2–1.1)
						Duration (years)			
						<1	5	6	0.8 (0.2–2.7)
						≥1	7	16	0.4 (0.2–1.0)
						Any contraceptive Any use	9	22	0.4 (0.2–0.9)
						Duration (years)			
						<1	5	6	0.8 (0.2–2.7)
						≥1	4	16	0.2 (0.1–0.7)

Table 10 (contd)

Reference	Location/period/age	Source of controls	Ascertainment of use	Participation (%)		Type/measure of therapy	No. of subjects		OR (95% CI)
				Cases	Controls		Cases	Controls	
WHO Collaborative Study (1988); Rosenblatt *et al.* (1991)	Seven countries/Jan. 1979–Feb. 1988/ <60 years	Hospital patients	Personal interviews	87	93	*Combined*			
						No use	118	687	Referent
						Combined only	14	149	0.5 (0.3–1.0)
						Any contraceptive			
						No use	118	655	Referent
						Any use	12	180	0.5 (0.2–1.1)
						Combined			
						Any contraceptive			
						No use	182	1 072	Referent
						High			
						Progestogen content			
						Duration (months)			
						1–24	1	85	0.1 (0.0–0.7)
						≥25	2	69	0.2 (0.0–0.8)
						Recency (months)			
						1–120	1	61	0.1 (0.0–0.8)
						≥121	2	93	0.2 (0.0–0.7)
						Low			
						Duration (months)			
						1–24	8	69	1.0 (0.5–2.4)
						≥25	1	56	0.1 (0.0–1.1)
						Recency (months)			
						1–120	2	72	0.3 (0.0–1.1)
						≥121	7	54	1.1 (0.5–2.8)
Koumantaki *et al.* (1989)	Athens, Greece/1984/ 40–79 years	Hospital patients	Personal interviews	80	95	*Not specified*			
						No use, ≤6 months' use	80	151	Referent
						>6 months' use	3	13	0.6 (0.2–2.0)[d]
Levi *et al.* (1991)	Canton of Vaud, Switzerland/ Jan 1988–July 1990/ 32–75 years	Hospital patients	Personal interviews	85[a]	85[a]	*Combined*			
						No use	105	227	Referent
						Any use	17	82	0.5 (0.3–0.8)
						Duration (years)			
						<2	9	19	1.0 (0.5–2.3)
						2–5	3	18	0.5 (0.1–1.2)
						5	5	45	0.3 (0.1–0.7)
						Recency (years)			
						<10	4	30	0.3 (0.1–0.9)
						10–19	7	37	0.4 (0.2–1.0)
						>19	5	15	0.8 (0.3–2.2)

Table 10 (contd)

Reference	Location/period/age	Source of controls	Ascertainment of use	Participation (%) Cases	Participation (%) Controls	Type/measure of therapy	No. of subjects Cases	No. of subjects Controls	OR (95% CI)
Shu et al. (1991)	Shanghai, China/April 1988–Jan. 1990/ 18–74 years	General population	Personal interviews	91	96	*Not specified*			
						No use (any birth control)	84	72	Referent
						Any use	32	46	0.8 (0.4–1.8)
						Duration (years)			
						≤ 2	NR	NR	1.4 (0.6–3.0)
						> 2	NR	NR	0.4 (0.1–1.2)
Stanford et al. (1993)	Five US areas/June 1987–May 1990/ 20–74 years	General population	Personal interviews	87	66	*Combined*			
						No use	321	187	Referent
						Any use	81	107	0.4 (0.3–0.7)
						Duration (years)			
						< 1	27	21	0.7 (0.3–1.4)
						1–2	16	33	0.3 (0.1–0.6)
						3–4	12	16	0.3 (0.1–0.8)
						5–9	14	15	0.7 (0.3–1.6)
						≥ 10	7	19	0.2 (0.1–0.5)
						Recency (years)			
						< 10	6	18	0.1 (0.0–0.3)
						10–14	15	27	0.3 (0.1–0.7)
						15–19	24	32	0.4 (0.2–0.8)
						≥ 20	33	27	0.7 (0.4–1.3)
						By duration (years)			
						< 3			
						Recency (years)			
						< 15	7	15	0.2 (0.1–0.6)
						15–19	10	16	0.3 (0.1–0.8)
						≥ 20	26	23	0.6 (0.3–1.3)
						≥ 3			
						Recency (years)			
						< 15	14	30	0.2 (0.1–0.5)
						15–19	12	16	0.4 (0.2–1.0)
						≥ 20	7	4	0.8 (0.2–3.3)
Jick et al. (1993)	Washington State, USA, Group Health Cooperative/1979–1989/50–64 years	Members of health maintenance organization	Mailed form and pharmacy database	83	79	*Not specified*			
						No use	110	737	Referent
						Any use	26	270	0.5 (0.3–0.9)
						Duration (years)			
						1	7	65	0.4 (0.1–1.4)
						2–5	11	90	0.8 (0.3–1.7)
						≥ 6	8	115	0.3 (0.1–0.9)

Table 10 (contd)

Reference	Location/period/age	Source of controls	Ascertainment of use	Participation (%) Cases	Participation (%) Controls	Type/measure of therapy	No. of subjects Cases	No. of subjects Controls	OR (95% CI)
Jick et al. (1993) (contd)						*Recency (years)*			
						1–10	5	67	0.4 (0.1–1.1)
						11–15	6	82	0.4 (0.1–1.2)
						16–20	4	57	0.5 (0.1–1.8)
						≥ 21	9	54	0.6 (0.2–2.1)
Voigt et al. (1994)[c]	Washington State, USA/1975–77 and 1985–87/40–59 years	General population	Personal interviews	83	95 and 73[f]	*Combined*			
						No use, < 1 year's use	117	284	Referent
						Recency (years)			
						> 10			
						Duration (years)			
						1–5	14	30	0.9 (0.4–1.9)
						> 5	4	16	0.4 (0.1–1.2)
						≤ 10			
						Duration (years)			
						1–5	7	28	1.0 (0.4–2.4)
						> 5	7	74	0.3 (0.1–0.6)
						Progestogen content[g]			
						Low			
						Duration (years)			
						1–5	10	22	1.1 (0.5–2.6)
						> 5	3	32	0.2 (0.1–0.8)
						High			
						Duration (years)			
						1–5	3	14	0.8 (0.2–3.1)
						> 5	3	28	0.3 (0.1–0.9)
Kalandidi et al. (1996)	Athens, Greece/1992–94/< 59–≥ 70 years	Hospital patients	Personal interviews	83	88	*Not specified*			
						No use	143	293	Referent
						Any use	2	5	1.3 (0.2–7.7)

OR, odds ratio; CI, confidence interval; NR, not reported; NA, not applicable

[a] Responses reported for case and control women combined
[b] Crude odds ratio and 95% confidence interval calculated from data provided in the published paper by exact methods
[c] Methods state that less than 2% of eligible case and control women refused an interview.
[d] 90% confidence interval
[e] Includes women from the study of Weiss & Sayvetz (1980)
[f] Response for controls identified 1985–1987
[g] Classified according to subnuclear endometrial vacuolization

(b)   *Cohort studies*

A questionnaire to derive information on oral contraceptive use was sent to approximately 97 300 married women aged 25–57 in eastern Massachusetts, United States, in 1970, who were identified from the 1969 Massachusetts residence lists (Trapido, 1983). The age-adjusted rate ratio for women who had ever used oral contraceptives relative to non-users was 1.4; there was no consistent pattern of a decreasing or increasing rate ratio with longer or more recent use (Table 9). Among nulliparous women, the age-adjusted rate ratio for oral contraceptive users relative to non-users was 2.4 (95% CI, 0.6–9.2), whereas the analogous rate ratio for parous women was 1.4 (95% CI, 0.8–2.4). Among women who also reported any use of post-menopausal oestrogen therapy, the age-adjusted rate ratio for oral contraceptive users relative to non-users was 2.0 (95% CI, 0.9–4.3). No distinction was made between sequential and combined oral contraceptive use, and both preparations were available to the cohort before and during the study follow-up.

Beral *et al.* (1999) followed-up approximately 23 000 oral contraceptive users and a similar number of non-users identified in 1968 and 1969 by the Royal College of General Practitioners. Use of oral contraceptives (not otherwise specified) and the occurrence of uterine cancer were both determined from physicians' reports. Uterine corpus cancer (i.e. excluding the cervix) was diagnosed in two of the oral contraceptive users and 16 of the non-users, resulting in a rate ratio of 0.2 (95% CI, 0.0–0.7) after adjustment for age, parity, smoking, social class, number of previously normal Papanicolaou ('Pap') smears and history of sexually transmitted disease. In a 25-year follow-up of deaths in the cohort, there were eight deaths from endometrial cancer, two of women who had ever used oral contraceptives and six of women who had never used them (rate ratio, 0.3; 95% CI, 0.1–1.9).

The study of the Oxford Family Planning Association included 17 032 married white women identified at 17 family planning clinics in England and Scotland (Vessey & Painter, 1995) who had used oral contraceptives (not otherwise specified), a diaphragm or an intrauterine device for at least five months. Information on contraceptive history and any hospital referrals was obtained from physicians or from the women themselves (for those who stopped attending the clinics) during the study follow-up. A total of 15 292 women remained under observation until the age of 45; only those who had never used oral contraceptives (5881) or had used them for eight years or more (3520) were followed from then on. Endometrial cancer was diagnosed in 15 women, only one of whom had used oral contraceptives (age-adjusted rate ratio, 0.1; 95% CI, 0.0–0.7). In a previous analysis of mortality in this cohort (Vessey *et al.*, 1989b), none of the oral contraceptive users but two of those using a diaphragm or an intrauterine device (the comparison group) had died from uterine corpus cancer.

(c)   *Case–control studies*

Weiss and Sayvetz (1980) compared 117 women identified from a population-based cancer registry with 395 control women in the general population of western Washington State, United States. Women who had used combined oral contraceptives for one year or more had half the risk for endometrial cancer of women who were either non-users or had used oral contraceptives for less than one year, after adjustment for age and use of post-menopausal oestrogen therapy (odds ratio, 0.5; 95% CI, 0.1–1.0). No further difference in the duration of use was seen between case and control women. In stratified analyses, the reduced risk was present only for women who had never used post-menopausal oestrogen therapy (odds ratio, 0.4; 95% CI, 0.1–1.1) or who had used it for two years or less (odds ratio, 0.1; 95% CI, 0.01–1.1); no reduction was noted among women who had used it for three years or more (odds ratio, 1.3; 95% CI, 0.3–6.6).

Among 154 women with endometrial cancer and 525 control women in a hospital-based study in the United States and Canada (Kaufman *et al.*, 1980), a 60% reduction in risk was seen among women who used combined oral contraceptives relative to non-users, after adjustment for use of non-contraceptive hormones, parity, body mass, menopausal status, age at menopause, ethnic group, diabetes, education, age and area of residence. The risk for endometrial cancer declined with increasing duration of use, and a sustained reduction in risk was suggested for women who had stopped using oral contraceptives in the previous five or more years. A reduction in risk was noted for women who had used combined oral contraceptives but had never used non-contraceptive oestrogens (odds ratio, 0.4; 95% CI, 0.2–0.8), but not for the women who had ever used both oral contraceptives and non-contraceptive oestrogens (odds ratio, 0.6; 95% CI, 0.3–1.6), although the lack of information on the duration of non-contraceptive oestrogen use makes it difficult to interpret this estimate.

Kelsey *et al.* (1982) studied women admitted to seven hospitals in Connecticut, United States. The 167 newly diagnosed cases of endometrial cancer were compared with 903 control women admitted for non-gynaecological surgical services. Among the study participants aged 45–55 years—the women who had had the opportunity to use oral contraceptives—those who had used oral contraceptives for 2.5 years or more had a 50% decrease in risk.

Among 79 women treated at a hospital in North Carolina, United States, for endometrial cancer, 6.3% had used combined oral contraceptives for six months or more, whereas 15.3% of the 203 control women from 52 counties in the State (the main referral area for the hospital) had done so (Hulka *et al.*, 1982). Since only 15% of the control women reported use of combined oral contraceptives, the risk estimates for more detailed aspects of oral contraceptive use are fairly imprecise (Table 10). There is a suggestion that the risk was lower with longer use (≥ 5 years), with previous use and with use of 'progestogen-predominant' (based on the relative proportions of oestrogens and progestogens in their chemical composition) oral contraceptives. When oral contraceptive use was stratified by use of post-menopausal oestrogens, both users of at least six months' duration (0 cases, 6 controls) and non-users (odds ratio, 0.6 [95% CI not provided]) of post-menopausal oestrogens appeared to have a reduced risk associated with use of oral contraceptives.

Henderson *et al.* (1983a) identified 127 women with endometrial cancer from the population-based cancer registry for Los Angeles County and matched them to control women of similar age who lived in the same neighbourhood as the matched case. The risk for endometrial cancer decreased with increasing duration of use of combined oral contraceptives, and this pattern remained after further adjustment for parity, current weight, infertility and amenorrhoea. Neither the recency of use of oral contraceptives nor the relative oestrogen and progestogen content of the oral contraceptives had a clear impact on the risk, beyond that explained by the duration of use (data not shown). When the analysis was stratified by body weight, a reduction in risk with longer duration of use was seen among women whose current weight was less than 170 lbs [77 kg] but not among women whose current weight was greater.

In a population-based study conducted by the Centers for Disease Control and the National Institute of Child Health and Human Development in the United States, women with newly diagnosed endometrial cancer, who were 20–54 years of age, were identified from eight cancer registries (Atlanta, Detroit, San Francisco, Seattle, Connecticut, Iowa, New Mexico, and four urban counties in Utah) in the United States Surveillance, Epidemiology and End Results (SEER) Program; 3191 controls were selected from the general population (Centers for Disease Control and the National Institute of Child Health and Human Development, Cancer and Steroid Hormone Study, 1987). Women who had used only combination oral contraceptives had half the risk for endometrial cancer of non-users (age-adjusted odds ratio, 0.5; 95% CI, 0.4–0.6). The risk generally decreased with increasing duration of oral contraceptive use, the greatest reduction in risk being seen among women who had used combined oral contraceptives for two years or more. The strength of the association was similar after adjustment for age alone and after multivariate adjustment for age, parity, education, body mass, menopausal status, geographic region, exogenous oestrogen use and infertility. The risk for endometrial cancer did not vary with recency of use of oral contraceptives or time since first use; both women who had ceased use of oral contraceptives 15 years or more before the study interview and women who had first used oral contraceptives more than 20 years before interview had a lower risk than non-users (age-adjusted odds ratios, 0.3 (95% CI, 0.2–0.6) and 0.4 (95% CI, 0.2–0.7), respectively). When the analysis was stratified by the formulation of the oral contraceptive, all formulations that had been used for at least six months or more were associated with a decreased risk for endometrial cancer. Nulliparous women who had used combined oral contraceptives for one year or more had a larger reduction in risk than non-users (age-adjusted odds ratio, 0.2; 95% CI, 0.1–0.5), but women of high parity had little difference in risk, the age-adjusted odds ratio for women who had had five or more births being 0.8 (95% CI, 0.4–1.9). No difference in risk was reported with body mass, smoking, alcohol consumption, use of exogenous oestrogens or menopausal status (data not shown) or for the different histological subtypes of endometrial cancer (adenocarcinoma, adenoacanthoma and adenosquamous carcinoma).

In a hospital-based study in the area of greater Milan, Italy, La Vecchia *et al.* (1986) compared the use of combined oral contraceptives by women admitted for endometrial cancer and women admitted for traumatic, orthopaedic, surgical and other conditions.

Seven (4%) of the 170 case women and 178 (14%) of the 1282 control women reported use of combined oral contraceptives, resulting in an odds ratio of 0.6 (95% CI, 0.2–1.3) after adjustment for age, marital status, education, parity, age at menarche, age at first birth, age at menopause, body mass index, cigarette smoking and use of non-contraceptive female hormones.

Pettersson *et al.* (1986) studied 254 women residing in the health care region of Uppsala (Sweden) who were referred to the Department of Gynaecologic Oncology with a newly diagnosed endometrial malignancy; each case was matched by age and county of residence to one control woman identified from a population registry. Use of combined oral contraceptives was analysed for women aged 60 or less, resulting in 108 cases and 113 controls. Women who had ever used these contraceptives for one year or more had a lower risk than non-users (odds ratios, 0.5 (95% CI, 0.2–1.1) and 0.4 (95% CI, 0.2–1.0), respectively). Among the women who had used combined oral contraceptives only for contraception, the reductions were slightly greater: odds ratios for any use versus none, 0.4 (95% CI, 0.2–0.9), and for one year versus none, 0.2 (95% CI, 0.1–0.7). It is unclear from the published paper if the estimates were adjusted for potentially confounding factors.

A hospital-based study was conducted in Australia, Chile, China, Colombia, Israel, Kenya, Mexico, the Philippines and Thailand to compare the use of combined oral contraceptives by 140 women with endometrial cancer and 910 women admitted to units other than obstetrics and gynaecology in each centre between 1979 and 1986 (WHO Collaborative Study of Neoplasia and Steroid Contraceptives, 1988). Women who had used only combined oral contraceptives had a lower risk for endometrial cancer than non-users (odds ratio, 0.5; 95% CI, 0.3–1.0), after adjustment for hospital, age, calendar year of interview and race. A reduction in risk was suggested at each level of the factors examined, including gravidity (odds ratios, 0.7 (95% CI, 0.3–1.5) for < 5 pregnancies and 0.3 (95% CI, 0.1–1.5) for ≥ 5 pregnancies), history of infertility (odds ratios, 0.6 (95% CI, 0.3–1.2) for none and 0.4 (95% CI, 0.0–7.3) for a positive history) and use of oestrogens for any other reason except menopausal symptoms (data not shown). The numbers of cases (total, 220) and control women (total, 1537) in this study continued to accrue through 1988 and were then further evaluated by Rosenblatt *et al.* (1991). Among the women who used combined oral contraceptives for contraception only, those who used formulations with a relatively 'high' dose of progestogen (on the basis of the ability of the preparation to induce subnuclear vacuolization in human endometrium) had a lower risk than non-users, regardless of the relative oestrogen dose (odds ratios, 0.2 (95% CI, 0.0–0.5) for high dose and 0 (95% CI, 0.0–1.1) for low dose). In contrast, women who used formulations with a relatively low dose of progestogen had little, if any, reduction in risk, regardless of the relative oestrogen dose (odds ratios, 1.1 (95% CI, 0.1–9.1) for high dose and 0.6 (95% CI, 0.3–1.3) for low dose). Additionally, the reduction in risk did not vary appreciably by the duration or recency of use for the women who used formulations with a relatively high dose of progestogen, whereas the women who used formulations with a relatively low dose of progestogen had a reduction in risk with longer duration of use (odds ratio, 0.1 (95% CI, 0.0–1.1) for ≥ 2 years' use versus none) or with more recent use (odds ratio, 0.3 (95% CI, 0.1–1.1) for use within the last 10 years versus none). Similar results were seen for first use of oral contraceptives within the previous 14 years. All of these estimates were adjusted for age, gravidity, age at menarche, centre and year of diagnosis.

Koumantaki *et al.* (1989) studied women with endometrial cancer admitted to two hospitals in Athens, Greece, and control women admitted to the Athens Hospital for Orthopaedic Disorders. Only three (4%) of the 83 case women and 13 (8%) of the 164 controls had used oral contraceptives for six or more months (odds ratio, 0.6; 90% CI, 0.2–2.0, adjusted for age, parity, age at menarche, age at menopause, menopausal oestrogen use, years of smoking, height and weight).

Among 122 women treated at a major referral hospital in the Canton of Vaud (Switzerland) for endometrial cancer, 14% had used combined oral contraceptives, as had 27% of the 309 control women admitted to the same hospital for non-neoplastic, non-gynaecological conditions (Levi *et al.*, 1991). The risk decreased from 1.0 (95% CI, 0.5–2.3) for use for less than two years to 0.5 (95% CI, 0.1–1.2) for use for two to five years to 0.3 (95% CI, 0.1–0.7) for use for more than five years. Oral contraceptive use within the previous 10 years (odds ratio, 0.3; 95% CI, 0.1–0.9) or within the previous 10–20 years (odds ratio, 0.4; 95% CI, 0.2–1.0) and first use before the age of 30 (odds ratio, 0.3; 95% CI, 0.1–0.7) were all associated with a reduction in the risk for endometrial cancer. Women who had used oral contraceptives for five years or more had a reduction in risk even if use had occurred 20 or more years previously. The risk estimates were adjusted for age, area of residence, marital status, education, parity, body mass, cigarette smoking and use of post-menopausal oestrogen therapy. Little variation in risk was seen by categories of body mass (odds ratios, 0.6 (95% CI, 0.3–1.0) for < 25 kg/m^2 and 0.2 [95% CI not provided] for ≥ 25 kg/m^2) or cigarette smoking (odds ratios, 0.5 (95% CI, 0.2–1.2) for ever smoked and 0.6 (95% CI, 0.3–1.3) for never smoked). Stratification by use of post-menopausal oestrogen therapy was also presented (odds ratios, 0.4 (95% CI, 0.1–1.2) for ever use and 0.5 (95% CI, 0.3–1.0) for never use), but duration of post-menopausal oestrogen therapy was not analysed. While no reduction in risk was noted for nulliparous women (6 cases and 14 controls) who used oral contraceptives (age-adjusted odds ratio, 0.8; 95% CI, 0.2–2.9), the parous oral contraceptive users (11 cases and 68 controls) did have a reduced cancer risk (age-adjusted odds ratio, 0.3; 95% CI, 0.1–0.7).

Shu *et al.* (1991) studied 268 women with endometrial cancer identified from the population-based Shanghai (China) Cancer Registry and 268 age-matched control women identified from the Shanghai Residents Registry. The risk for endometrial cancer varied little between users of oral contraceptives (not otherwise specified) and women who had never used any type of contraception, after adjustment for age, gravidity and weight (odds ratio, 0.8; 95% CI, 0.4–1.8). When the duration of use was evaluated, there was a suggestion that oral contraceptive use for more than two years was associated with a reduction in risk (odds ratio, 0.4; 95% CI, 0.1–1.2).

In the United States, 405 women with endometrial cancer diagnosed at seven hospitals (in Chicago, Illinois; Hershey, Pennsylvania; Irvine and Long Beach, California;

Minneapolis, Minnesota; and Winston-Salem, North Carolina) and 297 age-, race- and residence-matched control women from the general population agreed to be interviewed (Stanford *et al.*, 1993). Use of combined oral contraceptives was reported by 20% of the case women and 36% of the control women (odds ratio, 0.4; 95% CI, 0.3–0.7, after adjustment for age, education, parity, weight and use of post-menopausal oestrogen therapy). There was no clear pattern of a decreasing risk with increasing duration of use (Table 10). Relative to non-users, a strong reduction in risk was noted for women who had used these preparations within the last 10 years (odds ratio, 0.1; 95% CI, 0.0–0.3) and for those who had used them first less than 15 years previously (odds ratio, 0.1; 95% CI, 0.0–0.4); both of these effects waned with more distant oral contraceptive use. The risk estimates varied little by age at first use (< 25, 25–29, 30–34, ≥ 35). When duration and recency were evaluated jointly, use within the previous 20 years was more strongly predictive of a risk reduction than longer duration of use (≥ 3 years). In a joint evaluation with other possible modifying factors, three or more years of combination oral contraceptive use were associated with a reduced risk for endometrial cancer among women of high parity (odds ratio for women with five or more births, 0.2; 95% CI, 0.0–0.6), women who weighed less than 150 lbs [68 kg] (odds ratio, 0.4; 95% CI, 0.2–0.9) and women who had never (odds ratio, 0.2; 95% CI, 0.1–0.6) or briefly (< 3 years) (odds ratio, 0.8; 95% CI, 0.2–3.2) used post-menopausal oestrogen therapy. No reduction and perhaps even an increase in risk was noted for use of combined oral contraceptives of three years or more by women who were nulliparous (odds ratio, 1.9; 95% CI, 0.3–11), weighed more than 200 lbs [91 kg] (odds ratio, 2.7; 95% CI, 0.8–8.5) or had used post-menopausal oestrogen therapy for three years or more (odds ratio, 4.1; 95% CI, 0.4–38). The estimates did not vary appreciably by history of smoking, infertility or menopausal status.

Jick *et al.* (1993) studied women who were members of a large health maintenance organization in western Washington State, United States. Women in whom endometrial cancer had been diagnosed (*n* = 142) were identified from the organization's tumour registry; the 1042 control women were also members of the organization. Both groups included only women who used the pharmacies of the organization and who had previously completed a questionnaire sent to all female members for a mammography study. Use of oral contraceptives (not otherwise specified), determined from the questionnaire, was reported by 18% of case women and 26% of controls, for an odds ratio of 0.5 (95% CI, 0.3–0.9), adjusted for age, enrolment date in the organization, body mass, age at menopause, parity and current use of post-menopausal oestrogen therapy. In comparison with non-users, the reduced risk for endometrial cancer was most pronounced for women who had used oral contraceptives for six or more years (odds ratio, 0.3; 95% CI, 0.1–0.9) or within the last 10 years (odds ratio, 0.4; 95% CI, 0.1–1.1).

Voigt *et al.* (1994) combined the study population described in the study of Weiss and Sayvetz (1980) with a similar study population identified between 1985 and 1987 in western Washington State, United States. The study included 316 cases and 501 controls. When oral contraceptive use was stratified by use of unopposed oestrogen, women who had used combined oral contraceptives for one year or more and who had also used unopposed oestrogens for three years or more had no reduction in risk relative to women who had not used oral contraceptives or women who had used them for less than one year (odds ratio, 1.1; 95% CI, 0.4–2.6), whereas a reduction was noted for women who had never used unopposed oestrogens or had used them for less than three years and had used combined oral contraceptives for more than one year (odds ratio, 0.5; 95% CI, 0.3–0.9). Thus, further analyses were restricted to women who had used unopposed oestrogens never or for less than three years. When duration and recency of use of combined oral contraceptives were evaluated jointly, longer use (> 5 years) was associated with a reduced risk for endometrial cancer irrespective of recency (last use, ≤ 10 years ago versus > 10 years ago). When duration and the relative potency of the progestogens in the formulation were evaluated jointly, a longer duration of use (> 5 years), and not progestogen dosage, was most predictive of a reduced risk.

Kalandidi *et al.* (1996) studied 145 women with endometrial cancer admitted to two hospitals in Athens, Greece, and 298 control women admitted to the major accident hospital in Athens with bone fractures or other orthopaedic disorders. Only two (1%) of the case women and five (1.7%) of the controls had ever used oral contraceptives (not otherwise specified). Although a multivariate-adjusted risk estimate was presented (odds ratio, 1.3; 95% CI, 0.2–7.9), no useful inferences can be drawn from this small study.

(d)   *Summary*

In general, women who have taken combined oral contraceptives have about one-half the risk for endometrial cancer of non-users (Kaufman *et al.*, 1980; Weiss & Sayvetz, 1980; Hulka *et al.*, 1982; Kelsey *et al.*, 1982; La Vecchia *et al.*, 1986; Pettersson *et al.*, 1986; Centers for Disease Control and the National Institute of Child Health and Human Development, Cancer and Steroid Hormone Study, 1987; WHO Collaborative Study of Neoplasia and Steroid Contraceptives, 1988; Koumantaki *et al.*, 1989; Levi *et al.*, 1991; Jick *et al.*, 1993; Stanford et al., 1993; Vessey & Painter, 1995; Beral *et al.*, 1999). The reduction first appears after two to five years of use (Kaufman *et al.*, 1980; Hulka *et al.*, 1982; Henderson *et al.*, 1983a; Pettersson *et al.*, 1986; Centers for Disease Control and the National Institute of Child Health and Human Development, Cancer and Steroid Hormone Study, 1987; Levi *et al.*, 1991; Shu *et al.*, 1991; Jick *et al.*, 1993; Stanford *et al.*, 1993; Voigt *et al.*, 1994) and continues to decrease as the duration of oral contraceptive use increases (Kaufman *et al.*, 1980; Henderson *et al.*, 1983a; Centers for Disease Control and the National Institute of Child Health and Human Development, Cancer and Steroid Hormone Study, 1987; Levi *et al.*, 1991; Stanford *et al.*, 1993). Some studies have shown a greater reduction in risk with more recent use (Levi *et al.*, 1991; Jick *et al.*, 1993; Stanford *et al.*, 1993), but others have found no difference (Kaufman *et al.*, 1980; Henderson *et al.*, 1983a; Centers for Disease Control and the National Institute of Child Health and Human Development, Cancer and Steroid Hormone Study, 1987; WHO Collaborative Study of Neoplasia and Steroid Contraceptives, 1988). When duration and recency of use were evaluated jointly, longer use (≥ 5 years) was associated with a reduced risk, irrespective of recency (Voigt *et al.*, 1994), whereas another study showed that recency (use within the last 15 years) and not duration of use was most predictive of a reduced risk (Stanford *et al.*, 1993). Some studies found that the reduction in risk may be greatest with use of oral contraceptives in which progestogen effects predominate (Hulka *et al.*, 1982) or that contain higher doses of progestogen (Rosenblatt *et al.*, 1991), but another study found that a longer duration of use (≥ 5 years), and not progestogen dose, was most predictive of a reduced risk (Voigt *et al.*, 1994).

While no reduction in risk was found for women in the highest categories of body weight in two studies (Henderson *et al.*, 1983a; Stanford *et al.*, 1993), two others found a reduced risk regardless of weight or body mass (Centers for Disease Control and the National Institute of Child Health and Human Development, Cancer and Steroid Hormone Study, 1987; Levi *et al.*, 1991). Although one study noted a reduced risk only among oral contraceptive users who were nulliparous (Centers for Disease Control and the National Institute of Child Health and Human Development, Cancer and Steroid Hormone Study, 1987), three others found that the reductions were strongest among parous women (Levi *et al.*, 1991) or women of higher parity (≥ 5 births) (WHO Collaborative Study of Neoplasia and Steroid Contraceptives, 1988; Stanford *et al.*, 1993). In comparison with women who did not use oral contraceptives, oral contraceptive users who had also used post-menopausal oestrogen therapy for three or more years showed no reduction in risk in two studies (Stanford *et al.*, 1993; Voigt *et al.*, 1994). While four other studies did find a reduced risk among oral contraceptive users who had ever used post-menopausal oestrogen therapy (Kaufman *et al.*, 1980; Hulka *et al.*, 1982; Centers for Disease Control and the National Institute of Child Health and Human Development, Cancer and Steroid Hormone Study, 1987; Levi *et al.*, 1991), the inclusion of women who had used this therapy for fewer than two or three years could have obscured any altered relationship with longer duration of use.

2.2.2   *Sequential oral contraceptives*

(a)   *Case reports*

In the mid-1970s, case reports appeared in the United States of endometrial abnormalities—ranging from proliferative lesions to severe atypical hyperplasia (Lyon & Frisch, 1976; Kaufman *et al.*, 1976; Cohen & Deppe, 1977) to endometrial cancer (Lyon, 1975; Silverberg & Makowski, 1975; Silverberg *et al.*, 1977)—among women who had used a sequential oral contraceptive preparation, Oracon®, containing 0.1 mg ethinyl-oestradiol and 25 mg dimethisterone (Weiss & Sayvetz, 1980). In response to these reports, sequential preparations were removed from the consumer market in the United States and Canada in 1976, but the impact of exposure to these preparations continued to be evaluated in epidemiological studies.

(b)   *Case–control studies*

The epidemiological studies of sequential oral contraceptive use and endometrial cancer are summarized in Table 11. Weiss and Sayvetz (1980) reported a seven-fold elevation in risk with use of Oracon®, but not with other types of sequential preparations, after adjustment for age, use of combined oral contraceptives and post-menopausal

Table 11. Case–control studies of use of sequential oral contraceptive pills and risk for endometrial cancer

Reference	Location/period/ages	Source of controls	Ascertainment of use	Participation (%)		Type/measure of therapy	No. of subjects		Odds ratio (95% CI)
				Cases	Controls		Cases	Controls	
Weiss & Sayvetz (1980)	Washington State, USA/Jan. 1975–Dec. 1977/36–55 years	General population	Personal interviews	83	96	No use Oracon® Other	110 6 1	376 8 11	Referent 7.3 (1.4–39) 0.3 (0.0–2.9)
Kaufman et al. (1980)	USA and Canada/July 1976–Dec. 1979/ < 60 years	Hospital patients	Personal interviews	96[a]	96[a]	No use Any use Oracon®	152 2 1	516 9 3	Referent [0.8 (0.2–2.8)][b] [1.1 (0.2–6.0)][b]
Henderson et al. (1983a)	Los Angeles county, USA/Jan. 1972–Dec. 1979/< 45 years	General population	Telephone interviews	81	NR	No use Duration (years) < 2 ≥ 2	116 2 9	121 5 1	Referent 0.4 (NR) 4.6 (NR)
Cancer and Steroid Hormone Study (1987)	Eight US areas/ Dec. 1980–Dec. 1982/ 20–54 years	General population	Personal interviews	73	84	No use Only sequential	250 7	1147 64	Referent 0.6 (0.3–1.3)
WHO Collaborative Study (1988)	Seven countries/Jan. 1979–Feb. 1986/ < 60 years	Hospital patients	Personal interviews	87	93	No use Only sequential	118 1	687 5	Referent 0.9 (0.1–8.3)

CI, confidence interval; NR, not reported
[a] Responses reported for case and control women combined
[b] Crude odds ratio and 95% CI calculated from data provided in published paper using exact methods

oestrogen therapy, among 117 women with endometrial cancer identified from a population-based cancer registry and 395 women from the general population in western Washington State, United States.

Henderson *et al.* (1983a) evaluated oral contraceptive use among 127 white case–control pairs matched for age (in five-year age groups) and area of residence; the case women were identified from the population-based University of Southern California Cancer Surveillance Program and controls from the case's neighbourhood of residence. An almost fivefold increase in risk was found with the use of any type of sequential oral contraceptive for two years or more on the basis of use by nine case women and one control. [The particular brand of sequential oral contraceptive, or the combination of brands, used is not clear from the published paper.]

A study in the United States (Atlanta, Georgia; Detroit, Michigan; San Francisco, California; Seattle, Washington; Connecticut, Iowa, New Mexico and four urban areas of Utah; Centers for Disease Control and the National Institute of Child Health and Human Development, Cancer and Steroid Hormone Study, 1987) found that only seven of 433 case women and 64 of 3191 controls had exclusively used sequential oral contraceptives, resulting in an age-adjusted odds ratio of 0.6 (95% CI, 0.3–1.3). Among the larger group of women with any use of sequential oral contraceptives (26 cases and 152 controls), the risk for endometrial cancer for women who had used them in the previous three to 12 years, for three years or more or who had used Oracon® was 1.5 times that of other sequential oral contraceptive users. No estimates of the risk for these women relative to that of non-users was provided in the published paper.

Two other studies found neither an excess nor a decreased risk among small numbers of women who had used sequential oral contraceptives. In a hospital-based study in several metropolitan areas in the United States and Canada, Kaufman *et al.* (1980) reported that only two (1.3%) of the 154 case women and nine (1.7%) of the 525 control women had reported use of any type of sequential oral contraceptive during personal interviews; one of the case women and three control women reported using Oracon®.

In the international hospital-based study described on p. 120, only one of the 140 case women and five of the 910 control women had exclusively used sequential oral contraceptives (crude odds ratio, 0.9; 95% CI, 0.1–8.3); the specific preparations were not reported (WHO Collaborative Study of Neoplasia and Steroid Contraceptives, 1988).

In summary, the case reports that preceded the epidemiological studies were important in indicating that the risk for endometrial cancer was potentially elevated among users of sequential oral contraceptives and specifically among users of a particular brand, which contained a relatively potent oestrogen, ethinyloestradiol, and a weak progestogen, dimethisterone. In contrast, it was not clear from the case–control studies whether the increase in risk was restricted to users of this brand or included users of other sequential preparations. This was largely due to the low prevalence of sequential oral contraceptive use in these study populations: only 6% or less of the control women in all of the studies. When the analyses were further stratified by specific preparations, the numbers of women in each category were too small for useful inferences to be drawn from most of these studies.

2.3 Cervical cancer

2.3.1 *Methodological considerations*

(a) *Stage of disease and classification*

Cervical cancer is a particularly difficult disease to study with respect to use of oral contraceptives. It is generally accepted that invasive cervical cancer results from a series of changes in the cervical epithelium, from normal epithelial structure to various grades of pre-invasive changes and then on to invasive cervical carcinoma. As oral contraceptives could act at any stage in this process to enhance progression to the next stage, studies should include separate assessment of the effects of steroid contraceptives on risk at different stages of the neoplastic process. Early studies of oral contraceptives and cervical neoplasia included a mixture of lesion types, and these are not considered in this review. In the studies of specific types of preneoplastic lesions, there is considerable variation in the definition of the cases included. In addition, the systems used to classify precancerous cervical lesions histologically and cytologically have changed over time. Early studies included cervical dysplasia (sometimes sub-classified into mild, moderate and severe) and carcinoma *in situ*. In more recent studies, cases have been classified as cervical intraepithelial neoplasia (CIN), with a grading system of I–III to designate the severity of the lesion. Lesions have also been referred to histologically as squamous intra-epithelial neoplasia and similarly graded on a scale of I–III to indicate severity. In general, the higher grades correspond roughly to carcinoma *in situ* and severe dysplasia, and the lower grades correspond roughly to mild and moderate dysplasia. In reviewing the literature on non-invasive cervical neoplasia, the terms used by the authors have been retained.

The two generally recognized histological types of invasive cervical carcinoma are squamous-cell carcinoma and adenocarcinoma. In many studies of invasive cervical cancer, these histological types have not been distinguished. In this review, such studies are usually classified with those of squamous-cell carcinoma, because squamous-cell carcinoma was the more common type at the time and in the places where the studies that did not distinguish them were conducted.

(b) *Confounding and effect-modifying variables*

Another difficulty in assessing the effect of oral contraceptives on the risk for cervical cancer is that the disease is caused by several types of human papillomavirus (HPV) (IARC, 1995). These viruses are sexually transmitted, and women with cervical neoplasia tend to be those whose sexual behaviour is conducive to the acquisition of sexually transmitted diseases, or who are married to men who have engaged in extramarital sexual relationships conducive to the acquisition of sexually transmitted agents. In some cultures, women who use oral contraceptives tend also to be women whose sexual behaviour is conducive to the acquisition of sexually transmitted agents. Under such circumstances, a spurious association between use of oral contraceptives and cervical neoplasia could be observed, if sexual practices are not controlled for either in the study design or in the statistical analysis. Unless otherwise stated, studies in which the sexual behaviour of the subjects has not been taken into consideration have been excluded from this review.

In recent studies, attempts have been made to control for HPV infection when assessing possible associations between use of oral contraceptives and cervical neoplasia. To date, however, all attempts to do so have been limited by technical deficiencies. It is generally accepted that cervical neoplasia results from persistent infection with an oncogenic type of HPV. If a woman clears her infection, then she is unlikely to develop a cervical neoplasm. If oral contraceptives were to enhance the risk for cervical cancer by increasing the likelihood that an HPV infection will become persistent, women should be classified according to whether they have persistent infection with an oncogenic HPV. In a case–control study, this would require an adequate serological test for markers of HPV persistence; to date, no such test has been developed. Another approach would be to conduct a prospective follow-up study of a large group of women who have recently acquired an oncogenic HPV type for the development of cervical neoplasia. This approach has several limitations: one is that women could be monitored only until they developed mild or moderate intraepithelial lesions, since it would be unethical not to treat such lesions and allow them to progress to more severe disease; the second problem is that such studies require large numbers of women and a long duration of follow-up. Studies of mild intraepithelial lesions are under way, but the results in relation to use of hormonal contraceptives to date are limited; furthermore, the results of studies of mild lesions may not indicate a relationship between use of oral contraceptives and more severe disease.

Another possibility is that oral contraceptives enhance the risk for cervical cancer in women with persistent HPV infection. In order to address this issue in case–control studies, analyses have been restricted to cases and controls with evidence of HPV DNA in cervical scrapings. In such studies that have been conducted to date, few controls have been found to have HPV, and the relative risk estimates are therefore imprecise.

(c)   *Studies of oral contraceptives and human papillomavirus infection*

Because oncogenic forms of HPV are involved in the etiology of cervical carcinoma, a number of investigations have been conducted to determine whether infection with HPV is associated with the use of oral contraceptives. It has been clearly shown that the sensitivity and specificity of methods for detecting HPV differ significantly. Methods involving the polymerase chain reaction (PCR) of DNA have been found to be the most sensitive and specific when compared with other methods such as filter *in situ*, dot–blot and Southern blot hybridization (IARC, 1995); and epidemiological studies of cervical carcinoma in which methods other than PCR have been used to detect HPV should be interpreted with the understanding of potential misclassification of HPV status. Studies on younger women have given inconsistent results for an association between the prevalence of HPV infection and oral contraceptive use. The following section is limited to studies in which PCR-based techniques were used.

Hildesheim *et al.* (1993) investigated the risk factors for HPV infection in 404 cytologically normal low-income women in Washington DC, United States, of a median age of 26 years. The prevalence of HPV infection was found to be higher among current users of oral contraceptives (42.9%) than among women who had never used them (33.3%). Former users (prevalence, 40%) were also at increased risk of having a current HPV infection (difference in prevalence, 2.6%; 95% CI, -10.2–15.5), although these findings were not significant.

Ley *et al.* (1991) found an increased risk for HPV infection with oral contraceptive use in their study of 467 university women of a mean age of 23 years. A higher prevalence of HPV infection was associated with both past (crude odds ratio, 3.0; 95% CI, 1.8–5.0) and current use (crude odds ratio, 3.3; 95% CI, 2.1–5.3).

Bauer *et al.* (1993) examined factors associated with HPV prevalence among 483 cytologically normal women of a median age of 34 years. The prevalence in non-users, former users and current users of oral contraceptives was 5.3, 12.8 and 34.0%, respectively, but this difference, after adjusting for confounding factors, could have occurred by chance.

Burk *et al.* (1996) studied 439 sexually active women in Brooklyn, New York, United States, of an average age of 31 years. Women who had ever used oral contraceptives but were not current users had a higher prevalence of HPV infection (21.9%) than those who had never used them (17.1%); current users had a 14.8% rate of HPV PCR-DNA positivity.

Wheeler *et al.* (1993) found that oral contraceptive use was not associated with HPV infection among 357 cytologically normal university women in New Mexico, United States, of a median age of 23 years. The prevalences of HPV infection in former users (43.9%) and current users (41.8%) were not significantly different from that in women who had never used them (50%) after control for other confounding factors.

Muñoz *et al.* (1996) investigated the association between HPV DNA positivity and risk factors among 810 middle-aged women who were controls in case–control studies of cervical cancer conducted in Spain, Colombia and Brazil. The mean age of these women differed by site: 41.7 years in Spain, 42.8 years in Colombia and 52.7 years in Brazil. Use of oral contraceptives was not significantly associated with HPV DNA positivity. When compared with non-users, women who had used contraceptives for three years or less (odds ratio, 0.7; 95% CI, 0.4–1.4) and more than three years (odds ratio, 0.6; 95% CI, 0.3–1.2) were not at increased risk for HPV infection.

Ho *et al.* (1998), investigating the risk factors for the acquisition of HPV infection in university women, found that oral contraceptive use was not significantly associated.

In a follow-up study of 393 women with normal cervical cytology, Hildesheim *et al.* (1994) found no evidence that persistence of HPV infection was associated with use of oral contraceptives.

The inconsistent results of these studies could be due to differences in the sexual behaviour of oral contraceptive users and non-users in the studies. In the aggregate, they do not provide direct evidence that oral contraceptives interact with HPV to cause cervical cancer. Some are, nevertheless, consistent with a role for oral contraceptives in the genesis of cervical cancer, either by enhancing the likelihood of infection or persistence of infection by oncogenic types or by some direct, synergistic mechanism of HPV and oral contraceptives.

(*d*)   *Influence of screening*

A third problem in assessing the effect of hormonal contraceptives on the risk for cervical cancer is the influence of the results of Pap smears. If the cases detected at screening are those more likely to be studied, and if women are more likely to have Pap smears if they have used oral contraceptives, then the women who are studied may be more likely to have used oral contraceptives than other cases in the population. This could lead to spuriously elevated relative risks in relation to oral contraceptive use in case–control studies, particularly for studies of intraepithelial lesions, which are largely asymptomatic and frequently detected at screening. Because of this potential bias, studies of intraepithelial lesions in which both the cases and the controls came from the same screening programme (the preferred design) are distinguished in this review from those in which they were not.

Screening with Pap smears may also influence the results of studies of invasive disease. If having a Pap smear protects against invasive disease, fewer cases will have used oral contraceptives than in the general population, which could result in a spuriously low relative risk. The influence of prior Pap smears must therefore be considered in assessing the risk for both intraepithelial and invasive cervical neoplasms in relation to oral contraceptive use.

2.3.2   *Descriptive studies*

Doll (1985) noted that mortality rates from cervical cancer in Britain increased in women born after 1935, corresponding to some change that took place in about 1960. This is approximately when oral contraceptives came into use, but it is also when women began to change their sexual behaviour, so that the trend could be the result of increased rates of HPV infection.

Peters *et al.* (1986a) reported an increase in the proportion of all newly diagnosed cervical adenocarcinomas in non-Hispanic white women under the age of 35 in Los Angeles County, United States, between 1972 and 1982. There was no increase in the risk for adenocarcinoma in older women, and there was a decreased prevalence incidence ratio for invasive squamous-cell cervical carcinoma in women of all ages during the same time period. The authors hypothesized that the trends were due to the introduction of oral contraceptives, which might preferentially increase the risk for adenocarcinomas over that for squamous-cell carcinomas. Schwartz and Weiss (1986) analysed data from the United States SEER Program and also noted an increase in the risk for adenocarcinomas between 1973 and 1982 in women under the age of 35. No comparable increase in the risk for adenocarcinomas was observed in older women, and no increase in the risk for adeno-squamous carcinomas or squamous-cell carcinomas was observed for the same period. In fact, the rates of squamous-cell carcinomas had decreased in all age groups during those same years. The results of this study are thus consistent with those of Peters *et al.* (1986a) and are not inconsistent with the hypothesis that use of oral contraceptives is associated with an increase in the risk for adenocarcinomas. Chilvers *et al.* (1987) reported, however, an increased risk for both adenocarcinoma and squamous-cell carcinoma in women under the age of 35 in three regions of England between 1968 and 1982, which would argue against a particularly strong increase in risk for adenocarcinomas associated with use of oral contraceptives.

Trends in the incidence rates of adenocarcinoma and adenosquamous carcinoma during the period 1973–91 were examined by Vizcaino *et al.* (1998) in 60 population-based registries in 25 countries. Consistent with the results of Doll (1985), they found a significant increase in the incidence of this condition in many countries between 1973 and 1991. The authors suggested that the increase was due in part to increased transmission of HPV; they also suggested that it was due in part to improvements in screening. With the introduction of the cyto-brush, more cervical adenocarcinomas *in situ* are being detected in some populations, which could result in a decline in the rates of invasive cervical adenocarcinoma. The patterns of the temporal changes across countries do not appear to be explained by variations in the patterns of use of oral contraceptives among these populations; and the observation that the rates of squamous and adenocarcinoma of the cervix are highly correlated among the populations studied suggests that oral contraceptives do not preferentially enhance the risk for adeno-carcinomas over that for squamous-cell carcinomas.

2.3.3   *Cohort studies*

    (a)   *Studies of cervical dysplasia and carcinoma* in situ *in the absence of assays for human papillomavirus DNA*

Peritz *et al.* (1977) reported the results of a cohort study of 17 942 women, 18–58 years of age, who received health examinations at the Kaiser Permanente Medical Center in Walnut Creek, California, United States, between 1968 and 1972. They did not provide serial Pap smears but, between 1973 and 1975, all women in the health plan who developed dysplasia or carcinoma *in situ* of the cervix were identified from medical records. After controlling for age, education, marital status, number of Pap smears before entry into the cohort, smoking and selected infections, the relative risk for either cervical dysplasia or carcinoma *in situ* was found to increase with the duration of oral contraceptive use. Carcinoma *in situ* and cervical dysplasia were combined in the estimates of relative risk, but the inclusion of squamous dysplasia in the analyses reduced the strength of the association, suggesting that the association was stronger for carcinoma *in situ* than for dysplasia.

Between 1970 and 1972, approximately 32 000 15–39-year-old women were re-cruited for a study in Ljubljana, Yugoslavia, through family planning and gynaecological clinics (Andolsek *et al.*, 1983). Attempts were made to collect Pap smears from women in the cohort annually, but large numbers of women were lost during the seven-year follow-up period. After adjustment for years of follow-up, age at first pregnancy and number of Pap smears, there was no significant increase in the risk for either carcinoma *in situ* or severe dysplasia in women who had used oral contraceptives. When the two conditions were combined, there was no trend of increase in risk with duration of use.

The results of three cohort studies that specifically assessed the risk for cervical dysplasia in relation to oral contraceptive use are summarized in Table 12. The study of

Table 12. Cohort studies of use of oral contraceptives and cervical dysplasia

Reference (date cohort started)	Comparison groups	No. of cases	Relative risk (95% CI)	Comments
Zondervan et al. (1996) (1968–74)	No use	35	1.0	– adjusted for social class,
	Any use	124	1.1 (0.7–1.7)	smoking, age at first birth,
	Current use	59	1.7 (1.0–2.8)	diaphragm use, condom use;
	Months of use			– p value of test for trend = 0.2;
	1–12	5	0.8 (0.3–2.1)	– 22 years of follow-up;
	13–24	5	0.7 (0.2–1.9)	– no increase in risk after
	25–48	11	0.5 (0.3–1.1)	12 months since last use
	49–72	34	1.8 (1.0–3.0)	
	73–96	26	1.2 (0.7–2.2)	
	≥ 97	43	1.1 (0.6–1.8)	
New Zealand Contraception and Health Study Group (1994) (1980–86)	IUD	92	1.0	– adjusted for smoking, age at first intercourse, number of partners, use of depot medroxyprogesterone acetate;
	Use	125	1.2 (0.9–1.6)	– 5.5 years of follow-up
Gram et al. (1992) (1979–80)	No use	NR	1.0	– adjusted for marital status,
	Past use	NR	1.4 (1.0–1.8)	age group, smoking, alcohol
	Current use	NR	1.5 (1.1–2.1)	abuse, oral contraceptive use;
	Age started			– 7 years' mean follow-up of
	> 24		1.1 (0.7–1.8)	users;
	20–24		1.5 (1.1–2.0)	– p value of test for trend = 0.05
	< 20		1.3 (0.9–1.9)	– 354 women with CIN grade I or II, 44 with CIN grade III, and 3 with carcinoma; results not altered when analysis restricted to grade I or II

IUD, intrauterine device; NR, not reported; CIN, cervical intraepithelial neoplasia

the Oxford Family Planning Association (Zondervan et al., 1996) covered 17 032 women who were recruited at 17 large family planning clinics in England and Scotland between 1968 and 1974. The most recent results represent 22 years of follow-up. No increase in the risk for cervical dysplasia was observed with duration of oral contraceptive use. A small increase in risk, of borderline statistical significance, was observed for current users; however, this possible increase did not persist 12 months after last use.

The New Zealand Contraception and Health Study Group (1994) followed a cohort of 7199 women who had initially had two Pap smears showing no dysplasia for an average of 5.5 years of follow-up. The women were screened annually for cervical abnormalities. When the cohort was established, 2469 women were using oral contraceptives, 2072 women were using an intrauterine device and 1721 women were using depot medroxyprogesterone acetate. In comparison with women who had used an intrauterine device, women who had used oral contraceptives were not at increased risk for cervical dysplasia. The women in the cohort had used oral contraceptives for an average of 2.5 years.

Between 1979 and 1980, 6622 women between the ages of 20 and 49 in Tromsø, Norway, were interviewed and subsequently followed-up for 10 years (Gram *et al.*, 1992) by linking the cohort to computerized information in the pathology registry at the University of Tromsø. Serial Pap smears were not taken from all women, although at least one cytological smear was recorded for 96% of the women in the registry between 1980 and 1989. As most of the cases were CIN-I or -II, this study is summarized in Table 12 with the two studies that provide information on dysplasia. The risk for disease was significantly increased among women who were using oral contraceptives when the cohort was established; it was somewhat lower and of borderline statistical significance for past users. Women who first used oral contraceptives before the age of 24 were at slightly greater risk than were women who began using them later. The difference is not, however, statistically significant and could be due to differences in duration of use among women who began using oral contraceptives at different ages. No information on duration of use was reported.

Table 13 shows the results of two cohort studies of oral contraceptives and cervical carcinoma *in situ*. In the study of the Oxford Family Planning Association (Zondervan *et al.*, 1996), the risk of women who had used oral contraceptives for more than 96 months was significantly increased, but no significant trend of increasing risk with duration of use was observed. The risk was also increased in current users of oral contraceptives but not in women who had stopped use for more than one year.

The study of the Royal College of General Practitioners (Beral *et al.*, 1988) was begun in 1968. Over 23 000 women who were taking oral contraceptives at the time and an approximately equal number of women who had never taken oral contraceptives were recruited by 1400 general practitioners throughout the United Kingdom, who reported details of oral contraceptive use and the health status of each woman in the study twice each year. After 17–19 years of follow-up, a significantly increased risk for cervical carcinoma *in situ* was found for women who had ever used oral contraceptives. The risk was also observed to increase with duration of use.

It should be noted that information on the number of sexual partners was collected only by the New Zealand Contraception and Health Study Group. All of the associations summarized in Tables 12 and 13 could, therefore, be due to residual confounding by sexual variables. It should also be noted that all of the risk estimates for current users were increased and that the risk decreased after cessation of use. These observations are consistent with a screening bias: women taking oral contraceptives may be more likely to have Pap smears than women who are not. On balance, the results of the cohort studies do not provide strong evidence that cervical dysplasia or carcinoma *in situ* is causally related to use of oral contraceptives.

Table 13. Cohort studies of use of oral contraceptives and cervical carcinoma *in situ*

Reference (date cohort started)	Comparison groups	No. of cases	Relative risk (95% CI)	Comments
Zondervan *et al.* (1996) (1968–74)	No use	22	1.0	– adjusted for social class, smoking, age at first birth, diaphragm use, condom use;
	Any use	99	1.7 (1.0–3.0)	
	Current use	45	2.2 (1.2–4.1)	
	Months of use			– *p* value of test for trend = 0.2;
	1–12	4	1.4 (0.5–4.4)	– 22 years of follow-up;
	13–24	7	1.8 (0.7–4.6)	– no significant increase in risk
	25–48	20	1.7 (0.8–3.5)	after 12 months since last use
	49–72	18	1.5 (0.7–3.0)	
	73–96	11	1.2 (0.5–2.6)	
	≥ 97	39	2.5 (1.3–4.7)	
Beral *et al.* (1988) (1968–70)	No use	34	1.0	– adjusted for age, parity, smoking, social class, number of prior normal Pap smears;
	Any use	173	2.9 (2.0–4.1)	
	Years of use			
	< 5	84	2.4	– *p* value of test for trend, < 0.001;
	5–9	66	3.6	– follow-up through 1987
	≥ 10	23	4.8	(17–19 years)

CI, confidence interval

(b)   *Studies of cervical dysplasia in which assays for human papilloma-virus DNA were performed*

Three cohort studies of a different design from those summarized in Tables 12 and 13 have been conducted. Koutsky *et al.* (1992) followed-up a cohort of 241 women with normal cervical cytology by cytological and colposcopic examinations every four months for approximately two years. HPV DNA was detected by dot–filter hybridization and Southern blot hybridization for confirmation. The risk for CIN-II or -III was not associated with use of oral contraceptives.

Liu *et al.* (1995) assembled a cohort of 206 women with cervical dysplasia who had been recruited into a randomized trial of the effect of folic acid supplementation on the course of cervical dysplasia; they had provided two to four cervical smears, which were tested for HPV-16 by Southern blotting. Follow-up examinations were conducted every two months for a total of six months. The risk for progression from low- to high-grade dysplasia was not associated with past or current use of oral contraceptives: the relative risk for progression in HPV-16-negative women was 1.6 (95% CI, 0.8–3.1) for past users versus never users and 1.4 (95% CI, 0.7–2.7) for current versus never users, whereas the comparable relative risks in HPV-16-positive women were 0.8 (95% CI, 0.6–1.1) and 0.8 (95% CI, 0.6–1.0), respectively. Although the differences in relative risk estimates for HPV-16-negative and -positive women could have occurred by chance, they are consistent with the hypothesis that oral contraceptives enhance progression of dysplasia in the absence of HPV-16.

In a study of similar design (Ho *et al.*, 1995), 70 women with cervical dysplasia were followed at three-month intervals for 15 months. HPV DNA was assayed by PCR techniques. The risk for persistent dysplasia was not associated with oral contraceptive use after HPV status was taken into account; results stratified by HPV status were not presented.

(c) Studies of invasive cervical carcinoma

The results of two cohort studies of the risk for invasive cervical carcinoma in relation to oral contraceptive use are summarized in Table 14. HPV status was not considered in either study. The study of the Oxford Family Planning Association (Zondervan *et al.*, 1996) found an increased risk for invasive cervical carcinoma in women who had ever used oral contraceptives that was of borderline statistical significance. The risk was particularly enhanced for women who had used oral contraceptives within the past two years. There was no trend of increase in risk with duration of use.

The study of the Royal College of General Practitioners (Beral *et al.*, 1988) also showed an increase in risk for invasive cervical carcinoma of borderline statistical significance among women who had ever used oral contraceptives and an increase in risk with duration of use. Beral *et al.* (1999) also found an increase in risk for deaths due to cervical carcinoma. On the basis of 25 years of follow-up and 172 deaths, the relative risk for

Table 14. Cohort studies of use of oral contraceptives and invasive cervical carcinoma

Reference (date cohort started)	Comparison groups	No. of cases	Relative risk (95% CI)	Comments
Zondervan *et al.* (1996) (1968–74)	No use	2	1.0	– adjusted for social class,
	Any use	31	4.4 (1.0–32)	smoking, age at first birth,
	Use in past 2 years	21	6.8 (1.6–49)	diaphragm use, condom use;
	Months of use			– *p* value of test for trend, 0.8;
	1–24	4	5.5 (0.8–51)	– 22 years of follow-up;
	25–72	6	2.8 (0.5–23)	– no significant increase in
	≥ 73	21	4.7 (1.1–33)	risk after 24 months since last use
Beral *et al.* (1988) (1968–70)	No use	16	1.0	– adjusted for age, parity,
	Any use	49	1.8 (1.0–3.3)	smoking, social class, number
	Years of use			of prior normal Pap smears;
	< 5	21	1.3	– *p* value of test for trend,
	5–9	17	2.0	< 0.001;
	≥ 10	11	4.4	– follow-up through 1987 (17–19 years)

CI, confidence interval

dying from cervical cancer among women who had ever used oral contraceptives was 1.7 (95% CI, 0.9–3.2). The relative risk increased with duration of use (p value for trend, 0.03) and was 4.1 (95% CI, 1.6–11) for users of 10 or more years' duration. The risk decreased with time since cessation of use and was not significantly increased 10 years after exposure.

Because these results are for invasive cervical cancer, they are unlikely to be due to preferential screening of women taking oral contraceptives. They could, however, be due to incomplete control of the confounding influence of sexual behaviour, since in neither of these studies was a detailed sexual history obtained.

2.3.4   Case–control studies

(a)   Studies of cervical intraepithelial neoplasia not based on screening programmes

Ten case–control studies of CIN in relation to use of oral contraceptives are summarized in Table 15. In all of these studies, the cases were selected from clinics, hospitals or tumour registries, and controls were selected from clinics, hospitals or the general population. HPV status was not assessed in any of these investigations. Because the cases and controls were not selected from the same screening programme, these studies are more likely than studies based on screened populations to be influenced by screening bias. Nevertheless, an attempt was made in all of the studies to control for both sexual variables and prior screening, and they therefore provide useful information on the possible association between CIN and oral contraceptive use. A study by Hellberg *et al.* (1985) is omitted from Table 15 because the controls were pregnant women and, as such, were not representative of the population from which the cases came with respect to contraceptive factors. Furthermore, no relative risk estimates were provided in the report of that study.

The study by Harris *et al.* (1980) was conducted at two hospitals in Oxford, England, between 1974 and 1979. After adjustment for pregnancy outside marriage, cigarette smoking and numerous sexual partners, the risk for carcinoma *in situ* or dysplasia was found to increase significantly with duration of oral contraceptive use.

Clarke *et al.* (1985) studied women attending the dysplasia clinic of the Toronto General Hospital, Canada, between 1979 and 1981 who had histologically confirmed cervical dysplasia. The controls were selected from the same neighbourhood as the corresponding cases. After controlling for number of sexual partners, the relative risk for women who had ever used oral contraceptives was estimated to be 1.7 ($p = 0.14$). Age at first sexual intercourse, smoking status and years of education were also considered as potential confounders. No information was presented on risk in relation to duration of use.

Irwin *et al.* (1988) identified women with carcinoma *in situ* from the population-based cancer registry of Costa Rica between 1982 and 1984. The controls were selected from a national survey. After adjustment for age, history of sexually transmitted disease or pelvic inflammatory disease, gravidity, age at first intercourse, number of sexual partners and history of Pap smears before 1982, a significant trend of increased risk with duration of use was observed. The risk was highest for women who had used oral

Table 15. Case-control studies of use of oral contraceptives and cervical intraepithelial neoplasia (CIN) in which cases and controls were not selected from the same screening programme

Reference	Definition of cases	No. of subjects		Relative risk (95% CI)[a]		Long-term use		Comments
		Cases	Controls	Ever	Current	Duration (years)	RR (95% CI)	
Harris et al. (1980)	Carcinoma in situ or dysplasia	237	422	Not reported		≥ 10	2.1 (significant trend, p = 0.003)	Cases from 2 hospitals, controls largely from gynaecological clinics of the same hospitals
Clarke et al. (1985)	Dysplasia	250	500	1.7		Not reported		Cases from dysplasia clinics, neighbourhood controls
Irwin et al. (1988)	Carcinoma in situ	583	938	1.6 (1.2–2.2)	2.3 (1.5–3.5)	≥ 10	2.0 (1.0–3.6) (p for trend = 0.04)	Cases from tumour registry, general population controls
Brock et al. (1989)	Carcinoma in situ	117	196	1.5 (0.4–6.6)	1.8 (0.4–8.6)	≥ 6	2.3 (0.5–11) (p for trend = 0.05)	Cases from 2 hospitals, controls from case's family physician's files or files of university-affiliated general practitioners
Jones et al. (1990)	Carcinoma in situ	293	801	Not reported	1.8 (1.0–3.4)	≥ 10	1.4 (0.8–2.7) (p for trend = 0.04)	Cases from clinics, general population controls
Cuzick et al. (1990)	CIN-I CIN-II CIN-III	110 103 284	833 833 833	Not reported		> 9 > 9 > 9	1.8 (NS) 2.5 (NS) 1.3 (NS)	Cases from many clinics, controls from general practitioners and family planning clinics
Coker et al. (1992)	CIN-II/-III	103	258	0.7 (0.3–1.6)	1.2 (0.5–2.8)	≥ 5	0.6 (0.2–1.4)	Cases from dysplasia referral clinic, controls from single family practice centre
De Vet et al. (1993)	Dysplasia	257	705	Not reported		> 10	2.3 (1.2–4.6)[b]	Cases from 40 municipalities, controls from populations of 6 of these municipalities

Table 15 (contd)

Reference	Definition of cases	No. of subjects		Relative risk (95% CI)[a]		Long-term use		Comments
		Cases	Controls	Ever	Current	Duration (years)	RR (95% CI)	
Kjaer et al. (1993)	Carcinoma in situ	586	614	1.4 (0.9–2.1)	1.5 (1.0–2.4)	≥ 10	1.7 (1.0–2.7) (p for trend = 0.01)	Cases from tumour registry, controls from general population
Ye et al. (1995)	Carcinoma in situ	231	8 364	1.0 (0.8–1.4)	1.2 (0.8–1.9)	> 5	1.5 (1.0–2.3) (p for trend = 0.13)	Hospitalized cases and controls; analyses restricted to cases with vaginal bleeding to minimize screening bias

CI, confidence interval; RR, relative risk; NS, not significant

[a] Controlled for various potentially confounding variables except human papillomavirus

[b] Among current users

contraceptives within the past year (current users); the relative risk was not increased after five years since cessation of use.

Brock *et al.* (1989) recruited women with histologically confirmed carcinoma *in situ* which had been diagnosed in two hospitals in Sydney, Australia, between 1980 and 1983. The controls were selected from the same clinics from which the cases came. After adjustment for number of sexual partners, age at first sexual intercourse and smoking, the risk for carcinoma *in situ* of women who had ever used oral contraceptives was estimated to be 1.5. The risk was somewhat higher for current users, and a trend of increasing risk with duration of use was observed which was of borderline statistical significance.

Jones *et al.* (1990) recruited cases of cervical carcinoma *in situ* from 24 participating hospitals in five United States cities. Controls from the same communities were ascertained through random-digit dialling. After control for age, race, interval since last Pap smear, number of abnormal smears, number of sexual partners, history of non-specific genital infection or sores and years of cigarette smoking, the relative risk was found to increase slightly with duration of oral contraceptive use. The risk was particularly high for current users of oral contraceptives (borderline statistical significance) and was not significantly elevated in former users.

Cuzick *et al.* (1990) recruited women referred to the Royal Northern Hospital in London, England, by their local general practitioners for evaluation of an abnormal cervical smear which was histologically classified as CIN-I, -II or -III. The controls came largely from one general practice and one family planning clinic. The relative risks for CIN were not significantly increased after more than nine years of oral contraceptive use, and no significant trends of increasing risk with duration of use were observed. The relative risk estimates were adjusted for age, social class, age at first intercourse, number of partners, parity and age at first birth. No information was provided on the risk of current users or risk in relation to time since last use.

Coker *et al.* (1992) recruited cases of CIN-II or CIN-III from a dysplasia clinic; controls were selected from a family practice centre [which might have biased the results with respect to hormonal contraceptive use]. No increase in risk was observed in relation to the features of oral contraceptive use considered, although the highest relative risk was observed for current users.

De Vet *et al.* (1993) studied women with dysplasia who were referred from 40 municipalities in the Netherlands to participate in a randomized clinical trial of the effects of β-carotene on cervical dysplasia. The controls were selected from the general population of six of these municipalities. After adjustment for the number of sexual partners, number of cigarettes smoked per day, marital status, number of children, age at first intercourse, current frequency of intercourse and age, the risk for dysplasia was found to be increased in current users of oral contraceptives who had used these products for over 10 years. The risk was not increased for current users who had used them for a shorter period or for former users.

Kjaer *et al.* (1993) recruited women with cervical carcinoma *in situ* who were living in the greater Copenhagen area between 1985 and 1986 through the Danish Cancer

Registry. The controls were recruited from the general population of Copenhagen. After control for age, years of smoking, number of sexual partners, proportion of sexually active life without use of barrier contraceptives, years of use of an intrauterine device, number of births, age at first episode of genital warts and ever having a Pap smear, the relative risk for cervical carcinoma *in situ* was found to increase significantly with duration of oral contraceptive use. The risk was also increased in current users of oral contraceptives and declined with years since last use, so that the relative risk was 1.0 after nine years since last exposure.

Ye *et al.* (1995) analysed data from the WHO Collaborative Study of Neoplasia and Steroid Contraceptives. Women hospitalized for treatment of carcinoma *in situ* were recruited from one centre each in Mexico and Chile and three centres in Thailand. The controls were women from the same hospitals as the cases but with diseases not considered to be associated with hormonal contraceptive use. Overall, women who had ever used oral contraceptives had a relative risk for cervical carcinoma *in situ* of 1.3 (95% CI, 1.2–1.5) and a strong trend of increasing risk with months of use: the relative risk of women who had used oral contraceptives for more than five years was 2.0 (95% CI, 1.7–2.5; p for trend < 0.001). The risk was also increased for women who had last used oral contraceptives within the previous 12 months (relative risk, 1.7) but not for women who had used them in the more distant past (relative risk, 1.2). To minimize any potential influence of screening bias, additional analyses were restricted to cases that presented with vaginal bleeding and were presumably not diagnosed by screening. In this subset (shown in Table 15), the risk was not significantly increased for women who had ever used oral contraceptives, and no significant trend of risk with duration of use was observed; there was also no increase in the risk of current users. These relative risk estimates were adjusted for age, hospital, marital status, number of pregnancies, history of induced abortion, number of Pap smears six months before the reference date, use of injectable contraceptives and use of condoms. Other potentially confounding variables that were considered but not found to be confounders included use of an intrauterine device or diaphragm, douching after intercourse, age at first sexual relationship, age at menarche, menopausal status, number of visits to a doctor for vaginal discharge, number of sexual relationships, history of any venereal disease or of gonorrhoea or syphilis, tubal ligation, ectopic pregnancy, stillbirth, miscarriage, prior dilatation and curettage, chest X-ray and family history of cancer.

Some consistencies among the results of the studies summarized in Table 15 are generally higher relative risk estimates for current users than for ever users and a tendency for the relative risks to decline with time since use. These findings suggest a bias due to screening in many of these studies. Nonetheless, most of the studies also found that the relative risk estimates were higher among long-term than short-term users of oral contraceptives, and, in many instances, a significant trend of increasing use with duration of use was observed. This too, however, could be due to selective factors. The longer a woman uses oral contraceptives, the more likely she is to have a Pap smear and to be diagnosed with CIN. The study of Ye *et al.* (1995) provides evidence that this kind of bias can occur.

(b)   *Studies of cervical intraepithelial neoplasia based on screening programmes*

The case–control studies of CIN summarized in Table 16 are those in which the cases and controls were selected from the same screening programme. Thomas (1972) compared women with carcinoma *in situ*, dysplasia and any abnormal Pap smear (class III, IV or V) with women whose Pap smears were normal. All of the subjects were residents of Washington County, Maryland (United States). No increase in the risk for these conditions in relation to ever having used oral contraceptives was observed. These estimates were not appreciably altered by controlling for age, circumcision status of the husband, use of barrier contraceptives, smoking status, frequency of church attendance, evidence of tricho-monas on the index smear, history of vaginal discharge, education, having been divorced or separated, having a husband who had previously been married, number of live births, conception of first child before marriage and age at first pregnancy. The risk in relation to duration of use was not reported, but the cases and controls did not differ with respect to mean cumulative dose of oestrogen or of progestogen received. They also did not differ with respect to time since first use of oral contraceptives or current use of oral contra-ceptives. The mean duration of use of oral contraceptives was slightly, but not significantly, higher for controls (21 months) than for the cases (20 months).

Worth and Boyes (1972) selected cases of carcinoma *in situ* from the British Columbia Screening Programme in Canada. The controls were women in the same medical practices as the cases who had negative Pap smears. The proportions of cases and controls who had ever used oral contraceptives were similar [the age-adjusted relative risk was 1.1], and the mean length in months of oral contraceptive use did not differ between the two groups (25.7 and 21.5 for cases and controls aged 20–24 and 33.9 and 32.0 months for women aged 25–29, respectively). Although the relative risk estimate was not controlled for other potential confounders, it is unlikely that doing so would have increased the relative risk estimate to a significant level. The results of these two early studies, although reassuring, are limited by the short duration of use and a short duration of follow-up.

Molina *et al.* (1988) recruited women with cervical carcinoma *in situ* who were referred from a screening programme to any one of three hospitals in Santiago, Chile. The controls were women with normal Pap smears who were selected from the same screening programme. After adjustment for total number of pregnancies, history of induced abortion, pay status (an indicator of socioeconomic status), age at first inter-course, number of sexual partners, history of vaginal discharge and frequency of prior Pap smears, no increase in the risk for cervical carcinoma *in situ* was observed in women who had ever used oral contraceptives, and no trend in risk with duration of use was observed. An increase in the risk of current users was found, but no increase in risk was observed for previous users.

Parazzini *et al.* (1992) recruited women with CIN from screening clinics in Milan, Italy. The controls were women with normal cervical smears selected from the same screening clinics. No increase in the risk for either CIN-I and -II or CIN-III was observed in women who had ever used oral contraceptives. No information was presented on

Table 16. Case–control studies of use of oral contraceptives and cervical intraepithelial neoplasia (CIN) in which the cases and controls were selected from the same screening programme

Reference	Definition of cases	No. of subjects		Relative risk (95% CI)[a]		Long-term use		Comments
		Cases	Controls	Ever	Current	Duration (years)	RR (95% CI)[a]	
Thomas (1972)	Carcinoma in situ	104	302	0.58 (NS)			Not reported	Mean duration of use and cumulative doses of oestrogen and progestogen not higher in cases than controls
	Dysplasia	105	302	1.24 (NS)				
	Pap III, IV, V (all cases)	324	302	0.91 (NS)				
Worth & Boyes (1972)	Carcinoma in situ	310	682	[1.1] (NS)[b]				Low response rates; no adjustment for confounders; RR calculated for age group 25–29 years
Molina et al. (1988)	Carcinoma in situ	133	254	1.0 (0.6–1.7)	3.2 (1.1–9.8)	> 6	0.7 (0.2–2.0)	
Negrini et al. (1990)	Low-grade SIL	208	1 423	0.9	0.8	≥ 5	0.5	Results similar in subset tested for and adjusted for HPV infection
	High-grade SIL	19	1 423	2.7	4.7	≥ 5	4.6	
Parazzini et al. (1992)	CIN I and II	124	323	0.9 (0.6–1.4)[b]			Not reported	No adjustment for confounders
	CIN III	138	323	1.0 (0.7–1.4)[b]				
Schiffman et al. (1993)	CIN	443	439	Not reported	1.3 (0.6–2.8)		Not reported	Adjusted for HPV infection
Muñoz et al. (1993)	CIN III							Adjusted for HPV infection
	Spain	249	242	1.3 (0.7–2.3)		≥ 5	1.8 (0.8–3.7)	
	Colombia	276	270	1.0 (0.6–1.6)		≥ 5	0.9 (0.5–1.5)	
Becker et al. (1994)	High-grade dysplasia	374	651	0.4 (0.2–0.9)	0.4 (0.2–1.0)	≥ 10	0.6 (0.2–1.4)	Adjusted for HPV infection

CI, confidence interval; RR, relative risk; Pap, Papanicolaou smear; NS, not significant; SIL, squamous intraepithelial neoplasia; HPV, human papillomavirus

[a] Controlled for various potentially confounding variables except HPV, unless otherwise stated

[b] Adjusted only for age

duration of use or time since last use; however, because the cases were recruited between 1981 and 1990, it can be assumed that some of the women who had used oral contraceptives had done so for a considerable time.

The remaining four studies summarized in Table 16 differ from the others and from the studies in Table 15 in that the investigators attempted to make some adjustment for HPV status. In the study of Negrini *et al.* (1990), women with cervical intraepithelial lesions were selected from among women who received their diagnosis in 13 clinics associated with three hospitals in the Washington DC area (United States). Women with normal Pap smears were selected from the same clinics to serve as controls. Cervical scrapings were assayed for specific types of HPV by Southern blot analysis. No increase in the risk for low-grade cervical intraepithelial lesions was observed with respect to any use of oral contraceptives, current use or long-term use. While the study was based on small numbers, after adjustment for age, interval since last Pap smear and lifetime number of sexual partners, the risk for high-grade squamous intraepithelial neoplasia was found to be increased for women who had ever used oral contraceptives, for long-term users and for current users. The only estimate that had a 95% CI that included unity was that for women who had used oral contraceptives for more than five years. The results for both low-grade and high-grade squamous intraepithelial neoplasia were not appreciably different from those shown in the Table after stratification on HPV status.

Schiffman *et al.* (1993) selected cases of CIN from a cytological screening programme at Kaiser Permanente in Portland, Oregon (United States). The controls were women with a normal Pap smear. Specific types of HPV DNA were assayed in cervical vaginal lavage specimens by PCR techniques. After adjustment for age and HPV infection, the risk for CIN was not significantly increased in women who had used oral contraceptives in the past or were using them currently. No information was provided on risk in relation to duration of use.

Muñoz *et al.* (1993) selected women with CIN-III from hospitals, pathology laboratories and screening clinics in Spain and Colombia and selected controls from the same place of recruitment as the corresponding case but among women who had normal cytological results on the same date as the case was detected. HPV DNA in cervical scrapings was assayed by PCR. The risk for CIN-III was not increased among women who had ever used oral contraceptives in either Spain or Colombia after adjustment for age, centre, number of sexual partners, age at first intercourse, HPV infection, *Chlamydia trachomatis* infection, husband's sexual partners (in Spain) and smoking status (in Colombia). The risk was also not significantly increased for women who had used oral contraceptives for more than five years, and in neither country was there a significant trend of increasing risk with duration of use. In Spain, however, the risk was somewhat increased in long-term users and the *p* of the test for trend was 0.08.

Becker *et al.* (1994) recruited women with high-grade dysplasia through the University of New Mexico Women's Health Care and Maternal and Infant Care clinics in the United States. Women who were referred to the University of New Mexico colposcopy clinic and found to have high-grade dysplasia were compared with controls with normal

Pap smears selected from the same clinics from which the cases came. In this study, the term 'high-grade dysplasia' was used to cover moderate dysplasia, severe dysplasia and carcinoma *in situ* combined. Cervical smears were assayed for specific types of HPV DNA by dot–blot hybridization and PCR techniques. The relative risk estimates were adjusted for age, age at first intercourse, lifetime number of sexual partners, ethnicity and HPV infection as identified by PCR. The relative risks for high-grade dysplasia were not increased among women who had ever used oral contraceptives, were current users or were long-term users.

In the aggregate, the results of the eight studies summarized in Table 16 do not provide convincing evidence that use of oral contraceptives enhances the risk for cervical intraepithelial lesions. The large relative risks in the study of Negrini *et al.* (1990) are based on small numbers, and the increase in the risk of current users suggests that the results were influenced by screening bias. With this exception, the results of the studies summarized in the Table are consistent with no influence of oral contraceptives on the risk for these lesions.

(c)   Hospital-based studies of invasive squamous-cell cervical carcinoma

Table 17 summarizes the results of seven hospital-based case–control studies of invasive squamous-cell cervical carcinoma. The case group in the study of Ebeling *et al.* (1987) consisted of 129 women with invasive cervical carcinoma treated at a university hospital or city hospital in Leipzig, Germany. The controls were selected from among women admitted to the same hospitals for skin diseases or orthopaedic conditions. After adjustment for number of pregnancies, age at first pregnancy, number of sexual partners, age at first intercourse, history of vaginal discharge, smoking and months since last Pap smear, the relative risk for invasive squamous-cell carcinoma decreased from 2.1 to 1.5 and was no longer statistically significant. In addition, the trend in risk with duration of use was reduced after adjustment to a non-significant level. The risk was higher for current users than for previous users (1.2; 95% CI, 0.6–2.5). The risk was particularly high for women who had begun use before the age of 25, but, after additional adjustment for age at first use, the relative risk of women who had used oral contraceptives for more than seven years was further reduced to 1.3. The risk of women who had first used oral contraceptives before the age of 25 remained statistically significant at 2.6 after adjustment for duration of use.

Parazzini *et al.* (1990) recruited 367 women under the age of 60 with invasive cervical cancer (assumed to be largely squamous-cell) from among women admitted to four large teaching and general hospitals in Milan, Italy. The controls were patients admitted for acute conditions to one of the hospitals in Milan and to several specialized Milan University clinics. The relative risk of women who had ever used oral contraceptives was 1.9 (95% CI, 1.0–3.1) after control for age, marital status, education, parity, number of sexual partners, age at first intercourse, cigarette smoking, history of Pap smears and use of barrier methods of contraception. The risk was further increased for women who had used oral contraceptives for more than two years, and there was a significant trend of

Table 17. Case–control studies of use of oral contraceptives and invasive squamous-cell cervical carcinoma: hospital controls

Reference	No. of subjects		Relative risk (95% CI)[a]		Long-term use			Comments
	Cases	Controls	Ever	Current	Duration (years)	RR (95% CI)[a]	p for trend	
Ebeling et al. (1987)	129	275	1.5 (0.8–2.9)	2.0 (1.0–4.1)	≥ 7	1.8 (1.0–3.8)	≥ 0.10	– includes 4 adenocarcinomas; – conducted in eastern Germany; – RR for women who first used oral contraceptives at ≤ 24 years, 3.0 (1.1–8.1)
Parazzini et al. (1990)	367	323	1.9 (1.0–3.1)	Not reported	> 2	2.5 (1.2–5.1)	0.007	Histological type not reported
Brinton et al. (1990)	667	1 429	1.1 (0.8–1.5)	1.3 (0.9–1.9)	≥ 10	1.1 (0.6–2.0)	Not reported	– conducted in 4 Latin American countries; – hospital and population controls; – RR estimates controlled for HPV 16/18 status
WHO Collaborative Study (1993)	2 361	13 644	1.3 (1.2–1.5)	1.0 (0.8–1.3)	> 8	2.2 (1.8–2.7)	< 0.001	Conducted in 11 centres in 9 countries
Eluf-Neto et al. (1994)	197	218	Not reported		≥ 5	2.5 (0.9–7.3)	0.11	– 9 adenocarcinomas, 9 adeno-squamous carcinomas and 3 undifferentiated carcinomas; – conducted in Brazil; – RR estimate controlled for HPV status

Table 17 (contd)

Reference	No. of subjects		Relative risk (95% CI)[a]		Long-term use			Comments
	Cases	Controls	Ever	Current	Duration (years)	RR (95% CI)[a]	p for trend	
Chaouki et al. (1998)	107	147	1.1 (0.4–3.4)	Not reported	> 5	6.4 (1.3–31)	0.004	– 107 cases and 56 controls with unknown use of oral contraceptives not included; – includes 16 adeno- and adenosquamous carcinomas; – conducted in Morocco; – RR estimate adjusted for HPV infection
Ngelangel et al. (1998)	323	380	Not reported		≥ 4	2.0 (0.5–7.6)	(not significant)	– conducted in the Philippines; – RR estimate adjusted for HPV infection

CI, confidence interval; RR, relative risk; HPV, human papillomavirus
[a] Controlled for various potentially confounding variables except HPV, unless otherwise stated

increasing risk with duration of use. The risk decreased slightly with time since last use, from 1.7 (95% CI, 0.8–3.7) for women who had last used oral contraceptives within the past five years to 1.5 (95% CI, 0.9–2.7) for women who had most recently used oral contraceptives more than five years previously.

Brinton *et al.* (1990) conducted a case–control study in selected hospitals in Panama, Costa Rica, Bogota, Colombia, and Mexico City, Mexico, with two age-matched controls selected for each case. In Panama and Costa Rica, one community and one hospital control were selected for each case, while in Bogota and Mexico City, both controls were selected from the same hospital from which the case was recruited. Cervical scrapings from all study subjects were tested for HPV DNA by filter in-situ hybridization. This method is now known to be of low sensitivity and specificity, so that if HPV was found to be associated with use of combined oral contraceptives, there could be residual confounding by HPV infection. After adjustment for age, number of sexual partners, age at first intercourse, interval since last Pap smear, number of births, HPV-16/-18 infection status and education, no increase in risk was seen for women who had ever used oral contraceptives. There was also no trend of increasing risk with increasing duration of use. There was, however, an increased relative risk of 1.7 (95% CI, 1.1–2.6) for women who had used oral contraceptives for more than five years and who had used them most recently within the past three years. The risk for users of this duration who had last used these compounds more than three years previously was not increased. These results are based on 667 cases of squamous-cell carcinoma and 61 cases of adeno-carcinoma. When the analyses were restricted to women with squamous-cell carcinoma, the results were not appreciably different.

The cases in the WHO Collaborative Study of Neoplasia and Steroid Contraceptives (1993) were of invasive cervical squamous-cell carcinoma and were recruited from one or more hospitals in Australia, Chile, Colombia, Israel, Kenya, Mexico, Nigeria and the Philippines. The controls were selected from among women admitted to the same hospitals as the cases for conditions not believed to be associated with the use of hormonal contraceptives. All of the relative risk estimates were controlled for age, centre, number of pregnancies and number of prior Pap smears. Control for additional variables obtained at interview did not appreciably alter the estimated relative risks. The risk of women who had ever used oral contraceptives was estimated to be 1.3 (95% CI, 1.2–1.5). A significant trend of increasing risk with duration of use was observed. Women who had used oral contraceptives in the past year (but not current users) were at increased risk, but a trend of decreasing risk with time since last use was observed. The increase in risk with duration of use was evident four to five years after first exposure, and the risk declined to that of non-users eight years after discontinuation of use.

Eluf-Neto *et al.* (1994) recruited 199 cases of invasive cervical cancer from seven hospitals in São Paulo, Brazil, and 225 controls from the same hospitals. HPV DNA was assayed in cervical scrapings from the study participants by PCR-based methods. After control for HPV status, a nonsignificantly increased risk was observed with duration of oral contraceptive use.

In a study in Rabat, Morocco, Chaouki *et al.* (1998) recruited 214 cases of invasive cervical cancer from a single cancer hospital and 203 controls from the same hospital or a nearby general hospital. HPV DNA was assayed in cervical specimens by a PCR-based assay. On the basis of 107 cases and 147 controls with a known history of use of oral contraceptives, no increase in the risk for cervical cancer was observed among women who had ever used oral contraceptives, after control for HPV status. A significant trend of increasing risk with duration of use was observed, however.

Ngelangel *et al.* (1998) recruited cases of invasive cervical cancer and controls from a single hospital in Manila, the Philippines. PCR-based assays for HPV DNA were performed on cervical scrapings from the study subjects. After control for HPV DNA status, a significant trend of increasing risk with duration of hormonal contraceptive use was observed.

(d)   Population-based studies of invasive squamous-cell cervical carcinoma

The results of seven case–control studies of invasive squamous-cell cervical carcinoma in which population controls were used are summarized in Table 18. Peters *et al.* (1986b) identified 200 cases of invasive squamous-cell cervical carcinoma from the Los Angeles Cancer Registry, United States, and compared them with 200 neighbourhood controls. No trend of increasing risk with increasing duration of oral contraceptive use was observed in univariate analyses. No information on risk in relation to features of use other than duration was reported.

Celentano *et al.* (1987) identified 153 cases of invasive squamous-cell cervical cancer in women who had been admitted to Johns Hopkins Hospital in Baltimore, Maryland (United States) between 1982 and 1984. The controls were selected from among women residing in the same neighbourhood as the cases. No increase in risk was seen for women who had ever used oral contraceptives after control for use of other methods of contraception (condom, intrauterine device, diaphragm and vaginal spermicides), age at first intercourse, years of smoking cigarettes, frequency of Pap smears, use since last Pap smear and having visited an obstetrician–gynaecologist. No additional information was provided on risk in relation to various features of oral contraceptive use.

In a case–control study in the United States (Brinton *et al.*, 1986, 1987), cases were recruited from 24 participating hospitals in Birmingham, Chicago, Denver, Miami and Philadelphia between 1982 and 1984. The controls were selected by random-digit dialling from the same populations from which the cases came. After control for age, ethnic origin, number of sexual partners, age at first intercourse, education, interval since last Pap smear and history of a non-specific genital infection or sore, the relative risk for invasive squamous-cell cervical carcinoma among women who had used oral contraceptives for more than 10 years was estimated to be 1.6 (95% CI, 0.9–2.9). This result is based on 417 women with squamous-cell carcinomas; when they were combined with 62 women with adenocarcinomas or adenosquamous carcinomas, the risk increased with duration of use. Analyses of both histological types indicated a higher risk for women

Table 18. Case–control studies of use of oral contraceptives and invasive squamous-cell cervical carcinoma: population controls

Reference	No. of subjects		Relative risk (95% CI)[a]		Long-term use			Comments
	Cases	Controls	Ever	Current	Duration (years)	RR (95% CI)[a]	p for trend	
Peters et al. (1986b)	200	200	Not reported		≥ 10	1.1 (0.5–2.7)	NS	– conducted in Los Angeles, USA; – risk relative to no use and use of < 2 years – univariate analysis only
Celentano et al. (1987)	153	153	0.7 (0.3–1.9)		Not reported			Conducted in Maryland, USA
Brinton et al. (1986)	417	789			≥ 10	1.6 (0.9–2.9)		Conducted in 5 US cities
Irwin et al. (1988)	129	631	0.8 (0.5–1.3)	0.3 (0.1–0.8)	≥ 5	0.9 (0.5–1.6)	NS	Conducted in Costa Rica
Bosch et al. (1992)	432	376	1.3 (0.9–2.0)					– conducted in Colombia and Spain; – RR estimates controlled for HPV status assessed by PCR; – risk increased with duration of use in HPV DNA-positive women only; in comparison with HPV-positive controls, RR = 8.9 (1.1–72)
Kjaer et al. (1993)	58	607	1.3 (0.5–3.3)	1.3 (0.5–3.7)	≥ 6	1.3 (0.5–3.5)	0.38	Conducted in Copenhagen, Denmark
Daling et al. (1996)	221	466	1.0 (0.6–1.6)		≥ 5	1.3 (0.7–2.2)	NS	– conducted in Washington State, USA; – RR, 2.3 (95% CI, 1.4–3.9) in women who used oral contraceptives before the age of 17, controlling for HPV-16 antibody status

RR, relative risk; CI, confidence interval; NS, not significant; HPV, human papillomavirus; PCR, polymerase chain reaction
[a] Controlled for various potentially confounding variables except HPV, unless otherwise stated

who had used oral contraceptives within the past year than for those who had used them in the more distant past.

In the study conducted in Costa Rica by Irwin *et al.* (1988), described above, 129 women with invasive cervical cancer (assumed to be squamous-cell) were compared with 631 controls selected from the general population of Costa Rica. No increase in risk was seen for women who had ever used oral contraceptives, and no trend of increasing risk with duration of use was found. Women who had used oral contraceptives within the past year were actually at reduced risk for disease, the estimate being 0.3 (95% CI, 0.1–0.8), but this estimate was based on only seven cases and 102 controls. No trend in risk with time since last use was observed. All of the estimates were adjusted for age, history of sexually transmitted disease or pelvic inflammatory disease, gravidity, age at first intercourse, number of sexual partners and history of prior Pap smears.

In a study of risk factors for cervical cancer in Colombia and Spain, Bosch *et al.* (1992) identified 436 women with histologically confirmed squamous-cell carcinoma and selected 387 controls from the general population in which the cases arose. No increase in risk was observed for women who had ever used oral contraceptives. Cervical scrapings from the study subjects were assayed for type-specific HPV DNA by PCR. No trend of increasing risk with duration of use was observed for women who had no HPV DNA, but a trend was observed for women who had HPV DNA, and this observation was statistically significant (p for trend = 0.027). This observation is, however, based on very small numbers of HPV DNA-positive controls: 17 among women who had never used oral contraceptives and one woman each who had used oral contraceptives for 1–9 and 10 or more years. The numbers of cases in these three categories were 110, 12 and 35, respectively. The relative risks in relation to non-users were estimated to be 3.0 (95% CI, 0.3–28) for users of oral contraceptives for 1–9 years and 8.9 (95% CI, 1.1–72) for users of more than 10 years' duration.

Kjaer *et al.* (1993) recruited 59 women with invasive cervical cancer and living in the greater Copenhagen area from the Danish Cancer Registry; the controls were selected from the general female population of greater Copenhagen. The risk for invasive squamous-cell cervical cancer was not significantly increased among women who had ever used oral contraceptives, and no significant trend of increasing risk with duration of use was observed. The relative risk of women who had used oral contraceptives within the past two years was 1.7 (95% CI, 0.6–4.7). The risk decreased to 1.0 for women who had last used oral contraceptives more than two years previously (p for trend = 0.002). The relative risks in this study were adjusted for age, years of school attendance, number of sexual partners, proportion of sexually active life without use of barrier contraceptives, ever having had gonorrhoea and ever having had a Pap smear.

In a population-based case–control study conducted in Washington State, United States, Daling *et al.* (1996) interviewed 221 women with invasive squamous-cell cervical carcinoma and 466 control women selected by random-digit dialling. Serum from most of the study subjects was tested for HPV-16 capsid antibodies. After adjustment for age, number of Pap smears in the last decade and lifetime number of sexual partners, the risk was not increased for women who had ever used oral contraceptives, and no trend of increasing risk with duration of use was observed. After control for HPV antibody status, the risks relative to that of women who first began using oral contraceptives after the age of 20 were 1.6 (95% CI, 1.0–2.4) for women who had first used them between the ages of 18 and 19 and 2.3 (95% CI, 1.4–3.8) for women who had first begun using them at age 17 or younger. No information was given on risk in relation to time since last use of oral contraceptives.

The results of the studies summarized in Tables 17 and 18 are not totally consistent, but some generalizations can be made cautiously. If the risk is increased in women who have ever used oral contraceptives, then the increase in risk is likely to be modest. Most of the studies do show a small increase in risk for 'ever users', but the risks are small, and the 95% CIs of the estimates in most instances include unity. The relative risk estimates for long-term users are generally higher in the hospital-based studies (Table 17) than in the population-based studies (Table 18), but the estimates are not consistently higher or lower in hospital-based studies in which HPV DNA status was considered than in such studies in which it was not. The higher relative risks in hospital-based than in population-based studies are therefore probably not due to differences in confounding.

None of the studies indicates that risk is increased long after initial exposure to oral contraceptives. The only possible exception is the study of Daling *et al.* (1996), in which it was found that the risk for women who were first exposed to oral contraceptives before the age of 17 was increased. This observation requires independent confirmation.

In the three studies in which risk was considered in relation to use of oral contraceptives among women with and without other risk factors for cervical cancer (Brinton *et al.*, 1986; Parazzini *et al.*, 1990; WHO Collaborative Study of Neoplasia and Steroid Contraceptives, 1993), there was some suggestion that the risk in relation to oral contraceptives might be greater in women with than without such sexual risk factors as a history of non-specific genital infection or sore (Brinton *et al.*, 1986), absence of use of barrier contraceptives (Brinton *et al.*, 1986; Parazzini *et al.*, 1990), having had multiple sexual partners (Parazzini *et al.*, 1990), a history of sexually transmitted diseases and presence of herpes simplex virus-II antibodies (WHO Collaborative Study of Neoplasia and Steroid Contraceptives, 1993). These observations are consistent with the idea that oral contraceptives enhance risk in the presence of a sexually transmitted oncogenic agent such as certain strains of HPV.

Table 19 summarizes the results of the four studies (described above) in which the risk for invasive squamous-cell cervical cancer in relation to oral contraceptive use was estimated on the basis of a comparison of cases and controls with evidence of HPV DNA in cervical cells. In each study, the relative risk estimates for women with HPV DNA were increased, and evidence for a trend of increasing risk with duration of use of combined oral contraceptives is provided from three of the studies. These results should be interpreted with caution, however, because few controls were found to be HPV-positive and all of the estimates therefore have wide confidence limits. In addition, three of the four studies shown in Table 19 are hospital-based.

Table 19. Case–control studies of use of oral contraceptives and invasive squamous-cell cervical cancer in which analyses were restricted to women with human papillomavirus (HPV) DNA in cervical scrapings

Reference	Use of oral contraceptives	All subjects			HPV-positive subjects		
		No. of subjects		RR (95% CI)[a]	No. of subjects		RR (95% CI)[a]
		Cases	Controls		Cases	Controls	
Bosch et al. (1992)	Never	291	270	1.0	110	17	1.0
	Ever	141	106	1.3 (0.9–2.0)	50	2	6.5 (1.3–31)
Eluf-Neto et al. (1994); Bosch et al. (1995)	Years of use						
	None	125	152	1.0	97	21	1.0
	1–4	39	44	1.3 (0.7–2.3)	30	9	1.2 (0.4–4.2)
	≥ 5	33	22	2.7 (1.4–5.2)	27	2	9.0 (1.4–57)
Chaouki et al. (1998)	Years of use						
	< 1	8	25	1.0	20	7	1.0
	1	14	14	1.4 (0.2–8.1)			
	2–5/2–4[b]	32	35	2.8 (0.6–13)	21	6	1.0 (0.2–6.6)
	> 5/≥ 5[b]	39	42	6.4 (1.3–31)	37	3	16 (2.2–115)
Ngelangel et al. (1998)	Years of use						
	None	258	277	1.0	NR	NR	1.0
	1–3	40	80	0.3 (0.1–0.7)	NR	NR	0.3 (0.1–0.8)
	≥ 4	25	23	2.0 (0.5–7.6)	NR	NR	2.8 (0.2–30)
	Total	323	380	–	303	35	–

RR, relative risk; CI, confidence interval; NR, not reported
[a] Controlled for various potentially confounding variables
[b] Years of use in HPV-positive subjects

In summary, if there is an increased risk for squamous-cell cervical carcinoma in relation to use of oral contraceptives, it is more likely to be found in relation to invasive rather than in-situ disease. The available evidence indicates that the effect of oral contraceptives on risk probably requires the presence of HPV DNA in the cervical epithelium.

(e)   Studies of invasive cervical adeno- and adenosquamous carcinomas

An early case–control study in Milan, Italy (Parazzini *et al.*, 1988), showed a relative risk of 0.8 (95% CI, 0.2–2.4) for cervical adenocarcinoma among women who had ever used combined oral contraceptives. Five case–control studies have been conducted to assess the risk of adenocarcinomas and adenosquamous carcinomas in relation to duration of use of oral contraceptives (Table 20). The study of Brinton *et al.* (1990), described previously, included 41 women with adenocarcinoma and 20 women with adeno-squamous carcinoma. The risk for either neoplasm among women who had ever used oral contraceptives was estimated to be 2.4 (95% CI, 1.3–4.6). No trend of increasing risk with duration of use was observed. The relative risk estimates were adjusted for age, number of sexual partners, age at first sexual intercourse, interval since last Pap smear, number of births, HPV-16/-18 infection status and education.

Thomas *et al.* (1996) analysed data from the WHO Collaborative Study of Neoplasia and Steroid Contraceptives, described previously. A total of 271 women with adeno-carcinoma and 106 women with adenosquamous carcinoma were included in the study. The risk of women who had ever used oral contraceptives was increased for adeno-carcinoma but not for adenosquamous carcinoma. A significant trend of increasing risk for adenocarcinoma was observed with duration of oral contraceptive use; no similar trend was observed for women with adenosquamous carcinoma, but, when both histo-logical types were combined, a significant trend of increasing risk was observed. The risk for adenocarcinoma was highest among women who had used these products within the past year and generally declined with time since last use. These trends were strongest for neoplasms that developed in women under the age of 35. The association with risk was also somewhat stronger for formulations with high-potency progestogens than for low-potency products.

Brinton *et al.* (1986, 1987) analysed data from the population-based case–control study conducted in five US cities described previously to assess the risks for adeno-carcinoma, adenosquamous carcinoma and both. As in the study of Thomas *et al.* (1996), the risk of long-term users of oral contraceptives was more strongly related to adeno-carcinoma than to adenosquamous carcinoma.

Between 1977 and 1991, Ursin *et al.* (1994) identified 195 cases of adenocarcinoma and adenosquamous carcinoma from the Los Angeles Cancer Registry, United States, which were compared with 386 neighbourhood controls. After adjustment for education, household income, number of sexual partners before the age of 20, number of episodes of genital warts, months of diaphragm use and weight gain between the age of 18 and the time of diagnosis, the relative risk of women who had ever used oral contraceptives was

Table 20. Case–control studies of use of oral contraceptives and cervical adeno- and adenosquamous carcinomas

Reference	Type of case	No. of subjects		Ever use	Long-term use			Comments
		Cases	Controls	RR (95% CI)[a]	Duration (years)	RR (95% CI)[a]	p for trend	
Brinton et al. (1990)	Adenocarcinoma and adenosquamous carcinoma	61	1 429	2.4 (1.3–4.6)	≥ 10	1.8 (0.5–6.5)	NS	– hospital and population controls; – conducted in 4 Latin American countries
Thomas et al. (1996)	Adenocarcinoma	271	2 084	1.6 (1.2–2.1)	≥ 8	2.4 (1.4–4.0)	0.003	– hospital controls; – conducted in 10 centres in 8 countries
	Adenosquamous carcinoma	106	803	1.1 (0.7–1.8)	≥ 8	1.6 (0.6–4.1)	NS	
	Both	377	2 887	1.5 (1.1–1.9)	≥ 8	2.2 (1.4–3.5)	0.003	
Brinton et al. (1986, 1987)	Adenocarcinoma	40	801		≥ 10	2.4[b]	0.15	– population controls; – conducted in 5 US cities; – separate analyses of adenocarcinoma and adenosquamous cancer based on very small numbers of women who used oral contraceptives for 10 years or longer (5 and 2, respectively)
	Adenosquamous carcinoma	23	801		≥ 10	1.3[b]	0.77	
	Both	62	789		≥ 10	3.0 (1.1–8.2)		
Ursin et al. (1994)	Adenocarcinoma and adenosquamous carcinoma	195	386	2.1 (1.1–3.8)	≥ 12	4.4 (1.8–11)	0.04	– population controls; – conducted in Los Angeles, USA – 150 cases were adenocarcinomas; 15 were adenosquamous; no pathological confirmation of the other cases
Ngelangel et al. (1998)	Adenocarcinoma or adenosquamous carcinoma	33	380	Not given	≥ 4	4.3 (0.3–57)	NS	– hospital controls; – conducted in the Philippines; – RR adjusted for HPV infection; – RR based on 4 exposed cases and 23 exposed controls only; – use of all hormonal contraceptives reported, but largely represents use of combined oral contraceptives

RR, relative risk; CI, confidence interval; NS, not significant; HPV, human papillomavirus

[a] Controlled for various potentially confounding variables except HPV, unless otherwise stated

[b] RR adjusted only for age and race

estimated to be 2.1 (95% CI, 1.1–3.8). The risk increased significantly with duration of use. The relative risk of current users of contraceptives was 1.8 (95% CI, 0.6–5.7) and was close to unity for women who had used oral contraceptives more than one year in the past. These results did not change when the analysis was limited to the 150 cases of adenocarcinoma.

In the study in the Philippines (Ngelangel *et al.*, 1998) summarized above, data for 33 cases of adenocarcinoma or adenosquamous carcinoma indicated an increased risk for women who had used oral contraceptives for four years or more. The estimate is based on only three exposed cases, however, and the confidence limits of the estimates are wide and include unity.

In the aggregate, the results of the five studies summarized in Table 20 suggest that long-term use of oral contraceptives increases the risk for cervical carcinomas with adenomatous elements, although confounding by HPV infection cannot be ruled out. The association with use of oral contraceptives appears to be somewhat stronger for adeno-carcinoma than for adenosquamous carcinoma.

It has also been suggested that use of oral contraceptives is more strongly related to adenocarcinoma than to squamous-cell carcinoma of the cervix. The results summarized in Tables 17, 18 and 20 are inconsistent in this regard. The study conducted in four Latin American countries (Brinton *et al.*, 1990) provided estimates for users of more than 10 years of 1.1 for squamous-cell carcinoma and 1.8 for adenocarcinoma or adenosqua-mous carcinoma. The studies in Los Angeles provide estimates of 1.1 for squamous-cell carcinoma in users of more than 10 years' duration (Peters *et al.*, 1986b) and 4.4 for adeno-carcinoma or adenosquamous carcinoma combined in users of more than 12 years' duration (Ursin *et al.*, 1994); these results, however, are based on different study popu-lations. The study in the Philippines (Ngelangel *et al.*, 1998) found relative risks of 2.0 and 4.3 in users of four years' or more duration for squamous and adenomatous carcinomas, respectively. The WHO Collaborative Study of Neoplasia and Steroid Contraceptives (1993) provided an estimate of 2.2 for both squamous-cell carcinoma and tumours with adenomatous elements (adenocarcinoma and adenosquamous carcinoma combined; Thomas *et al.*, 1996) in women who had used oral contraceptives for more than eight years. In the study conducted in five United States cities (Brinton *et al.*, 1986, 1987), the risks for adenocarcinoma and adenosquamous carcinoma combined of users of more than 10 years' duration was estimated to be 3.0, while the estimate for squamous-cell carcinoma was 1.6. The estimate for squamous-cell carcinoma adjusted only for age and race was 1.2. For adenocarcinoma and adenosquamous carcinoma separately, the relative risks adjusted for age and race were 2.4 and 1.3, respectively. The results of these studies thus do not resolve the question of whether use of oral contraceptives is more strongly related to adenocarci-noma and adenosquamous carcinoma than to squamous-cell carcinoma.

Another method that has been used to address the issue of the relative strength of the association between oral contraceptives and various histological types of cervical carci-noma is comparison of use by women with squamous and adenomatous cervical lesions. Persson *et al.* (1987) compared the oral contraceptive use of 23 women with adenocarcinoma with that of 46 women with squamous-cell carcinoma. The proportions of women who had used oral contraceptives in each group were similar, and the duration of use did not differ. Jones and Silverberg (1989) similarly compared 18 cases of endo-cervical adenocarcinoma with an equal number of cases of squamous-cell carcinoma; both groups included both *in situ* and invasive disease. The proportions of women in the two groups who had used oral contraceptives did not differ significantly. Honoré *et al.* (1991) compared each of 99 women with cervical adenocarcinoma with three comparable women with squamous-cell carcinoma, with matching on age, year of diagnosis and clinical stage. The women in the two groups did not differ with respect to any use of oral contraceptives and, among users, the two groups did not differ with respect to age at start of use, age at discontinuation of use or months of use of oral contraceptives. Hopkins and Morley (1991) compared 61 women with adenocarcinoma and 206 women with squamous-cell carcinoma who were under the age of 40. Thirty-three per cent of the women with adeno-carcinomas and 31% of those with squamous-cell carcinomas had ever used oral contra-ceptives. The results of these clinical studies do not support the hypothesis that use of oral contraceptives is more strongly related to the development of adenocarcinoma than squamous carcinoma of the uterine cervix.

On balance, there appears to be insufficient evidence to conclude firmly that use of oral contraceptives is related to adenocarcinoma of the uterine cervix. The associations observed could be due to residual confounding by HPV infection, and a firm conclusion about the risk for adenocarcinoma of users of oral contraceptives must await the results of investigations that adequately control for HPV infection.

2.4   Ovarian cancer

2.4.1   *Descriptive studies*

Younger women in several developed countries have experienced substantial declines in the incidence and mortality rates of ovarian cancer. Cohort analyses based on data from Switzerland (Levi *et al.*, 1987), England and Wales (Beral *et al.*, 1988; dos Santos Silva & Swerdlow, 1995), Great Britain (Villard-Mackintosh *et al.*, 1989), Sweden (Adami *et al.*, 1990) and the Netherlands (Koper *et al.*, 1996) and a systematic analysis of mortality trends in 16 European countries (La Vecchia *et al.*, 1992, 1998) showed that women born after 1920—i.e. the generations that have used combined oral contraceptives—have consis-tently reduced ovarian cancer rates. The downward trends were greater in countries where combined oral contraceptives have been most widely used (La Vecchia *et al.*, 1998).

Thus, descriptive data on the incidence and mortality rates of ovarian cancer are consistent with the hypothesis of a favourable effect of combined oral contraceptive use on subsequent ovarian cancer rates.

2.4.2   *Cohort studies*

The results of cohort studies on use of combined oral contraceptives and ovarian cancer are summarized in Table 21. Most of the evidence refers to epithelial neoplasms, unless otherwise specified. Three cohort studies conducted in the United States and the

Table 21. Selected cohort studies on use of combined oral contraceptives and ovarian cancer, 1980–97

Reference	No. of cases (age, years)	Relative risk (95% CI)		Comments
		Any use	Longest use	
Ramcharan et al. (1981a), USA	16 (18–64)	0.4 (0.1–1.0)	–	Adjusted for age only; Walnut Creek Study on Contraception
Beral et al. (1988), UK	30 (≥ 25)	0.6 (0.3–1.4)	≥ 10 years, 0.3	Royal College of General Practitioners' cohort
Vessey & Painter (1995), UK	42 (all)	0.4 (0.2–0.8)	> 8 years, 0.3 (0.1–0.7)	Oxford Family Planning cohort
Hankinson et al. (1995), USA	260 (30–65)	1.1 (0.8–1.4)	≥ 5 years, 0.7 (0.4–1.1)	Nurses' Health Study

CI, confidence interval

United Kingdom provided data on a total of about 100 cases of epithelial ovarian cancer. In the Walnut Creek Study in the United States (Ramcharan *et al.*, 1981a), 16 cases of ovarian cancer were registered between 1968 and 1977, corresponding to an age-adjusted relative risk of 0.4 for any use of combined oral contraceptives.

The Royal College of General Practitioners' study was based on 47 000 women recruited in 1968 in 1400 British general practices (Beral *et al.*, 1988): 30 cases of ovarian cancer were observed up to 1987, corresponding to multivariate relative risks of 0.6 (95% CI, 0.3–1.4) for any use of combined oral contraceptives and of 0.3 for 10 years of use or more. Allowance was made in the analysis for age, parity, smoking and social class. In a subsequent follow-up study of mortality in that cohort up to the end of 1993 (Beral *et al.*, 1999), 55 deaths from ovarian cancer were reported; there was a statistically significantly reduced mortality rate from ovarian cancer among women who had ever used oral contraceptives (relative risk, 0.6; 95% CI, 0.3–1.0).

The study of the Oxford Family Planning Association was based on 17 032 women enrolled between 1968 and 1974 from various family planning clinics in the United Kingdom (Vessey & Painter, 1995). Up to October 1993, 42 cases of ovarian cancer were registered, corresponding to relative risks of 0.4 (95% CI, 0.2–0.8) for any use of combined oral contraceptives and 0.3 (95% CI, 0.1–0.7) for more than eight years of use. Adjustment was made for age and parity.

In the Nurses' Health study, based on 121 700 registered nurses aged 30–55 in 1976, 260 cases of ovarian cancer were observed prospectively between 1976 and 1988 (Hankinson *et al.*, 1995). The multivariate relative risk for any use, which essentially reflected former use, was 1.1 (95% CI, 0.8–1.4) but declined to 0.7 (95% CI, 0.4–1.1) for use for five years or more. Adjustment was made for age, tubal ligation, age at menarche, age at menopause, smoking and body mass index.

2.4.3 *Case–control studies*

The epidemiological evidence from case–control studies on use of combined oral contraceptives and ovarian cancer is well defined and consistent: at least 20 out of 21 studies published between 1980 and 1997 found relative risks below unity, the sole apparent outlier being a study conducted in China (Shu *et al.*, 1989).

Table 22 gives the main results of case–control studies of ovarian cancer published between 1980 and 1997 which included information on use of combined oral contraceptives. Table 23 gives age-specific relative risks and 95% CIs, while Table 24 gives the relative risks related to time since last use for studies that provided the relevant information. The findings of two pooled analyses of case–control studies on the issue are also included. These were conducted on 971 cases and 2258 controls in three European countries (Franceschi *et al.*, 1991a) and on 2197 cases and 8893 controls in white women from 12 studies in the United States (Whittemore *et al.*, 1992), for a total of over 3100 cases and 11 000 controls.

In a pooled analysis of individual data from three hospital-based European studies (Franceschi *et al.*, 1991a), the multivariate relative risk was 0.6 (95% CI, 0.4–0.8) for any

Table 22. Selected case–control studies of use of oral contraceptives and ovarian cancer, 1980–97

Reference, location	Type of study	No. of cases (age, years)	Relative risk (95% CI)			Comments
			Any use	Longest use	Duration (years)	
Willett et al. (1981), USA	Nested in a cohort	47 (< 60)	0.8 (0.4–1.5)	0.8 (0.3–2.1)	> 3	Prevalent cases from the Nurses' Health cohort study; adjusted for age
Hildreth et al. (1981), USA	Hospital-based	62 (45–74)	0.5 (0.1–1.7)	Not reported		Adjusted for age and parity; odds ratio based on 3 cases with use of oral contraceptives
Weiss et al. (1981a), USA	Population-based	112 (36–55)	0.6 (not reported)	0.4 (0.2–1.3)	≥ 9	Adjusted for age, demographic factors and parity
Franceschi et al. (1982), Italy	Hospital-based	161 (19–69)	0.7 (0.4–1.1)	Not reported		Adjusted for age
Cramer et al. (1982), USA	Population-based	144 (< 60)	0.4 (0.2–1.0)	0.6	> 5	Adjusted for age and parity
Rosenberg et al. (1982), USA	Hospital-based	136 (< 60)	0.6 (0.4–0.9)	0.3 (0.1–0.8)	≥ 5	Protection by use of combined and sequential oral contraceptives; independent of parity; adjusted for several variables
Risch et al. (1983), USA	Population-based	284 (20–74)	[0.5] (not reported)	Not reported		Multivariate odds ratio approximately 0.9 per year of use
Tzonou et al. (1984), Greece	Hospital-based	150 (all ages)	0.4 (0.1–1.1)	Not reported		Adjusted for age, parity, age at menopause and use of oestrogen replacement therapy
Cancer and Steroid Hormone Study (1987), USA	Population-based	492 (20–54)	0.6 (0.5–0.7)	0.2 (0.1–0.4)	≥ 10	Consistent results by type of combined oral contraceptive
Harlow et al. (1988), USA	Population-based	116 (20–79)	0.4 (0.2–0.9)	0.4 (0.2–1.0)	> 4	Borderline malignancy; adjusted for age and parity

Table 22 (contd)

Reference, location	Type of study	No. of cases (age, years)	Relative risk (95% CI)		Duration (years)	Comments
			Any use	Longest use		
Wu et al. (1988), USA	Hospital- and population-based	299 (18–74)	0.7 (0.5–1.1)	0.4 (0.2–0.7)	> 3	Combination of two studies conducted in the 1970s and 1980s
Shu et al. (1989), China	Population-based	229 (18–70)	1.8 (0.8–4.1)	1.9 (0.4–9.3)	> 5	Only 23 cases and 12 controls had ever used combined oral contraceptives
WHO Collaborative Study (1989a), 7 countries	Hospital-based	368 (< 62)	0.8 (0.6–1.0)	0.5 (0.3–1.0)	> 5	Similar results in developed and developing countries
Hartge et al. (1989a), USA	Hospital-based	296 (20–79)	1.0 (0.7–1.7)	0.8 (0.4–1.5)	> 5	Data collected between 1978 and 1981
Booth et al. (1989), UK	Hospital-based	235 (< 65)	0.5 (0.3–0.9)	0.1 (0.01–1.0)	> 10	Consistent results in strata of parity
Parazzini et al. (1991a), Italy	Hospital-based	505 (22–59)	0.7 (0.5–1.0)	0.5 (0.3–0.9)	≥ 2	Protective effect present in strata of major risk factors for ovarian cancer
Parazzini et al. (1991b), Italy	Hospital-based	91 (23–64)	0.3 (0.2–0.6)	0.2 (0.1–0.6)	≥ 2	Borderline malignancy; adjusted for age, parity, education, age at menopause and oral contraceptive use
Polychronopoulos et al. (1993), Greece	Hospital-based	189 (< 75)	0.8 (0.2–3.7)	Not reported		Multivariate RR; only three cases and seven controls had ever used combined oral contraceptives
Rosenberg et al. (1994), USA	Hospital-based	441 (< 65)	0.8 (0.6–1.0)	0.5 (0.2–0.9)	≥ 10	Association persisted as long as two decades after stopping and was not confined to any type of oral contraceptive formulation

Table 22 (contd)

Reference, location	Type of study	No. of cases (age, years)	Relative risk (95% CI)		Duration (years)	Comments
			Any use	Longest use		
Risch et al. (1994, 1996), Canada	Population-based	450 (35–79)	0.5 (0.4–0.7)	0.3 (0.2–0.6)	≥ 10	The inverse relationship was stronger for non-mucinous (RR, 0.9) for each year of use than for mucinous tumours (RR, 1.0); trend per year of use, 0.9 among all subjects
Purdie et al. (1995), Australia	Population-based	824 (18–79)	0.5 (0.4–0.7)	0.3 (0.2–0.4)	≥ 1	Adjusted for parity
Pooled analyses						
Franceschi et al. (1991a), Greece, Italy, UK	Three hospital-based studies	971 (< 65)	0.6 (0.4–0.8)	0.4 (0.2–0.7)	≥ 5	Protection was still present ≥ 15 years after stopping use (odds ratio, 0.5).
Whittemore et al. (1992), USA	Pooled analysis of 12 US population- and hospital-based case–control studies	2197 (all)	0.7 (0.6–0.8)	0.3 (0.2–0.4)	≥ 6	Invasive epithelial neoplasms in white women; protection present in population- and hospital-based studies
Harris et al. (1992), USA	Same pooled analysis as Whittemore et al. (1992)	327	0.8 (0.6–1.1)	0.6 (0.4–0.9)	> 5	Epithelial tumours of low malignant potential in white women
John et al. (1993), USA	Pooled analysis of 7 of the 12 studies in the pooled analysis of Whittemore et al. (1992)	110	0.7 (0.4–1.2)	0.6 (0.2–1.6)	≥ 6	Epithelial ovarian cancers in black women

CI, confidence interval; RR, relative risk

Table 23. Selected case–control studies on use of combined oral contraceptives and ovarian cancer, 1980–97; age-specific relative risks

Reference	Age group (years)	Relative risk (95% CI)
Willett et al. (1981)	< 35	0.3 (0.1–1.3)
	35–44	1.1 (0.4–3.2)
	≥ 45	1.3 (0.4–3.9)
Rosenberg et al. (1982)	18–29	0.4
	30–39	0.6
	40–49	0.5
	50–59	0.7
Centers for Disease Control	20–29	0.3 (0.1–1.4)
(1983b)	30–39	0.8 (0.3–2.0)
	40–49	0.6 (0.4–1.1)
	50–54	0.6 (0.3–1.1)
Parazzini et al. (1991a)	< 35	0.4 (0.2–0.9)
	35–44	0.8 (0.4–1.4)
	45–54	0.7 (0.4–1.3)
	55–59	0.8 (0.1–7.6)
Rosenberg et al. (1994)	< 45	0.5 (0.3–0.8)
	45–65	0.7 (0.4–1.2)
Pooled analysis		
Franceschi et al. (1991a)	< 45	0.6 (0.3–1.0)
	45–54	0.5 (0.3–1.0)
	55–64	0.6 (0.4–0.9)

CI, confidence interval

use and 0.4 (95% CI, 0.2–0.7) for longest (≥ 5 years) use. Allowance was made in the analysis for age, other socio-demographic factors, menopausal status and parity. The protection persisted for at least 15 years after use had ceased.

In a pooled analysis of individual data from 12 studies in the United States (Whittemore *et al.*, 1992), the corresponding values were 0.7 (95% CI, 0.6–0.8) for any use and 0.3 (0.2–0.4) for use for more than six years in the population-based studies. Adjustment was made for age, study and parity. The results were similar when the hospital-based and population-based studies were considered separately: the relative risks were 0.7 in both types of study for any use of combined oral contraceptives, 0.6 in hospital-based studies and 0.3 in population-based studies for longest use (> 6 years) and 0.95 (not significant) and 0.90 ($p < 0.001$), respectively, per added year of use.

An inverse association was also observed in a further analysis of seven studies of 110 cases and 251 controls in black women in the United States. The relative risk was 0.7 for any use and 0.6 for use for six years or more (John *et al.*, 1993). The United States pooled

Table 24. Selected case–control studies on use of combined oral contraceptives and ovarian cancer, 1980–97; results according to time since last use

Reference	Time since last use (years)	Relative risk (95% CI)
Cramer et al. (1982)	< 2	2.1 (NR)
	2–< 6	0.7 (NR)
	6–< 10	0.7 (NR)
	≥ 10	0.3 (NR)
Rosenberg et al. (1982)	< 1	0.3 (NR)
	1–4	0.4 (NR)
	5–9	0.8 (NR)
	≥ 10	0.5 (NR)
Centers for Disease Control (1983b)	< 1	1.0 (0.4–2.2)
	1–4	0.6 (0.3–1.1)
	5–9	0.5 (0.3–0.9)
	≥ 10	0.5 (0.3–0.9)
Harlow et al. (1988)	≤ 5	0.3 (0.1–0.9)
	> 5	0.6 (0.3–1.4)
WHO Collaborative Study (1989a)	< 0.5	0.9 (0.5–1.8)
	0.5–< 5	0.9 (0.5–1.5)
	5–< 10	0.8 (0.5–1.4)
	≥ 10	0.5 (0.3–0.9)
Hartge et al. (1989a)	< 1	0.5 (0.1–1.6)
	1–9	0.9 (0.5–1.6)
	≥ 10	1.4 (0.7–2.6)
Parazzini et al. (1991a)	< 10	0.5 (0.3–0.8)
	≥ 10	0.9 (0.5–1.5)
Rosenberg et al. (1994)	< 15	0.4 (0.2–0.8)
	15–19	0.5 (0.3–1.0)
	≥ 20	0.8 (0.4–1.5)

CI, confidence interval; NR, not reported

analysis also included data on 327 cases of epithelial ovarian neoplasms of borderline malignancy in white women. The relative risks were 0.8 (95% CI, 0.6–1.1) for any use of combined oral contraceptives and 0.6 (0.4–0.9) for five years of use or more (Harris et al., 1992).

The most convincing aspect of the inverse relationship between use of combined oral contraceptives and risk for ovarian cancer is the consistency of the results, independently of the type of study (hospital- or population-based), geographical area (Australia, Europe, North America and developing countries) and type of analysis, including allowance for covariates which differed from study to study, although more variables tended to be included in most recent ones. Likewise, the inverse relationship between use of combined oral contraceptives and ovarian cancer was observed for most types of formulations considered, including those with low doses (Cancer and Steroid Hormone Study of the Centers for Disease Control and the National Institute of Child Health and Human Development, 1987; Rosenblatt et al., 1992; Rosenberg et al., 1994).

The overall estimate of protection for any use is approximately 40%, and a steady inverse relationship exists with duration of use. The decrease in risk was over 50%, and probably around 60% for use for more than five years; however, in contrast to the findings of the Cancer and Steroid Hormone Study of the Centers for Disease Control and the National Institute of Child Health and Human Development (1987), no protection was evident after very short-term use, i.e. three to six months, in an analysis of factors associated with the short-term use of oral contraceptives by Gross et al. (1992) on the data of the above study.

Willett et al. (1981) conducted a case–control study of 47 cases of ovarian cancer and 470 controls nested in the Nurses' Health Study cohort (based on 121 964 registered nurses aged 30–55 in 1986 and residing in 11 large American states). They found an age-adjusted relative risk of 0.8 (95% CI, 0.4–1.5) for any use of combined oral contra-ceptives and 0.2 (95% CI, 0.1–1.0) for women aged 35 or younger, who were more likely to be current users.

Hildreth et al. (1981) considered 62 cases of epithelial ovarian cancer and 1068 hospital controls aged 45–74 in Connecticut, United States, that had been diagnosed between 1977 and 1979. The response rate was 71% for both cases and controls. The multivariate relative risk for any use of combined oral contraceptives, after allowance for age and parity, was 0.5 (95% CI, 0.2–1.7).

Weiss et al. (1981a), in a population-based case–control study of 112 cases diagnosed between 1975 and 1979 in Washington and Utah, United States, found a relative risk (adjusted for age, demographic factors and parity) of 0.6 for any use and 0.4 (95% CI, 0.2–1.3) for longest use, which was of borderline statistical significance (p = 0.04). The response rate was 66% for cases and 92% for controls.

Franceschi et al. (1982) considered data on 161 cases of epithelial ovarian cancer and 561 hospital controls in women interviewed in Milan, Italy, in 1979–80. The age-adjusted relative risk for ever use was 0.7 (95% CI, 0.4–1.1).

Cramer et al. (1982) conducted a case–control study of 144 cases and 139 population controls in 1978–81 in the Greater Boston area (United States) and found a relative risk, adjusted for age and parity, of 0.4 (95% CI, 0.2–1.0) for any use of combined oral contraceptives, in the absence of a consistent duration–risk relationship (relative risk, 0.6 for > 5 years). The latter may be due to the small number of cases. The response rates were around 50% for both cases and controls.

Rosenberg et al. (1982), in a hospital-based case–control study of 136 cases and 539 controls collected between 1976 and 1980 from various areas of the United States and Canada, found an age-adjusted relative risk of 0.6 (95% CI, 0.4–0.9) for any use and 0.3 for use for five years or more. The response rates were 94% for both cases and controls, and the results were not materially modified by multivariate analysis.

Risch *et al.* (1983) provided data from a case–control study of 284 cases and 705 controls from Washington and Utah (United States) diagnosed between 1975 and 1979, giving a significant multivariate relative risk estimate of 0.9 per year for use of combined oral contraceptives. The response rates were 68% for cases and 95% for controls.

In a case–control study conducted in 1980–81 on 150 cases and 250 hospital controls in Athens, Greece, Tzonou *et al.* (1984) found a multivariate relative risk (adjusted for age, parity, age at menopause and use of post-menopausal oestrogen therapy) of 0.4 (95% CI, 0.1–1.1). The lack of significance may be due to the low frequency of use of combined oral contraceptives in this study, which was only 2.7% in cases and 7.2% in controls.

The Centers for Disease Control Cancer and Steroid Hormone Study (1983b) and the Cancer and Steroid Hormone Study of the Centers for Disease Control and National Institute of Child Health and Human Development (1987) was a population-based investigation conducted between December 1980 and December 1982 in eight areas of the United States on 546 women 20–54 years of age with ovarian cancer and 4228 controls. The response rates were 71% for cases and 83% for controls. The multivariate relative risk, adjusted for age and parity, for any use of combined oral contraceptives was 0.6 (95% CI, 0.5–0.7), which decreased to 0.2 (0.1–0.4) for use for10 years or more. The results were consistent when specific formulations of combined oral contraceptives were considered separately.

Harlow *et al.* (1988) provided information on use of combined oral contraceptives in 116 cases of epithelial ovarian cancers of borderline malignancy diagnosed between 1980 and 1985 and 158 controls. The relative risk for any use, adjusted for age and parity, was 0.4, in the absence, however, of a consistent duration–risk relationship.

Wu *et al.* (1988), in a hospital-based case–control study of 299 cases diagnosed in 1983–85 and 752 hospital controls and 259 population-based controls from the San Francisco Bay area, United States, found a relative risk, adjusted for parity, of 0.7 (95% CI, 0.5–1.1) for any use and 0.4 (95% CI, 0.2–0.7) for more than three years of use. The overall relative risk per year of use was 0.9 (95% CI, 0.8–0.9). The response rate was about 70% for both cases and controls.

Shu *et al.* (1989), in a case–control study conducted during 1984–86 in Shanghai, China, on 229 ovarian cancer cases (172 epithelial) and an equal number of controls, found a relative risk (adjusted for education, parity, ovarian cysts and age at menarche) of 1.8 (95% CI, 0.8–4.1) for any use of combined oral contraceptives. Only 23 cases and 12 controls had ever used such preparations. The response rates were 89% for cases and 100% for controls. In China, use of combined oral contraceptives might have been an indication of a westernized life style.

The WHO Collaborative Study of Neoplasia and Steroid Contraceptives (1989a) included data on 368 cases of histologically confirmed cases of epithelial ovarian cancer and 2397 hospital controls. The patients were interviewed between 1979 and 1986 in seven countries, with response rates of 73% for cases and 94% for controls. The multivariate relative risk (adjusted for age, centre, year of interview and parity) for any use of combined oral contraceptives was 0.8 (95% CI, 0.6–1.0) and decreased to 0.5 (95% CI,

0.3–1.0) for five years of use or more. The reduction in risk was of a similar magnitude in developed and developing countries (Thomas, 1991).

In a case–control study conducted in 1978–81 in the Washington DC area of the United States with 296 patients with epithelial ovarian cancer and 343 hospital controls, Hartge et al. (1989a) found relative risks (adjusted for age and race) of 1.0 (95% CI, 0.7–1.7) for any use of combined oral contraceptives and 0.8 (95% CI, 0.4–1.5) for use for more than five years. The response rates were 74% for cases and 78% for controls.

Booth et al. (1989), in a hospital-based case–control study of 235 patients and 451 controls interviewed between 1978 and 1983 in London and Oxford, England, found multivariate relative risks of approximately 0.5 (95% CI, 0.3–0.9) for any use and 0.1 (0.01–1.0) for use for more than 10 years. They reported a significant inverse trend in risk with duration of use. Allowance was made for age, social class, gravidity and duration of unprotected intercourse.

Parazzini et al. (1991a) provided data on 505 cases of epithelial ovarian cancer in women under 60 years of age and 1375 hospital controls interviewed between 1983 and 1989 in northern Italy. The multivariate relative risk (adjusted for age, sociodemographic factors, parity, age at menarche, lifelong menstrual pattern, menopausal status and age at menopause) for any use of combined oral contraceptives was 0.7 (95% CI, 0.5–1.0), which decreased to 0.5 (0.3–0.9) for two years of use or more, with a significant inverse trend in risk with duration. The response rate was 98% for both cases and controls.

Parazzini et al. (1991b) also considered 91 patients with epithelial ovarian cancer of borderline malignancy and 237 hospital controls who were interviewed between 1986 and 1990 in northern Italy. The multivariate relative risk (adjusted for age, education, parity and age at menopause) for any use of combined oral contraceptives was 0.3 (95% CI, 0.2–0.6), and that for two years of use or more was 0.2 (0.1–0.6). The response rate was 98% for both cases and controls.

In a case–control study of 189 cases and 200 controls conducted in 1989–91 in greater Athens, Greece (Polychronopoulou et al., 1993), only three cases and seven controls had any use of combined oral contraceptives, corresponding to a multivariate relative risk of 0.8 (95% CI, 0.1–3.7). The response rate for cases was about 90%.

Rosenberg et al. (1994) updated their 1982 report, providing data collected between 1977 and 1991 on 441 cases of epithelial ovarian cancer and 2065 hospital controls from various areas of the United States. The response rate was 94% for both cases and controls. The multivariate relative risk for any use (adjusted for parity, hysterectomy, monolateral oophorectomy, tubal ligation, family history of ovarian cancer and sociodemographic factors) was 0.8 (95% CI, 0.6–1.0). No significant protection was observed with up to three years of use, but the relative risk declined to 0.5 (95% CI, 0.2–0.9) for 10 years of use or more. The risk estimates were similar for various types of combined oral contraceptive formulations.

Risch et al. (1994, 1996) provided data on 450 cases of epithelial ovarian cancer in women aged 35–79 diagnosed between 1989 and 1992 and 564 controls in Ontario, Canada. The response rates were 71% for cases and 65% for controls. The odds ratio, adjusted for age and parity, for any use of oral contraceptives was 0.5 (95% CI, 0.4–0.7); after 10 or more years of use, it was 0.3 (0.2–0.6). The overall multivariate odds ratio per each year of use of combined oral contraceptives, adjusted for age, parity, lactation, use of postmenopausal oestrogen therapy, tubal ligation, hysterectomy and family history of breast cancer, was 0.90 (95% CI, 0.86–1.0), and the protection was stronger for serous and endometrioid cancers than for mucinous neoplasms.

Purdie *et al.* (1995) in a population-based study of 824 cases diagnosed between 1990 and 1993 and 860 controls in three Australian states found a relative risk of 0.6 (95% CI, 0.5–0.7) for any use, which declined to 0.3 (0.2–0.4) for 10 years of use or more. The response rates were 90% for cases and 73% for controls. Allowance was made in the analysis for sociodemographic factors, family history of cancer, talc use, smoking and reproductive and hormonal factors.

Parity is a well-recognized protective factor for ovarian cancer (Parazzini *et al.*, 1991c) and is a correlate of the use of combined oral contraceptives, i.e. a potentially relevant confounder. The inverse relationship between use of combined oral contraceptives and ovarian cancer was also observed, however, after adequate allowance had been made for parity and was reproduced consistently in several studies across separate strata of parity, age and other potential covariates, including marital status, education, menopausal status, other types of contraceptive use and other selected menstrual and reproductive factors.

The association between oral contraceptive use and the risk for ovarian cancer has been assessed in women with germ-line mutations in the *BRCA-1* or *BRCA-2* gene (Narod *et al.*, 1998). Thus, 207 women with such mutations and ovarian cancer were compared with 53 of their sisters who had one of these mutations. The relative risk for ovarian cancer was estimated to be 0.4 (95% CI, 0.2–0.7) for women who had ever used oral contraceptives and 0.3 (0.1–0.7) for women who had used oral contraceptives for six or more years.

At least two studies (Harlow *et al.*, 1988; Parazzini *et al.*, 1991b) and the pooled analysis of 12 United States studies (Harris *et al.*, 1992) also considered epithelial ovarian tumours of borderline malignancy. An inverse relationship was seen for these neoplasms, suggesting that combined oral contraceptives exert protection against the whole process of epithelial ovarian carcinogenesis.

Little information is available on the different histological types of epithelial ovarian cancer. In a Canadian study (Risch *et al.*, 1996), the inverse association was apparently stronger for non-mucinous (odds ratio per year of use, 0.9; 95% CI, 0.85–0.93) than for mucinous (odds ratio per year of use, 0.97; 0.93–1.04) tumours. This observation, however, requires confirmation.

In the case of non-epithelial ovarian cancers, 38 germ-cell neoplasms and 45 sex-cord-stromal neoplasms were identified from the collaborative analysis of four United States case–control studies (Horn-Ross *et al.*, 1992). The multivariate relative risks for any use of combined oral contraceptives were 2.0 (95% CI, 0.8–5.1) for germ-cell cancers and 0.4 (0.2–0.8) for sex-cord-stromal neoplasms. The data were inadequate to evaluate duration of use or any other time–risk relationship. Similarly, the few available data indicate a consistent inverse association between use of combined oral contraceptives and benign epithelial tumours (ovarian cysts) (Parazzini *et al.*, 1989; Booth *et al.*, 1992) but not benign ovarian teratomas (Westhoff *et al.*, 1988; Parazzini *et al.*, 1995).

The favourable effect of use of combined oral contraceptives on the risk for epithelial ovarian cancer seems to persist for at least 10–15 years after use of the contraceptives has ceased (Cancer and Steroid Hormone Study of the Centers for Disease Control and National Institute of Child Health and Human Development, 1987; Franceschi *et al.*, 1991a; Whittemore *et al.*, 1992; Rosenberg *et al.*, 1994) and is not confined to a particular formulation (Rosenblatt *et al.*, 1992; Rosenberg *et al.*, 1994). There is some suggestion that formulations with lower doses of oestrogen are slightly less protective: in the WHO Collaborative Study on Neoplasia and Steroid Contraceptives (Rosenblatt *et al.*, 1992), the relative risk for ovarian cancer associated with any use of combined oral contraceptives was 0.7 (95% CI, 0.4–1.1) for high-dose preparations and 0.8 (95% CI, 0.5–1.3) for low-dose ones. The available data do not provide definite evidence of an inverse association between use of combined oral contraceptives with low-dose oestrogen and ovarian cancer for longer periods or in relation to recency of use.

The suppression of ovulation induced by oral contraceptives has been suggested to explain the inversion association, since it protects the ovarian epithelium from recurrent trauma and contact with follicular fluid (Fathalla, 1971; Casagrande *et al.*, 1979; Parazzini *et al.*, 1991c). Combined oral contraceptives may also protect against ovarian cancer by reducing exposure to pituitary gonadotropins, which stimulate the growth of cell lines derived from human ovarian carcinoma (Simon *et al.*, 1983). The lack of apparent protection by post-menopausal oestrogen therapy, however, does not support the existence of a favourable role of gonadotropin stimulation on ovarian carcinogenesis.

Since the incidence of ovarian cancer is already appreciable in middle age, and survival from the disease is unsatisfactory, the protection attributable to use of oral contraceptives is important and is therefore one of the major issues in any risk–benefit, public health evaluation of the use of combined oral contraceptives (Gross & Schlesselman, 1994; La Vecchia *et al.*, 1996).

2.5   Cancers of the liver and gall-bladder

The vast majority of primary liver cancers are hepatocellular carcinomas. Chronic infection with hepatitis B (HBV) or C virus causes hepatocellular carcinoma, the relative risk exceeding 50 in many studies (IARC, 1994). Drinking of alcoholic beverages also causes liver cancer (IARC, 1988). Cholangiocarcinoma is much less common, although it is frequent in parts of South-East Asia and can be caused by infection with liver flukes (Parkin *et al.*, 1991).

2.5.1   *Descriptive studies*

Forman *et al.* (1983) analysed the rates of mortality from primary liver cancer among men and women in England and Wales between 1958 and 1981. The age-standardized death rate in women aged 20–39 increased from 0.9 per million in 1970–75 to 1.8 per million in 1976–81 ($p < 0.005$), whereas changes in death rates between these periods among women aged 40–54 and among men were small and not statistically significant. The authors suggested that the change was consistent with the idea that oral contraceptives caused some cases of liver cancer, but noted that no such trend was apparent in Australia, western Germany, the Netherlands or the United States, other countries where oral contraceptive use had been similar to that in England and Wales. In an analysis of subsequent secular trends in mortality in England and Wales, Mant and Vessey (1995) concluded that the rate of mortality from liver cancer had remained constant in women in age groups that had had major exposure to oral contraceptives, and Waetjen and Grimes (1996) found no evidence for an effect of oral contraceptive use on secular trends in liver cancer death rates in Sweden or the United States.

2.5.2 *Cohort studies*

Colditz *et al.* (1994) studied a cohort of 121 700 female registered nurses aged 30–55 in the United States in 1976 who were followed-up for deaths until 1988. Women who reported angina, myocardial infarct, stroke and cancer (other than non-melanoma skin cancer) at baseline were excluded, leaving 116 755 women for follow-up. Of these, 55% reported having used oral contraceptives, and 5% reported current use. It was estimated that 98% of the deaths were ascertained. Incidence rates with person–months of follow-up were used as the denominator and oral contraceptive use at recruitment as the exposure. The relative risks were adjusted for age and for potential confounders including smoking but not alcohol consumption. There were 2879 deaths after 1.4 million women–years of follow-up. The risks associated with any use of oral contraceptives relative to no use, adjusted for age, smoking, body mass index and follow-up interval, were 0.93 (95% CI, 0.85–1.0) for death from any cause and 0.9 (0.8–1.0) for death from any cancer. There were 10 deaths from primary liver or biliary-tract cancer during the 12 years of follow-up, two of which were among women who had used oral contraceptives, with a relative risk of 0.4 (95% CI, 0.1–2.4). No information was provided on infection with hepatitis viruses.

Hannaford *et al.* (1997) described the relationships between use of oral contraceptives and liver disease in two British prospective studies by the Royal College of General Practitioners and the Oxford Family Planning Association. In the first study, 46 000 women, half of whom were using combined oral contraceptives, were recruited in 1968–69 and followed-up until they changed their general practitioner or until 1995. Cancer diagnoses were categorized according to the woman's contraceptive status at the time. There were five cases of liver cancer, comprising one hepatocellular carcinoma in a woman who had never used oral contraceptives, three cholangiocarcinomas in women who had formerly used oral contraceptives and one cholangiocarcinoma in a woman who had never used oral contraceptives. The risk for cholangiocarcinoma associated with former use of oral contraceptives in relation to no use was 3.2 (95% CI, 0.3–31). In a study of mortality in the same cohort after 25 years of follow-up, there were five deaths from liver cancer among women who had used combined oral contraceptives and one in a woman who had never used them, for a relative risk of 5.0 (95% CI, 0.6–43) (Beral *et al.*, 1999). In the study of the Oxford Family Planning Associaiton, 17 032 women were recruited between 1968 and 1974, and most were followed-up until 1994. Three liver cancers were reported, comprising two hepatocellular carcinomas and one cholangiocarcinoma, all in women who had formerly used oral contraceptives. No information on infection with hepatitis viruses was provided.

2.5.3 Case–control studies

(a) Benign neoplasms of the liver

Edmondson *et al.* (1976) interviewed by telephone 34 of 42 eligible women who had undergone surgery for hepatocellular adenoma in Los Angeles, United States, between 1955 and 1976. One age-matched friend control was interviewed for each case. Twenty-eight of the 34 cases (82%) and 19 of 34 controls (56%) had used oral contraceptives for more than 12 months. The risks relative to use of oral contraceptives for less than 12 months were 1.3 for 13–36 months of use, 5.0 for 61–84 months, 7.5 for 85–108 months and 25 for 109 months and longer.

Rooks *et al.* (1979) interviewed 79 of 89 eligible in women aged 16–50 in whom hepatocellular adenoma had been diagnosed between 1960 and 1976 at the Armed Forces Institute of Pathology, Washington DC, United States. Three age-matched neighbourhood controls were sought for each case, and 220 were interviewed. Seventy-two of the 79 cases (91%) and 99 of 220 controls (45.0%) had used oral contraceptives for more than 12 months. The risks relative to use of oral contraceptives for less than 12 months were 9 for 13–36 months of use, 116 for 37–60 months, 129 for 61–84 months and 503 for 85 months and longer.

(b) Malignant tumours of the liver

The studies on malignant tumours of the liver described below are summarized in Table 25.

Henderson *et al.* (1983b) studied women in Los Angeles County, United States, in whom liver cancer had been diagnosed and confirmed histologically during 1975–80 when they were 18–39 years of age. Two neighbourhood controls were sought for each case and matched on age and ethnic group. Twelve cases of liver cancer were identified, and interviews were obtained with 11 of the patients: eight with hepatocellular carcinoma, one with a giant-cell carcinoma, one with a sclerosing duct-forming carcinoma and one with a papillary carcinoma. Four out of 22 identified controls refused to be interviewed and were replaced, giving a response rate among those first selected of 82%; the true response rate was probably lower because the census information used to identify controls could not be obtained for 4.3% of the houses surveyed. Three patients, two with hepatocellular carcinoma, were interviewed in person by telephone; next-of-kin respondents were used for the others. None of the patients or controls reported a prior history of hepatitis or jaundice; none of the four cases had antigens to HBV surface antigen (HBsAg);

Table 25. Case–control studies of use of combined oral contraceptives and cancers of the liver

Reference and study area (period of diagnosis)	Cancer type	Combined oral contraceptives Use	No. of cases	No. of controls	Relative risk (95% CI)	Comments
Henderson et al. (1983b) USA (1975–80)	Hepatocellular	Never	1[a]	8	[1.0]	No association with alcohol use; none of the 4 cases tested had antibodies to HBV surface antigen
		Ever	7	8	[7.0 (0.7–71)] [unmatched analysis]	
	Other	Never	0	1		
		Ever	3	5		
Neuberger et al. (1986) UK (1976–85)	Hepatocellular	*Total group*		*Expected no.*		No information on alcohol use
		Never	8	7.3	1.0	
		Ever	18	18.7	1.0 (0.4–2.4)	
		< 4 years	4	11.4	0.3 (0.1–1.1)	
		4–7 years	5	5.0	0.9 (0.3–3.4)	
		≥ 8 years	9	2.3	4.4 (1.5–13)	
		Excluding HBV-positive		*Expected no.*		
		Never	5	5.9	1.0	
		Ever	17	16.1	1.5 (0.5–4.4)	
		< 4 years	4	9.8	0.5 (0.1–1.9)	
		4–7 years	5	4.5	1.5 (0.4–6.3)	
		≥ 8 years	8	1.8	7.2 (2.0–26)	
Forman et al. (1986) UK (1979–82)	Hepatocellular	Never	4	68	1.0	No information on alcohol use; cases with hepatitis or cirrhosis excluded; no information on HBV status
		Ever	15	79	3.8	
		< 4 years	8	56	3.0	
		4–7 years	4	19	4.0	
		≥ 8 years	3	4	20	
	Cholangio-carcinoma	Never	8	68	1.0	
		Ever	3	79	0.3	
		< 4 years	1	56	0.1	
		≥ 4 years	2	23	0.9	

Table 25 (contd)

Reference and study area (period of diagnosis)	Cancer type	Combined oral contraceptives			Relative risk (95% CI)	Comments
		Use	No. of cases	No. of controls		
Palmer et al. (1989) USA (1977–85)	Hepatocellular	Never	1	29	[1.0]	No information on alcohol use or HBV status; one case of hepatocellular carcinoma had cirrhosis
		Ever	8	16	[14 (1.7–126)]	
		< 2 years	1	7	–	
		2–4 years	4	4	20 (2.0–190)	
		≥ 5 years	3	5	20 (1.6–250)	
	Cholangio-carcinoma	Never	0	8		
		Ever	2	2		
WHO Collaborative Study Group (1989b) Chile, China, Colombia, Israel, Kenya, Nigeria, Philippines, Thailand (1979–86)	Hepatocellular	Never	29	197	1.0	No significant difference in alcohol drinking habits between cases and controls; no information on HBV status, but all centres except one were in endemic areas
		Ever	7	69	0.6 (0.2–1.6)	
		≤ 2 years	6	45	0.8 (0.3–2.2)	
		> 2 years	1	24	0.2 (0.0–1.9)	
	Cholangio-carcinoma	Never	19	162	1.0	
		Ever	11	72	1.2 (0.5–3.1)	
		≤ 2 years	6	41	1.2 (0.4–3.7)	
		> 2 years	5	30	1.3 (0.4–4.1)	
Kew et al. (1990) South Africa (< 1989)	Hepatocellular	Never	39	84	1.0	Association unaltered by adjustment for alcohol use; 19 cases had antibodies to HBV surface antigen
		Ever	7	8	1.9 (0.6–5.6)	
		< 4 years	3	3	2.1 (0.4–11)	
		4–8 years	1	1	2.0 (0.1–33)	
		> 8 years	3	4	1.5 (0.3–7.2)	
Vall Mayans et al. (1990) Spain (1986–88)	Hepatocellular	Never	23	54	1.0	Association unaltered by adjustment for alcohol use; none of the oral contraceptive users had antibodies to HBV surface antigen
		Ever	6	3	[4.7 (1.1–20)]	

Table 25 (contd)

Reference and study area (period of diagnosis)	Cancer type	Combined oral contraceptives			Relative risk (95% CI)	Comments
		Use	No. of cases	No. of controls		
Yu et al. (1991) USA (1984–90)	Hepatocellular	Never	12	40	1.0	Association unaltered by adjustment for alcohol; 7 cases had antibodies to HBV or HCV: exclusion of these increased the association with oral contraceptives
		Ever	13	18	3.0 (1.0–9.0)	
		< 1 year	4	7	2.3 (0.5–11)	
		1–5 years	3	7	1.7 (0.3–9.1)	
		> 5 years	6	4	5.5 (1.2–25)	
Hsing et al. (1992) USA (1985–86)	Hepatocellular	*All subjects*				Adjusted for alcohol use; subjects with cirrhosis were excluded; no information on HBV status
		Never	33	306	1.0	
		Ever	39	243	1.6 (0.9–2.6)	
		< 5 years	16	121	1.2 (0.6–2.4)	
		5–9 years	13	61	2.0 (1.0–4.4)	
		≥ 10 years	8	41	2.0 (0.8–4.8)	
		Spouse or parent respondent				
		Never	17	211	1.0	
		Ever	35	180	2.7 (1.4–5.3)	
		< 5 years	15	93	2.1 (0.9–4.6)	
		5–9 years	13	48	3.9 (1.6–9.6)	
		≥ 10 years	7	26	4.8 (1.7–14)	
	Cholangio-carcinoma	*Spouse or parent respondent*				
		Never	7	211	1.0	
		Ever	6	180	0.8 (0.3–2.7)	
		< 5 years	2	93	0.5 (0.1–2.7)	
		5–9 years	1	48	0.6 (0.1–5.4)	
		≥ 10 years	3	26	3.3 (0.7–16)	

Table 25 (contd)

Reference and study area (period of diagnosis)	Cancer type	Combined oral contraceptives			Relative risk (95% CI)	Comments
		Use	No. of cases	No. of controls		
Tavani et al. (1993b) Italy (1984–92)	Hepatocellular	Never	34	173	1.0	Association unaltered by adjustment for alcohol use; no information on HBV status; relative risk, 4.3 (1.0–18) > 10 years after last use
		Ever	9	21	2.6 (1.0–7.0)	
		≤ 5 years	5	17	1.5 (0.5–5.0)	
		> 5 years	2	4	3.9 (0.6–25)	
Collaborative MILTS Project Team (1997) France, Germany, Greece, Italy, Spain, UK (1990–96)	Hepatocellular	All subjects				Association unaltered by adjustment for alcohol
		Never	145	693	1.0	
		Ever	148	1 086	0.8 (0.5–1.0)	
		1–2 years	26	238	0.8 (0.5–1.3)	
		3–5 years	26	201	0.6 (0.3–1.1)	
		≥ 6 years	90	638	0.8 (0.5–1.1)	
		No cirrhosis or HBV or HCV				
		Never	16	250	1.0	
		Ever	35	324	[1.7 (0.9–3.1)] [unmatched analysis]	
		1–2 years	5	74	1.3 (0.4–4.0)	
		3–5 years	5	57	1.8 (0.5–6.0)	
		≥ 6 years	25	193	2.8 (1.3–6.3)	

CI, confidence interval; HBV, hepatitis B virus; HCV, hepatitis C virus
a This case had received injections of hormones of undetermined type for nine months.

none of the patients reported exposure to any known hepatotoxin such as vinyl chloride, and there was no difference in the frequency of alcohol consumption between cases and controls. Smoking histories were not reported. Ten of the 11 patients (seven of the eight cases of hepatocellular carcinoma) had used oral contraceptives, and the eleventh had received hormone injections of an undetermined type; 13 of the 22 controls had used oral contraceptives. The average duration of use of oral contraceptives was 64.7 months for the patients and 27.1 months for the controls (one-sided matched $p < 0.005$). [The relative risk for any use of oral contraceptives was 7.0 (95% CI, 0.7–71) for hepatocellular carcinoma and 6.9 (0.7–64) for all liver cancers (unmatched analyses).]

Neuberger *et al.* (1986) studied 26 women in whom hepatocellular carcinoma had been diagnosed and confirmed histologically in a non-cirrhotic liver when they were under the age of 50. The cases were referred from all over Britain to the Liver Unit at King's College School of Medicine and Dentistry, London, between 1976 and 1985. The controls were 1333 women who were hospital controls in a case–control study of breast cancer and had been interviewed during 1976–80; the response rate was not given. The source of information on the exposures of the cases is not specified, but may have been interviews. The results were not adjusted for smoking or alcohol use. Eighteen of the 26 case women had taken oral contraceptives. The controls were used to calculate the expected numbers of cases for each duration of pill use, within age and calendar groups. The expected number of women who had ever used oral contraceptives was 18.7, giving a relative risk of 1.0 (95% CI, 0.4–2.4). The relative risks for durations of use were 0.3 (95% CI, 0.1–1.1) for < 4 years, 0.9 (0.3–3.4) for 4–7 years and 4.4 (1.5–13) for ≥ 8 years. None of the case women had HBsAg, but one had antisurface antibodies and three had anticore antibodies. Exclusion of these four cases changed the relative risks associated with oral contraceptive use to 1.5 (95% CI, 0.5–4.4) for any use, 0.5 (0.1–1.9) for < 4 years, 1.5 (0.4–6.3) for 4–7 years and 7.2 (95% CI, 2.0–26) for ≥ 8 years. Three cases in this study were also included in the study of Forman *et al.* (1986), described below.

Forman *et al.* (1986) identified all women certified to have died from liver cancer at the age of 20–44 in England and Wales between 1979 and 1982. Deaths from secondary liver cancer or from benign liver tumours were excluded. Two controls were selected for each case from among women who had died from cancer of the kidney, cancer of the brain or acute myeloid leukaemia, and, for 1982 only, two further controls were selected for each case from among women who had died as a result of a road traffic accident. Information on exposure was obtained from a questionnaire sent to the general practitioners of cases, and information was obtained for 46 of 85 (54.1%) potential cases and for 147 of 233 (63.1%) eligible controls. Further information, including pathological data, was sought for potential cases and resulted in 35 confirmed cases of primary liver cancer, of which 24 were hepatocellular carcinoma and 11 were cholangiocarcinoma. Five of the deaths from hepatocellular carcinoma were excluded from the analysis, two because they had had chronic active hepatitis, two because they had had severe alcoholic disease and associated liver cirrhosis and one because she had had Down's syndrome, which might have prejudiced the prescription of oral contraceptives. Eighteen of the 30 case women

(15 of the 19 with hepatocellular carcinoma) had used oral contraceptives, compared with 79 of the 147 controls. Information on smoking and alcohol habits was not available. The relative risks, adjusted for age and year of birth, were: for hepatocellular carcinoma, 3.8 for any use, 3.0 for use for < 4 years, 4.0 for 4–7 years and 20.1 for ≥ 8 years; for cholangiocarcinoma, 0.3 for any use, 0.1 for < 4 years and 0.9 for ≥ 4 years. [The published relative risks were adjusted for age and year of birth, but confidence intervals were not given. The unadjusted relative risks and 95% confidence intervals, calculated from the published data, were: hepatocellular carcinoma, any use, 3.2 (95% CI, 1.0–10); < 4 years, 2.4 (0.7–8.5); 4–7 years, 3.6 (0.8–16); and ≥ 8 years, 13 (2.1–78); cholangiocarcinoma, any use, 0.3 (95% CI, 0.1–1.3); < 4 years, 0.2 (0.0–1.3); ≥ 4 years, 0.7 (95% CI, 0.2–3.7).] There was no information on infection with hepatitis viruses. Three cases in this study were also included in the study of Neuberger *et al.* (1986), described above.

Palmer *et al.* (1989) conducted a hospital-based case–control study of women in whom liver cancer had been diagnosed when they were 19–54 years of age in five United States cities in 1977–85. They identified 12 cases of liver cancer, of which nine were hepatocellular carcinoma, two were cholangiocarcinoma and one was undetermined. None of the case women reported a history of hepatitis, nor was there mention in their hospital discharge summaries of HBV infection; liver cirrhosis was discovered at the time of surgery in one case of hepatocellular carcinoma. Five controls were selected for each case and matched on hospital, age and date of interview; the diagnoses of controls were trauma for 16, eight herniated discs, five acute respiratory infections and 31 eye, ear and gastrointestinal conditions. Information on exposure was obtained from case and control women at interview. Overall, 95% of the subjects approached were interviewed. Smoking status was not reported, but alcohol intake was similar in cases and controls. Eleven of the 12 case women (eight of the nine cases of hepatocellular carcinoma) and 20 of the 60 controls had used oral contraceptives. The risk for hepatocellular carcinoma relative to women who had used oral contraceptives for < 2 years was 20 (95% CI, 2.0–190) for 2–4 years of use and 20 (1.6–250) for ≥ 5 years of use. [The unmatched relative risk for any use was 15 (95% CI, 1.7–126).]

The WHO Collaborative Study of Neoplasia and Steroid Contraceptives (1989b) was a hospital-based case–control study conducted in eight countries. The eligible cases were those of women in whom liver cancer was diagnosed between 1979 and 1986 and who were born after 1924 or 1929. A total of 168 eligible cases were identified; 122 (72.6%) of the diagnoses were confirmed, and these women were interviewed. Histological typing was available for 69 cases: 36 were hepatocellular carcinoma, 29 were cholangiocarcinoma, one was an adenocarcinoma and three were other types. Controls were selected from among individuals admitted to the same hospitals as the cases with conditions not thought to be related to use of oral contraceptives. The aim was to select two controls for each case, but controls were not individually matched to cases; there was thus a pool of over 14 000 controls, from whom up to eight were selected for each case of liver cancer, matched on age, study centre and year of interview. The overall response rate of controls was 94.3%. All case and control women were interviewed. Information on smoking was not collected; there was no statistically significant difference between case and control women in alcohol consumption, 17.2% of the cases and 26% of the controls having ever drunk alcohol. The finding that 25 of the 122 cases (20.5%) and 216 of the 802 controls (26.9%) had used oral contraceptives gave relative risks, adjusted for number of live births and occupation, of 0.7 (95% CI, 0.4–1.2) for any use, 0.8 (0.4–1.5) for use for 1–12 months, 0.7 (0.3–1.7) for 13–36 months and 0.7 (0.3–1.7) for ≥ 37 months. The relative risks for any use by histological subtype were 0.6 (95% CI, 0.2–1.6) for hepatocellular carcinoma, 1.2 (0.5–3.1) for cholangiocarcinoma and 0.5 (0.2–1.3) for a clinical diagnosis with no histological confirmation. Information on prior infection with hepatitis viruses was not collected, but all except one of the study centres were in countries with high rates of liver cancer and where HBV infection is endemic.

Kew *et al.* (1990) conducted a hospital-based case–control study in Johannesburg, South Africa, among patients in whom histologically confirmed hepatocellular carcinoma was diagnosed when they were aged 19–54. Two controls per case were selected and matched on age, race, tribe, rural or urban birth, hospital and ward. Patients with diseases in which contraceptive steroids might be causally implicated were not considered eligible as controls. All of the subjects were interviewed, but the response rates were not given. Smoking and alcohol intake were associated with the risk for liver cancer, but inclusion of these variables in the analysis did not alter the results. Seven of 46 cases (15.2%) and eight of 92 controls (8.7%) had used oral contraceptives, giving an overall relative risk of 1.9 (95% CI, 0.6–5.6). The relative risks were 2.1 (95% CI, 0.4–11) for use for < 4 years, 2.0 (0.1–33) for 4–8 years and 1.5 (95% CI, 0.3–7.2) for > 8 years. Nineteen of the 46 cases were HBsAg-positive, 25 had evidence of past infection with HBV, and two had never been infected. The relative risk for hepatocellular carcinoma in HBsAg-negative patients who used contraceptive steroids of any type was 0.4 (95% CI, 0.2–1.0).

Vall Mayans *et al.* (1990) conducted a hospital-based case–control study in Catalonia, north-eastern Spain, where 96 patients admitted to the Liver Unit of the University Hospital in Barcelona between 1986 and 1988 were identified, 74 of whom had histo-logically or cytologically confirmed hepatocellular carcinoma. Liver cirrhosis was present in 83 (86.5%) cases. For the 29 cases in women, two controls were selected per case and matched on sex, age, hospital and time of admission. Patients with diagnoses related to use of oral contraceptives were considered ineligible as controls. One control was excluded from the analysis because of later confirmation of liver cirrhosis. Serum from all patients was tested for HBsAg, antibody to hepatitis B core antigen and antibody to hepatitis surface antigen. All patients were interviewed, but the response rates were not given. Smoking was not associated with risk, and adjustment for alcohol intake did not alter the results. Six of the 29 female cases (20.7%) and three of the 57 female controls (5.3%) had used oral contraceptives [unmatched relative risk, 4.7 (95% CI, 1.1–20)]. Overall, 9.4% of cases and 2.1% of controls were HBsAg-positive, and all of the users of oral contraceptives were HBsAg-negative.

Yu *et al.* (1991) used a population-based cancer registry to identify cases of histo-logically confirmed hepatocellular carcinoma diagnosed in black or white non-Asian women residents aged 18–74 in Los Angeles County, United States, between 1984 and 1990. Two neighbourhood controls were sought for each case and matched on sex, year of birth and race. Eighty-four of 412 eligible patients (20.4%) were interviewed (70.6% died before contact could be made), of which 10 were excluded from the analysis because the diagnosis of hepatocellular carcinoma was not confirmed. The response rate among the controls first selected was 71%. Adjustment for smoking and alcohol did not alter the results. Thirteen of the 25 case women (52%) and 18 of the 58 controls (31%) had used oral contraceptives. The relative risks were 3.0 (95% CI, 1.0–9.0) for any use, 2.3 (0.5–11) for use for ≤ 12 months, 1.7 (95% CI, 0.3–9.1) for 13–60 months and 5.5 (95% CI, 1.2–25) for ≥ 61 months. For the 11 case women who had formerly used oral contraceptives, the mean time since last use was 14.5 years. Seven case women had antibodies to one or more markers of hepatitis viral infection; when these cases were excluded, the association between use of oral contraceptives and the risk for hepatocellular carcinoma became stronger.

Hsing *et al.* (1992) studied deaths from primary liver cancer among women aged 25–49 in the United States (except Oregon) in 1985 and in the National Mortality Followback Survey in 1986. Of the 203 deaths from liver cancer identified, 52 cases not specified as primary, four cases of chronic liver disease and 29 cases with a history of liver cirrhosis were excluded. This left 98 cases for analysis, of which 76 were primary liver cancer and 22 were cholangiocarcinoma. Controls were selected from among women in the National Mortality Followback Study who had died in 1986 from causes other than liver cancer and whose next-of-kin returned the questionnaire. Potential controls with evidence of chronic liver disease or whose causes of death were thought to be associated with oral contraceptive use were excluded, leaving 629 controls for analysis. Information on exposure was obtained from next-of-kin by postal questionnaire. The results were presented both for all subjects and for subjects for whom the respondent was the spouse or parent (thought to be more reliable). The relative risks were adjusted for smoking and alcohol use. For all subjects with complete data, 39 of 72 cases (54.2%) and 243 of 549 controls (44.3%) had ever used oral contraceptives; the relative risks were 1.6 (95% CI, 0.9–2.6) for any use, 1.2 (0.6–2.4) for use for < 5 years, 2.0 (1.0–4.4) for 5–9 years and 2.0 (0.8–4.8) for ≥ 10 years. For subjects whose spouse or parent responded, the relative risks were 2.7 (95% CI, 1.4–5.3) for any use, 2.1 (0.9–4.6) for use for < 5 years, 3.9 (1.6–9.6) for 5–9 years and 4.8 (1.7–14) for ≥ 10 years. When the four Asian cases and 10 controls, from populations presumed to have a higher prevalence of HBV infection, were excluded from the analysis, higher risk estimates were seen for any use (2.8; 95% CI, 1.4–5.5) and for long-term (≥ 10 years) use (5.2; 1.7–15). The relative risks for the 13 cases of cholangiocarcinoma were 0.8 (95% CI, 0.3–2.7) for any use, 0.5 (0.1–2.7) for < 5 years of use, 0.6 (0.1–5.4) for 5–9 years and 3.3 (0.7–16) for ≥ 10 years.

Tavani *et al.* (1993b) conducted a hospital-based case–control study of women with histologically or serologically confirmed hepatocellular carcinoma diagnosed at the age of 28–73 in the greater Milan area, Italy, between 1984 and 1992. The controls were women admitted to hospital for acute non-neoplastic diseases (37% traumas, 13% other orthopaedic disorders, 40% acute surgical conditions, 10% other). Since none of the women aged 60 or over had ever used oral contraceptives, the analysis was restricted to women under that age. All of the participating subjects were interviewed; the response rates were not given but were close to 100% in other reports of this study. The results were not adjusted for smoking or alcohol use. Nine of the 43 cases (20.9%) and 21 of the 194 controls (10.8%) had ever used oral contraceptives. The relative risks, adjusted for age, education and parity, were 2.6 (95% CI, 1.0–7.0) for any use, 1.5 (0.5–5.0) for use for ≤ 5 years and 3.9 (0.6–25) for use for > 5 years. In relation to time since oral contraceptives were last used, the relative risks were 1.1 (95% CI, 0.3–4.6) for ≤ 10 years and 4.3 (1.0–18) for > 10 years. There was no information on infection with hepatitis viruses.

The Multicentre International Liver Tumour Study (Collaborative MILTS Project Team, 1997) included women with hepatocellular carcinoma diagnosed before the age of 65 between 1990 and 1996 in seven hospitals in Germany and one each in France, Greece, Italy, Spain and the United Kingdom. The diagnoses were based on histological examination or on imaging and increased α-fetoprotein concentration. An average of four controls was sought for each case: two general hospital controls without cancer, one hospital control with an eligible tumour diagnosis and one population control. The controls were frequency matched for age, and living controls were obtained for cases who had died. Of the 368 eligible cases, 317 (86.1%) were included in the study, although 24 of these were excluded from the analysis because of missing information on confounding factors. Information was obtained at interview, except for 136 case women (42.9%) who had died or who could not be interviewed for other reasons, for whom a next-of-kin was interviewed. The overall response rate for controls was not given, but that for hospitalized patients (cases and hospital controls) varied from 68 to 100% between centres, whereas the response rate for population controls varied from 60 to 80% between countries. Smoking and alcohol use were considered as confounders but were not included in the models presented. Oral contraceptive use was reported for 148 of the 293 cases (50.5%) and 1086 of the 1779 controls (61.0%). The relative risk for any use of oral contraceptives was 0.8 (95% CI, 0.5–1.0), and those for durations of use were 0.8 (0.5–1.3) for 1–2 years, 0.6 (0.3–1.1) for 3–5 years and 0.8 (95% CI, 0.5–1.1) for ≥ 6 years. For use of oral contraceptives containing cyproterone acetate, the relative risks were 0.9 (95% CI, 0.5–1.6) for any use, 0.9 (0.4–2.4) for use for 1–2 years, 0.9 (0.3–2.4) for 3–5 years and 0.9 (95% CI, 0.4–2.0) for ≥ 6 years. When the analysis was restricted to the 51 cases without liver cirrhosis or evidence of infection with hepatitis viruses, the relative risks were 1.3 (95% CI, 0.4–4.0) for use of any oral contraceptives for 1–2 years, 1.8 (0.5–6.0) for 3–5 years and 2.8 (1.3–6.3) for ≥ 6 years.

(c)   Gall-bladder

Yen *et al.* (1987) studied extrahepatic bile-duct cancers in Massachusetts and Rhode Island, United States, between 1975 and 1979 in 27 women with histologically confirmed bile-duct cancer and 152 controls, who were patients with a variety of other cancers. All of the subjects were interviewed. Of the women under 60 years of age, four of 10 cases and six of 76 controls reported use of combined oral contraceptives (age-adjusted relative risk, 7.8; 95% CI, 2.0–30).

The relationship between use of combined oral contraceptives and risk for primary gall-bladder cancer was examined in 58 case and 355 control women who were participating in an international hospital-based case–control study during 1979–86 (WHO Collaborative Study of Neoplasia and Steroid Contraceptives, 1989c). Any use of combined oral contraceptives was not associated with risk, adjusted for age and history of gall-bladder disease (relative risk, 0.6; 95% CI, 0.3–1.3), and no increase in risk was seen among women who had taken combined oral contraceptives for more than three years (0.6; 0.2–2.2) or more than 12 years before cancer diagnosis (0.6; 0.2–1.8).

2.6   Colorectal cancer

2.6.1   Cohort studies

The Walnut Creek Contraceptive Drug Study (1981) showed no association between use of combined oral contraceptives and all cancers of the digestive tract (age-adjusted relative risk, 0.9; 95% CI, 0.4–2.0). [The majority of these cancers were probably colorectal cancers.] The results of cohort studies that specifically addressed colorectal cancers are shown in Table 26.

Reports on the association between use of combined oral contraceptives and the risk for colorectal cancer were made from the the Nurses' Health Study (Chute *et al.*, 1991; Martinez *et al.*, 1997). Follow-up until 1992 of 89 448 nurses for over 1 million person–years, with 501 incident cases of colorectal cancer, showed a relative risk adjusted for age, body mass index, exercise, family history of cancer, aspirin use, alcohol use, smoking, meat intake and reproductive factors of 0.8 (95% CI, 0.7–1.0). Women who had used combined oral contraceptives for 96 months or more were at significantly lower risk (0.6; 95% CI, 0.4–0.9). The results for colon cancer were similar to those for rectal cancer.

In the Iowa Women's Health Study cohort (Bostick *et al.*, 1994), described in the monograph on 'Post-menopausal oestrogen therapy', the prevalence of any use of combined oral contraceptives was 17% among women with colon cancer and 19% among women without colon cancer. Any use was associated with a relative risk, adjusted for age, height, parity, energy intake and vitamin intake, of 1.0 (95% CI, 0.7–1.4).

Beral *et al.* (1999) reported on a 25-year follow-up of 46 000 women who were recruited in 1968-69 by general practitioners throughout Britain. At recruitment, 49% of the women were using combined oral contraceptives; by the end of the follow-up, 63% had used them at some time, the median duration of use being four years. The relative risk for death from colorectal cancer among women who had ever used combined oral contraceptives, adjusted for age, parity, social class and smoking, was 0.6 (95% CI, 0.4–0.9). The trend in risk by duration of use was not significant. The relative risk of women who had last used combined oral contraceptives 15 years or more previously was 1.0 (95% CI, 0.5–2.0) and that for death from all cancers combined for any use was 1.0 (95% CI, 0.8–1.1).

Table 26. Cohort studies of use of combined oral contraceptives and colorectal cancer

Reference	Country	Study population (follow-up) no. of cancers	RR (95% CI) (any versus no use)			Duration of use	Adjustment/comments
			Colon–rectum	Colon	Rectum		
Martinez et al. (1997) (Nurses Health Study)	USA	89 448 (12 years) 501	0.8 (0.7–1.0)	0.6 (0.4–1.0)	0.8 (0.5–1.2)	Significant trend (RR for ≥ 8 years' use, 0.6; 95% CI, 0.4–0.9)	Age, body mass index, exercise, family history of cancer, aspirin use, alcohol use, smoking, meat intake and reproductive factors Prevalence of combined oral contraceptive use, 32%; mostly past use
Bostick et al. (1994)	Iowa, USA	35 215 (4 years) 212	–	1.0 (0.7–1.4)	–	Not reported	Adjusted for age, height, parity, energy and vitamin intake Prevalence of combined oral contraceptive use, 19%
Beral et al. (1999)	United Kingdom	46 000 (25 years) 170 deaths	0.6 (0.4–0.9)	–	–	No trend	Mortality rates, adjusted for age, parity, social class and smoking RR for ≥ 10 years of use, 0.3 (0.1–1.2); RR for last use ≥ 15 years previously, 1.0 (0.5–2.0)

RR, relative risk; CI, confidence interval

2.6.2   *Case–control studies*
   (*a*)   *Colorectal polyps*

In a study by Jacobson *et al.* (1995) in New York City, United States, described in detail in the monograph on 'Post-menopausal oestrogen therapy', a lower frequency of any use of combined oral contraceptives was found among cases of colorectal polyps (72/280) than among control women (19/126) (relative risk, 0.6; 95% CI, 0.3–1.1).

Potter *et al.* (1996) in a study in Minnesota, United States, described in detail in the monograph on 'Post-menopausal oestrogen therapy', found similar proportions of women who had ever used combined oral contraceptives among women with and without polyps; the risk associated with ≥ 5 years of use relative to that of women who had not undergone colonoscopy was 0.8 (95% CI, 0.5–1.4) and that relative to community controls was 1.1 (0.6–1.8).

   (*b*)   *Colorectal cancer*

Several of the case–control investigations on use of combined oral contraceptives and colorectal cancer risk are also described in the monographs on 'Post-menopausal oestrogen therapy' and 'Post-menopausal oestrogen–progestogen therapy', and are summarized only briefly here. Table 27 lists the studies summarized below.

Weiss *et al.* (1981b), in a study in the United States described in detail in the monograph on 'Post-menopausal oestrogen therapy', reported that any use of combined oral contraceptives was commoner among cases (33%) than among controls (23%), but the difference was not significant. The age-adjusted relative risks were 1.3 (95% CI, 0.5–3.1) for < 5 years of use and 2.0 (0.7–5.2) for ≥ 5 years of use. The relative risks for any use were 1.0 for colon cancer and 2.6 ($p = 0.09$) for rectal cancer.

Potter and McMichael (1983), in Adelaide, Australia, found that use of combined oral contraceptives was slightly less common among cases of colon cancer than among controls, with a relative risk adjusted for reproductive variables of 0.5 (95% CI, 0.3–1.2) for any versus no use. The relative risk for rectal cancer was 0.7 (95% CI, 0.3–1.8), with a trend of decreasing risk with increasing duration of use (relative risk for ≥ 25 months of use, 0.2; 95% CI, 0.0–1.0).

In the case–control study of Furner *et al.* (1989) described in detail in the monograph on 'Post-menopausal oestrogen therapy', the crude relationship between colorectal cancer and the use of combined oral contraceptives was 0.6 (95% CI, 0.3–1.3); only nine case and 32 control women had ever used combined oral contraceptives.

A case–control study conducted by Kune *et al.* (1990) in Melbourne, Australia, between 1980 and 1981 included all local incident cases of colorectal cancer (108 colon and 82 rectum) and 200 age-matched female controls representing a random sample of local population. The relative risks, adjusted for reproductive factors, of women who had ever used combined oral contraceptives were 1.2 (95% CI, 0.6–2.3) for colon and 2.0 (95% CI, 1.0–4.1) for rectal cancer. The relative risks associated with more than nine years' duration of use, however, were 0.7 for colon and 0.9 for rectal cancer [confidence intervals not given].

Table 27. Case–control studies of use of combined oral contraceptives and colorectal cancer

Reference	Country	Cases : controls (type of controls)	RR (95% CI) (any versus no use)			Duration of use	Recency of use	Adjustments/Comments
			Colon–rectum	Colon	Rectum			
Weiss et al. (1981b)	Washington, USA	143 : 707 (population)	≤ 5 years, 1.3 (0.5–3.1) ≥ 5 years, 2.0 (0.7–5.2)	1.0	2.6 (p = 0.09)	No significant trend	Not reported	Age; Prevalence of combined oral contraceptive use was about 30% (22% for ≥ 5 years' use)
Potter & McMichael (1983)	Adelaide, Australia	155 : 311 (population)	–	0.5 (0.3–1.2)	0.7 (0.3–1.8)	Inverse trend (RR for > 2 years' use, 0.20; 95% CI, 0.0–1.0)	Not reported	Reproductive variables (diet was influential); Prevalence of combined oral contraceptive use among controls, 18%
Furner et al. (1989)	Chicago, USA	90 : 208 (spouses)	0.6 (0.3–1.3)	–	–	Not reported	Not reported	Unadjusted; Prevalence of combined oral contraceptive use among controls, 6%
Kune et al. (1990)	Melbourne, Australia	190 : 200 (population)	–	1.2 (0.6–2.3)	2.0 (1.0–4.1)	No effect (RR for > 9 years use, 0.7 for colon and 0.9 for rectum; not significant)	Not reported	Age, parity and age at birth of first child; Prevalence of combined oral contraceptive use among controls, 20%
Fernandez et al. (1998a)	Italy	1232 : 2793 (hospital)	0.6 (0.5–0.9)	0.7 (0.5–0.9)	0.7 (0.5–1.1)	No effect	Stronger protection from recent use (RR for < 10 years, 0.4; 95% CI, 0.3–0.7)	Age, education, cancer family history, body mass index, oestrogen replacement therapy, parity, menopause and energy intake; Prevalence of use of combined oral contraceptives among controls, 12%

Table 27 (contd)

Reference	Country	Cases : controls (type of controls)	RR (95% CI) (any versus no use)			Duration of use	Recency of use	Adjustments/Comments
			Colon–rectum	Colon	Rectum			
Peters et al. (1990)	Los Angeles, USA	327 : 327 (neighbours)	–	**< 5 years:** 1.0 (0.6–1.8); right colon, 1.4 (0.6–3.3); left colon, 0.7 (0.3–1.5) **≥ 5 years:** 1.1 (0.4–2.9); right colon, 1.3 (0.3–5.5); left colon, 1.0 (0.2–4.8)	–	No effect	Not reported	Family history of cancer, parity, exercise, fat, alcohol and calcium intake / Prevalence of combined oral contraceptive use among controls, 19%
Franceschi et al. (1991b)	North-eastern Italy	89 : 148 (hospital)	0.2 (0.0–2.0)	–	–	Not reported	Not reported	Unadjusted / Only 1 case and 9 controls had ever used combined oral contraceptives
Wu-Williams et al. (1991)	North America and China	395 : 1112 (neighbours)	–	North America: 1.2 ($p = 0.67$); China: 0.6 ($p = 0.27$)	North America: 0.4 ($p = 0.04$); China: 0.7 ($p = 0.34$)	No trend	Not reported	Unadjusted (but unaltered by exercise, saturated fat and years in the USA) / Prevalence of combined oral contraceptive use among controls, 16% in North America and 12% in China
Jacobs et al. (1994)	Seattle, USA	193 : 194 (population)	–	1.2 (0.7–1.9); right colon, 1.2 (0.7–2.3); left colon, 1.1 (0.6–2.1)	–	No trend	Not reported	Age, age at birth of first child and vitamin intake / Prevalence of combined oral contraceptive use among controls, 27%

Table 27 (contd)

Reference	Country	Cases : controls (type of controls)	RR (95% CI) (any versus no use)			Duration of use	Recency of use	Adjustments/Comments
			Colon–rectum	Colon	Rectum			
Kampman *et al.* (1997)	USA	894 : 1120 (members of medical care programme)	–	0.9 (0.7–1.1)	–	Not reported	Not reported	Age, family history of colorectal cancer, aspirin use, energy intake, post-menopausal oestrogen therapy and exercise Prevalence of combined oral contraceptive use among controls, 25%

RR, relative risk; CI, confidence interval

Franceschi *et al.* (1991b) carried out a case–control study in north-eastern Italy which included a very few users of combined oral contraceptives (one case and nine controls). The crude relative risk was 0.2, but the 95% CI (0.0–2.0) was very broad.

A pooled analysis of a case–control study from Milan (Negri *et al.*, 1989; Fernandez *et al.*, 1996) and a multicentre study from Italy (Talamini *et al.*, 1998) which involved 803 cases of colon cancer, 429 of rectal cancer and 2793 hospital controls (Fernandez *et al.*, 1998) provided a relative risk estimate (adjusted for age, education, family history of cancer, body mass index, parity, menopause, use of post-menopausal oestrogen therapy and energy intake) of 0.6 (95% CI, 0.5–0.9) for colon cancer and 0.7 (0.4–1.0) for rectal cancer for women who had ever used combined oral contraceptives. Increasing duration of use was related to a decreasing risk for colon cancer. The relative risk for recent users (< 10 years since last use) was 0.4 (95% CI, 0.3–0.7). Similar patterns of risk were found for various strata of age, educational level, parity, family history of colorectal cancer and body mass index.

In the case–control study of Peters *et al.* (1990) in Los Angeles, United States, described in detail in the monograph on 'Post-menopausal oestrogen therapy', use of combined oral contraceptives was not associated with an increased risk for colon cancer. The relative risk, adjusted for family history of cancer, parity, exercise and fat, alcohol and calcium intake, was 1.1 (95% CI, 0.4–2.9) for ≥ 5 years of use. This estimate was based on very few long-term users (13 cases and 15 controls).

The study by Wu-Williams *et al.* (1991), among Chinese women in North America and China, also described in the monograph on 'Post-menopausal oestrogen therapy', included small proportions of women who had ever used combined oral contraceptives: 16% in North America and 12% in China. The crude relative risks for rectal cancer were 0.4 ($p = 0.04$) in North America and 0.7 ($p = 0.34$) in China, and those for colon cancer were 1.2 ($p = 0.67$) and 0.55 ($p = 0.27$), respectively.

In the study of Jacobs *et al.* (1994) in Seattle, United States, described in the monograph on 'Post-menopausal oestrogen therapy', any use of combined oral contraceptives was reported by about 25% of both women with colon cancer and controls. The relative risk, adjusted for age and vitamin intake was 1.2 (95% CI, 0.7–1.9).

Kampman *et al.* (1997), in a study described in the monograph on 'Post-menopausal oestrogen therapy', did not find a significant association between the risk for colon cancer and use of combined oral contraceptives, which was reported by about 25% of cases and controls. The relative risk, adjusted for age, family history of colorectal cancer, aspirin use and energy intake, was 0.9 (95% CI, 0.7–1.1).

2.7   Cutaneous malignant melanoma

2.7.1   *Cohort studies*

In the late 1960s, three large cohort studies of users of combined oral contraceptives were begun (Table 28). All three provided information on the risk for cutaneous malignant melanoma according to use of combined oral contraceptives, but were based on small numbers of observed cases. Furthermore, it was not possible in any of the studies

Table 28. Cohort studies of use of combined oral contraceptives and risk for cutaneous malignant melanoma

Reference	Country, study	Population (follow-up), no. of cancers	RR (95% CI) any versus no use	Duration of use	Recency of use	Adjustments/comments
Hannaford et al. (1991)	United Kingdom, Oxford Family Planning Association	17 032 (15 years) 32	0.8 (0.4–1.8)	No trend (RR for ≥ 10 years' use, 1.0; 95% CI, 0.2–1.6)	No effect	Age, parity, social class and smoking No increase in risk for any combined oral contraceptive formulation
	United Kingdom, Royal College of General Practitioners	23 000 (20 years) 58	0.9 (0.6–1.5)	No trend (RR for ≥ 10 years' use, 1.8; 95% CI, 0.8–3.9)	No effect	Age, parity, social class and smoking No risk increase for any combined oral contraceptive formulation
Ramcharan et al. (1981b)	California, USA, Walnut Creek Contraceptive Drug Study	17 942 (8 years) 20	3.5 (1.4–9.0)	No trend	Not reported	Age
Bain et al. (1982)	USA, Nurses' Health Study	121 964 (at start) 141	0.8 (0.5–1.3) women < 40 years, 1.4 (0.8–2.5)	No trend	No effect	Age, parity, height and hair dye use Nested case–control investigation (141 non-fatal cutaneous malignant melanomas and 2820 age-matched controls)

RR, relative risk; CI, confidence interval

to make allowance for major determinants of cutaneous malignant melanoma such as solar exposure and phenotypic characteristics.

Between 1968 and 1974, 17 032 white married women aged 25–39 were recruited at 17 family planning clinics in the United Kingdom, in the framework of a study by the Oxford Family Planning Association (Adam *et al.*, 1981; Hannaford *et al.*, 1991). On entry, 56% of women were taking oral contraceptives, 25% were using a diaphragm and 19% were using an intrauterine device. Since, during the course of the study, each woman's oral contraceptive status could change, users of these preparations might have contributed periods of observation for either current or former users. After 266 866 woman–years of follow-up, 32 new cases of cutaneous malignant melanoma were recorded, 17 of which were among women who had ever used oral contraceptives (relative risk, 0.8; 95% CI, 0.4–1.8). None of the rates observed in any category of duration of use was materially different from that seen in women who had never used these preparations. The relative risks, adjusted for age, parity, social class and smoking, were 0.6 (95% CI, 0.2–1.6) for < 5 years of use, 1.0 (0.4–2.6) for 5–9 years and 1.0 (0.2–3.1) for ≥ 10 years. There was no relationship between time since stopping use of oral contraceptives and the risk for cutaneous malignant melanoma. None of the formulations resulted in a specific risk pattern. The distribution of cutaneous malignant melanomas by site was similar in users and non-users of oral contraceptives.

Between 1968 and 1969, 1400 general practitioners throughout the United Kingdom recruited 23 000 women who were using oral contraceptives and a similar number of age-matched women who had never used them, in the framework of the study of the Royal College of General Practitioners (Kay, 1981; Hannaford *et al.*, 1991). After 482 083 woman–years of follow-up, 58 new cases of cutaneous malignant melanoma had been recorded, 31 of which were among women who had ever used combined oral contraceptives; the relative risk, adjusted for age, parity, social class and smoking, was 0.9 (95% CI, 0.6–1.5). No significant trend of increasing risk with duration of use was seen, the relative risk for 10 years or more of use being 1.8 (95% CI, 0.8–3.9), and the relative risk did not vary according to recency of use, the oestrogen or progestogen content of the contraceptives or the site of cutaneous malignant melanoma.

A cohort study of 17 942 women who were members of the Kaiser-Permanente Health Plan, in California, United States, aged 18 and older, was established in 1970 within the Walnut Creek Contraceptive Drug Study. Ramcharan *et al.* (1981b) updated the preliminary findings of Beral *et al.* (1977) to approximately eight years of follow-up and observed 20 cases of cutaneous malignant melanoma (age-adjusted relative risk, 3.5; 95% CI, 1.4–9.0). All five cases in women 18–39 years of age occurred among users of combined oral contraceptives. The influence of duration and recency of use was not assessed. The percentage distribution of hours of exposure to the sun by current, past or no use of combined oral contraceptives was similar.

In a postal survey of 121 964 registered nurses in the United States in 1976 (Bain *et al.*, 1982), no overall relationship was found between risk for cutaneous malignant melanoma and use of combined oral contraceptives among 141 women with non-fatal cutaneous malignant melanoma and 2820 age-matched control women. The relative risk, adjusted for age, parity, height and hair dye use, was 0.8 (95% CI, 0.5–1.3). No significant trends emerged with duration of use or time since first use. For women who were under the age of 40 at the time cutaneous malignant melanoma was diagnosed, the relative risk was 1.4 (95% CI, 0.8–2.5). For women under 40 who had used combined oral contraceptives for more than two years at least 10 years before diagnosis of cutaneous malignant melanoma, the relative risk was 2.3 (95% CI, 0.8–6.9). An analysis restricted to the 84 histologically documented cases of cutaneous malignant melanoma showed similar results [not shown].

2.7.2 Case-control studies

These studies are summarized in Table 29.

Adam *et al.* (1981) investigated 169 cases of cutaneous malignant melanoma in women aged 15–49 years that had been notified to the cancer registries of south-western England during 1971–76, and 507 age-matched control women drawn from the lists of the same general practitioners as the cases. Data were obtained from the general practitioners' records and for about 70% of the study women from postal questionnaires. The risk for cutaneous malignant melanoma was not significantly increased among women who had ever used combined oral contraceptives, the unadjusted relative risk being 1.3 (95% CI, 0.9–2.0) from the practitioners' records and 1.1 (95% CI, 0.7–1.8) from the postal questionnaires.

In an Australian investigation by Green and Bain (1985), described in detail in the monograph on 'Post-menopausal oestrogen therapy', there was no increased risk for cutaneous malignant melanoma in relation to use of combined oral contraceptives, with an age-adjusted relative risk of 0.7 (95% CI, 0.4–1.5), and no trend of increasing risk with increasing duration of use, the relative risk for > 4 years' use being 0.4 (95% CI, 0.2–1.1). The risk was also not elevated among women who had first used combined oral contraceptives 10 or more years before diagnosis of cutaneous malignant melanoma, with a relative risk of 0.9 (95% CI, 0.4–2.2).

In the case–control study of Holly *et al.* (1983) in Seattle, United States, described in detail in the monograph on 'Post-menopausal oestrogen therapy', use of combined oral contraceptives for five years or more was commoner among cases than controls, with age-adjusted relative risks of 1.5 for 5–9 years of use and and 2.1 for ≥ 10 years' duration (not significant). This relationship was seen only with long-term use of combined oral contraceptives among women with superficial spreading melanoma, with relative risks of 2.4 for 5–9 years and 3.6 for ≥ 10 years of use, and a highly significant trend ($p = 0.004$) with increasing duration of use. Adjustment was not made for the pattern of exposure to the sun.

In the study of Lew *et al.* (1983), in Massachusetts, United States, described in detail in the monograph on 'Post-menopausal oestrogen therapy', no data were given on hormonal treatment, but it was reported that cases and controls did not differ with respect to use of combined oral contraceptives.

Table 29. Case–control studies of use of combined oral contraceptives and malignant melanoma

Reference	Country	Cases : controls (type of controls)	Subgroup	RR (95% CI) any versus no use	Duration of use	Recency of use	Adjustment/Comments
Adam et al. (1981)	England	169 : 507 (same general practitioner)	General practitioners' records, postal questionnaires	1.3 (0.9–2.0) 1.1 (0.7–1.8)	No significant trend (RR for ≥ 5 years, 1.6; 95% CI, 0.8–3.0)	No effect	Unadjusted Responses to postal questionnaire (response rate about 70%) did not show an association between use of combined oral contraceptives and exposure to the sun
Green & Bain (1985)	Queensland, Australia	91 : 91 (population)		0.7 (0.4–1.5)	No trend (RR for > 4 years' use, 0.4; 95% CI, 0.2–1.1)	No effect for use ≥ 10 years before diagnosis, 0.9; 95% CI, 0.4–2.2)	Age After allowance for phenotypic characteristics and solar exposure, RR for > 4 years' use, 0.4 (95% CI, 0.1–2.0)
Holly et al. (1983)	Seattle, USA	87 : 863 (population)	1–4 years 5–9 years ≥ 10 years	1.0 1.5 (NS) 2.1 (NS)	Significant trend only for SSM (RR ≥ 10 years use, 3.6)	Increased risk for ≥ 12 years since first use: 4.4 (95% CI, 2.0–9.7)	Age No data on solar exposure
Lew et al. (1983)	Massachusetts USA	111 : 107 (friends of cases)	–	–	–	–	No difference in combined oral contraceptive use
Beral et al. (1984)	Sydney, Australia	287 : 574 (hospital and population)		1.0 (NS)	No significant trend	No significant effect	Unadjusted (but altered by education, phenotype, history of sunburn and solar exposure) Increased risk for women who had begun taking combined oral contraceptives at least 10 years before and with ≥ 5 years' duration of use: 1.5 (95% CI, 1.0–2.1). No difference by location, thickness or type of CMM

Table 29 (contd)

Reference	Country	Cases : controls (type of controls)	Subgroup	RR (95% CI) any versus no use	Duration of use	Recency of use	Adjustment/Comments
Helmrich et al. (1984)	United States and Canada	160 : 640 (hospital)		0.8 (0.5–1.3)	No trend (RR for ≥ 10 years' use, 1.0; 95% CI, 0.4–2.9 [only age-adjusted])	No effect of time since first use (RR for first use ≥ 10 years previously, 1.1; 95% CI, 0.7–1.8)	Age, area, religion, education and hormone-related variables
Holman et al. (1984)	Western Australia	276 : 276	CMM SSM	1.0 (0.6–1.6) 1.1 (0.6–2.2)	No significant trend (RR for ≥ 5 years use, 1.1; 95% CI, 0.6–2.0)	No effect (RR for ≥ 10 years' use before diagnosis, 1.1; 95% CI, 0.7–1.7)	Age and residence
Gallagher et al. (1985)	Canada	361 : 361 (members of health plans)	CMM < 1 year 1–4 years ≥ 5 years SSM < 1 year 1–4 years ≥ 5 years	 1.0 0.9 0.8 1.1 1.1 0.9	No trend	No effect (RR for use ≥ 10 years prior to diagnosis, 1.0)	Age, education, phenotype and freckling Allowance for phenotypic characteristics
Østerlind et al. (1988)	Denmark	280 : 536	CMM SSM	0.8 (0.5–1.2) 0.9 (0.6–1.3)	No trend (RR for ≥ 10 years' use, 1.0; 95% CI, 0.6–1.7)	No effect (RR for use ≥ 10 years before diagnosis, 1.3; 95% CI, 0.7–2.2)	Age, phenotype and sunbathing No difference according to type and potency of combined oral contraceptives
Zanetti et al. (1990)	Northern Italy	186 : 205 (population)	CMM SSM	1.0 (0.5–1.9) 1.3 (0.4–4.5)	No trend (RR for ≥ 3 years' use, 1.0; 95% CI, 0.5–2.7)	No effect	Age, education, phenotype and sunbathing Risk did not change according to CMM type or location, age or combined oral contraceptive potency

Table 29 (contd)

Reference	Country	Cases : controls (type of controls)	Subgroup	RR (95% CI) any versus no use	Duration of use	Recency of use	Adjustment/Comments
Augustsson et al. (1991)	Sweden	69 : 196 (population)			Not reported		No difference in combined oral contraceptive use
Lê et al. (1992)	France	91 : 149 (hospital)	< 10 years ≥ 10 years	1.1 (0.6–2.0) 2.1 (0.7–5.9)	No significant trend	No effect of use 15–20 years before diagnosis (RR, 1.9; 95% CI, 0.8–4.5)	
Palmer et al. (1992)	Philadelphia and New York, USA	615 : 2107	Severe Not severe	1.1 (0.8–1.5) 1.5 (1.1–2.4)	No trend (RR for not severe for ≥ 10 years' use, 2.0; 95% CI, 0.9–4.3)	No effect (RR for first use ≥ 20 years before severe CMM, 1.1; 95% CI, 0.7–1.8)	Age, education, body mass index, menopause and phenotype Elevated risk among not severe cases of CMM was attributed to surveillance bias; similar RR for different types
Zaridze et al. (1992)	Moscow, Russian Federation	96 : 96		0.04 (0.0– 0.5)	Not reported	Not reported	Phenotype, naevi and sunbathing Only one case and seven controls
Holly et al. (1995)	San Francisco, USA	452 : 930 (population)	CMM SSM	0.7 (0.5–0.9) 0.7 (0.5–1.0)	No trend (RR for ≥ 10 years' use: CMM, 0.8; 95% CI, 0.5–1.3; SSM, 1.0; 95% CI, 0.6–1.6)	No effect (RR for use ≥ 17 years before diagnosis, 0.6; 95% CI, 0.4–0.7)	Age (unaltered by education, phenotype and solar exposure)

Table 29 (contd)

Reference	Country	Cases : controls (type of controls)	Subgroup	RR (95% CI) any versus no use	Duration of use	Recency of use	Adjustment/Comments
Westerdahl et al. (1996)	Sweden	180 : 292 (population)		1.6 (0.9–2.8)	No effect (RR for > 8 years' use, 1.0; 95% CI, 0.5–2.0)	No effect	Phenotype, naevi and sunburns Age at use and timing of use in relation to first child did not influence risk
Ocular melanoma							
Hartge et al. (1989b)	Wilmington and Philadelphia, USA	238 : 223 (detached retina)		0.9 (0.4–1.7)	No trend (RR for ≥ 10 years' use, 0.2; NS)	No effect	Age

RR, relative risk; CI, confidence interval; NS, not significant; CMM, cutaneous malignant melanoma; SSM, superficial spreading melanoma

In the study of Beral *et al.* (1984) in Sydney, Australia, described in detail in the monograph on 'Post-menopausal oestrogen therapy', women who had ever used combined oral contraceptives were not at increased risk for cutaneous malignant melanoma (relative risk, 1.0). There was, however, an increased risk for women who had used these formulations for five years or more and who had begun use at least 10 years before diagnosis of cutaneous malignant melanoma, with a relative risk of 1.5 (95% CI, 1.0–2.1). The increase in risk persisted after control for phenotypic characteristics, number of moles and measures of exposure to ultraviolet light. The risk did not vary according to the location, thickness or type of melanoma.

In a case–control study carried out in several parts of the United States and Canada between 1976 and 1982 (Helmrich *et al.*, 1984), the case series consisted of 160 women aged 20–59 years with a recent histological diagnosis of cutaneous malignant melanoma, and the controls were 640 women aged 20–59 years admitted to hospital for trauma or orthopaedic and surgical conditions. The age-adjusted relative risk for those who had ever used combined oral contraceptives was 0.8 (95% CI, 0.5–1.3), and there was no trend in risk with increasing duration of use, the relative risk for ≥ 10 years of use being 1.0 (95% CI, 0.4–2.9). For the 40 case and 140 control women who had first used combined oral contraceptives at least 10 years previously, the relative risk was 1.1 (95% CI, 0.7–1.8) and for women with more advanced cutaneous malignant melanoma (i.e. Clark's level IV and V), the relative risk was 0.6 (95% CI, 0.2–2.3).

In the study of Gallagher *et al.* (1985), in Canada, described in detail in the monograph on 'Post-menopausal oestrogen therapy', no association was seen between the risk for cutaneous malignant melanoma and use of combined oral contraceptives in 361 cases and an equal number of controls aged 20–69. The relative risks for < 1, 1–4 and ≥ 5 years' use, adjusted for age, phenotypic characteristics and freckling, were 1.0, 0.9 and 0.8, respectively. No association was seen between type of superficial spreading melanoma and duration of use or years since last use, the relative risk for women who had used combined oral contraceptives 10 or more years before diagnosis of cutaneous malignant melanoma being 1.0.

In the Danish study of Østerlind *et al.* (1988), described in detail in the monograph on 'Post-menopausal oestrogen therapy', use of oral contraceptives was not related to the risk for cutaneous malignant melanoma (relative risk adjusted for age, phenotypic characteristics and sunbathing, 0.8; 95% CI, 0.5–1.2) or superficial spreading melanoma (relative risk, 0.9; 95% CI, 0.6–1.3), and there was no evidence of a dose–response relationship, the relative risk for ≥ 10 years' use being 1.0 (95% CI, 0.6–1.7). No specific risk pattern was seen with the type of oral contraceptive, such as sequential, progestogen only and high-potency combined oral contraceptives, assessed separately, but there were few women in each group.

Zanetti *et al.* (1990) carried out a case–control study in Turin, northern Italy, between 1984 and 1987 of 186 women aged 19–92 with histologically confirmed cutaneous malignant melanoma out of 211 identified from the Turin Cancer Registry and 205 control women aged 17–92 drawn from the National Health Service Registry (out of the 300 initially contacted). Use of combined oral contraceptives, analysed only in women aged 60 or younger, was not associated with cutaneous malignant melanoma, the relative risk adjusted for age, education, phenotypic characteristics and sunbathing being 1.0 (95% CI, 0.5–1.9); no association was seen with superficial spreading melanoma (relative risk, 1.3; 95% CI, 0.4–4.5). Similarly, the longest duration of use ($\geq$ 3 years: 1.0; 95% CI, 0.5–2.7) or use that had started 10 or more years before the diagnosis of cutaneous malignant melanoma was not associated with an increased risk. The relative risks were identical for use of combined oral contraceptives containing high oestrogen doses ($\geq$ 50 μg) and low oestrogen doses.

Augustsson *et al.* (1991) studied 69 cases of cutaneous malignant melanoma in Swedish women aged 30–50 and compared them with 196 controls drawn from the same population. Skin type, phenotypic characteristics, number of naevi and dysplastic naevi were taken into account. Although the relative risk was not reported, no difference in the use of combined oral contraceptives was reported between cases and controls.

Lê *et al.* (1992) assessed the effect of use of combined oral contraceptives on the risk for cutaneous malignant melanoma risk in France between 1982 and 1987. The cases were those of 91 white women under 45 years of age who had new, histologically confirmed melanomas, and the controls were 149 women consulting for diagnosis or treatment of diseases unrelated to use of combined oral contraceptives, including skin diseases. No significant association was found between the total duration of use of combined oral contraceptives (relative risk, adjusted for age at menarche for $\geq$ 10 years' use, 2.1; 95% CI, 0.7–5.9) or the time since first use (relative risk 15–20 years since first use, 1.9; 95% CI, 0.8–4.5) and the risk for cutaneous malignant melanoma, and no difference was found between superficial spreading melanoma and other types of cutaneous malignant melanoma. The relative risk for 49 case women and 78 matched controls who were aged 30–40 and had used oral contraceptives for 10 or more years, however, was significantly increased: 4.4 (95% CI, 1.1–17). In a subgroup of 57 case women and 65 controls for whom allowance could be made for phenotypic characteristics and solar exposure, the relative risks were similar.

A case–control study on cutaneous malignant melanoma was carried out between 1979 and 1991 in Philadelphia and New York, United States (Palmer *et al.*, 1992), in which the cases were in 615 women under the age of 70 (median age, 40) who had recently received a first diagnosis of cutaneous malignant melanoma. Patients with melanoma *in situ* were not included. Two control groups of white women with a median age of 41 years with other malignancies (610 patients) or non-malignant illnesses (1497 patients) judged to be unrelated to use of combined oral contraceptives were selected. In order to address the possibility of selection bias due to differential surveillance of combined oral contraceptive users and non-users, the cases were subdivided by severity. For severe cases (thickness $\geq$ 0.75 mm, or Clark's level IV or V), the relative risks adjusted for age, education, menopause and phenotypic characteristics were 1.1 (95% CI, 0.8–1.5) for any use, 1.1 (0.6–2.1) for $\geq$ 10 years' use and 1.1 (0.7–1.8) for $\geq$ 20 years' use. For non-severe cases, increased risks were found for any use (1.5; 95% CI, 1.1–2.2) and for $\geq$ 10 years' use (2.0; 0.9–4.3). The relative risks did not vary by type of cutaneous malignant melanoma. According to the authors, the increased risks seen for non-severe cases of cutaneous malignant melanoma were probably due to greater surveillance of combined oral contraceptive users.

Zaridze et al. (1992) evaluated risk factors in 96 cases of cutaneous malignant melanoma in Moscow, Russian Federation. Controls matched by age were recruited from among persons visiting cancer patients. Use of combined oral contraceptives could be analysed for 54 women with cutaneous malignant melanoma and 54 controls and showed a strong inverse association: the relative risk, adjusted for phenotypic characteristics, naevi and sunbathing, was 0.04 (95% CI, 0.0–0.5). Only one case and seven controls, however, had ever used combined oral contraceptives.

In the study of Holly et al. (1995), described in detail in the monograph on 'Post-menopausal oestrogen therapy' (Holly et al., 1994), 72% of the cases of cutaneous malignant melanoma and 79% of the control subjects in San Francisco, United States, reported ever having used combined oral contraceptives. The age-adjusted relative risk was 0.7 (95% CI, 0.5–0.9) for all cutaneous malignant melanoma and 0.7 (95% CI, 0.5–1.0) for superficial spreading melanoma. Examination by latency and duration of use showed no significant trend. The relative risk for ≥ 10 years' use was 0.8 (95% CI, 0.5–1.3) for all cutaneous malignant melanoma and 1.0 (95% CI, 0.6–1.6) for superficial spreading melanoma. Use beginning ≥ 17 years before diagnosis was associated with relative risks of 0.6 (95% CI, 0.4–0.7) for cutaneous malignant melanoma and 0.6 (95% CI, 0.4–0.8) for superficial spreading melanoma.

In the Swedish study of Westerdahl et al. (1996), described in the monograph on 'Post-menopausal oestrogen therapy', any use of combined oral contraceptives (40% of cases and 37% of controls) was associated with a non-significantly elevated risk of 1.6 (95% CI, 0.9–2.8) after adjustment for phenotypic characteristics, naevi and sunburns. No trend in risk was seen with duration of use (relative risk for > 8 years' use, 1.0; 95% CI, 0.5–2.0), age at first use or age at last use.

A meta-analysis of 18 published case–control studies on cutaneous malignant melanoma and use of combined oral contraceptives, including 17 of the papers reviewed here and that of Beral et al. (1977), showed a pooled relative risk of 1.0 (95% CI, 0.9–1.0) (Gefeller et al., 1997). The data for 3796 cases and 9442 controls showed no significant heterogeneity of the effect of combined oral contraceptives in the different studies, and analysis of various subgroups, defined by the design characteristics of the studies, did not materially alter this result.

2.8   Retinal melanoma

In a case–control study of ocular melanoma in the United States (Hartge et al., 1989b), described in the monograph on 'Post-menopausal oestrogen therapy', use of combined oral contraceptives was reported by about 13% in both cases and controls, to give an age-adjusted relative risk of 0.9 (95% CI, 0.4–1.7). The estimated risk was not related to duration of use (relative risk for ≥ 10 years' use, 0.2; 95% CI, 0.3–1.2) or to the interval since first or last use.

2.9   Thyroid cancer

None of the cohort studies provided information on use of combined oral contraceptives and the risk for thyroid cancer. The case–control studies are summarized in Table 30.

In the case–control study of McTiernan *et al.* (1984), in Seattle, United States, described in detail in the monograph on 'Post-menopausal oestrogen therapy', the use of combined oral contraceptives (prevalence: 93/141 cases and 130/219 controls) was associated with a slightly increased risk for thyroid cancer (1.6; 95% CI, 1.0–2.5). The magnitude of the excess risk did not increase with increasing duration of use (relative risk for > 3 years' duration, 1.2). The risk was higher among women with follicular thyroid cancer (3.6; 95% CI, 1.1–12.8) and among those women who discovered their own tumours as compared with those whose tumour was found by a physician.

Preston-Martin *et al.* (1987) evaluated the risk factors for thyroid cancer in women aged 40 or less in Los Angeles, United States, between 1980 and 1981. The cases were in 108 white women with papillary, follicular or mixed thyroid cancer (out of 135 identified through Southern California Cancer Surveillance Program) and controls were 108 age-matched women who lived near the case women (neighbourhood controls). More cases (67/78) than controls (76/106) had ever used combined oral contraceptives (unadjusted relative risk, 2.4; 95% CI, 1.1–5.7). Cases and controls did not differ with respect to age at first use. There was no trend of increasing risk with increasing duration of use, the relative risk for > 5 years' duration of use being 2.4 (95% CI, 0.9–6.9).

In a study conducted in Connecticut, United States (Ron *et al.*, 1987), described in the monograph on 'Post-menopausal oestrogen therapy', similar proportions of cases (55/109) and controls (110/208) had ever used combined oral contraceptives, the relative risk adjusted for age, parity, radiotherapy to the head and neck and benign thyroid disease being 0.8 (not significant). For women under the age of 35 at the time of diagnosis, the relative risk was 1.8 (not significant). Duration and latency of use were not assessed.

Franceschi *et al.* (1990) found relatively few users of combined oral contraceptives among cases of thyroid cancer in Italy (23/165 cases and 28/214 controls). The age-adjusted relative risks were 1.1 (95% CI, 0.5–2.4) for use for < 24 months and 1.1 (95% CI, 0.4–3.0) for use for ≥ 24 months.

In a case–control study in Hawaii (Kolonel *et al.*, 1990), described in the monograph on 'Post-menopausal oestrogen therapy', women who had ever used combined oral contraceptives (43% among controls) showed no increased risk for thyroid cancer. The relative risk, adjusted for age and ethnic group was 0.9 (95% CI, 0.5–1.5). The effects of duration and latency of use were not reported.

Levi *et al.* (1993), in study in Switzerland, described in detail in the monograph on 'Post-menopausal oestrogen therapy', found a prevalence of any use of combined oral contraceptives of 56% among thyroid cancer cases and 44% among control women; the relative risk, adjusted for age and a history of benign thyroid disease, was 1.2 (95% CI, 0.7–2.3). There was no trend of increasing risk with increasing duration of use, the relative risk for ≥ 5 years' use being 1.4 (95% CI, 0.7–2.7). Analyses restricted to women under 45 years of age or to cases of papillary thyroid cancer yielded similar risk estimates.

Table 30. Case–control studies on use of combined oral contraceptives and thyroid cancer

Reference	Country	Cases : controls (type of controls)	RR (95% CI), any versus no use	Duration of use	Adjustment/comments
McTiernan et al. (1984)	Seattle, USA	141 : 319 (population)	1.6 (1.0–2.5)	No trend (RR for > 3 years' use, 1.2)	Age Greatest risk increase seen for follicular thyroid cancer (RR, 3.6; 95% CI, 1.1–13)
Preston-Martin et al. (1987)	Los Angeles, USA	108 : 108 (population)	2.4 (1.1–5.7)	No trend (RR for > 5 years' use, 2.4; 95% CI, 0.9–6.9)	Unadjusted. Only women aged 40 or less
Ron et al. (1987)	Connecticut, USA	109 : 208 (population)	0.8	Not reported	Age, parity, radiotherapy to the head and neck and benign thyroid diseases RR for women < 35 was 1.8 (not significant)
Franceschi et al. (1990)	Italy	165 : 214 (hospital)	< 2 years, 1.1 (0.5–2.4) ≥ 2 years, 1.1 (0.4–3.0)	No effect	Age and area of residence
Kolonel et al. (1990)	Hawaii, USA	140 : 328 (population)	0.9 (0.5–1.5)	Not reported	Age and ethnic group Increased risk for women with difficulty in conceiving (RR, 1.8; 95% CI, 1.0–3.1) and those who used fertility drugs (RR, 4.2; 95% CI, 1.5–11)
Levi et al. (1993)	Vaud, Switzerland	91 : 306 (hospital)	1.2 (0.7–2.3)	No trend (RR for ≥ 5 years' use, 1.4; 95% CI, 0.7–2.7)	Age and history of benign thyroid disease Similar risk estimates for women under 45 and for papillary thyroid cancer
Preston-Martin et al. (1993)	Shanghai, China	207 : 207 (population)	1.7 (1.0–3.1)	No trend (RR for > 5 years' use, 0.9; 95% CI, 0.4–2.4)	Age
Wingren et al. (1993)	South-eastern Sweden	93 : 187 (population)	No risk (RR not reported)	Not reported	Only papillary carcinomas

Table 30 (contd)

Reference	Country	Cases : controls (type of controls)	RR (95% CI), any versus no use	Duration of use	Adjustment/comments
Hallquist et al. (1994)	Northern Sweden	123 : 240 (population)	All, 0.8 (0.5–1.4) Papillary, 0.6 (0.3–1.2)	No trend	Age Risk did not vary by timing in relation to age at first pregnancy
Galanti et al. (1996)	Sweden and Norway	191 : 341 (population)	0.9 (0.6–1.5)	No trend (> 2 years' use RR, 0.8; 95% CI, 0.5–1.3)	Age and parity

RR, relative risk; CI, confidence interval

Preston-Martin *et al.* (1993) carried out a study in Shanghai, China, between 1981 and 1984, which included 207 women aged 18–54 listed in the Shanghai Cancer Registry as having a histologically confirmed thyroid cancer; 20% of the cases were reviewed by a pathologist. The 207 control women, matched to the cases by year of birth, were chosen randomly from the Shanghai Residents' Registry; over 90% of the eligible subjects were interviewed. Few women had used combined oral contraceptives (43/207 cases and 29/207 controls), but any use of such formulations was associated with a marginally increased risk (unadjusted relative risk, 1.7; 95% CI, 1.0–3.1). Among users, however, there was no trend in risk with the duration of use, the relative risk for > 5 years' use being 0.9 (95% CI, 0.4–2.4).

Wingren *et al.* (1993) studied 93 cases of thyroid cancer and 187 controls aged 20–60 in south-east Sweden and reported that use of combined oral contraceptives was not associated with an increased risk. No data were shown.

Hallquist *et al.* (1994), in Sweden, reported that 42/123 cases and 92/240 controls had reported any use of combined oral contraceptives, giving an age-adjusted relative risk of 0.8 (95% CI, 0.5–1.4). The corresponding relative risk for papillary thyroid cancer was 0.6 (95% CI, 0.3–1.2). The risk did not vary by duration of use, being 0.6 (95% CI, 0.2–1.5) for ≥ 7 years' use, or by timing of use in relation to age at first pregnancy.

Galanti *et al.* (1996), in a study in Sweden and Norway described in the monograph on 'Post-menopausal oestrogen therapy', reported that 98/179 cases and 180/334 controls had used combined oral contraceptives. No relation was found between use and the risk for thyroid cancer; the age- and parity-adjusted relative risk for any use was 0.9 (95% CI, 0.6–1.5). Use for > 2 years was associated with a relative risk of 0.8 (95% CI, 0.5–1.3).

2.10   Other cancers

A 25-year follow-up of 46 000 women in Great Britain in the framework of a study on oral contraceptives by the Royal College of General Practitioners did not show significant excess mortality from lung cancer (relative risk, 1.2; 95% CI, 0.8–1.8) or any other cancer (Beral *et al.*, 1999).

In a study by La Vecchia *et al.* (1994), from Milan, Italy, described in detail in the monograph on 'Post-menopausal oestrogen therapy', use of combined oral contraceptives was not related to the risk for gastric cancer. Six of 229 cases and 19 of 614 controls had ever used such formulations, giving a relative risk adjusted for age, education, a family history of cancer and dietary habits of 1.3 (95% CI, 0.5–3.5).

Chow *et al.* (1995) in a study in Minnesota, United States, described in detail in the monograph on 'Post-menopausal oestrogen therapy', found no relation between use of combined oral contraceptives and the risk for renal-cell cancer; the relative risk, adjusted for age, smoking and body mass index was 0.8 (95% CI, 0.4–1.3). For use longer than 10 years, the relative risk was 0.3 (95% CI, 0.1–1.0).

The risk for renal-cell cancer and use of combined oral contraceptives was also evaluated in an international study by Lindblad *et al.* (1995), described in detail in the monograph on 'Post-menopausal oestrogen therapy'. Any use of combined oral contraceptives was associated with a relative risk, adjusted for age, smoking and body mass index, of 0.7 (95% CI, 0.5–0.9). There was an inverse trend in risk with increasing duration of use, the relative risk for > 10 years' use being 0.5 (95% CI, 0.3–0.9).

3. Studies of Cancer in Experimental Animals

In this section, only relevant studies on oestrogens and progestogens alone and in combination that were published subsequent to or not included in Volume 21 of the IARC Monographs (IARC, 1979) are reviewed in detail. Studies reviewed previously are summarized briefly.

3.1   Oestrogen–progestogen combinations
3.1.1   *Studies reviewed previously*
Mouse

The results of studies reviewed previously (Committee on Safety of Medicines, 1972; IARC, 1979) on the carcinogenicity of combinations of oestrogens and progestogens in mice are as follows:

Chlormadinone acetate in combination with mestranol tested by oral administration to mice caused an increased incidence of pituitary adenomas in animals of each sex. Oral administration of chlormadinone acetate in combination with ethinyloestradiol to mice resulted in an increased incidence of mammary tumours in intact and castrated males.

After oral administration of ethynodiol diacetate and mestranol to mice, increased incidences of pituitary adenomas were observed in animals of each sex. The combination of ethynodiol diacetate plus ethinyloestradiol, tested by oral administration to mice, increased the incidences of pituitary adenomas in animals of each sex and of malignant tumours of connective tissues of the uterus.

Lynoestrenol in combination with mestranol was tested in mice by oral administration. A slight, nonsignificant increase in the incidence of malignant mammary tumours was observed in females which was greater than that caused by lynoestrenol or mestranol alone.

The combination of megestrol acetate plus ethinyloestradiol, tested by oral administration to mice, caused an increased incidence of malignant mammary tumours in animals of each sex.

Noresthisterone acetate plus ethinyloestradiol, tested by oral administration to mice, increased the incidences of pituitary adenomas in animals of each sex, but the incidences were comparable to those induced by ethinyloestradiol alone. The combination of norethisterone plus ethinyloestradiol was also tested in mice by oral administration; an increased incidence of pituitary adenomas was observed in females. Norethisterone plus mestranol increased the incidences of pituitary adenomas in animals of each sex.

Norethynodrel in combination with mestranol was tested by oral administration in mice. Increased incidences of vaginal or cervical tumours were found in female mice and of pituitary adenomas in males and females. In female mice, an increased incidence of malignant mammary tumours was observed, but the incidence was not greater than that seen with norethynodrel alone. In castrated male mice, the combined treatment resulted in an increased incidence of mammary tumours.

The combination of norgestrel plus ethinyloestradiol was tested in mice by oral administration; no increase in the incidence of tumours was observed.

Rat

The results of studies reviewed previously (Committee on Safety of Medicines, 1972; IARC, 1979) on the carcinogenicity in rats of several combinations are as follows:

Ethynodiol diacetate plus ethinyloestradiol was tested for carcinogenicity by oral administration to rats. The incidence of malignant mammary tumours was increased in animals of each sex. In combination with mestranol, the incidence of mammary tumours was increased in one study but not in another.

Lynoestrenol in combination with mestranol was tested in female rats by oral administration. No increase in tumour incidence was observed.

Megestrol acetate plus ethinyloestradiol was tested by oral administration to rats. The incidence of benign liver tumours was increased in animals of each sex, but not to a level greater than that observed with ethinyloestradiol alone. In male rats, there was a small increase in the incidence of benign and malignant mammary tumours; females showed a small increase in the incidence of malignant mammary tumours.

The combination of noresthisterone acetate plus ethinyloestradiol, tested by oral administration to rats, increased the incidences of benign mammary tumours and liver adenomas in males. Norethisterone plus mestranol increased the incidence of malignant mammary tumours in female rats and increased the incidence of liver adenomas in males.

Norethynodrel in combination with mestranol was tested by oral administration to rats. In males, increased incidences of liver adenomas, pituitary adenomas and benign and malignant mammary tumours were observed, but the incidences were no greater than those with norethynodrel alone. In females, the incidences of pituitary adenomas and malignant mammary tumours were increased.

Norgestrel plus ethinyloestradiol, tested for carcinogenicity in rats by oral administration, caused a small increase in the incidence of benign mammary tumours in males.

Dimethisterone and oestradiol were tested in dogs, with no increase in the incidence of mammary tumours

3.1.2   *New studies*
(a)   *Oral administration*
Rat

Schuppler and Gunzel (1979) summarized data from a study by the Committee on Safety of Medicines (1972) in the United Kingdom on the incidence of hepatocellular adenomas in groups of 24–124 male and female rats [strain not specified] treated orally with combinations of various oestrogens and progestogens at doses up to 400 times the human contraceptive dose. The statistically significant increases indicated in their report are indicated by a '+' in Table 31.

Table 31. Effects of progestogen–oestrogen combinations on the incidence of hepatocellular adenomas in rats

Progestogen	Oestrogen	Ratio	Males	Females
Norethynodrel	Mestranol	66:1	+	–
		25:1	–	–
Norethisterone	Mestranol	20:1	+	–
Lynestrenol	Mestranol	33:1	Not tested	–
Megestrol acetate	Ethinyloestradiol	5:1	+	–
		80:1	+	–

From Schuppler & Gunzel (1979)

Groups of 10 female Sprague-Dawley rats, seven weeks of age, were treated with Enovid E (100 μg mestranol + 25 mg norethynodrel) in the diet for nine months, with daily intakes of 0.02–0.03 and 0.5–0.75 mg/kg bw. The numbers of altered γ-glutamyl transpeptidase (γ-GT)-positive hepatic foci, considered to be preneoplastic lesions, were counted at autopsy. A statistically significant ($p < 0.001$) increase in the number of foci (2.8 foci/cm²) was observed in comparison with untreated controls (0.2 foci/cm²). No increase in the incidence of hepatic nodules or carcinomas was observed at this time (Yager & Yager, 1980).

Female Wistar rats, 15–17 weeks of age, were treated with quingestanol acetate plus quinestrol, which are 3-cyclopentyl ether derivatives of norethisterone acetate and ethinyloestradiol, respectively, as a 2:1 mixture suspended in sesame oil containing piperidine (0.05% v/w) by stomach tube. A group of 75 rats was treated once weekly with 30 mg/kg bw, 60 rats were treated with 1.2 mg/kg bw per day, and 75 rats were used as vehicle controls; all treatments were given for 50 weeks, followed by 30 weeks of observation for reversibility of any lesions. Groups of 10 animals were killed at 25 and 50 weeks; at 66 weeks, five rats from each treatment group and three vehicle controls were killed, and at 80 weeks all survivors in the treated groups and 10 vehicle controls were killed. Treatment was associated with irreversible hair loss, a reversible decrease in body weight and reversible ataxia. The only treatment-related tumours were mammary masses and adenocarcinomas: at 40–50 weeks, the incidences of adenocarcinomas were 10/33 in rats at 30 mg/kg bw, 15/27 in those at 1.2 mg/kg bw and 1/12 in vehicle controls [statistics not specified]. After treatment was suspended, the incidences of mammary adenocarcinomas were reduced, with 1/8 at weeks 51–66 and 0/12 at weeks 67–80 in animals at 30 mg/kg bw, 3/7 and 2/8 at those times in animals at 1.2 mg/kg bw and 0/10 and 1/13 in vehicle controls (Lumb et al., 1985).

Male and female Wistar rats, four weeks old, were given ethinyloestradiol (0.075 mg) + norethisterone acetate (6 mg) dissolved in olive oil by gavage daily, ethinyloestradiol +

norethisterone acetate + 10% ethanol in the drinking-water on five days a week, olive oil + ethanol or olive oil alone. The animals were treated for up to 12 months, with interim kills at two, four, six, eight and 12 months, when the livers were analysed for the presence of hepatocellular carcinomas and hyperplastic nodules. In females, ethinyloestradiol + norethisterone acetate induced a 100% incidence of hyperplastic nodules by four months and hepatocellular carcinomas in 2/25 animals at 12 months. Ethanol increased the incidence of hepatocellular carcinoma at 12 months to 9/22; no hyperplastic nodules or hepatocellular carcinomas were seen in the controls receiving ethanol alone. In males, ethinyloestradiol + norethisterone acetate induced hyperplastic nodules in 6/20 animals at 12 months but no hepatocellular carcinomas. Ethanol increased the incidence of hyperplastic nodules to 100%, beginning at four months, and that of hepatocellular carcinomas to 2/17 at 12 months. Again, ethanol alone had no effect on the incidences of hyperplastic nodules or hepatocellular carcinoma, but it enhanced nuclear and cytosolic oestrogen receptors and DNA adduct formation, as detected by ^{32}P-postlabelling (Yamagiwa et al., 1991, 1994).

Monkey

Norlestrin (50:1 norethisterone acetate + ethinyloestradiol) was given to groups of 15–17 young adult female rhesus (Macaca mulatta) monkeys weighing 2.8–5.7 kg at the beginning of the study. Norlestrin powder was blended with soft fruit and vegetables and was administered over 10 years as 21 consecutive daily doses followed by seven days without treatment. The daily doses were 0, 0.051, 0.51 and 2.55 mg/kg bw which represented 0, 1, 10 and 50 times the human contraceptive dose. There were no effects on survival and no treatment-related alterations in coagulation or other clinical parameters. Only a few tumours appeared but were found in all groups (Fitzgerald et al., 1982).

(b)　Administration with known carcinogens

Mouse

Groups of 20 female B6AF$_1$ mice, 12 weeks of age, were treated with 3-methylcholanthrene by insertion of an impregnated silk thread into the cervical canal and through the uterine wall; a control group was treated with silk thread not impregnated with 3-methylcholanthrene. Pellets containing steroids were then implanted subcutaneously and renewed every three weeks for 15 weeks. The doses given every three weeks were 15 mg norethynodrel and 0.5 mg mestranol per mouse, alone and in combination. No tumours developed in mice that had not received 3-methylcholanthrene, but the steroids caused some histopathological changes in the mucosa of the cervix, uterus and vagina. The incidences of uterine adenoacanthomas were increased ($p < 0.01$) by all three treatments: control, 5/35; mestranol, 10/19; norethynodrel, 11/14; mestranol + norethynodrel, 10/18. Squamous-cell carcinomas of the cervix were observed in all groups, but the incidences were not statistically significantly increased in those receiving steroids (Blanzat-Reboud & Russfield, 1969).

The effects of two formulations, Ovral, consisting of 0.05 mg ethinyloestradiol + 0.5 mg norgestrel, and Noracycline, consisting of 0.05 mg ethinyloestradiol + 1 mg lynoestrenol, on carcinomas of the uterine cervix induced by 3-methylcholanthrene were studied in groups of 10–30 Swiss albino female mice, eight to nine weeks of age. The mice treated with 3-methylcholanthrene received a sterile cotton thread impregnated with beeswax containing approximately 300 μg of the carcinogen into the uterine cervix. The oral contraceptive combinations were administered orally at doses of 1/2000th of a pill (0.025 μg ethinyl-oestradiol + 0.25 μg norgestrel), 1/200th of a pill (0.25 μg ethinyloestradiol + 2.5 μg nor-gestrel) and 1/20th of a pill (2.5 μg ethinyloestradiol + 25 μg norgestrel) of Ovral, and 1/2000th of a pill (0.025 μg ethinyloestradiol + 0.5 μg lynoestrol), 1/200th of a pill (0.25 μg ethinyloestradiol + 5 μg lynoestrol) and 1/20th of a pill (2.5 μg ethinyloestradiol + 50 μg lynoestrol) of Noracycline. Treatment was for 30, 60 or 90 days. Animals that did not receive 3-methylcholanthrene did not develop cervical tumours at any dose of oral contra-ceptive. In contrast, treatment with either formulation caused dose-dependent, biphasic effects on the incidence of squamous-cell carcinomas induced by 3-methylcholanthrene. At the two lower doses, they were protective in comparison with treatment with the carcinogen alone ($p < 0.05$), while at the high dose they enhanced carcinogenesis: The incidence of squamous-cell carcinomas was 6/23 with 3-methylcholanthrene alone and 8/17 with the high dose of Ovral at 90 days, although the difference was not indicated as being statistically significant. With Noracycline, the enhancement was statistically significant after both 60 days (13/24 versus 2/23, $p < 0.05$) and 90 days (12/19 versus 6/23, $p < 0.05$). At all doses and at all times, both formulations also significantly enhanced the incidence of cervical hyperplasia (Hussain & Rao, 1992).

In a more recent study with the same model, Ovral was administered to Swiss mice at the same two lower doses as the previous study, with 3-methylcholanthrene at a higher dose of 600 μg. The cotton thread was inserted into the right uterine horn. After 90 days, the incidence of tumours in the uterine endometrium was 8/15 in mice receiving the carcinogen alone and 1/16 in the group receiving the carcinogen + the 1/2000th dose of Ovral ($p < 0.05$). No tumours were seen in the group treated with 3-methylcholanthrene + Ovral at the 1/200th dose (Chhabra et al., 1995).

Rat

Groups of 9–10 female Sprague-Dawley rats, seven weeks of age, were initiated by treatment with 5 mg/kg bw N-nitrosodiethylamine (NDEA) 24 h after partial hepa-tectomy. Twenty-four hours later they were fed a diet containing mestranol + nore-thynodrel at concentrations providing 0.02–0.03 and 0.5–0.75 mg/kg bw per day, respectively. After nine months, a statistically significant ($p < 0.001$) increase in the number of γ-GT-positive altered hepatic foci was observed (7.3 versus 0.3 foci/cm^2), with no significant increase in the incidence of nodules or carcinomas (Yager & Yager, 1980).

Groups of female weanling Wistar rats received an intraperitoneal injection of 0 or 200 mg/kg bw NDEA. One month later, half the animals in each group (5–6 rats) received 1/10th of a tablet of Ovulen-50 (5 μg ethinyloestradiol + 100 μg ethynodiol diacetate) daily orally in 0.1 mL propylene glycol for 60 weeks; the other half of the rats in each group received the vehicle. The livers were examined histochemically for γ-GT-positive foci and histologically. None of the rats developed liver tumours. In rats that had not been initiated with NDEA, Ovulen-50 increased the incidences of γ-GT-positive foci and of microscopic hyperplastic nodules in all five rats; such foci and nodules were not seen in other groups. The authors speculated that the absence of foci and nodules in NDEA-initiated rats with and without treatment with Ovulen-50 may have been due to an interplay of the drug-metabolizing enzymes and that the Ovulen-50 steroids were more rapidly metabolized by the NDEA-initiated rats (Annapurna *et al.*, 1988). [The Working Group noted that opposite effects, i.e. enhancement of foci and nodules in initiated livers by oral contraceptive steroids, have been seen in many other studies and that the results of this study must be considered an exception to the general finding and that they lack a mechanistic explanation.]

The results of the previous and new studies on oestrogen–progestogen combinations are summarized in Tables 32 and 33.

3.2   Oestrogens used in combined oral contraceptives

3.2.1   *Studies reviewed previously*

Mouse

Ethinyloestradiol administered to mice increased the incidence of pituitary adenomas and malignant mammary tumours in animals of each sex and the incidences of uterine and cervical tumours in females.

Mestranol increased the incidences of pituitary adenomas and malignant mammary tumours in animals of each sex.

Rat

When ethinyloestradiol was tested for carcinogenicity in rats, the incidences of liver adenomas were increased in animals of each sex and that of liver carcinomas in females.

Administration of mestranol increased the incidence of malignant mammary tumours in females in one of two treated groups.

3.2.2   *New studies*

(a)   *Oral administration*

Mouse

Schuppler and Gunzel (1979) summarized data on the incidence of hepatic adenomas in groups of 40–120 male and female mice of three strains after oral administration of ethinyloestradiol or mestranol for 20 months at up to 400 times the human contraceptive dose. Only mice of strain BDH-SPF showed a small increase in incidence after receiving ethinyloestradiol.

Rat

Schuppler and Gunzel (1979) reported that the study of the Committee on Safety of Medicines (1972) found no increase in the incidence of liver adenoma in female rats

Table 32. Effects of combinations of various progestogens and oestrogens on tumour incidence in mice

| Combination | Pituitary adenomas | | Mammary tumours | | | Uterine tumours | Cervical/vaginal tumours |
	Male	Female	Benign (males)	Malignant Male	Malignant Female		
Chlormadinone acetate + mestranol	+	+					
Chlormadinone acetate + ethinyloestradiol			+/c				
Ethynodiol diacetate + mestranol	+	+					
Ethynodiol diacetate + ethinyloestradiol	+	+				+	
Lynoestranol + mestranol				+/-			
Lynoestranol + ethinyloestradiol + 3-methylcholanthrene							+[a]
Megestrol acetate + ethinyloestradiol				+	+		
Norethisterone acetate + ethinyloestradiol	+/?	+/?					
Norethisterone + ethinyloestradiol		+					
Norethisterone + mestranol	+	+					
Norethynodrel + mestranol	+	+	c			+	+
Norethynodrel + mestranol + 3-methylcholanthrene				+/?			–
Norgestrel + ethinyloestradiol + 3-methylcholanthrene							+[a]

+, increased tumour incidence; +/-, slightly increased tumour incidence; +/c, increased tumour incidence in intact and castrated animals; c, increased tumour incidence in castrated animals; +/?, increased tumour incidence, but not greater than that with the oestrogen or progestogen alone

[a] Protection at doses 1/2000th and 1/200th that of a pill for women; enhancement at a dose of 1/20th that of a pill for women

Table 33. Effects of combinations of various progestogens and oestrogens on tumour incidence in rats

Combination	Pituitary adenomas		Mammary tumours			Liver					
	Male	Female	Benign (males)	Malignant		Adenoma		Carcinoma		Foci (females)	
				Male	Female	Male	Female	Male	Female		
Ethynodiol diacetate + ethinyloestradiol				+	+						
Ethynodiol diacetate + mestranol				?	?						
Megestrol acetate + ethinyloestradiol			+/−	+/−	+/−	+/?	+/?				
Norethisterone acetate + ethinyloestradiol			+			+		−	+		
Norethisterone + mestranol					+	+	−				
Norethynodrel + mestranol	+/?	+	+/?	+/?	+	+/?	−	−	−	+	
Norethynodrel + mestranol + N-nitrosodiethylamine							−	−	−	+	
Norgestrel + ethinyloestradiol			+/−								

+, increased tumour incidence; +/−, slighly increased tumour incidence; +/?, increased tumour incidence, but not greater than that with the oestrogen or progestogen alone; ? conflicting; −, no effect

treated orally with mestranol. Of four studies on the incidences of hepatocellular adenoma and carcinoma in groups of 40–120 male and female rats treated orally with ethinyl-oestradiol at doses up to 400 times the human contraceptive dose, only one showed a statistically significant increase in the incidence of hepatocellular adenoma in males (0% controls, 15.3% treated) and in females (8% controls, 23.5% treated); the incidence of hepatocellular carcinoma was significantly increased only in females (0% controls, 7.4% treated).

Groups of female Sprague-Dawley rats received ethinyloestradiol or mestranol in the diet from about seven weeks of age at concentrations of 0.1 or 0.5 mg/kg diet (ppm) mestranol for nine and 12 months or 0.5 ppm ethinyloestradiol for nine months. The ingested doses were approximately equivalent to 6 or 30 µg/kg bw per day or 3–15 times the human contraceptive dose. Ethinyloestradiol caused a statistically significant ($p < 0.05$) increase in the number of γ-GT-positive, altered hepatic foci, but not in the volume percentage of liver occupied by foci, after nine months. No increase in the incidence of nodules or carcinomas was observed. The high dose of mestranol had similar effects after nine months, but after 12 months, mestranol caused a statistically significant ($p < 0.05$) increase in both the number of altered hepatic foci, and the volume percentage of the liver occupied by foci showed a significant ($p < 0.05$) dose–response relationship. Furthermore, after 12 months, the high dose of mestranol caused a significant ($p < 0.05$) increase in the incidence of hepatic nodules and carcinomas combined (4/16 compared with 0/15 in controls) (Yager et al., 1984).

Female Wistar rats, four weeks of age, were treated with 0 (control), 75 or 750 µg ethinyloestradiol in 0.5 mL olive oil by gavage daily for various times up to 12 months. By four months, the incidence of glutathione S-transferase-positive, altered hepatic foci, considered to be preneoplastic lesions, was 100% in both groups. At 12 months, hepato-cellular carcinomas were found in 2/23 rats at 75 µg ethinyloestradiol and 10/26 at 750 µg, with none in 24 controls. This response correlated with increased oxidative damage to liver nuclear DNA. Antioxidant vitamins (vitamins C and E and β-carotene) slightly reduced the oxidative DNA damage, significantly reduced the number of altered hepatic foci and reduced the hepatocellular carcinoma incidence (Ogawa et al., 1995).

Dog

Groups of 15 female beagles, 10–14 months of age at the start of the experiment, received mestranol at a dose of 0.02 or 0.05 mg/kg bw per day for cycles of 21 days followed by seven days with no drug; a group of 18 bitches served as controls. All of the animals were hysterectomized at two years of age. No mammary tumours were detected after five years (Kwapien et al., 1980).

(b)   Subcutaneous implantation

Rat

Holtzman (1988) studied the effects of retinyl acetate on ethinyloestradiol-induced mammary carcinogenesis. A group of 24 female ACI rats aged 59–65 days received subcutaneously implanted ethinyloestradiol in cholesterol pellets (1 mg/20 mg pellet). All treated rats developed pituitary tumours, and 21/24 developed mammary gland carcinomas within 25 weeks. Retinyl acetate did not significantly decrease the mammary tumour incidence but reduced the tumour multiplicity by about 50%.

Hamster

A group of 15 male Syrian golden hamsters weighing 90–100 g received 20-mg pellets of ethinyloestradiol in the shoulder region. The pellets were replaced at three-month intervals and oestrogen treatment was continued for seven to eight months. Three animals developed microscopic renal-cell carcinomas. It was also reported that all 10 castrated male hamsters receiving similar treatment but fed 0.2% α-naphthoflavone developed hepatocellular carcinomas compared with 0/10 hamsters receiving only α-naphthoflavone in the diet (Li & Li, 1984).

(c)   Administration with known carcinogens
Liver models

Mouse: Lee *et al.* (1989) compared the effects of several promoters, including ethinyl-oestradiol, in three strains of NDEA-initiated male mice. Six-week-old C3H/HeN (C3H), C57BL/6N (C57) and BALB/cA (BALB) mice underwent a two-thirds hepatectomy, followed 20 h later by an intraperitoneal injection of 20 mg/kg bw NDEA; 6 h later, the animals were given a diet containing phenobarbital at a concentration of 50 mg/kg diet (ppm), clofibrate at 1000 ppm and ethinyloestradiol at 10 ppm. The animals were killed after 20 weeks for detection of glucose 6-phosphatase-deficient, altered hepatic foci. The mouse strains differed widely with regard to the mean liver volume occupied by foci after receiving NDEA and in their sensitivity to promotion. The most sensitive strain was C3H. The mean volume ($\times 10^6$ μm^3) of the liver foci was 13.2 ± 1.8 in 18 mice that received NDEA only, 460 ± 72 in 20 mice given phenobarbital and 28 ± 6 in 20 mice given clofibrate; 11 mice given ethinyloestradiol showed no effect, the mean liver volume being 12 ± 10. When the data were expressed as total volume of foci/cm^3 liver $\times 10^6$ μm^3, ethinyloestradiol was seen to be protective, reducing the value of 710 ± 128 in 18 controls to 34 ± 22. Similar results were found in C57 and BALB mice.

Female B6C3F$_1$ mice, 12 days of age, were treated with 5 mg/kg bw NDEA by intra-peritoneal injection. At five to seven weeks of age, the mice were randomly assigned to groups of 12 which were exposed by inhalation to unleaded gasoline at 0, 292 or 2056 ppm for 6 h per day on five days per week for 16 weeks, to ethinyloestradiol in the diet at a concentration of 1 ppm or to 1 ppm ethinyloestradiol + 2056 ppm unleaded gasoline. Altered hepatic foci were determined in standard histological sections. The percentage of the liver volume occupied by foci was significantly reduced in ethinyloestradiol-treated mice, from 1.1 ± 0.7 in NDEA controls to 0.26 ± 0.31; however, the volume of foci was significantly increased by the high dose of unleaded gasoline, to 4.31 ± 2.51, and further increased to 18 ± 5 by ethinyloestradiol + the high dose of unleaded gasoline (Standeven *et al.*, 1994).

Rat: Ethinyloestradiol and mestranol promoted the appearance of altered hepatic foci and the development of hepatic nodules (adenomas) and carcinomas in initiated male and female rats (Wanless & Medline, 1982; Mayol *et al.*, 1991; Hallstrom *et al.*, 1996; Yager & Liehr, 1996). On the basis of dose and time responses, these synthetic oestrogens are strong promoters of hepatocarcinogenesis (Yager *et al.*, 1991). Selected studies that support this conclusion are summarized below.

Groups of 12–18 female Sprague-Dawley rats, approximately seven weeks of age, were subjected to a two-thirds partial hepatectomy to induce cell proliferation and initiated by intraperitoneal injection of 20 mg/kg bw NDEA; 24 h later, they were fed a semi-purified diet containing mestranol at a concentration of 0.1 or 0.5 ppm for 9 or 12 months or ethinyloestradiol at 0.5 ppm for nine months. The daily intakes of mestranol were approximately 6 and 30 μg/kg bw or 3–15 times the human contraceptive dose. All survivors were killed at 9 or 12 months, and the livers were evaluated for γ-GT-positive foci and the presence of nodules (adenomas) and carcinomas. By nine months, ethinyloestradiol and mestranol had caused a significant ($p < 0.05$) increase in the number of γ-GT foci but no increase in the incidence of nodules or hepatocellular carcinoma. Mestranol induced a significant, dose-dependent increase in the incidence of hepatocellular carcinomas by 12 months, with incidences of 6/15 animals given NDEA alone, 7/17 animals given NDEA plus mestranol at 0.1 ppm and 11/14 animals given NDEA + 0.5 ppm mestranol. A similar number of foci developed in rats fed 0.5 ppm mestranol and in rats fed a diet containing 50 ppm phenobarbital (Yager *et al.*, 1984).

Ovariectomized Sprague-Dawley rats, 70 days of age, were given a single intra-peritoneal injection of 200 mg/kg bw NDEA; beginning on day 80 and every 28 days thereafter for various periods, the rats were treated with subcutaneous implants of Silastic tubing containing a mixture of ethinyloestradiol and cholesterol. The doses of ethinyloestradiol delivered were calculated to be 0, 16, 37, 90 and 230 μg/kg bw per day. After 30 weeks, the proportion of the liver volume occupied by γ-GT-positive, altered hepatic foci showed a linear increase with dose. The increase was statistically significant at 90 and 230 μg/kg bw per day. In initiated rats treated with ethinyloestradiol at 90 μg/kg bw per day, the incidences of hepatic tumours (adenomas + carcinomas) were significantly greater ($p < 0.05$) than in NDEA-initiated controls with cholesterol implants after 30, 40 and 60 weeks of promotion (Campen *et al.*, 1990).

Female Sprague-Dawley rat pups, five days of age, were initiated by an intra-peritoneal injection of 10 mg/kg bw NDEA or received no treatment. At weaning, groups of 8–12 rats were fed a semi-synthetic basal diet (controls) or basal diet containing mestranol at a concentration of 0.02 or 0.2 mg/kg (0.02 and 0.2 ppm, respectively) for eight months. When administered alone, mestranol did not induce the appearance of placental glutathione *S*-transferase-positive foci; however, in NDEA-initiated rats, mestranol at a concentration of 0.2 ppm significantly increased ($p < 0.05$) the percentage of the liver volume occupied by foci over that in NDEA-initiated rats fed basal diet. No increase was observed at 0.02 ppm (Dragan *et al.*, 1996).

Three studies have been conducted to determine whether ethinyloestradiol and mestranol initiate carcinogenesis in the liver.

Female Sprague-Dawley rats fed a semi-purified diet underwent a two-thirds hepatectomy and 24 h later, at the peak of regenerative DNA synthesis, groups of 10 rats were treated by gavage with corn oil or mestranol at a dose of 100 or 500 mg/kg bw. A positive control group was injected intraperitoneally with 10 mg/kg bw NDEA. After another 24 h, the rats were transferred to a diet containing 0.05% phenobarbital to promote any hepatocytes that had been initiated. The rats were killed four months later and their livers analysed for γ-GT-positive foci. NDEA initiation caused a more than 10-fold increase in the number of foci/cm^2, but the number was not significantly increased in rats treated with 100 mg/kg bw mestranol. While there was an approximately fivefold increase in the number of foci in the group fed 500 mg/kg bw, the effect was not statistically significant (Yager & Fifield, 1982).

Male Fischer 344 rats weighing 130–165 g were given various oestrogens and progestogens by intraperitoneal injection approximately 18 h after a two-thirds hepatectomy. Positive controls were treated with N-nitrosomorpholine. Two weeks later, the rats were given 0.02% 2-acetylaminofluorene in the diet for two weeks and carbon tetrachloride by gavage at the end of the first week. The animals were then killed, and the numbers of γ-GT-positive foci were determined in 9–15 rats per group. Ethinyloestradiol at a dose of 0.05 mg/kg bw did not increase the number of γ-GT-positive foci over that in controls (Schuppler et al., 1983).

Groups of 12 female Sprague-Dawley rats weighing 140–160 g were fed a semi-purified diet containing ethinyloestradiol at a concentration of 10 ppm for six weeks and then returned to basal diet; controls received basal diet alone. On day 7, all rats were given a two-thirds hepatectomy to increase cell proliferation. After one week on basal diet (week 6–7), the rats were given 0.02% 2-acetylaminofluorene in the diet for two weeks with carbon tetrachloride by gavage at the end of the first week to induce regenerative growth and rapid growth of any initiated foci. The rats were then killed and the numbers of γ-GT-positive foci determined. Ethinyloestradiol caused a significant ($p < 0.01$) fourfold increase in the number of foci/cm^2 and a sixfold increase in focal area as a percentage of liver volume (Ghia & Mereto, 1989). [The Working Group noted that ethinyloestradiol was administered for five weeks as opposed to a single treatment, as in the previous two studies.]

Prostate models

Ethinyloestradiol has been used in experimental models of prostate cancer to cause reversible atrophy of the prostate. When treatment is withdrawn, the prostate undergoes regrowth and DNA synthesis, setting the stage for initiation by chemical carcinogens. Shirai et al. (1986, 1990), Takai et al. (1991) and Mori et al. (1996) used this protocol. [The Working Group was aware of these studies but did not consider them relevant for evaluating the carcinogenicity of ethinyloestradiol or combinations containing it.]

Kidney models

Rat: Groups of 19–27 male Fischer 344 rats, six weeks of age, were fed diets containing 0.05% N-nitrosobis(2-hydroxypropyl)amine (NDHPA), 0.1% N-nitrosoethyl-N-hydroxyethylamine (NEHEA), 0.03% N-nitrosopiperidine (NPip), 0.02% 2-acetyl-aminofluorene or 0.5% N-nitrosobutyl-N-(4-hydroxybutyl)amine (NBHBA) for two weeks, followed by 0.001% (10 ppm) ethinyloestradiol for 49 weeks. At that time, ethinyloestradiol was found to have enhanced the incidences of liver hyperplastic nodules in rats initiated with NDHPA, NEHEA, 2-acetylaminofluorene or NPip and to have enhanced the incidence of hepatocellular carcinoma in rats initiated with NEHEA compared with controls; this nitrosamine also enhanced the incidence of kidney ade-nomas and renal-cell carcinomas. Tumorigenesis was inhibited in the lungs and urinary bladder of rats initiated with NDHPA or NBHBA. Ethinyloestradiol alone had no tumori-genic effect (Shirai *et al.*, 1987).

Hamster: Syrian golden hamsters, five weeks of age, were separated into groups of 30 animals that received four weekly subcutaneous injections of 10 mg/kg bw N-nitrosobis(2-oxopropyl)amine (NBOPA) to initiate renal tumorigenesis. These groups then received either control diet or a diet containing 1 ppm ethinyloestradiol for 27 weeks. An additional group of animals was fed the diet containing ethinyloestradiol. Ethinyloestradiol alone did not cause renal tumours or dysplasia. Initiation with NBOPA alone caused the appearance of nephroblastoma in 1/21 animals and 469 dysplastic tubules. Ethinyloestradiol increased the incidence of renal tumours in NBOPA-initiated animals to 4/27 (adenomas) compared with 1/21 (a nephroblastoma) and significantly ($p < 0.001$) increased the number of dys-plastic tubules (1602 compared with 469) (Mitsumori *et al.*, 1994).

The results of previous and new studies on oestrogens in mice and rats are summarized in Tables 34 and 35.

3.3 Progestogens used in combined oral contraceptives

3.3.1 *Studies reviewed previously*

Mouse

Chlormadinone acetate tested by oral administration to mice slightly increased the incidence of benign liver tumours in treated males.

Oral administration of ethynodiol diacetate to mice increased the incidence of benign liver tumours in males and increased the incidence of mammary tumours in castrated males.

Lynoestrenol increased the incidence of benign liver tumours in males and that of malignant mammary tumours in females.

Megestrol acetate increased the incidence of malignant mammary tumours in females.

Norethisterone acetate increased the incidence of benign liver tumours in males.

Norethisterone increased the incidences of benign liver tumours in males and of pituitary adenomas in females.

Oral administration of norethynodrel increased the incidences of pituitary adenomas in animals of each sex, of mammary tumours in castrated males and of malignant mammary tumours in females.

Table 34. Effects of ethinyloestradiol and mestranol alone and with known carcinogens on tumour incidence in mice

Oestrogen	Pituitary adenoma		Malignant mammary tumours		Uterine tumours	Vaginal/ cervical tumours	Liver			
							Adenoma		Foci (females)	
	Male	Female	Male	Female			Male	Female		
Ethinyloestradiol	+	+	+	+	+	+	+	+		
Mestranol	+	+	+	+			–	–		
Ethinyloestradiol + N-nitrosodiethylamine									Protective	
Ethinyloestradiol + N-nitrosodiethylamine + unleaded gasoline									+	

+, increased tumour incidence; –, no effect

Table 35. Effects of ethinyloestradiol and mestranol alone and with known carcinogens on tumour incidence in rats

Oestrogen	Pituitary adenoma (females)	Malignant mammary tumours (females)	Liver Adenoma		Carcinoma		Foci (females)	Kidney Adenoma (males)	Carcinoma (females)
			Male	Female	Male	Female			
Ethinyloestradiol	+	+	+	+		+	+		
Mestranol		+				+/−	+		
Ethinyloestradiol + N-nitrosoethyl-N-hydroxyethylamine					+			+	
Ethinyloestradiol + N-nitroso-diethylamine			+	+	+	+	+[a]		+
Mestranol + N-nitrosodiethylamine			+	+	+	+	+		

+, increased tumour incidence; −, no effect; +/−, slightly increased tumour incidence

[a] In one of three studies, ethinyloestradiol initiated hepatocarcinogenesis

After oral administration of norgestrel to mice, no increase in tumour incidence was observed.

Rat

In rats, oral administration of chlormadinone acetate, megestrol acetate or norgestrel did not increase the incidence of any tumour type.

Ethynodiol diacetate, tested by oral administration to rats, increased the incidence of benign mammary tumours in males.

Lynoestrenol slightly increased the incidence of malignant mammary tumours in females.

Norethisterone increased the incidence of benign liver tumours in males and caused small increases in the incidences of benign and malignant mammary tumours in males and of malignant mammary tumours in females.

Norethynodrel increased the incidences of benign and malignant liver-cell tumours, pituitary adenomas and benign and malignant mammary tumours in males and increased the incidence of benign liver tumours in females.

3.3.2   *New studies*
         (a)   *Oral administration*

Mouse

Schuppler and Gunzel (1979) summarized data from the study of the Committee on Safety of Medicines (1972) in the United Kingdom and from additional studies on the hepatocarcinogenicity of the progestogens, norgestrel, norethisterone acetate, norethisterone, chlormadione acetate, ethynodiol diacetate, norethynodrel, megestrol acetate and lynoestrenol, in mice. Increased incidences of liver tumours were detected in groups of 40–80 male CF-LP mice treated with norethisterone acetate, norethisterone, chlormadinone acetate or ethynodiol diacetate and in groups of 40–80 female CF-LP mice treated orally with norethynodrel for 20 months, but the increases were not significant at the 5% level. It was also reported that megestrol acetate given orally at up to 400 times the human contraceptive dose caused a statistically significant increase in the incidence of hepatocellular adenoma in females, from approximately 1% (25 mice) to 5% (73 mice) ($p < 0.05$). Groups of 120 male and female mice [strain not indicated] were treated orally with lynoestrenol at doses up to 400 times the human contraceptive dose for 20 months. The incidence of hepatocellular adenomas was significantly ($p < 0.05$) increased (from approximately 1 to 8%) in males. The incidences induced by megestrol acetate and lynoestrenol were given only as the average for three dose groups, making it impossible to determine a dose–response relationship. There were no statistically significant effects on liver tumour incidence in males or females treated orally with dl-norgestrel alone for 20 months (Schuppler & Gunzel, 1979). [The Working Group noted discrepancies in the numbers of animals and tumour incidences in these two reports but was unable to resolve the differences in the absence of the original data.]

Groups of 40 male and 40 female C57BL/10J mice, seven weeks of age, were fed a diet containing cyproterone acetate obtained by grinding 50-mg tablets of Androcur™ and mixing the powder into the diet at a concentration of 800 mg/kg (ppm) (calculated intake, 125 mg/kg bw per day) for 104 weeks. A control group consisted of eight males and eight females. Cyproterone acetate increased the mortality rate in both males and females after 40 weeks on test: no females survived past 97 weeks, and only four males survived to 104 weeks. The weight of the liver was increased in animals of each sex, and the increase in males was in excess of 100%. In addition, weight gain was reduced such that, at the end of a separate 13-week treatment period, the cyproterone acetate-treated mice weighed 33% less than controls. The causes of death were uterine enlargement in female mice and neoplastic diseases in males. The liver tumour incidences are shown in Table 36. Overall, hepatocellular tumours developed in 44% of the males and 22% of the females. In addition, 85% of the animals developed adenomatous polyps of the pyloric antrum and pancreatic islet hyperplasia (Tucker & Jones, 1996; Tucker et al., 1996). [The Working Group noted that this study has been criticized since the dose of cyproterone acetate administered clearly exceeded the maximum tolerated dose (Schauer et al., 1996).]

Table 36. Effects of cyproterone acetate (CPA) on liver tumour incidence in C57BL/10J mice

Liver tumour	Males		Females	
	Control	CPA	Control	CPA
Hepatocellular adenoma	0/8	7/39	0/8	2/37
Hepatocellular carcinoma	0/8	12/39	0/8	8/37

From Tucker & Jones (1996); Tucker et al. (1996)

Rat

Schuppler and Gunzel (1979) summarized data from the study of the Committee on Safety of Medicines (1972) on the hepatocarcinogenicity in rats of a number of progestogens. Rats [strain unspecified] were treated orally with the progestogens for two years at doses up to 400 times the human contraceptive dose. Table 37 summarizes the results presented in their paper, which indicate statistically significant increases. Cyproterone acetate at doses 200–400 times the human contraceptive dose did not increase the incidence of hepatocellular adenomas in another study in this report. In a further study, groups of 35 male and 35 female rats were treated orally with cyproterone acetate at doses of 250, 1250 or 6250 times the human contraceptive dose and were observed for 20 months. In males, a significant ($p < 0.01$) increase in the incidence of liver adenomas occurred only at 6250 times the human contraceptive dose, while in females a significant ($p < 0.01$) increase was observed at both 1250 and 6250 that dose (Schuppler et al., 1977; Schuppler & Gunzel, 1979).

**Table 37. Effects of various progestogens on the
incidence of hepatocellular adenomas in rats**

Progestogen	Males	Females
Norgestrel	–	–
Norethisterone	+	–
Chlormadinone acetate	–	–
Ethynodiol diacetate	–	–
Norethynodrel	+	+
Lynoestrenol	–	–
Megestrol acetate	–	–

From Committee on Safety of Medicines (1972)

Albino Sprague-Dawley-derived rats were fed diets containing 7.5 or 75 ppm nore-thisterone acetate, which provided intakes approximately 10 and 100 times the human contraceptive dose. The actual progestogen intake was stated to be 0.303 mg/kg bw for males and 0.397 mg/kg bw for females at the low dose and 3.18 mg/kg bw for males and 4.15 mg/kg bw for females at the high dose. Survival over the two-year study was greater in the treated (22%) than in control (10%) rats. Dose-related effects were seen in liver enlargement, numbers of altered hepatic foci and liver neoplastic nodules (adenomas or regenerative nodules) and the incidence of uterine polyps [details not reported]. No statistically significant increase in the incidence of malignant tumours was observed in the liver or other organs (Schardein, 1980).

Male Fischer 344 rats weighing 130–150 g were subjected to a partial hepatectomy 18 h before treatment with a microcrystalline suspension of cyproterone acetate (purity analytically confirmed) in saline as a single intraperitoneal injection of 100 mg/kg bw. Thirteen days later, the rats were fed a diet containing 0.02% 2-acetylaminofluorene to inhibit normal hepatocyte growth, and seven days later, the rats were given 2 mL/kg bw carbon tetrachloride to cause hepatocyte necrosis and stimulate regenerative growth. One week later, the rats were killed and their livers analysed for γ-GT-positive foci. Cyproterone acetate did not significantly increase the number of γ-GT-positive foci over control values (Schuppler et al., 1983). [The Working Group noted the use of a single dose and only male rats.]

The tumour initiating activity of cyproterone acetate was tested in groups of six female Sprague-Dawley rats, 22 days of age at the start of treatment, given 0 (vehicle control), 25, 50 or 100 mg/kg bw orally in olive oil on five consecutive days. One week after the last treatment, the rats were given 10 mg/kg bw Clophen A50 (a technical mixture of polychlorinated biphenyls) as a tumour promoter twice weekly for 11 weeks. One group of four animals was untreated. The livers were analysed for the presence of ATPase-deficient and γ-GT-positive foci. The numbers and area of these foci were significantly increased in a dose-dependent manner by cyproterone acetate (Deml et al., 1993).

Dog

Groups of 16 young pure-bred beagle bitches received lynoestrenol orally in tablet form at a dose representing 10, 50 and 125 times the human contraceptive dose daily for 364 weeks; controls received a placebo tablet. The results are summarized in Table 38. A biphasic dose–response effect on mammary tumorigenesis was seen: at the low dose, lynoestrenol appeared to protect against the development of mammary tumours, but at the intermediate and high doses, it was associated with increased incidences of mammary nodules and carcinomas [statistics not specified] (Misdorp, 1991).

Table 38. Effects of lynoestrol on mammary tumour incidence in beagle bitches

Treatment	Nodule incidence	Nodule latency (weeks)	Carcinoma incidence
Control	5/16	323	1/16
10 × HCD	0/16*		[0]
50 × HCD	16/16	191**	3/16 [NR]
125 × HCD	16/16	152**	7/16 [NR]

From Misdorp (1991); HCD, human contraceptive dose; [NR], statistical analysis not reported
*Significantly lower than in other groups ($p < 0.05$)
**Significantly earlier than in controls ($p < 0.05$)

In a study to determine the six-month toxicity of the progestogen STS 557, levonorgestrel was administered as control to four female and four male beagles, 7–12 months of age, at a dose of 1 mg/kg bw orally seven times a week for six months. Mammary hyperplasia but no nodules or malignant tumours was observed (Hoffmann *et al.*, 1983). [The Working Group noted the short duration of the study.]

    (*b*)   *Administration with known carcinogens*

Mouse

Groups of 20 female $B6AF_1$ mice, 12 weeks of age, received a silk thread impregnated with 3-methylcholanthrene inserted into the cervical canal and passed through the uterine wall; a control group received unimpregnated silk thread. Pellets containing 15 mg per mouse norethynodrel and 0.5 mg per mouse mestranol, alone and in combination, were then implanted subcutaneously and were renewed every three weeks for a total of 15 weeks. No tumours developed in the mice that did not receive 3-methylcholanthrene, but the steroids caused various histopathological changes in the mucosa of the cervix, uterus and vagina. Norethynodrel alone promoted the incidence of uterine tumours (11/14 compared with 5/35 in controls) but not of cervical or vaginal tumours (Blanzat-Reboud & Russfield, 1969).

Rat

Female Sprague-Dawley rats, seven weeks of age, were initiated with NDEA 24 h after partial hepatectomy; 24 h later, they were fed a diet containing norethynodrel, providing intakes of 0.5–0.75 mg/kg bw per day for nine months. After four months, a statistically significant ($p < 0.05$), sixfold increase in the number of γ-GT-positive, altered hepatic foci was observed in comparison with rats given NDEA alone. At nine months, the number of foci was reduced and significantly greater than with NDEA alone only when one norethynodrel-treated rat with a large number of foci was deleted from the analysis. No significant increase in the incidence of nodules or carcinomas was observed after nine months (Yager & Yager, 1980).

Male Fischer 344 rats, weighing 130–150 g, were subjected to a partial hepatectomy and 18 h later were given norethynodrel or norethisterone acetate (purity confirmed analytically) by intraperitoneal injection of 100 mg/kg bw as a microcrystalline suspension in saline; 13 days later, the rats were fed a diet containing 0.02% acetylaminofluorene to inhibit normal hepatocyte growth, and seven days later the rats were given 2 mL/kg bw carbon tetrachloride to cause hepatocyte necrosis and stimulate regenerative growth. One week later, the rats were killed and their livers were analysed for γ-GT-positive foci. Neither norethynodrel nor norethisterone acetate significantly increased the number of γ-GT-positive foci over control values (Schuppler *et al.*, 1983).

Hamster: Groups of 30 Syrian golden hamsters, five weeks of age, received four weekly subcutaneous injections of *N*-nitrosobis(2-oxypropyl)amine (NBOPA) at a dose of 10 mg/kg bw to initiate renal tumorigenesis and then received either control diet or a diet containing 10 mg/kg diet (ppm) levonorgestrel for 27 weeks. A third group of animals was not treated with the nitrosamine but was fed the diet containing levonorgestrol. Levonorgestrel alone did not cause renal tumours or dysplasia. Initiation with NBOPA caused nephroblastoma in 1/21 animals and 469 dysplastic tubules. Levonorgestrel did not significantly enhance the incidence of renal tumours in initiated animals (2/27 nephroblastomas and 2/27 renal adenomas) or increase the total number of dysplastic tubules (747) (Mitsumori *et al.*, 1994).

The results of previous and new studies on progestogens are summarized in Tables 39–41.

4. Other Data Relevant to an Evaluation of Carcinogenicity and its Mechanisms

4.1   Absorption, distribution, metabolism and excretion

The disposition of various formulations of oral contraceptives used in humans differs. In general, both the oestrogenic and progestogenic compounds in combined oral contraceptives are absorbed by the gut and metabolized largely in the liver. A fraction of the absorbed dose of ethinyloestradiol and several progestogens is excreted in the bile during

Table 39. Effects of various progestogens alone and with a known carcinogen on tumour incidence in mice

Progestogen	Pituitary adenoma		Mammary tumours		Uterine tumours	Vaginal/ cervical tumours	Liver			
	Male	Female	Benign (males)	Malignant (females)			Adenoma		Carcinoma	
							Male	Female	Male	Female
Chlormadinone acetate							+/-			
Cyproterone acetate							+[a]	+/–[a]	+[a]	+[a]
Ethynodiol diacetate			c				+/-			
Lynoestrenol				+			+			
Megestrol acetate				+				+		
Norethisterone acetate							+/-			
Norethisterone		+					+/-			
Norethynodrel	+	+	c	+				+/-		
Norethynodrel + 3-methyl-cholanthrene					+	–				

+, increased tumour incidence; +/–, slightly increased tumour incidence; –, no effect; c, increased incidence in castrated males
[a] Dose exceeded the maximum tolerated daily dose

Table 40. Effects of various progestogens alone and with a known carcinogen on tumour incidence in rats

Progestogen	Pituitary adenoma (males)	Mammary tumours			Liver				
		Benign (males)	Malignant		Adenoma		Carcinoma (males)	Foci	
			Male	Female	Male	Female		Male	Female
Cyproterone acetate					+[a]	+[a]			+[b]
Ethynodiol diacetate		+							
Lynoestrenol				+/-					
Norethisterone acetate					+	+		+	+ or −[c]
Norethisterone		+/-	+/-	+/-	+				
Norethynodrel		+	+		+	+	+		−[c]
Norethynodrel + N-nitrosodiethylamine	+								+

+, increased tumour incidence; +/-, slightly increased tumour incidence; −, no effect
[a] Liver adenomas detected only at high doses
[b] Tested for initiating activity; the results were positive in one study in which it was administered for five days and negative when administered as a single dose
[c] Tested as a single dose for initiating activity

Table 41. Effects of various progestogens on mammary tumour incidence in bitches

Progestogen	Benign	Malignant
Chlormadinone acetate	+	+
Lynoestrenol	+[a]	+[a]
Megestrol acetate	+	+

+, increased tumour incidence
[a] In this study, lynoestrenol had a biphasic effect, with protection at the low dose (10 times the human contraceptive dose) and enhancement at 50 and 125 times the human contraceptive dose.

its first transit through the liver. Although some of these compounds are partially re-absorbed via the enterohepatic circulation, a fraction may be lost in this 'first pass', reducing the overall bioavailability. The absorption rates are usually rapid, peak serum values being observed between 0.5 and 4 h after intake. Serum concentrations rise faster with multiple treatments than single doses and achieve higher steady-state levels, which are still punctuated by rises after each daily dose. The rise in steady-state levels with multiple doses may reflect the inhibitory effect of both oestrogens and progestogens on cytochrome P450 metabolic enzyme activities. Alternatively, oestrogens may induce the production of sex hormone-binding globulin, which may increase the capacity of the blood to carry progestogens. Binding of progestogen to the sex hormone-binding globulin may displace oestrogens and androgens, which may then cause adverse androgenic side-effects and alter serum lipid concentrations. The metabolism of progestogens and ethinyloestradiol typically involves oxidative modifications. In some cases, metabolism converts an inactive pro-drug into a hormonally active compound. Oxidized metabolites are typically conjugated as glucuronides or sulfates, and most are eliminated rapidly, with half-lives of 8–24 h.

Kopera (1985) reviewed the drug interactions associated with administration of progestogens to patients receiving other medications. Progestogens adversely affect the metabolism of various drugs and, in turn, the metabolism of progestogens is affected by the other drugs. These effects occur presumably as a consequence of effects on the induction of metabolic enzymes or on competition for metabolic pathways or for binding to serum carrier proteins.

Thomas *et al.* (1993) studied a single menstrual cycle in 25 pre-menopausal women who smoked five or more cigarettes per day and 21 non-smoking women to compare the plasma concentrations of luteinizing hormone, follicle-stimulating hormone, oestradiol, progesterone, testosterone, androstenedione, dehydroepiandrosterone sulfate and sex hormone-binding globulin and urinary excretion of oestradiol, oestriol and oestrone. No significant differences were found between the two groups for these parameters or in the lengths of the follicular and luteal phases.

Kuhnz and Löfberg (1995) evaluated the ratio of 6β-hydroxycortisol to cortisol excreted in urine as a measure of drug metabolizing activity. Groups of 12–15 women received combined oral contraceptives containing levonorgestrel, gestodene or cyproterone acetate in combination with ethinyloestradiol, or levonorgestrel or gestodene alone. Little or no difference in the ratio was observed between groups.

Coenen et al. (1996) gave groups of 22 women oral monophasic combined contraceptives containing 35, 30, 30 or 20 µg ethinyloestradiol with 250 µg norgestimate, 75 µg gestodene, 150 µg desogestrel or 150 µg desogestrel, respectively. Each woman received a dose once a day for 21 days of a 28-day cycle for six cycles. All of the steroidal serum parameters tested (total testosterone, free testosterone, dihydrotestosterone, androstenedione) were significantly decreased, and the concentrations of the steroid-binding proteins, sex hormone-binding globulin and cortisol-binding globulin were significantly increased, irrespective of the oral contraceptive preparation used. Differences between the groups were observed only in dehydroepiandrosterone sulfate and cortisol-binding globulin.

4.1.1   Ethinyloestradiol

(a)   Humans

Goldzieher and Brody (1990) reviewed information about the pharmacokinetics of ethinyloestradiol and mestranol given in a dose of 35 and 50 µg, respectively, in combination with 1 mg norethisterone. A group of 24 women received ethinyloestradiol and 27 women received mestranol. Serum ethinyloestradiol concentrations were measured after treatment with either oestrogen. Both treatments produced equal average serum concentrations of about 175 pg/mL, but there was wide inter-individual variation. The maximal serum concentrations were achieved in about 1–2 h, and the half-life for elimination ranged from 13 to 27 h. Intra-individual variation in the plasma concentration of ethinyloestradiol derived from mestranol did not differ significantly from that observed after ethinyloestradiol treatment. The oral bioavailability of ethinyloestradiol was only 38–48%. The authors also reviewed their earlier studies of patterns of urinary conjugates, glucuronides and sulfates in women from Nigeria, Sri Lanka and the United States after oral administration of radiolabelled ethinyloestradiol. The proportions of glucuronides and sulfates were about 70 and 18%, respectively, in each population; however, the Nigerian women had the lowest concentrations of oxidative metabolites and the American women the highest. [The basis for this diversity, whether genetic, nutritional or environmental, was unclear.]

Hümpel et al. (1990) obtained serum samples from a group of 30 women during one cycle of a combined oral contraceptive containing ethinyloestradiol and desogestrel and from a group of 39 women taking ethinyloestradiol and gestodene. The mean serum concentrations were 186–226 nmol/L sex hormone-binding globulin, 89–93 mg/L cortisol-binding globulin and 280–281 µg/L cortisol. The serum concentrations of ethinyloestradiol reached mean maximum levels of 106–129 pg/mL 1.6–1.8 h after pill intake.

Kuhnz *et al.* (1990a) compared the pharmacokinetics of ethinyloestradiol given as a single dose in combination with either gestodene or desogestrel to 18 women. In contrast to previous reports that the bioavailability of ethinyloestradiol differed according to the associated progestogen, this study showed no significant difference. The maximum concentration of ethinyloestradiol was found 1.9 h after ingestion and reached 101 and 104 pg/mL for the two combinations, respectively. The values for maximum concentrations and for the integral of the serum concentration over time (area under the concentration curve) differed between individuals, but, for each individual, the concentration of ethinyloestradiol reached with the two contraceptives was usually about the same.

(b)   Experimental systems

Standeven *et al.* (1990) studied the metabolism of ethinyloestradiol in primary cultures of rat hepatocytes. At 4, 24 or 48 h after establishment in culture, the cells maintained their ability to metabolize up to 90% of ethinyloestradiol substrate (4 nmol/L or 2 µmol/L) to polar conjugates during a 4-h incubation. The metabolites formed were reported to differ both quantitatively and qualitatively from those formed in rats *in vivo*.

The major pathway of ethinyloestradiol metabolism in humans and animals is 2-hydroxylation, which is presumably catalysed by the 3A4 isoform of cytochrome P450 (Guengerich, 1988; Yager & Liehr, 1996). Like catechols of oestrone and oestradiol, hydroxylated metabolites of ethinyloestradiol can also undergo redox cycling and damage DNA (Yager & Liehr, 1996).

4.1.2   *Mestranol*

(a)   Humans

The pharmacokinetics of mestranol has been investigated (Goldzieher & Brody, 1990) and reviewed (Bolt, 1979; Kuhl, 1990).

Mestranol is a pro-drug that binds poorly to the oestrogen receptor until it is demethylated in the gastrointestinal tract to its active form, ethinyloestradiol; 54% of mestranol is converted to ethinyloestradiol (Bolt & Bolt, 1974). Since the demethylation is not complete, more mestranol than ethinyloestradiol must be administered to achieve the same effect. The pharmacokinetics of mestranol corresponds to that of ethinyloestradiol, except that the peak concentrations are lower. Since mestranol is more lipophilic than ethinyloestradiol, it can be stored in fatty tissues (Bolt, 1979).

In a study by Goldzieher and Brody (1990), 24 women received ethinyloestradiol and 27 were given mestranol, both in combination with norethisterone. The bioavailability and maximum concentration of mestranol were about 30% lower than those of ethinyloestradiol. A 50-µg oral dose of mestranol was bioequivalent to a 35-µg dose of ethinyloestradiol, both administered in combination with 1 mg norethisterone. Administration of 50 µg mestranol resulted in a mean maximum concentration of ethinyloestradiol of 175 pg/mL at 1.9 h. Intra-individual differences in the plasma concentration of ethinyloestradiol over 24 h were large, however, when the effects of single doses were compared in the same individual at different times. The metabolites of mestranol found in urine are, apart from ethinyloestradiol, 2-hydroxyethinyloestradiol, 2-methoxyethinyl-oestradiol and 2-hydroxyethinyloestradiol-3-methyl ether (reviewed by Bolt, 1979).

 (*b*) *Experimental systems*

Studies in rats have shown that metabolites of mestranol undergo enterohepatic circulation, which may be affected by antibiotics such as neomycin (Brewster *et al.*, 1977). Further metabolism of demethylated mestranol is species-specific; for example, 2-hydroxylation occurs in rats and D-homo-annulation in rabbits and guinea-pigs (Abdel-Aziz & Williams, 1969; Ball *et al.*, 1973).

4.1.3 *Chlormadinone acetate*

 (*a*) *Humans*

The pharmacokinetics of chlormadinone acetate has been reviewed by Kuhl (1990) and in previous *IARC Monographs* (IARC, 1974, 1979); no recent data are available in humans, probably because there has been no or limited use since the early 1970s.

After intravenous injection of radiolabelled chlormadinone acetate, the steroid and its metabolites have an initial rapid half-life of 2.4 h, followed by a slow half-life of 80.1 h. The mean metabolic clearance rate is 126 L/day for chlormadinone acetate and 42.6 L/day for chlormadinone acetate and its metabolites. The long half-life and slow elimi-nation rate are probably due to accumulation of the drug in fat tissue (Dugwekar *et al.*, 1973).

 (*b*) *Experimental systems*

The major metabolites of chlormadinone acetate are 2α-hydroxychlormadinone acetate and 3β-hydroxychlormadinone acetate. Incubation of chlormadinone acetate with human or rat liver microsomes produces mainly the 3β-hydroxy metabolite. In contrast, incubation with microsomes from phenobarbital-treated rats produces the 2α-hydroxy metabolite, indicating that the metabolite pattern is dependent on the hepatic mono-oxygenase state (Handy *et al.*, 1974).

4.1.4 *Cyproterone acetate*

 (*a*) *Humans*

A group of eight young women were treated with a single oral dose of 100 mg cypro-terone acetate followed by a single intramuscular dose of 300 mg four weeks later, and the plasma concentration of both parent compound and the 15β-hydroxy metabolite were quantified in seven of the women. The bioavailability of cyproterone acetate after oral administration was about 88%; the mean maximum serum concentration reached 255 ng/mL between 2 and 3 h, and thereafter decreased biphasically, reaching a terminal half-life of about 3.6 days. After intramuscular injection, the serum concentration reached 191 ng/mL after two to three days and then declined, with a half-life of about 4.3 days. The serum concentrations of the 15β-hydroxy metabolite exceeded those of the parent compound 6 h after oral administration and four days after intramuscular injection.

Thereafter, the concentration of the 15β-hydroxy metabolite decreased at a rate parallel to that of cyproterone acetate, indicating that the formation of this metabolite was the rate-limiting metabolic step (Huber *et al.*, 1988).

A group of 15 women was treated with a single oral dose of 2.0 mg cyproterone acetate plus 0.035 mg ethinyloestradiol. After one week, three cycles of multiple treatments were started with the same preparation. After the single dose, the maximum concentration of cyproterone acetate was 15.2 ng/mL, which decreased biphasically with half-lives of 0.8 and 54 h, respectively; 3.5% of the dose was free, while 96.5% was bound to serum proteins. During the multiple treatment cycles, a twofold higher accumulation of cyproterone acetate was observed, and its half-life increased to 78 h (Kuhnz *et al.*, 1993a).

In a study to determine the bioequivalence of one 100-mg and two 50-mg tablets and to compare two analytical methods for cyproterone acetate, 36 young men received one 100-mg dose followed three weeks later by two 50-mg tablets. The mean maximum concentrations of cyproterone acetate in serum were 200–260 ng/mL 2–3 h after dosing, followed by a second peak between 6 and 12 h. Thereafter, the concentrations decreased biphasically until 120 h after dosing, reaching a mean half-life of about 50 h (Baumann *et al.*, 1996).

(b) Experimental systems
No data were available to the Working Group.

4.1.5 Desogestrel
(a) Humans
McClamrock and Adashi (1993) reported that desogestrel is metabolized rapidly and completely in the liver and gut wall. It is metabolized to 3-keto-desogestrel, which mediates its progestogenic effects, and it is not metabolized further to another progestogen. The serum concentrations of 3-keto-desogestrel reached maximum levels within 2–3 h after oral administration of desogestrel and were subsequently cleared with a half-life of 12–24 h. In a review (Stone, 1995), it was reported that desogestrel reaches a steady-state serum concentration within 8–10 days. In serum, about 5% of desogestrel circulates freely, while 65% is bound to albumin and 30% to sex hormone-binding globulin.

Madden *et al.* (1990) studied the metabolism of desogestrel in microsomes from six human livers *in vitro*. The main metabolite formed was 3-keto-desogestrel; 3α-hydroxy-desogestrel and 3β-hydroxydesogestrel were also detected. The metabolism of desogestrel was inhibited by 50% by primaquine at a concentration of 30 μmol/L, but not by levonorgestrel at 250 μmol/L.

Nineteen women were given three cycles of a triphasic oral contraceptive with combinations of desogestrel and ethinyloestradiol at doses of 50 and 35 μg for the first seven days, 100 and 30 μg for days 8–14 and 150 and 30 μg for days 15–21, respectively, followed by seven days without hormone. Multiple blood samples were taken from the women throughout this interval, and serum concentrations of 3-keto-desogestrel, ethinyloestradiol and sex hormone-binding globulin were determined, together with the elimination half-life and dose proportionality. The concentration of 3-keto-desogestrel reached steady-state level at each desogestrel dose, and the pharmacokinetics was proportional to dose. The concentration of ethinyloestradiol also reached a steady state, and the pharmacokinetics was constant thereafter. The concentration of sex hormone-binding globulin was significantly increased between days 1 and 7 of the cycle but not between days 7, 14 and 21 (Archer *et al.*, 1994).

(b)   Experimental systems
No data were available to the Working Group.

4.1.6   Gestodene
(a)   Humans
Gestodene is an active progestogen that has an oral bioavailability of almost 100% and shows pharmacokinetics linear to dose. The serum concentrations are four times higher after multiple treatment cycles than after one cycle, and the area under the concentration curve increases by five- to eightfold after multiple cycles of gestodene plus ethinyloestradiol. Gestodene is metabolized primarily in the liver by P450 CYP 3A4, and it is a strong inducer of this enzyme. Although ethinyloestradiol is also metabolized by CYP 3A4, gestodene does not appear to inhibit its metabolism. Known metabolites of gestodene include dihydrogestodene, 3,5-tetrahydrogestodene and hydroxygestodene. After a single 75-µg dose of gestodene alone, 64% of the compound was bound to sex hormone-binding globulin in the serum, 34% was bound to albumin and about 1.3% was free. Clearance is dependent on the concentration of free gestodene. The half-life of clearance and elimination is 10–18 h and is higher after multiple doses than after a single dose of gestodene plus ethinyloestradiol. Monophasic preparations typically contain 75 µg gestodene plus 20 or 30 µg ethinyloestradiol, given for 21 days per 28-day cycle. Triphasic preparations contain 50, 70 or 100 µg of gestodene combined with 30, 40 and 30 µg ethinyloestradiol, respectively, in phases administered for weeks 1, 2, and 3 of a four-week cycle. Gestodene does not reduce the oestrogen-induced increases in the concentration of sex hormone-binding globulin and does not affect serum testosterone levels (Shoupe, 1994; Kuhl *et al.*, 1995; Wilde & Balfour, 1995). Täuber *et al.* (1990) found that orally administered gestodene is completely absorbed and exhibits dose-linear pharmacokinetics. The maximum serum concentrations reached 1, 3 and 5 ng/mL after single doses of 25, 75 and 125 µg, respectively. Only 0.6% was not bound to protein, while 75% was bound to sex hormone-binding globulin and 24% to albumin.

Kuhnz *et al.* (1990b) studied the binding of gestodene to serum protein in 37 women who had taken a combined oral contraceptive containing gestodene plus ethinyloestradiol for at least three months: 0.6% was free, while 24% was bound to albumin and 75% to sex hormone-binding globulin .

Kuhnz *et al.* (1991) examined the effects of single and multiple administrations of a triphasic combined oral contraceptive containing gestodene and ethinyloestradiol on the concentrations of ethinyloestradiol and testosterone in 10 women. After a single oral dose of 0.1 mg gestodene plus 0.03 mg ethinyloestradiol, the serum ethinyloestradiol concentration reached 100 pg/mL in about 1.9 h; thereafter, the concentration declined, with a half-life of 11 h. On day 21 of the treatment cycle, the maximum concentrations reached 140 pg/mL 1.6 h after pill intake. In comparison with pretreatment concentrations, those of total and free testosterone were reduced by about 60%.

Kuhnz *et al.* (1993b) treated 14 women with a combined oral contraceptive containing 0.1 mg gestodene plus 0.03 mg ethinyloestradiol as a single dose or for three months as a triphasic regimen. The maximum serum concentrations of gestodene were 4.3 ng/mL after a single dose, 15 ng/mL at the end of the first cycle and 14.4 ng/mL at the end of three cycles, reached 30 min after dosing. A half-life for clearance of 18 h was observed after a single treatment, the volume of distribution being 84 L. Multiple treatments increased the clearance half-life to 20–22 h and reduced the distribution volume to about 18 L. The serum sex hormone-binding globulin concentration increased with multiple treatments, presumably as an effect of ethinyloestradiol; this change in serum protein concentration is thought to account for the observed change in the distribution of gestodene, from 1.3% free, 69% bound to sex hormone-binding globulin and 29% bound to albumin after a single treatment, to 0.6% free, 81% bound to sex hormone-binding globulin and 18% bound to albumin after multiple treatments.

Heuner *et al.* (1995) treated 14 women with a combined oral contraceptive containing 0.1 mg gestodene plus 0.03 mg ethinyloestradiol as a single administration or for three months as a triphasic regimen. The serum concentrations of gestodene, ethinyloestradiol, cortisol-binding globulin, sex hormone-binding globulin and testosterone were followed after the single treatment and through cycles 1 and 3. The serum concentration of ethinyloestradiol reached a peak of about 65 pg/mL by 1.7 h after oral administration; after multiple treatments, the maximum was as high as 90 pg/mL, but the time to reach the maximum concentration was unchanged. The concentration of gestodene reached a maximum of 3.5 ng/mL within 0.7 h after a single dose and 8.7 ng/mL within 0.9 h after multiple doses. The clearance half-time for a single dose of gestodene also increased, from 12.6 h to nearly 20 h. There was a large increase in the concentration with time after multiple treatments. After a single dose, 1.3% of gestodene in serum was unbound, while 30% was bound to albumin and 68% was bound to sex hormone-binding globulin.

(*b*) *Experimental systems*

No data were available to the Working Group.

4.1.7 *Levonorgestrel* (see also the monograph on 'Hormonal contraceptives, progestogens only', section 4.1.2)

(*a*) *Humans*

The clinical pharmacokinetics and metabolic effects of levonorgestrel have been reviewed (Fotherby, 1995; Lachnit-Fixson, 1996). Lipid metabolism appears to be largely unaffected by three-phasic administration of levonorgestrel, most studies showing no significant change in the concentrations of high- or low-density lipoprotein or cholesterol. Effects on carbohydrate metabolism have been described, but the results are not consistent. Since levonorgestrel binds strongly to sex hormone-binding globulin, its pharmacokinetics is affected by the large number of factors that affect this globulin.

Stanczyk and Roy (1990) reviewed the metabolism of levonorgestrel in women treated orally with radioactively labelled compound. Levonorgestrel was found mostly untransformed in serum within 1–2 h after administration, but the concentrations of conjugated metabolites increased progressively between 4 and 24 h after ingestion. Most of the conjugates were sulfates and glucuronides. In addition to the remaining unconjugated levonorgestrel, considerable amounts of unconjugated and sulfate-conjugated forms of $3\alpha,5\beta$-tetrahydrolevonorgestrel were found; smaller quantities of conjugated and unconjugated $3\alpha,5\alpha$-tetrahydrolevonorgestrel and 16β-hydroxylevonorgestrel were also identified (Sisenwine et al., 1975a). About 45% of radioactively labelled levonorgestrel was excreted via the urine and about 32% via the faeces. The major urinary metabolites were glucuronides—most abundantly $3\alpha,5\beta$-tetrahydrolevonorgestrel glucuronide—and smaller quantities of sulfates (Sisenwine et al., 1975b).

Carol et al. (1992) evaluated the pharmacokinetics of levonorgestrel in groups of 11–20 women given single or multiple treatments with combined oral contraceptive preparations containing 125 µg levonorgestrel plus 30 or 50 µg ethinyloestradiol. The serum concentrations of levonorgestrel reached a maximum of about 4 ng/mL 1–2 h after a single treatment with either preparation. After 21 days of treatment, the peak and sustained concentrations of levonorgestrel were about twice as high as those after a single treatment. The serum concentration of sex hormone-binding globulin increased after treatment with both contraceptives but to a greater extent with the contraceptive containing 50 µg ethinyloestradiol, indicating the important role of the oestrogen in induction of this protein.

Kuhnz et al. (1994a) treated 14 women with a combined oral contraceptive containing 0.125 mg levonorgestrel plus 0.03 mg ethinyloestradiol as a single dose or for three months as a triphasic regimen. The serum concentration of free levonorgestrel reached a peak of 0.06–0.08 ng/mL about 1 h after treatment. In contrast, the calculated values of the area under the concentration curve more than doubled, from 0.32 to 0.75–0.77 ng × h/mL, during the first and third multiple treatment cycles. The serum concentrations of cortisol-binding globulin and sex hormone-binding globulin more than doubled after multiple treatments with the contraceptive. After a single dose, 1.4% of the levonorgestrel in serum was free, while 43% was bound to albumin and 55% to sex hormone-binding globulin. After multiple treatments, only 0.9–1.0% levonorgestrel in serum was free and 25–30% was bound to albumin, while the amount bound to sex hormone-binding globulin increased to 69–74%. The concentrations of free and total testosterone decreased from 3 and 460 pg/mL, respectively, before treatment to 1 and 270 pg/mL, respectively, at the end of one treatment cycle, but had increased again to 2 and 420 pg/mL by the first day of the third cycle.

Kuhnz et al. (1992) treated groups of eight to nine women with a combined oral contraceptive containing 0.15 mg levonorgestrel plus 0.03 mg ethinyloestradiol as a single dose or for three months on a monophasic regimen. The peak concentrations of levo-norgestrel were found 1 h after single or multiple treatments, but the peak serum concen-trations were 3.1 and 5.9 ng/mL, respectively. The area under the concentration curve increased by two- to fourfold for total and free levonorgestrel when a single dose was compared with multiple treatments. The distribution of free, albumin-bound and sex hormone-binding globulin-bound levonorgestrel was similar in women who had received one or multiple treatments, but the serum concentration of the globulin increased signifi-cantly after multiple treatments.

(b) Experimental systems

Kuhnz *et al.* (1995) studied aspects of the pharmacokinetics of levonorgestrel, nor-gestimate and levonorgestrel-oxime in rats, the last two compounds being pro-drugs of levonorgestrel. The maximum concentration of levonorgestrel was reached about 1 h after treatment and decreased thereafter. In animals treated with norgestimate or levonor-gestrel-oxime, the serum concentration of levonorgestrel increased up to about 8 h after treatment and decreased only slightly thereafter up to 24 h after treatment. The total dose ingested, measured as the area under the concentration curve, for levonorgestrel during a 24-h interval was related linearly to the administered dose of each compound.

In a trial of drugs for pregnancy maintenance, Kuhnz and Beier (1994) administered levonorgestrel at a dose of 10–300 µg/day or norgestimate at 30–1000 µg/day subcuta-neously to pregnant rats which had been ovariectomized on day 8 of pregnancy. These rats also received a daily dose of 1 µg oestrone. Doses of 300 µg/day of either compound fully maintained pregnancy. In serum samples collected from each animal, the concentration of levonorgestrel increased up to 2–8 h after administration and remained at a plateau thereafter up to 24 h. The area under the concentration curve during the 24-h interval after administration was linearly related to the administered dose of levonorgestrel.

4.1.8 Megestrol acetate

(a) Humans

After administration of megestrol acetate at 160 mg/day to post-menopausal women with advanced breast cancer, the maximum concentration in serum was reached within 2–4 h. Co-administration of megestrol acetate and aminoglutethimide decreased the serum concentration of megestrol acetate by 74% (Lundgren *et al.*, 1990).

Megestrol acetate is hydroxylated at various positions of the steroid molecule (Cooper & Kellie, 1968; Lundgren *et al.*, 1990). It is metabolized more slowly than pro-gesterone. The 17α-acetoxy group and the 6(7)-double bond are considered to provide resistance to metabolism by liver enzymes (Cooke & Vallance, 1965). The major route of elimination in humans is via the urine. After administration of 4–90 mg radiolabelled megestrol acetate to patients, 56–78% was excreted in the urine and only 7–30% in faeces; 5–8% of that in urine was present as metabolites (Cooper & Kellie, 1968).

(b)   *Experimental systems*
No data were available to the Working Group.

4.1.9   *Norethisterone* (see also the monograph on 'Hormonal contraceptives, progestogens only, section 4.1.3)

(a)   *Humans*

Although norethisterone is absorbed almost completely, it undergoes first-pass metabolism, which decreases its bioavailability to an average of 64%. There is wide interindividual variation in its absorption, which is estimated to be as high as three- to fivefold. Norethisterone is absorbed rapidly, achieving maximum serum concentrations within 1–4 h. After doses of 0.5, 1 and 3 mg, the serum concentrations peaked at 2–5, 5–10 and up to 30 ng/mL, respectively. When given in combination with ethinyloestradiol, norethisterone reaches higher serum levels, which also increase with multiple doses until they reach a steady state at high concentrations. The higher steady-state level has been attributed to a reduced rate of metabolism when norethisterone and ethinyloestradiol are combined. Furthermore, the oestrogen induces sex hormone-binding globulin which binds norethisterone and changes the relative distribution of free and albumin-bound norethisterone. The half-life for elimination is about 8–10 h. Norethisterone is stored in various target organs, and about 22% of the dose accumulates in fat (Kuhl, 1990).

The major metabolites of norethisterone are isomers of 5α-dihydronorethisterone and tetrahydronorethisterone, which are excreted largely as glucuronides. Because of steric hindrance of the bulky ethinyl group at position 17α, only a small percentage of norethisterone metabolites are conjugated at the 17β-hydroxy group. The ethinyl group remains intact in 90% of metabolites (Kuhl, 1990; Shenfield & Griffin, 1991).

(b)   *Experimental systems*
No data were available to the Working Group.

4.1.10   *Lynoestrenol, ethynodiol diacetate and norethynodrel*

(a)   *Humans*

Lynoestrenol, ethynodiol diacetate and norethynodrel are pro-drugs of norethisterone. Both lynoestrenol and norethynodrel are converted into the active steroids in the gastrointestinal tract and liver, and the conversion is so fast that, 30 min after ingestion, ethynodiol diacetate cannot be detected in serum. The metabolic pathways of lynoestrenol and ethynodiol diacetate involve ethynodiol as the intermediate. The disposition of the three progestogens is largely similar to that of norethisterone, except that the terminal half-life after ingestion of lynoestrenol is longer (Kuhl, 1990).

(b)   *Experimental systems*
No data were available to the Working Group.

4.1.11 *Norgestimate*

(*a*) *Humans*

Alton *et al.* (1984) studied the metabolism of ¹⁴C-labelled norgestimate in four women over two weeks. An average of 36.8% of the radiolabel was recovered in faeces and 46.8% in urine. Of the urinary metabolites, 57% was released by enzymatic hydrolysis while 12% was unconjugated. The metabolites were separated by chromatography and shown to include norgestrel, 16β-hydroxynorgestrel, 2α-hydroxynorgestrel, 3α,5β-tetrahydronorgestrel, 3,16-dihydroxy-5-tetrahydronorgestrel and an unidentified trihydroxylated metabolite of norgestrel.

McGuire *et al.* (1990) reviewed previous studies on norgestimate and noted that the ¹⁴C-labelled compound was rapidly absorbed and reached maximum levels in serum within 0.5–2 h. The estimated half-life for elimination was 45–71 h. The pattern of metabolites separated and identified by gas chromatography and mass spectroscopy indicated the progressive steps of metabolism: norgestimate undergoes hydrolysis at the 17 position, cleavage of the oxime at position 3, followed by reduction of the ketone, hydroxylation in the A and D rings, reduction of the double bond between carbons 4 and 5, and subsequent conjugation to a sulfate or glucuronide. In a study of 10 women who received one or multiple oral doses of 180 μg norgestimate plus 35 μg of ethinyloestradiol, norgestimate was found to be absorbed rapidly, with a maximum serum concentration of 100 pg/mL reached 1 h after treatment. The concentrations declined rapidly thereafter, and none was detectable by 5 h with the techniques used.

The metabolism of norgestimate was investigated in fragments of human colon and in microsomes isolated from human liver. Two hours after addition of labelled norgestimate to the colon tissue, 38% unaltered norgestimate, 49% 17-deacetylnorgestimate and 8.1% conjugated metabolites were found. Five hours after addition of norgestimate to human liver microsomes, there was some deacetylation of norgestimate to 17-deacetylnorgestimate in the absence of NADPH; in the presence of NADPH, only 30% unaltered norgestimate remained, with 39% 17-deacetylnorgestimate, less than 2% 3-ketonorgestimate, 10% norgestrel and 15% unidentified metabolites. The metabolism of 17-deacetylnorgestimate by human liver microsomes was NADPH- and oxygen-dependent and yielded norgestrel and other metabolites (Madden & Back, 1991).

Kuhnz *et al.* (1994b) treated 12 women with single doses of combined oral contraceptives containing either 250 μg levonorgestrel plus 50 μg ethinyloestradiol or 250 μg norgestimate plus 35 μg ethinyloestradiol. About 22% of the dose of norgestimate became available systemically as levonorgestrel.

(*b*) *Experimental systems*

Norgestimate is metabolized mainly to levonorgestrel. In rabbits, norgestimate had no greater androgenic activity than progesterone *in vivo* or *in vitro*. It showed very poor affinity for androgen receptors and did not bind to human sex hormone-binding globulin (Phillips *et al.*, 1992).

After subcutaneous administration of norgestimate to immature, castrated male rats and pregnant female rats, levonorgestrel was the principal metabolite. The progestational and androgenic pharmacological responses to treatment with norgestimate were equivalent to those observed at the concentrations of levonorgestrel achieved after that dose (Kuhnz & Beier, 1994).

4.1.12   *Norgestrel*

(*a*)   *Humans*

No data were available to the Working Group.

(*b*)   *Experimental systems*

Hussain *et al.* (1991) examined the effects of an oral contraceptive containing ethinyloestradiol at 50 µg and norgestrel at 0.5 mg, on hepatic cytochrome P450 and cytochrome b5 activity in microsomes and glutathione *S*-transferase activity in cytosol. Doses spanning two orders of magnitude (1/20th–1/2000th of the pill dose) were administered to mice daily for 15 days before the study *in vitro*. The intermediate doses significantly decreased cytochrome P450 and cytochrome b5 activity and increased the sulfhydryl group concentration but had no effect on glutathione *S*-transferase activity; the highest dose (1/20th of the pill), however, decreased the activity of this enzyme.

4.2   Receptor-mediated effects

4.2.1   *Combined oral contraceptives*

Anderson *et al.* (1989) obtained tissue from breast biopsies taken from 347 pre-menopausal women and determined the incorporation of tritiated thymidine into the DNA of epithelial cells. The labelling index (the percentage of cells that had incorporated tritiated thymidine) was higher in women who used combined oral contraceptives than in women who did not during the first 13 days and last seven days of the menstrual cycle. The difference was significant for days 6–13 (approximately 80% increase for 38–44 women per group) but not for days 21–28 (15–20% increase for 43–49 women per group). Multivariate analysis indicated that the effect of current oral contraceptive use increased cell proliferation significantly ($p < 0.01$); the effect appeared to be confined to nulliparous women ($p < 0.005$). The women reported use of at least 20 different brands of oral contraceptive, and the heterogeneity in response in terms of labelling index was statistically significant in the multivariate analysis. There was an apparent relation between ethinyloestradiol dose and labelling index, which increased from 0.66% (95% CI, 0.52–0.85; $n = 83$) and 0.89% (95% CI, 0.65–1.2; $n = 55$) for users of less than 35 µg per day to 1.3% (95% CI, 0.82–1.9; $n = 15$) for women taking 35 µg per day and 3.5% (95% CI, 3.2–3.9) for two women using 50 µg per day. There was no apparent effect of progestogen dose, which was associated with a labelling index of 0.97–0.98% in 21 women using low-progestogen doses, i.e. norgesterel or desogestrel, and 51 women using high-progestogen doses, i.e. norethisterone, lynoestrenol or ethynodiol acetate. This value was similar to the labelling index found in 36 women using triphasic oral contraceptives (0.94%). In a study by

Williams *et al.* (1991), of similar design, 49 oral contraceptive users were compared with 127 women who were not. The observation of an increased breast epithelial cell labelling index in users during the second week of the menstrual cycle was confirmed. Furthermore, throughout the menstrual cycle, fewer cells expressed oestrogen receptor in users than in non-users, the major difference also occurring during week 2. Two further studies did not, however, find an increased labelling index in breast epithelium of women using combined oral contraceptives (Anderson *et al.*, 1982; Going *et al.*, 1988). In a smaller study (Olsson *et al.*, 1996), breast epithelium staining for Ki-S5 antibody (a marker of DNA synthesis) was investigated in reduction mammoplasty samples from 58 women aged 17–47 years; 18 women were current users of oral contraceptives, 34 were past users, and six had never been exposed. There was no difference in labelling index in the three groups or between parous and nulliparous women. There was, however, a significant increase in labelling in 41 women who had used oral contraceptives before a first full-term pregnancy and in 31 who had used them before the age of 20 in comparison with the other women ($n = 17$ and 27, respectively). Taken together, these studies clearly demonstrate that combined oral contraceptive use increases breast epithelial cell proliferation; the study of Anderson *et al.* (1989) suggests that the dose of ethinyloestradiol influences the magnitude of this effect in the presence of progestogens.

4.2.2   *Ethinyloestradiol*

   (*a*)   *Humans*

Odlind *et al.* (1980) studied the effects of combined oral contraceptive use on the concentrations of sex hormone-binding globulin in five healthy pre-menopausal women. A dose of 35 µg per day ethinyloestradiol in combination with 0.5 mg per day nore-thisterone or a dose of 50 µg per day mestranol combined with 1 mg norethisterone given for the duration of one menstrual cycle increased the concentrations by approximately 100%. Administration of 60 µg ethinyloestradiol every other day in combination with 0.5 mg per day norethisterone caused a 50% increase, and a combination of 50 µg per day ethinyloestradiol with 3 mg norethisterone acetate or 2.5 mg lynoestrenol caused a 20% increase. The same dose of 50 µg per day ethinyloestradiol in combination with 1 mg per day lynoestrenol increased the concentration of sex hormone-binding globulin by approximately 80%.

   (*b*)   *Experimental systems*

The synthetic oestrogen ethinyloestradiol has been shown to bind to the oestrogen receptor of calf and rabbit uterus, rat liver and human oviduct (Kappus *et al.*, 1973; Eisenfeld *et al.*, 1978; Muechler & Kohler, 1980; Powell-Jones *et al.*, 1980; Aten & Eisenfeld, 1982; Lubahn *et al.*, 1985). Its relative binding affinity to the human oviductal receptor was about equal to that of oestradiol (Muechler & Kohler, 1980). Binding to the calf uterine receptor was 2–2.5 times higher than that of oestradiol (Lubahn *et al.*, 1985).

Ethinyloestradiol transiently enhanced replicative DNA synthesis (tritiated thymidine incorporation) in female rat liver. After subcutaneous implantation of time-release pellets providing 2.5 μg/rat ethinyloestradiol per day, DNA synthesis peaked between 24 and 72 h and slowly returned to control values within 7–14 days (Yager *et al.*, 1986). Similar findings were obtained with doses of 2 μg/kg per day to 3 mg/kg per day delivered by sub-cutaneous injection. A daily dose of 0.5 mg/kg (approximately 80 μg/rat) caused an increase in liver weight (by about 60% in comparison with pair-fed controls, the latter showing a 35% reduction in liver weight in comparison with control rats fed *ad libitum*) and in liver DNA content (by approximately 30% in comparison with pair-fed controls) (Ochs *et al.*, 1986). For these two effects, the relationship between dose and response was approximately log-linear over the range of doses tested (Ochs *et al.*, 1986; Schulte-Hermann *et al.*, 1988). Oral administration of ethinyloestradiol was less effective than subcutaneous injection (Ochs *et al.*, 1986). The effects at the lower doses are probably mediated by the oestrogen receptor, because the increase in DNA synthesis was inhibited by treatment with the anti-oestrogen tamoxifen (15 μg/rat per day), which by itself did not alter hepatic DNA synthesis (Yager *et al.*, 1986).

Prolonged exposure of female rats to ethinyloestradiol at a dose of 2.5 or 5 μg/rat per day from time-release pellets stimulated replicative DNA synthesis in the liver during the first week, but strongly inhibited this process after 28 days (72% inhibition) and 42 days (88% inhibition) of ethinyloestradiol treatment in comparison with untreated controls. Treatment with 5 μg/rat per day ethinyloestradiol for 21 days inhibited the regenerative growth response (tritiated thymidine incorporation) usually seen during the first four days after partial hepatectomy. Epidermal growth factor receptor levels were decreased after seven days of ethinyloestradiol treatment, but had returned to control levels after 21 days (Yager *et al.*, 1994).

Moser *et al.* (1996) treated 12-day-old B6C3F1 mice with a single intraperitoneal dose of 5 mg/kg bw NDEA followed four weeks later by administration of ethinyloestradiol at 1 mg/kg diet for 16 weeks. Treatment with NDEA and oestrogen did not change the DNA labelling index (0.4–0.8%; bromodeoxyuridine (BrdU) incorporation) observed in normal hepatocytes, but ethinyloestradiol reduced by approximately 70% the markedly increased labelling index (18%) caused by NDEA in hepatic foci of cellular alteration. This ethinyl-oestradiol-induced decrease in DNA synthesis in foci was accompanied by a decrease in the size of these foci and by a reduction in the number of foci with a decreased (as com-pared with normal hepatocytes) content of transforming growth factor (TGF)-β1 and of the mannose-6-phosphatase/insulin–like growth factor-II receptor, which is involved in acti-vation of latent TGF-β1.

Vickers *et al.* (1989) and Vickers and Lucier (1991, 1996) gave ovariectomized rats a single intraperitoneal dose of 200 mg/kg bw NDEA, followed by a daily dose of 90 μg/kg bw ethinyloestradiol by slow-release implant for 30 weeks. This treatment restored the decreased liver weights to the values in intact controls, increased the uterine weights above those of intact controls, and restored the decreased total nuclear and cytosolic oestrogen receptor concentrations and the nuclear hepatic oestrogen receptor occupancy in elutriated hepatic parenchymal cells to values greater than those in intact controls. Pretreatment with the chemical carcinogen slightly enhanced these effects of ethinyloestradiol (Vickers & Lucier, 1991). Very similar effects were found in isolated hepatic sinusoidal endothelial and Kupffer cells enriched by centrifugal elutriation. These cell fractions, derived from female rats treated with a single intraperitoneal dose of 200 mg/kg bw NDEA with or without ethinyloestradiol at 90 μg/kg bw per day for 30 weeks, showed a 5–6.5-fold increase in nuclear oestrogen receptor levels and a two- to three-fold increase in receptor occupancy (Vickers & Lucier, 1996).

In vitro, ethinyloestradiol at 15×10^{-6} mol/L induced mitogenesis in primary cultures of female rat hepatocytes, increasing tritiated thymidine incorporation by two- to three-fold 30 h after exposure (Shi & Yager, 1989; Ni & Yager, 1994a). Although ethinyl-oestradiol by itself therefore appeared to have only weak mitogenic effects on rat hepa-tocytes, as a co-mutagen with epidermal growth factor it strongly enhanced the induction of hepatic DNA synthesis when this factor was added during the last 12 h of the 30-h exposure to oestrogen. Thus, Shi and Yager (1989) demonstrated that 25 ng/mL epi-dermal growth factor increased tritiated thymidine incorporation by almost ninefold at an ethinyloestradiol concentration of 2.5 μmol/L, and almost 14-fold at 15 μmol/L. An 18-h exposure to 2 μmol/L ethinyloestradiol doubled the number of epidermal growth factor receptors per cell, providing a rational explanation for the increased sensitivity of ethinyloestradiol-exposed hepatocytes to epidermal growth factor. A similar effect occurred *in vivo* 24 h after a single 2.5-μg dose of ethinyloestradiol given to female rats: binding of radiolabelled epidermal growth factor started to increase after 8 h and reached twofold maximum enhancement after 18 h. The amount of epidermal growth factor receptor protein increased proportionally, and its half-life increased by 4.3-fold, while receptor mRNA synthesis was not affected by ethinyloestradiol. Thus, stabilization of the epidermal growth factor receptor protein appeared to be the mechanism by which ethinyloestradiol co-stimulated epidermal growth factor-induced mitogenesis in female rat hepatocytes. Epidermal growth factor-induced growth of male rat hepatocytes, however, was inhibited by oestrogen treatment (Francavilla *et al.*, 1989). Although this result suggests that marked sex differences exist in the mitogenic effects of epidermal growth factor and oestrogens on rat liver, the use of a different cell culture medium may also have played a role (Yager & Liehr, 1996).

In the presence of 30 nmol/L dexamethasone, ethinyloestradiol treatment at concen-trations of 1×10^{-5}–3×10^{-5} mol/L for five days induced γ-GT activity in cultured rat hepatocytes (Edwards & Lucas, 1985).

4.2.3   *Mestranol*

(a)   *Humans*

Odlind *et al.* (1980) studied the effects of combined oral contraceptive use on the plasma concentrations of sex hormone-binding globulin in five healthy pre-menopausal women. A dose of 50 μg/day mestranol in combination with 1.0 mg/day norethisterone given for the duration of one menstrual cycle to five pre-menopausal women increased the concentration of sex hormone-binding globulin by approximately 100%.

(b)   *Experimental systems*

Mestranol does not bind to the oestrogen receptor in rabbit uterus (Kappus *et al.*, 1973) but bound to those in calf uterus and human oviduct (Muechler & Kohler, 1980; Lubahn *et al.*, 1985), although its relative binding affinity was about two orders of magnitude less than that of oestradiol or ethinyloestradiol.

Mestranol caused a threefold increase in replicative DNA synthesis in female rat liver 24 h after the insertion of slow-release pellets delivering 2.5 or 5 μg/rat per day. This effect may be mediated by the oestrogen receptor because the increase in DNA synthesis induced by 2.5 μg per day mestranol was inhibited by concomitant treatment with 15 μg/rat per day tamoxifen, which by itself did not alter hepatic DNA synthesis (Yager *et al.*, 1986). The mestranol-induced increase in DNA synthesis was confirmed in experiments in which mestranol was given at a dose of 0.2 mg/kg diet to female rats for eight months. This treatment effectively promoted the induction of enzyme-altered foci in the liver by a single dose of NDEA, as judged from a threefold increase in the BdrU incorporation index in these preneoplastic foci relative to the labelling index in the surrounding normal hepatocytes, which was also increased (Dragan *et al.*, 1996).

In vitro, mestranol at doses of 10^{-8}–10^{-5} mol/L enhanced mitogenesis in HepG2 human hepatocarcinoma cells by up to 80% in comparison with control cells (Coezy *et al.*, 1987), and it was co-mitogenic at 10^{-6}–10^{-5} mol/L in primary female rat hepatocytes cultured in the presence of TGF-α (Ni & Yager, 1994b). In another study, however, mestranol inhibited the growth of Hep3B human hepatoma cells at 10^{-5} mol/L under conditions in which it did not significantly affect the growth of HepG2 cells (Jiang *et al.*, 1995). Tamoxifen at 10^{-6}–10^{-5} mol/L eliminated the mestranol-induced mitogenesis in oestrogen receptor-containing HepG2 carcinoma cells, which points to an oestrogen-mediated mechanism (Coezy *et al.*, 1987). In Hep3B hepatoma cells, which do not express oestrogen receptor, tamoxifen inhibits all cell growth. In the presence of mestranol, an additive inhibitory effect was observed, which suggests that the growth inhibition by mestranol observed in these cells is an oestrogen receptor-independent process (Jiang *et al.*, 1995).

Mestranol *per se* induced γ-GT activity in cultured rat hepatocytes at concentrations of 3×10^{-6}–10^{-4} mol/L in the presence of 30 nmol/L dexamethasone (Edwards & Lucas, 1985).

The combination of norethynodrel (0.5 or 5 mg/rat per day) and mestranol (7.5 or 75 μg/rat per day) given as a pellet implant to female Sprague-Dawley rats, starting at 45, 55, 65 or 75 days of age, caused changes in the mammary gland that resulted in protection against induction of mammary cancer by a single dose (80 mg/kg bw) of 7,12-dimethylbenz[*a*]anthracene (DMBA) (Russo *et al.*, 1989). The hormone treatment was given for 21 days, followed by 21 days' recovery, at which time some rats were killed to study mammary gland morphology, while others received DMBA. The hormone treatment at both doses decreased the number of terminal end-buds per mammary gland and increased the number of alveolar buds, but did not alter the number of terminal ducts; cell proliferation, measured as the DNA-labelling index, was reduced in the terminal ducts and alveolar buds but remained unchanged in the terminal end-buds (Russo *et al.*,

1989; Russo & Russo, 1991). In these experiments, a trend was observed for the hormonal treatment to produce less effect when initiated at a later age. The reduction in cell proliferation in terminal end-buds and terminal ducts, the target tissues for DMBA, may explain the protective effect of the hormone combination on the development of mammary cancer.

In a study with rhesus monkeys (Tavassoli *et al.*, 1988), mestranol alone at 0.02 or 0.1 mg/kg per day and combinations of mestranol and ethynerone, chlorethinyl norgestrel and anagestone acetate were given for 10 years in 28-day cycles consisting of 21 days of administration followed by seven days without treatment. Mestranol alone induced minimal to moderate proliferative and atypical alterations in the mammary gland in 8/34 animals, whereas minimal to mild changes occurred in 2/16 controls. With the various mestranol–progestogen combinations, mild to severe atypical hyperplasia was observed in 22–25/52 animals, about 12% in each group showing severe lesions that could not be distinguished from human mammary carcinoma *in situ*. Minimal to severe proliferative atypia were found in 11/15 animals given one of the progestogens, ethynerone; two of these animals had a severe lesion similar to carcinoma *in situ* and one had invasive breast cancer.

4.2.4 *Chlormadinone acetate*

  (*a*) *Humans*

No relevant data were available to the Working Group.

  (*b*) *Experimental systems*

The progestogen chlormadinone acetate inhibited the induction by ethinyloestradiol of nuclear and cytoplasmic progesterone receptor in human endometrium (Kreitmann *et al.*, 1979), and it has been found to bind strongly to the human uterine progesterone receptor, as determined in a competitive binding assay with the 20 000 × *g* supernatant fraction of human endometrium and myometrium (Briggs, 1975). It reduced the binding of oestradiol to rat uterine oestrogen receptor both *in vivo* and *in vitro* (Di Carlo *et al.*, 1983). Chlormadinone acetate did not have any detectable oestrogenic activity when tested for induction of alkaline phosphatase activity as an indicator of oestrogen response in oestrogen receptor-containing and oestrogen-sensitive Ishikawa human endometrial cancer cells (Botella *et al.*, 1995).

In vitro, chlormadinone acetate at 10^{-6} mol/L stimulated the growth of androgen-sensitive mouse mammary carcinoma Shionogi cells, with a reduction in doubling time of approximately 50%. This effect could be inhibited by a 5×10^{-6} mol/L excess of the androgen receptor-blocking anti-androgen hydroxyflutamide, which by itself did not stimulate the growth of these cells (Luthy *et al.*, 1988). Consistent with these observations, chlormadinone acetate weakly bound to the rat ventral prostate androgen receptor (Botella *et al.*, 1987).

The growth stimulatory effect of chlormadinone acetate on Shionogi cells was confirmed *in vivo* in DD/S mice: the tumour size was increased by more than threefold over that in controls after 21 days of treatment with two daily dose of 250 μg/mouse (Plante *et al.*, 1988). When tested in castrated male rats at a dose of 10 mg twice daily for 14 days, chlormadinone acetate increased ventral prostate weight by about 50% and stimulated the activity of the cell proliferation-related enzyme ornithine decarboxylase in the ventral prostate by almost 12-fold; effects of similar magnitude were found with 5α-dihydrotestosterone at a dose of 0.15 mg twice daily. Thus, chlormadinone acetate has weak androgenic activity, while no evidence for anti-androgenic activity was detected in these studies (Labrie *et al.*, 1987).

Studies with the human breast cancer cell line ZR-75-1, which contains functional oestrogen, progesterone and androgen receptors, suggested that chlormadinone acetate inhibited the growth of these cells by an interaction of androgen and progesterone receptor-mediated mechanisms (Poulin *et al.*, 1990).

Chlormadinone acetate inhibited the activity of microsomal oestrone sulfatase in human breast carcinoma tissue *in vitro*, suggesting that it may reduce the formation of biologically active oestrogen in human breast cancer cells *in vivo* (Prost-Avallet *et al.*, 1991). It also reduced the activity of 5α-reductase and increased the activity of hepatic 3α- and 3β-hydroxysteroid dehydrogenase in male and female rats (Lax *et al.*, 1984).

4.2.5   *Cyproterone acetate*

(*a*)   *Humans*

No relevant data were available to the Working Group.

(*b*)   *Experimental systems*

Cyproterone acetate is an anti-androgen that has been shown to act at the level of both the (peripheral) androgen receptor and the hypothalamus-pituitary, suppressing gonadotrophin release. Interestingly, it also had intrinsic androgenic activity when tested for its ability to increase the weight of the ventral prostate of castrated male rats (Poyet & Labrie, 1985). In comparison with 5α-dihydrotestosterone, however, it bound only weakly to the rat ventral prostate androgen receptor (Botella *et al.*, 1987). In a test system comprising steroid receptor-deficient CV-1 monkey kidney cells stably transfected with androgen receptor and a reporter plasmid containing the mouse mammary tumour virus promotor linked to the chloramphenicol acetyltransferase gene, transcriptional activation of chloramphenicol acetyltransferase has been used to show both androgenic activity of cyproterone acetate (Warriar *et al.*, 1993) and lack of androgenic activity (Fuhrmann *et al.*, 1992). The human androgen receptor was used in the former study and the rat androgen receptor in the latter, but it is not clear whether this difference was responsible for the discordant findings. In both studies, excess cyproterone acetate inhibited the effect of androgens.

Cyproterone acetate stimulated the growth of androgen-sensitive mouse mammary carcinoma Shionogi cells *in vivo* in DD/S mice; the tumour size was increased 11-fold over that in controls after 21 days of treatment with two daily doses of 250 μg/mouse (Plante *et al.*, 1988).

Cyproterone acetate did not stimulate and, indeed, even inhibited the growth of the original MCF-7 human breast cancer cell line at concentrations of 10^{-7}–10^{-5} mol/L, as measured by tritiated thymidine incorporation (Lippman $et~al.$, 1976). In a later study, stimulation of the growth of the oestrogen-sensitive breast cancer cell lines MCF-7 and EFM-19 was found at concentrations of 10^{-8}–10^{-6} mol/L cyproterone acetate. This effect was influenced by competition with 5α-dihydrotestosterone but not oestradiol, indicating involvement of the androgen receptor but not the oestrogen receptor (Hackenberg $et~al.$, 1988). In contrast, studies with the human breast cancer cell line ZR-75-1, which contains functional oestrogen, progesterone and androgen receptors, indicated that cyproterone acetate inhibits the growth of these cells, suggesting that this occurs via an interaction of androgen and progesterone receptor-mediated mechanisms (Poulin $et~al.$, 1990).

Cyproterone acetate is also a progestogen and has been demonstrated to bind to the progesterone receptor of human uterus (Grill $et~al.$, 1985) and MCF-7 human breast cancer cells (Bergink $et~al.$, 1983). Cyproterone acetate had oestrogenic activity in ovariectomized mice, as was evident from the observed vaginal keratinization and increases in uterine weight and protein content (Lohiya & Arya, 1981). It did not alter the uterine hyperplastic response to conjugated equine oestrogen in ovariectomized rats (Kumasaka $et~al.$, 1994).

Cyproterone acetate has considerable effects on the rodent liver: it stimulates the proliferation of hepatocytes, resulting in liver enlargement due to hyperplasia, in the absence of hepatotoxic effects. After three to six daily administrations by gavage of 40–130 mg/kg cyproterone acetate dissolved in oil to female and male rats, the increase in the ratio of liver weight:body weight reached a plateau at 1.5 times to more than twice the values in vehicle-treated controls, while the hepatic DNA content nearly doubled (Bursch $et~al.$, 1986; Schulte-Hermann $et~al.$, 1988; Roberts $et~al.$, 1995). A threshold dose of 5–10 mg/kg per day was found for these effects in female Wistar rats, male rats being less sensitive and showing less pronounced growth of the liver. With a lag of 12–14 h, replicative DNA synthesis was induced by cyproterone acetate in female Wistar rats, reaching a maximum 18–24 h after the first dose, with a predominant response of periportal hepatocytes (Schulte-Hermann $et~al.$, 1980a). Cyproterone acetate given at a dose of 125 mg/kg bw per day in the diet to C57BL/10J mice increased the BrdU nuclear labelling index in the liver, the effect being statistically significant in females (Tucker & Jones, 1996; Tucker $et~al.$, 1996). As many as 75% of all hepatocytes responded to cyproterone acetate with proliferation (Schulte-Hermann $et~al.$, 1980b). Several studies have demonstrated that after cessation of cyproterone acetate treatment, the liver regresses to its normal size, due to massive induction of apoptosis (Bursch $et~al.$, 1986; Roberts $et~al.$, 1995). Cyproterone acetate induced the synthesis of TGF-β1 which is possibly involved in the apoptotic response of hepatocytes after withdrawal of cyproterone acetate (Bursch $et~al.$, 1993; Oberhammer $et~al.$, 1996).

The mitogenic activity of cyproterone acetate in rat hepatocytes is apparently a direct effect, since the compound stimulated replicative DNA synthesis in female rat hepatocytes cultured in serum-free medium at non-cytotoxic concentrations of 10^{-7}–10^{-4} mol/L

(Parzefall *et al.*, 1989); however, proliferation of hepatocytes isolated from human surgical specimens was, on average, not increased by exposure to cyproterone acetate for 24 h at concentrations of 10^{-5} mol/L. This lack of effect was seen with and without subsequent addition of epidermal growth factor during 24 h. In contrast, cyproterone acetate and epidermal growth factor acted in an additive manner in stimulating DNA synthesis in rat hepatocytes, whereas epidermal growth factor *per se* enhanced the growth of both human and rat cultured liver cells (Parzefall *et al.*, 1991). The observations with human hepatocytes were limited to cells obtained from seven subjects; while in most cases no effect was observed, a dose-related increase in proliferation was induced by cyproterone acetate in hepatocytes from one of the subjects and a dose-related decrease in cells from another. More observations are therefore needed before a firm conclusion can be reached about the possible proliferative effects of cyproterone acetate on human liver.

Cyproterone acetate caused a shift of the cell cycle of cultured rat hepatocytes from G_0 to the G_1 phase (Duivenvoorden & Maier, 1994), with concomitant induction of c-*myc* and c-*fos* expression (Duivenvoorden *et al.*, 1995).

Female rats were subjected at six weeks of age to a carcinogenic regimen of a two-thirds hepatectomy followed 20 h later by gastric intubation with 30 mg/kg NDEA and, one week later, administration of 0.1% phenobarbital in the drinking-water for four to six months. In cultured hepatocytes derived from three rats, cyproterone acetate at 5×10^{-6} mol/L induced a fourfold increase in replicative DNA synthesis in putatively preneoplastic γ-GT-positive cells and a twofold increase in γ-GT-negative hepatocytes. These effects required the presence of both epidermal growth factor and insulin, which by themselves increased proliferation 10-fold over that in controls but did not differentially affect the proliferation of γ-GT-positive and γ-GT-negative cells (Neumann *et al.*, 1992). In the same series of experiments, stimulation of DNA repair synthesis by cyproterone acetate was observed in hepatocytes from both carcinogen-treated and untreated rats, and in medium without epidermal growth factor. This raises the possibility that cyproterone acetate has tumour-initiating potential. Cyproterone acetate *per se* at concentrations of 10^{-6}–10^{-5} mol/L induced γ-GT activity in cultured rat hepatocytes (Edwards & Lucas, 1985).

The exact mechanism by which cyproterone acetate induces liver-cell proliferation and hepatic hyperplasia is not understood. Although it stimulated incorporation of tritiated thymidine into cultured hepatocytes from carcinogen-treated female rats at concentrations of 2×10^{-6}–10^{-5} mol/L, another anti-androgen, flutamide, inhibited stimulation of hepatocyte proliferation induced by epidermal growth factor and insulin (Neumann *et al.*, 1992). These findings suggest that the hyperplastic effects of cyproterone acetate are not related to its anti-androgenic properties. It is, however, conceivable that the effects are, at least in part, related to the aforementioned androgenic properties of cyproterone acetate, possibly mediated by the androgen receptor. Unlike compensatory liver cell proliferation, which occurs in rats in response to surgical or toxic reduction of the liver mass, direct hepatic hyperplasia induced by cyproterone acetate *in vivo* did not involve up-regulation of the immediate–early response proto-oncogenes c-*fos*, c-*jun* and c-*myc* or induction of the transcription factors NF-κB and AP-1 (Coni *et al.*, 1993; Menegazzi *et al.*, 1997). *In vitro*, however, cyproterone acetate-induced hepatocyte proliferation was accompanied by increased expression of not only c-*fos* but also c-*myc* (Duivenvoorden *et al.*, 1995). These observations suggest that the stimulation of rat hepatocyte proliferation by cyproterone acetate *in vivo* may differ from that in culture.

Cyproterone acetate also increased the activity of 5α-reductase and decreased the activity of 3α- and 3β-hydroxysteroid dehydrogenases in the livers of male and female rats (Lax *et al.*, 1984).

4.2.6   *Desogestrel*
(*a*)   *Humans*
Ruokonen and Käär (1985) studied the effects of desogestrel at a dose of 125 μg per day for 60 days in 30 healthy pre-menopausal women with regard to the serum levels of ceruloplasmin and cortisol-binding globulin, as indicators of oestrogenic activity. The concentrations of these proteins were not affected by the treatment, indicating a lack of oestrogenic activity of desogestrel in these women. The serum concentration of sex hormone-binding globulin was markedly decreased by the treatment, to 70 and 60% of pre- and post-treatment values at 30 and 60 days, respectively.

(*b*)   *Experimental systems*
The progestogen desogestrel is converted to its unique, directly acting metabolite 3-keto-desogestrel, and this metabolite was used in all of the studies conducted *in vitro*. The relative binding affinity of 3-keto-desogestrel to the rabbit uterine progesterone receptor has been reported to be approximately equal to (Fuhrmann *et al.*, 1995) or nine times higher than that of progesterone (Phillips *et al.*, 1990).

The progestational activity of desogestrel *in vivo*, measured by inhibition of ovulation and endometrial stimulation in rabbits, was similar to that of progesterone (Phillips *et al.*, 1987).

The 3-keto metabolite of desogestrel also bound with high affinity to androgen and glucocorticoid receptors (Kloosterboer *et al.*, 1988; Juchem & Pollow, 1990; Phillips *et al.*, 1990; Fuhrmann *et al.*, 1995), but not to oestrogen or mineralocorticoid receptors (Juchem & Pollow, 1990; Fuhrmann *et al.*, 1995; Schoonen *et al.*, 1995a,b). The relative binding affinity for the rat ventral prostate androgen receptor was approximately 12% that of dihydrotestosterone (Phillips *et al.*, 1990). In *trans*-activation assays, 3-keto-desogestrel had clear androgenic activity and weak glucocorticoid activity, but no agonist or antagonist activity was found in assays that involved the mineralocorticoid receptor (Fuhrmann *et al.*, 1995).

In comparison with 5α-dihydrotestosterone, desogestrel had modest androgenic activity *in vivo*, as measured by stimulation of ventral prostate growth in castrated rats (Phillips *et al.*, 1987).

3-Keto-desogestrel stimulated the growth of most oestrogen-sensitive human mammary cancer cell lines tested (van der Burg *et al.*, 1992; Kalkhoven *et al.*, 1994;

Schoonen *et al.*, 1995a,b). MCF-7 cell proliferation was stimulated by 3-keto-desogestrel at a concentration of 10^{-6} mol/L, but only in the presence of insulin added to the medium at ≥ 10 ng/mL (van der Burg *et al.*, 1992). In experiments in which growth stimulation by 3-keto-desogestrel was compared in various cell lines, it did not appear to require insulin or epidermal growth factor. The growth stimulation was dose-dependent, beginning at concentrations of 10^{-7} mol/L for MCF-7 cells and 10^{-10} mol/L for T47D cells obtained from two different sources (Kalkhoven *et al.*, 1994). These dose–response results were confirmed in studies in which the same and two additional sub-lines of MCF-7 and one of the T47D cell lines were used, while the other T47D line did not respond to 3-keto-desogestrel (Schoonen *et al.*, 1995a,b). The experiments were performed with breast cancer cell lines grown in phenol red-free medium containing steroid-devoid (dextran-coated charcoal-stripped) serum (van der Burg *et al.*, 1992; Kalkhoven *et al.*, 1994; Schoonen *et al.*, 1995a,b). Under the conditions of these experiments, progesterone receptor expression in both MCF-7 and T47D cells was maintained and was 40-fold higher in the T47D than in the MCF-7 cells. Furthermore, expression of the progesterone-inducible gene encoding fatty acid synthase was more strongly up-regulated by 3-keto-desogestrel in T47D than in MCF-7 cells. By use of a reporter construct containing two progesterone response elements in front of the thymidine kinase promotor coupled to the chloramphenicol acetyltransferase gene transfected into both cell lines, progesterone receptor-mediated *trans*-activation was observed at a concentration of 3-keto-desogestrel as low as 10^{-9} mol/L (Kalkhoven *et al.*, 1994). In other experiments, the stimulating effects on cell growth of 3-keto-desogestrel at concentrations of 10^{-7}–10^{-6} mol/L were not blocked by simultaneous treatment of the cells with anti-progestogens such as RU486, whereas the anti-oestrogens 4-hydroxytamoxifen and ICI164,384 (at 10^{-7} mol/L) did inhibit this stimulation (van der Burg *et al.*, 1992; Schoonen *et al.*, 1995a,b). Growth stimulation of T47D cells by 3-keto-desogestrel at 10^{-10} mol/L was inhibited by RU486 and not by 4-hydroxytamoxifen (both at 10^{-7} mol/L) (Kalkhoven *et al.*, 1994). These findings suggest that stimulation of cell proliferation by 3-keto-desogestrel is mediated by the oestrogen receptor at high concentrations and by the progesterone receptor at low concentrations. This is apparently not related to effects at the level of receptor–ligand interaction: 3-keto-desogestrel causes *trans*-activation of reporter constructs containing oestrogen or progesterone response elements transfected into MCF-7 and T47D cells at 10^{-6} and 10^{-9} mol/L, respectively, while 4-hydroxytamoxifen, but not RU486, inhibited *trans*-activation of the oestrogen response element-containing construct, and RU486, but not 4-hydroxytamoxifen, inhibited *trans*-activation of the progesterone response element-containing construct. The expression of the oestrogen-inducible *pS2* gene in MCF-7 cells was slightly inhibited by 3-keto-desogestrel at 10^{-9} mol/L and was not affected at 10^{-6} mol/L (Kalkhoven *et al.*, 1994).

Oestradiol at concentrations of 10^{-10} mol/L and higher strongly induced the growth of the MCF-7 and T47D cell lines, regardless of the sub-line used (van der Burg *et al.*, 1992; Kalkhoven *et al.*, 1994; Schoonen *et al.*, 1995a,b). The growth stimulation of MCF-7 cells by oestrogen at 10^{-10} mol/L was inhibited by 3-keto-desogestrel at a concentration of

10^{-8} mol/L but not by the anti-progestogen RU38486 (Schoonen *et al.*, 1995a). Oestrogen-induced growth in T47D cells was not blocked by 3-keto-desogestrel at 10^{-6} mol/L in one sub-line (T47D-A) but was totally inhibited in another sub-line (T47D-S) at a concentration of 10^{-10}–10^{-8} mol/L. These two sub-lines differ considerably, in that RU38486, but not 4-hydroxytamoxifen or ICI164,384, blocked oestrogen-stimulated growth in the T47D-A cell line, while both anti-progestogens and anti-oestrogens inhibited T47D-S (Schoonen *et al.*, 1995b).

3-Keto-desogestrel at concentrations of 10–40 ng/mL inhibited the growth of endothelial cells derived from human decidual endometrium; the growth of these cells was stimulated by exposure to oestradiol at 5 ng/mL (Peek *et al.*, 1995).

3-Keto-desogestrel, but not the parent compound desogestrel, showed moderate affinity for and slow dissociation from sex hormone-binding globulin in human serum (Juchem & Pollow, 1990). Its strong interaction with this globulin could lead to displacement of testosterone and to an increased concentration of free testosterone; however, the decrease in serum sex hormone-binding globulin after progestogen treatment is probably more important in this respect (Nilsson & von Schoultz, 1989).

4.2.7 *Ethynodiol diacetate*

(a) *Humans*

No relevant data were available to the Working Group.

(b) *Experimental systems*

The progestogen, ethynodiol diacetate, binds with low affinity (K_i 1.3×10^{-7} mol/L) to both the oestrogen and the progesterone receptor in rabbit uterine cytosol (Tamaya *et al.*, 1977) but hardly at all to the human endometrial progesterone receptor (Briggs, 1975; Shapiro *et al.*, 1978). It also has been reported to have androgenic properties (Darney, 1995), but no information was available on its receptor-mediated effects.

4.2.8 *Gestodene*

(a) *Humans*

No relevant data were available to the Working Group.

(b) *Experimental systems*

The progestogen gestodene binds to the rabbit uterine progesterone receptor with a relative binding affinity reported to be similar (Fuhrmann *et al.*, 1995) or nine times higher than that of progesterone itself (Phillips *et al.*, 1990), and 8–10 times higher than that of progesterone in human endometrial, breast and liver tissue (Iqbal & Colletta, 1987).

Gestodene also bound with high to moderate affinity to the androgen, mineralo-corticoid and glucocorticoid receptors (Kloosterboer *et al.*, 1988; Juchem & Pollow, 1990; Phillips *et al.*, 1990; Fuhrmann *et al.*, 1995), but did not bind to the oestrogen receptor (Juchem & Pollow, 1990; Pollow *et al.*, 1990; Fuhrmann *et al.*, 1995). Oestrogen receptor binding of gestodene has, however, been reported to occur in malignant breast tissue with threefold higher affinity than that of oestradiol (Iqbal *et al.*, 1986). Oestradiol and tamoxifen did not interfere with gestodene binding, but gestodene in excess amounts could reduce oestradiol binding (Iqbal & Valyani, 1988). High-affinity binding of gestodene was found in all breast cancer cell lines tested, but not in endometrial carcinoma cells. Cytosolic gestodene binding could not be inhibited by excess oestradiol, although nuclear binding was abolished (Colletta *et al.*, 1989). On the basis of these observations, a novel binding site was postulated (Iqbal & Valyani, 1988; Colletta *et al.*, 1989). These findings should be re-evaluated in the light of the identification of the oestrogen receptor-β and current knowledge about oestrogen receptor action. The relative binding affinity of gestodene for the rat ventral prostate androgen receptor was approximately 15% that of dihydrotestosterone (Phillips *et al.*, 1990). In *trans*-activation assays, gestodene had clear androgenic activity and weak glucocorticoid activity, but antagonist activity was found for the mineralocorticoid receptor (Fuhrmann *et al.*, 1995).

Gestodene has been shown to be a potent competitor for binding of 5α-dihydrotestosterone to the androgen receptor in human foreskin fibroblasts, with activity similar to that of testosterone (Breiner *et al.*, 1986).

Gestodene stimulated the growth of most oestrogen-sensitive human mammary cancer cells lines tested (van der Burg *et al.*, 1992; Catherino *et al.*, 1993; Kalkhoven *et al.*, 1994; Schoonen *et al.*, 1995a,b). In one study, stimulation of cell proliferation by gestodene at a concentration of 10^{-6} mol/L was found in MCF-7 cells but only in the presence of insulin at ≥ 10 ng/mL (van der Burg *et al.*, 1992). In subsequent experiments, stimulation by gestodene was compared in various cell lines and appeared not to require insulin or epidermal growth factor. Furthermore, a dose-dependent stimulation of cell growth was observed, beginning at a concentration of 10^{-7} mol/L for MCF-7 cells and 10^{-10} mol/L for T47D cells obtained from two sources (Kalkhoven *et al.*, 1994). In other experiments with similar but not identical culture conditions, gestodene induced near-maximal growth stimulation of MCF-7 cells, at a concentration of 10^{-7} mol/L (Catherino *et al.*, 1993). These dose–response results were confirmed in studies with the same and two additional sub-lines of MCF-7; one of two T47D sub-lines tested did not respond to gestodene (Schoonen *et al.*, 1995a,b). All of the experiments were performed with breast cancer cell lines grown in phenol red-free medium which, except in one study (Catherino *et al.*, 1993), contained steroid-free (dextran-coated charcoal-stripped) serum (van der Burg *et al.*, 1992; Kalkhoven *et al.*, 1994; Schoonen *et al.*, 1995a,b). Under the conditions of these experiments, progesterone receptor expression in both cell types was maintained and was 20–40-fold higher in the T47D cells than in the MCF-7 cells (Kalkhoven *et al.*, 1994; see also Sutherland *et al.*, 1988). Furthermore, expression of the progesterone-inducible gene encoding fatty acid synthase was more strongly up-regulated by gestodene in T47D than in MCF-7 cells (Kalkhoven *et al.*, 1994). With reporter constructs containing two progesterone response elements in front of the *tk* promotor coupled to the chloramphenicol acetyltransferase gene transfected into both cell lines, *trans*-activation was observed at gestodene concentrations as low as 10^{-9} mol/L, clearly demonstrating expression of functional progesterone receptor in these cell lines without (Kalkhoven *et al.*, 1994) or with addition of oestradiol to the medium to boost receptor expression (Catherino *et al.*, 1993). The stimulating effects of gestodene at 10^{-7}–10^{-6} mol/L were not blocked, however, by simultaneous treatment of the cells with anti-progestogens such as RU38486, whereas they were inhibited by the anti-oestrogens 4-hydroxytamoxifen (10^{-7} mol/L) and ICI164,384 (10^{-7}–10^{-6} mol/L) (van der Burg *et al.*, 1992; Catherino *et al.*, 1993; Schoonen *et al.*, 1995a,b). Stimulation of the growth of T47D cells by gestodene at a lower concentration (10^{-10} mol/L) was inhibited by RU486 and not by 4-hydroxytamoxifen (both at 10^{-7} mol/L), suggesting that the cell proliferation-stimulating effects of gestodene are mediated via the oestrogen receptor at high concentrations and by the progesterone receptor at low concentrations (Kalkhoven *et al.*, 1994). This effect is apparently not related to effects at the level of receptor–ligand interaction, because gestodene causes *trans*-activation of reporter constructs containing oestrogen or progesterone response elements transfected into MCF-7 and T47D cells at 10^{-10}–10^{-6} mol/L. Furthermore, 4-hydroxytamoxifen and ICI164,384, but not RU486, inhibited *trans*-activation of the oestrogen response element-containing construct, while RU486, but not 4-hydroxy-tamoxifen or ICI164,384, inhibited *trans*-activation of the progesterone response element-containing construct (Catherino *et al.*, 1993; Kalkhoven *et al.*, 1994). The expression of the oestrogen-inducible *pS2* gene in MCF-7 cells was slightly inhibited by gestodene at a low concentration (10^{-9} mol/L), but was not affected at 10^{-6} mol/L (Kalkhoven *et al.*, 1994).

Oestradiol at concentrations of 10^{-10} mol/L and higher strongly induces the growth of the MCF-7 and T47D cell lines, regardless of the sub-line used (van der Burg *et al.*, 1992; Kalkhoven *et al.*, 1994; Schoonen *et al.*, 1995a,b). The growth stimulation of MCF-7 cells by oestrogen at 10^{-10} mol/L was inhibited by gestodene at a concentration of 10^{-8} mol/L, and this effect was not blocked by RU38486 (Schoonen *et al.*, 1995a). Oestrogen-induced growth in T47D cells was not blocked by gestodene at 10^{-6} mol/L in one sub-line (T47D-A) but was totally inhibited in another sub-line (T47D-S) at a concentration of 10^{-10}–10^{-8} mol/L. These two sub-lines differ considerably, in that RU38486, but not 4-hydroxytamoxifen or ICI164,384, blocked oestrogen-stimulated growth in the T47D-A cell line, while both anti-progestogens and anti-oestrogens were inhibitory for T47D-S (Schoonen *et al.*, 1995b).

Gestodene induced a large increase in secretion of TGF-β by T47D breast cancer cells, but not HEC-1B human endometrial cancer cells, and the inhibitory effect of gesto-dene on oestrogen-stimulated T47D cell proliferation was reduced by treatment with a polyclonal antiserum to TGF-β (Colletta *et al.*, 1991). Gestodene also inhibited oestrogen-stimulated T47D cell proliferation in sub-lines that had lost their sensitivity to TGF-β to the same extent as in sub-lines that retained their sensitivity to this growth inhibiting factor (Kalkhoven *et al.*, 1996); therefore, the involvement of TGF-β in the growth modulating effects of gestodene remains unclear.

Gestodene showed high affinity for and slow dissociation from sex hormone-binding globulin in human serum (Juchem & Pollow, 1990).

When given to female Wistar rats at a dose of 10 mg/kg per day for seven days, gestodene had a slight but significant growth-stimulating effect on the liver, as seen in a 10–15% increase in DNA content without a change in weight (Schulte-Hermann *et al.*, 1988).

4.2.9   *Levonorgestrel* (see also the monograph on 'Hormonal contraceptives, progestogens only', section 4.2.2)

   (*a*)   *Humans*

In the study of Ruokonen and Käär (1985), described in section 4.2.6, the serum concentrations of ceruloplasmin and cortisol-binding protein were not affected, indicating a lack of oestrogenic activity of levonorgestrel in these women. The serum concentration of sex hormone-binding globulin was markedly decreased, to 50–55% of pre- and post-treatment values at both 30 and 60 days.

Ten women were given 30 µg per day levonorgestrel orally on days 7–10 of the menstrual cycle, and endometrial biopsy samples were taken on the 11th day of the previous cycle and on the day after the last dose (also day 11 of the cycle). Levonorgestrel had no effect on the number of glandular and stromal cell mitoses, basal-cell vacuolation or the diameter and epithelial thickness of the endometrial glands (Landgren *et al.*, 1990).

   (*b*)   *Experimental systems*

Levonorgestrel binds with high affinity to progesterone receptors (Lemus *et al.*, 1992); its relative binding affinity has been reported to be 1.25 (Kuhnz *et al.*, 1995) to five times (Phillips *et al.*, 1990) higher than that of progesterone itself for the rabbit uterine progesterone receptor and 1.43 and 1.25 times higher for human uterine and recombinant progesterone receptors, respectively (Kuhnz *et al.*, 1995). Metabolites of levonorgestrel showed less or no binding to the progesterone receptor (Lemus *et al.*, 1992).

Levonorgestrel had clear progestational activity *in vivo*, both in a pregnancy maintenance test in female rats (Kuhnz & Beier, 1994) and as measured by inhibition of ovulation and endometrial stimulation in rabbits, indicating that it is slightly less active than progesterone (Phillips *et al.*, 1987).

Levonorgestrel also bound with high affinity to androgen, mineralocorticoid and glucocorticoid receptors (Kloosterboer *et al.*, 1988; Juchem & Pollow, 1990; Phillips *et al.*, 1990), but not to oestrogen receptors (Iqbal *et al.*, 1986; Juchem & Pollow, 1990; Lemus *et al.*, 1992). The relative binding affinity of levonorgestrel for the rat ventral prostate androgen receptor was approximately 20% that of 5α-dihydrotestosterone (Phillips *et al.*, 1990).

Levonorgestrel had moderate androgenic activity *in vivo*, in comparison with 5α-dihydrotestosterone, as measured by stimulation of ventral prostate growth in immature, castrated rats (Phillips *et al.*, 1987; Kuhnz & Beier, 1994).

Levonorgestrel stimulated the growth of oestrogen-sensitive human mammary cancer cells lines. MCF-7 cell proliferation was stimulated by levonorgestrel at a concentration of 10^{-6} mol/L, but only in the presence of insulin added to the medium at ≥ 10 ng/mL (van der Burg *et al.*, 1992). In experiments in which stimulation by levonorgestrel was compared in three sub-lines of MCF-7 and two of T47D cells, stimulation occurred at concentrations of 10^{-7} mol/L and higher in all cell lines except one of the T47D sub-lines (Schoonen *et al.*, 1995a,b). The experiments were performed with breast cancer cell lines grown in phenol red-free medium which contained steroid-free (dextran-coated charcoal-stripped) serum (van der Burg *et al.*, 1992; Schoonen *et al.*, 1995a,b). Under the conditions of these experiments, progesterone receptor expression in both cell types was maintained and was 20–40-fold higher in T47D cells than in MCF-7 cells (van der Burg *et al.*, 1992; Kalkhoven *et al.*, 1994). The stimulating effects of levonorgestrel at 10^{-7}–10^{-6} mol/L were not blocked by simultaneous treatment of the cells with anti-progestogens such as RU486, whereas the anti-oestrogens 4-hydroxytamoxifen (at 10^{-7} mol/L) and ICI164,384 (at 10^{-7}–10^{-6} mol/L) inhibited this stimulation (van der Burg *et al.*, 1992; Schoonen *et al.*, 1995a,b). These findings suggest that the cell proliferation-stimulating effects of levonorgestrel are not mediated via the progesterone receptor but via the oestrogen receptor (Kalkhoven *et al.*, 1994).

Levonorgestrel increased the reductive activity of 17β-hydroxysteroid dehydrogenase in an oestrogen- and progestogen-stimulated MCF-7 cell line in phenol red-free medium. This effect would increase the formation of oestradiol, indicating a possible mechanism by which this progestogen may increase breast cell proliferation *in vivo* (Coldham & James, 1990).

Levonorgestrel had oestrogenic activity at concentrations of 10^{-8}–10^{-6} mol/L when tested for induction of alkaline phosphatase activity as an indicator of oestrogen response in oestrogen receptor-containing and oestrogen-sensitive Ishikawa human endometrial cancer cells (Botella *et al.*, 1995).

Oestradiol at concentrations of 10^{-10} mol/L and higher strongly induced the growth of MCF-7 and T47D cell lines, regardless of the sub-line used (van der Burg *et al.*, 1992; Kalkhoven *et al.*, 1994; Schoonen *et al.*, 1995a,b). The growth stimulation of MCF-7 cells by 10^{-10} mol/L oestrogen was inhibited by 10^{-9} mol/L levonorgestrel in one sub-line, and the effect was not blocked by RU486; no effect was seen in another sub-line (Schoonen *et al.*, 1995a). Oestrogen-induced growth in T47D cells was not blocked by 10^{-6} mol/L levonorgestrel in one sub-line but was totally inhibited in another sub-line at concentrations of 10^{-10}–10^{-8} mol/L. These two T47D sub-lines differ considerably, in that RU486, but not 4-hydroxytamoxifen or ICI164,384, blocked oestrogen-stimulated growth in the former sub-line, while both anti-progestogens and anti-oestrogens inhibited the other (Schoonen *et al.*, 1995b).

Levonorgestrel at concentrations of 0.1–2 ng/mL inhibited the growth of decidual endothelial cells derived from human endometrium, the growth of which was stimulated by exposure to oestradiol at 5 ng/mL but inhibited by lower concentrations and not affected by higher concentrations (Peek *et al.*, 1995).

Levonorgestrel had high affinity for and slow dissociation from sex hormone-binding globulin in human serum (Juchem & Pollow, 1990). It displaced testosterone, thus at least theoretically resulting in an increase in free testosterone (Nilsson & von Schoultz, 1989).

Protein and mRNA expression of vascular endothelial growth factor was increased in the endometrium of cynomolgus monkeys treated with levonorgestrel for 20 days as compared with endometrial samples from luteal-phase monkeys. These effects were limited to stromal cells for protein expression detected by immunohistochemistry and to the vascular endothelial growth factor-189 isoform for mRNA expression (Greb *et al.*, 1997).

Levonorgestrel had no significant effect on the growth of the liver in female Wistar rats (Schulte-Hermann *et al.*, 1988).

4.2.10   *Lynoestrenol*

(*a*)   *Humans*

Maudelonde *et al.* (1991) studied the effects of lynoestrenol given at a dose of 10 mg/day on days 5–25 of each menstrual cycle for one to three months to 31 pre-menopausal women with biopsy-confirmed benign breast disease, by comparing them with a group of 16 untreated women with similar clinical characteristics. Fine-needle aspirates were obtained at the start of the study and at the end of the one- to three-month treatment. The mean percentage of cells staining positively for oestrogen receptor decreased from about 60 to 20%, while the number of cells staining positively for cathepsin D (as an indicator of oestrogenic activity) remained the same. The pre-treatment values for these two parameters were not significantly different from those found in the untreated controls. The reduction in the number of oestrogen receptor-positive cells was viewed by the authors as consistent with the anti-oestrogenic activity of lynoestrenol.

Ruokonen and Kään (1985) studied the effects of lynoestrenol at a dose of 5 mg/day for 60 days in 30 healthy pre-menopausal women on serum levels of ceruloplasmin and cortisol-binding globulin, as indicators of oestrogenic activity. The concentrations of these two proteins were slightly (10–20%) elevated after 30 and 60 days of treatment as compared with pre-treatment, but this was significant only 30 days after the start of treatment. Nevertheless, the results indicated weak oestrogenic activity of lynoestrenol in these women. The serum concentration of sex hormone-binding globulin was markedly decreased by the treatment, to 60 and 50% of pre-treatment values at 30 and 60 days, respectively.

In the study of Odlind *et al.* (1980), described in section 4.2.3, a dose of 1 mg/day lynoestrenol in combination with 50 µg/day ethinyloestradiol given for the duration of one menstrual cycle increased the concentration of sex hormone-binding globulin by approximately 100%, but a combination with a higher lynoestrenol dose of 2.5 mg/day caused only a non-significant, 17% increase.

(*b*)   *Experimental systems*

The progestogen lynoestrenol was found to bind with low affinity to both the oestrogen and the progesterone receptor in rabbit uterine cytosol (Tamaya *et al.*, 1977) and to the human endometrial progesterone receptor (Briggs, 1975).

Lynoestrenol has been reported to have oestrogenic activity *in vivo* (Lax, 1987). It enhanced the activity of microsomal oestrone sulfatase in human breast carcinoma tissue, suggesting that it could stimulate the formation of biologically active oestrogen in human breast cancer cells (Prost-Avallet *et al.*, 1991).

Lynoestrenol has also been reported to have androgenic properties (Darney, 1995).

4.2.11   *Megestrol acetate*

(a)   *Humans*

No relevant data were available to the Working Group.

(b)   *Experimental systems*

The progestogen megestrol acetate has been found to bind strongly to the human uterine progesterone receptor, as determined in a competitive binding assay with $20\ 000 \times g$ supernatants of human endometrium and myometrium (Briggs, 1975). Its 19-nor analogue nomegestrol acetate has very high affinity for the progesterone receptor in rat uterus (Botella *et al.*, 1990). Neither megestrol acetate nor nomegestrol acetate affected the growth of the mammary cancer cell lines, MCF-7 and T47D:A18, or *trans*-activated an oestradiol-responsive reporter construct containing oestrogen response elements (Catherino & Jordan, 1995). Nomegestrol acetate also had no oestrogenic activity, as demonstrated by the lack of induction of alkaline phosphatase activity in oestrogen receptor-containing and oestrogen-sensitive Ishikawa human endometrial cancer cells (Botella *et al.*, 1995).

In vitro, megestrol acetate stimulated the growth of androgen-sensitive mouse mammary carcinoma Shionogi cells, with a reduction in the doubling time of approximately 50% at a concentration of 10^{-6} mol/L. This effect was counteracted by a 5×10^{-6} mol/L excess of the androgen receptor blocking anti-androgen, hydroxyflutamide, which itself did not stimulate the growth of these cells (Luthy *et al.*, 1988). Consistent with these observations, megestrol acetate bound weakly to the rat ventral prostate androgen receptor, with an affinity approximately equal to that of testosterone (Botella *et al.*, 1987).

When tested in castrated male rats at a dose of 10 mg given subcutaneously twice daily for 14 days, megestrol acetate increased the ventral prostate weight by about 50% and induced a 13-fold stimulation of the activity of the cell proliferation-related enzyme ornithine decarboxylase in the ventral prostate; similar effects were found with a dose of 0.15 mg 5α-dihydrotestosterone twice daily (Labrie *et al.*, 1987). When castrated rats that had received testosterone re-substitution (via silastic implants) were treated with megestrol acetate at 20 mg/kg per day subcutaneously for 14 or 28 days, however, the prostate weights were reduced by 49 and 65%, respectively (Burton & Trachtenberg, 1986). Thus, megestrol acetate has weak androgenic activity in castrated male rats (Labrie *et al.*, 1987), while it has clear anti-androgenic activity in intact rats (Burton & Trachtenberg, 1986).

Megestrol acetate bound to the glucocorticoid receptor in human mononuclear leukocytes and induced glucocorticoid-like effects in these cells, including inhibition of proliferative responses to mitogenic stimuli (Kontula *et al.*, 1983).

Studies with the human breast cancer cell line ZR-75-1, which contains oestrogen, progesterone and androgen receptors, suggested that megestrol acetate inhibits the growth of these cells through an interaction of androgen and progesterone receptor-mediated mechanisms (Poulin *et al.*, 1990).

Megestrol acetate weakly inhibited the induction of angiogenesis by basic fibroblast growth factor and TGF-α in rabbit cornea *in vitro*. This anti-angiogenic activity was not correlated with its binding to glucocorticoid, progesterone or androgen receptors (Yamamoto *et al.*, 1994).

4.2.12   *Norethisterone*

(*a*)   *Humans*

In the study of Odlind *et al.* (1980), described in section 4.2.3, a dose of 0.5 or 1.0 mg/day norethisterone in combination with 35 μg/day ethinyloestradiol or 50 μg/day mestranol, respectively, given for the duration of one menstrual cycle increased the concentration of sex hormone-binding globulin by approximately 100% in both cases, but the daily dose of 0.5 mg norethisterone in combination with 60 μg ethinyloestradiol given every other day caused only a 45% increase. The dose of 3 mg/day norethisterone acetate in combination with 50 μg/day ethinyloestradiol increased the concentration of sex hormone-binding globulin by approximately 25%.

Ten women were given 300 μg/day norethisterone orally on days 7–10 of the menstrual cycle, and endometrial biopsy samples were taken on the 11th day of the previous cycle and on the day after the last dose (also day 11 of the cycle). The treatment reduced the number of glandular cell mitoses by 65% and markedly increased the number of vacuolated cells in the endometrium, from 0 to 5.5% (Landgren *et al.*, 1990).

(*b*)   *Experimental systems*

Norethisterone bound with an affinity close to that of the natural ligand to the progesterone receptor in rabbit uterine cytosol (Tamaya *et al.*, 1977) and to the nuclear and cytosolic progesterone receptors in human uterine endometrium and myometrium (Briggs, 1975; Shapiro *et al.*, 1978; Kasid & Laumas, 1981). It bound with low affinity to the nuclear and the cytosolic progesterone receptors in cultured MCF-7 human breast tumour cells (Kloosterboer *et al.*, 1988). In an assay of progestogen-specific stimulation of alkaline phosphatase activity in T47D human breast cancer cells, slightly less than full agonist activity was demonstrated for norethisterone in comparison with progesterone (Markiewicz & Gurpide, 1994). In human endometrial stromal cells in culture, however, norethisterone and progesterone were equally effective in stimulating protein and mRNA expression of insulin-like growth factor binding protein-2 (Giudice *et al.*, 1991).

In comparison with progesterone, norethisterone had weak to moderate mixed antagonist/agonist progestational activity; *in vivo* it effectively interfered with pregnancy in the post-nidation period in rats and somewhat less effectively in hamsters, but it also inhibited progesterone-supported pregnancy in ovariectomized rats (Reel *et al.*, 1979). Furthermore, it showed weak inhibitory activity on ovulation and endometrial stimulation in rabbits (Phillips *et al.*, 1987). In immature female rabbits, norethisterone induced increased expression of uteroglobin in both protein and mRNA (Cerbón *et al.*, 1990). This effect is mediated by the progesterone receptor, because it is abolished by RU486 (Pasapera *et al.*, 1995).

Norethisterone was found to bind with lower affinity than the natural ligand to the oestrogen receptor in rabbit uterine cytosol (Tamaya *et al.*, 1977) and rat uterine homogenate (van Kordelaar *et al.*, 1975). Norethisterone acetate inhibited specific binding of oestradiol in the cytosolic fraction of female rat liver at concentrations of 10^{-5}–10^{-4} mol/L, and injection of norethisterone acetate *in vivo* induced nuclear translocation of the oestrogen receptor, i.e. cytosol receptor depletion, in the livers of female rats (Marr *et al.*, 1980).

Norethisterone at concentrations of 10^{-7}–10^{-6} mol/L showed weaker oestrogenic activity than oestradiol when tested for its stimulatory effect on alkaline phosphatase activity in Ishikawa human endometrial cancer cells, which is an oestrogen-specific response inhibited by 4-hydroxytamoxifen (Markiewicz *et al.*, 1992; Botella *et al.*, 1995). Binding of oestradiol to rat uterine oestrogen receptors was reduced by norethisterone both *in vivo* and *in vitro* (Di Carlo *et al.*, 1983). In addition, several anti-oestrogenic effects were found *in vivo*: in ovariectomized rats treated subcutaneously with oestradiol valerate at 50 µg/rat once a week, norethisterone acetate at a daily dose of 1 mg was about equally effective as tamoxifen at a daily dose of 0.06 mg/rat in reducing the oestrogen-induced increase in uterine weight and serum prolactin (Spritzer *et al.*, 1995). Norethisterone also reduced the hyperplastic response of the uterus in ovariectomized rats after treatment with conjugated equine oestrogen; tamoxifen did not have this effect (Kumasaka *et al.*, 1994).

Norethisterone stimulated the growth of most oestrogen-sensitive human mammary cancer cells lines tested (Jeng & Jordan, 1991; Jeng *et al.*, 1992; Schoonen *et al.*, 1995a,b). It stimulated cell proliferation at concentrations of 10^{-8}–10^{-7} mol/L in studies with the oestrogen receptor-positive MCF-7 and T47D:A18 cell lines (Jeng *et al.*, 1992), and these results were confirmed in studies with three sub-lines of MCF-7 and two other T47D cell lines of different origin, except that one of the latter did not respond to norethisterone (Schoonen *et al.*, 1995a,b). All of these experiments were performed with cells grown in phenol red-free medium which contained steroid-free (dextran-coated charcoal-stripped) serum (Jeng *et al.*, 1992; Schoonen *et al.*, 1995a,b). Norethisterone induced *trans*-activation of reporter constructs containing an oestrogen response element coupled to the chloramphenicol acetyltransferase gene transfected into these cells (Jeng *et al.*, 1992); however, the cell growth-stimulating and reporter gene *trans*-activating effects of norethisterone at 10^{-6} mol/L were blocked by simultaneous treatment of the cells with the anti-oestrogens 4-hydroxytamoxifen (10^{-7} mol/L) and ICI164,384 (10^{-7}–10^{-6} mol/L), but not by anti-progestogens such as RU486 (Jeng & Jordan, 1991; Jeng *et al.*, 1992; Schoonen *et al.*, 1995a,b). This suggests that the stimulatory effects of norethisterone on cell proliferation are mediated via the oestrogen receptor, but not the progesterone receptor. Support for this notion was provided by studies indicating that norethisterone did not stimulate the growth of the oestrogen receptor-negative human breast cancer cell lines MDA-MB-231, BT-20 and T47D:C4 (Jeng et al., 1992). Furthermore, the stimulation of MCF-7 cell proliferation by norethisterone was accompanied by a marked decrease in TGF-β2 and TGF-β3 mRNA levels, while the level of TGF-β1 mRNA was not affected. The inhibitory effect on TGF-β2 and TGF-β3 mRNA could be blocked by addition of 4-hydroxytamoxifen (Jeng & Jordan, 1991).

Norethisterone increased the reductive activity of 17β-hydroxysteroid dehydrogenase in an oestrogen- and progestogen-stimulated MCF-7 cell line cultured in the absence of phenol red (Coldham & James, 1990), which indicates that this progestogen stimulates breast cell proliferation *in vivo* by increasing the formation of oestradiol.

Oestradiol at concentrations of 10^{-10} mol/L and higher strongly induced the growth of the MCF-7 and T47D cell lines, regardless of the sub-line used (van der Burg et al., 1992; Kalkhoven et al., 1994; Schoonen et al., 1995a,b). The stimulation of MCF-7 cell growth by oestrogen at 10^{-10} mol/L was not significantly inhibited by norethisterone at the concentrations tested (up to 10^{-6} mol/L) (Schoonen et al., 1995a). Oestrogen-induced growth in T47D cells was not blocked by norethisterone at 10^{-6} mol/L in one sub-line (T47D-A), but it was completely inhibited in another sub-line (T47D-S) at a concentration of 10^{-8} mol/L. These two sub-lines differ considerably, in that RU486, but not 4-hydroxytamoxifen or ICI164,384, blocked oestrogen-stimulated growth in the T47D-A cell line, while both anti-progestogens and anti-oestrogens were inhibitory for T47D-S (Schoonen et al., 1995b).

In vivo, norethisterone had no androgenic activity, as judged by the lack of stimulation of ventral prostate growth in castrated rats (Phillips et al., 1987); however, norethisterone reduced the activity of 5α-reductase in the livers of male and female rats and also decreased the activity of hepatic 3β-hydroxysteroid dehydrogenase in castrated male rats. These effects were not blocked by flutamide or oestradiol, suggesting that androgen receptor-mediation was not involved. The oestrogen-like activity of norethisterone, i.e. the suppression of 3β-hydroxysteroid dehydrogenase, can probably be ascribed to an effect of 'high oestrogen dose' (Lax et al., 1984).

Studies with the human breast cancer cell line ZR-75-1, which contains functional oestrogen, progesterone and androgen receptors, suggest that norethisterone inhibits the growth of these cells by a combined action of androgen and progesterone receptor-mediated mechanisms in the presence of oestrogens. In oestrogen-free medium, however, norethisterone stimulated the growth of these cells, an effect that was counteracted by the anti-oestrogen EM-139 (Poulin et al., 1990).

Norethisterone did not bind to the glucocorticoid receptor on human mononuclear leukocytes (Kontula et al., 1983). It showed moderate affinity for human sex hormone-binding globulin, which could only slightly increase the level of free testosterone (Nilsson & von Schoultz, 1989).

Norethisterone increased secretion of vascular endothelial growth factor by the human breast cancer cell line T47D to a similar extent (two- to threefold over basal levels) as progesterone. This effect, which was progestogen-specific and did not occur in

MCF-7, ZR-75 or MDA-MB-231 cells, suggests an angiogenic response of these cells to norethisterone (Hyder *et al.*, 1998).

4.2.13 *Norethynodrel*

(a) *Humans*

No relevant data were available to the Working Group.

(b) *Experimental systems*

Norethynodrel is metabolized *in vivo* to norethisterone, which binds the progesterone receptor in rabbit uterine cytosol and human uterine endometrium and myometrium, whereas no binding to the progesterone receptor was reported in cultured MCF-7 human breast tumour cells, as pointed out above in the section on norethisterone. Shapiro *et al.* (1978) reported that the binding affinity of norethynodrel itself to the human uterine progesterone receptor is 23% that of progesterone. Progestogen-specific stimulation of alkaline phosphatase activity in T47D human breast cancer cells revealed the full agonist activity of norethynodrel, which was as strong as that of progesterone (Markiewicz & Gurpide, 1994).

The affinity with which norethynodrel bound to the oestrogen receptor in whole rat uterine homogenate was closest to that of the natural ligand of all the progestogens tested (van Kordelaar *et al.*, 1975). Norethynodrel at concentrations of 10^{-8}–10^{-6} mol/L showed moderate oestrogenic activity in comparison with oestradiol when tested for its stimulatory effect on alkaline phosphatase activity in Ishikawa human endometrial cancer cells, which is an oestrogen-specific response inhibited by 4-hydroxytamoxifen (Markiewicz *et al.*, 1992; Botella *et al.*, 1995).

Norethynodrel stimulated the growth of the oestrogen receptor-positive human breast cancer cell lines MCF-7 and T47D-A18 at concentrations of 10^{-8}–10^{-7} mol/L in experiments performed with cells grown in phenol red-free medium which contained steroid-free (dextran-coated charcoal-stripped) serum. Norethynodrel induced *trans*-activation of reporter constructs containing an oestrogen response element coupled to the chloramphenicol acetyltransferase gene transfected into these cells; however, the cell growth-stimulating and reporter gene-*trans*-activating effects of norethynodrel at 10^{-7} mol/L were blocked by simultaneous treatment of the cells with the anti-oestrogens 4-hydroxytamoxifen (10^{-7} mol/L) and ICI164,384 (10^{-7}–10^{-6} mol/L), but not by anti-progestogens such as RU486. These findings suggest that the stimulation of cell proliferation by norethynodrel is mediated via the oestrogen receptor, not the progesterone receptor. Support for this notion is provided by studies indicating that norethynodrel does not stimulate the growth of the oestrogen receptor-negative human breast cancer cell lines MDA-MB-231, BT-20 and T47D:C4 (Jeng *et al.*, 1992).

The androgenic activity of norethynodrel has not been studied, but its metabolite norethisterone has androgenic activity *in vivo* (Phillips *et al.*, 1987; Duc *et al.*, 1995).

Norethynodrel increased the secretion of vascular endothelial growth factor by the human breast cancer cell line T47D to a similar extent (two- to threefold over basal

levels) as progesterone. This effect, which was progestogen-specific and did not occur in
MCF-7, ZR-75 or MDA-MB-231 cells, suggests an angiogenic cellular response to norethynodrel (Hyder *et al.*, 1998).

The combination of mestranol (7.5 or 75 μg/rat per day) and norethynodrel (0.5 or
5 mg/rat per day) given as a pellet implant to female Sprague-Dawley rats, starting at 45,
55, 65 or 75 days of age, caused changes in the developing mammary gland that resulted
in protection against induction of mammary cancer by a single dose (80 mg/kg bw) of
DMBA (Russo *et al.*, 1989). The hormone treatment was given for 21 days, followed by
21 days' recovery, at which time some rats were killed to study the morphology of their
mammary glands, while other rats received DMBA. The hormone treatment at both
doses decreased the number of terminal end-buds per mammary gland and increased the
number of alveolar buds but did not alter the number of terminal ducts; cell proliferation,
measured as the DNA-labelling index, was reduced in the terminal ducts and alveolar
buds but remained unchanged in the terminal end-buds (Russo *et al.*, 1989; Russo &
Russo, 1991). In these experiments, a trend was observed for the hormonal treatment to
produce less effect when initiated at a later age. The reduction in cell proliferation in
terminal end-buds and terminal ducts, the target tissues for DMBA, may explain the
protective effect of the hormonal combination on the development of mammary cancer.

Reboud and Pageaut (1977) administered norethynodrel by subcutaneous implantation of resin pellets to female BALB/C, B6AF1 and C57BL6 mice for two weeks at a
dose of 15 mg/mouse once a week and for nine weeks or eight months at 15 mg/mouse
every three weeks. Under each of the exposure conditions and in all strains, norethynodrel caused irregular hyperplasia of the vagina and exo-cervix similar to that
observed during oestrus, unlike progesterone which caused mucoid and dysplastic
cervical changes at the same dose. Progesterone, but not norethynodrel, is a cervical
tumour promoter in mice treated with 3-methylcholanthrene.

Norethynodrel had a strong growth-stimulating effect on the livers of female Wistar
rats when given at a dose of 10–100 mg/kg bw for seven days, as was evident from a
15–25% increase in liver weight and an approximately 40% increase in hepatic DNA
content (Schulte-Hermann *et al.*, 1988).

Norethynodrel *per se* at concentrations of 3×10^{-6}–10^{-4} mol/L induced γ-GT activity
in cultured rat hepatocytes in the presence of 30 nmol/L dexamethasone (Edwards &
Lucas, 1985).

4.2.14   *Norgestimate*

(*a*)   *Humans*

No relevant data were available to the Working Group.

(*b*)   *Experimental systems*

The binding affinity of norgestimate for human and rabbit uterine progesterone
receptors has been reported to be 1–3% that of progesterone itself (Juchem *et al.*, 1993;
Kuhnz *et al.*, 1995). Other studies showed a 10-fold lower (Killinger *et al.*, 1985) or even

a somewhat higher binding affinity (Phillips *et al.*, 1990) relative to progesterone. The apparent discrepancies in the observed progesterone receptor binding may be due to the fact that metabolites of norgestimate, levonorgestrel (see above) and levonorgestrel-17-acetate, bind with approximately eight- and fourfold higher affinity, respectively, to this receptor in human myometrial tissue (Juchem *et al.*, 1993).

Norgestimate had clear progestational activity *in vivo*, both in a test for pregnancy maintenance in female rats (Kuhnz & Beier, 1994) and as measured by inhibition of ovulation and endometrial stimulation in rabbits (Killinger *et al.*, 1985; Phillips *et al.*, 1987). In these three endocrine bioassays, norgestimate was 3–10 times more active than progesterone (Phillips *et al.*, 1987).

In vivo, norgestimate had little or no androgenic activity in comparison with 5α-dihydrotestosterone, as measured by stimulation of ventral prostate growth in immature castrated rats (Phillips *et al.*, 1987, 1990; Kuhnz & Beier, 1994).

At concentrations as low as 10^{-10} mol/L, norgestimate up-regulated the expression of the prostate-specific antigen at the mRNA and protein level in T-47D human breast cancer cells. Expression of the antigen in these cells was also stimulated by other progestogens, androgens and corticosteroids (Zarghami *et al.*, 1997).

Norgestimate also bound with very low affinity to the androgen receptor but not at all to the oestrogen receptor (Juchem & Pollow, 1990; Phillips *et al.*, 1990). The relative binding affinity for the rat ventral prostate androgen receptor was approximately 0.3% that of 5α-dihydrotestosterone (Phillips *et al.*, 1990).

Norgestimate did not bind to sex hormone-binding globulin in human serum (Juchem & Pollow, 1990).

4.2.15 *Norgestrel*

(a) *Humans*

No relevant data were available to the Working Group.

(b) *Experimental systems*

Norgestrel binds strongly to the progesterone receptor in human uterus, with an affinity equal to 50 or > 90% that of progesterone (Briggs, 1975; Shapiro *et al.*, 1978). A similar result was reported for receptor binding in the chick oviduct (Haukkamaa *et al.*, 1980). Norgestrel bound with sixfold higher affinity than progesterone to the progesterone receptor in rabbit lung (Nielsen *et al.*, 1987).

In an assay of progestogen-specific stimulation of alkaline phosphatase activity in T47D human breast cancer cells, moderate agonist activity was demonstrated for norgestrel in comparison with progesterone (Markiewicz & Gurpide, 1994).

Norgestrel at concentrations of 10^{-8}–10^{-6} mol/L stimulated the growth of the oestrogen receptor-containing and oestrogen-sensitive mammary cancer cell lines MCF-7 and T47D:A18; this activity was inhibited by the anti-oestrogens ICI182,780 and ICI164,384 (at a concentration of 10^{-6} mol/L), but not by RU486 (at a concentration of 10^{-7} mol/L) (Jeng *et al.*, 1992; Catherino *et al.*, 1993; Catherino & Jordan, 1995). Norgestrel did not affect the growth of the oestrogen receptor-negative and oestrogen-independent mammary cancer cell lines MDA-MB-231, BT-20 and T47DC4 (Jeng et al., 1992). Progesterone receptor expression was maintained in both cell types. With reporter constructs containing two progesterone response elements in front of the tk promotor coupled to the chloramphenicol acetyltransferase gene transfected into the MCF-7 cell line, transcriptional activation was observed with norgestrel at a concentration of 10^{-6} mol/L, clearly demonstrating expression of functional progesterone. During these experiments, 10^{-10} mol/L oestradiol was present in the medium to boost receptor expression (Catherino et al., 1993). These findings suggest that the stimulating effects of norgestrel on cell proliferation are mediated via the oestrogen receptor. This is apparently not related to effects at the level of receptor–ligand interaction, because norgestrel at concentrations of 10^{-9}–10^{-6} mol/L causes trans-activation of reporter constructs containing oestrogen response elements (from the vitellogenin or pS2 gene) or progesterone response elements transfected into MCF-7 cells; ICI164,384, but not RU486, inhibited trans-activation of the oestrogen response element-containing constructs, while RU486, but not ICI164,384, inhibited trans-activation of the progesterone response element-containing construct (Catherino et al., 1993; Catherino & Jordan, 1995). Norgestrel also stimulated the protein expression of the progesterone receptor in MCF-7 cells at 10^{-6} but not at 10^{-8} mol/L (Catherino et al., 1993).

Norgestrel showed much weaker binding than the natural ligand to the oestrogen receptor in whole rat-uterine homogenate (van Kordelaar et al., 1975), while displacement of ^{3}H-oestradiol binding to the cytosolic fraction of female rat liver occurred only at norgestrel concentrations of 10^{-5}–10^{-4} mol/L (Marr et al., 1980). The binding of oestradiol to rat uterine oestrogen receptor was reduced, however, by norgestrel, both in vivo at 1 h after a single oral dose of 15 mg/kg bw and in vitro (Di Carlo et al., 1983). In vivo, norgestrel partially reversed the hyperplastic and metaplastic changes found in oestrogen-exposed rat uterus (White et al., 1982).

Norgestrel had much weaker oestrogenic activity than oestradiol at concentrations greater than 1×10^{-6} mol/L when tested for its stimulatory effect on alkaline phosphatase activity in Ishikawa human endometrial cancer cells, which is an oestrogen-specific response inhibited by 4-hydroxytamoxifen (Markiewicz et al., 1992; Markiewicz & Gurpide, 1994).

Norgestrel was shown to be a potent competitor for binding of 5α-dihydrotestosterone to the androgen receptor in human foreskin fibroblasts, with an activity similar to that of testosterone (Breiner et al., 1986).

Studies with the human breast cancer cell line ZR-75-1, which contains functional oestrogen, progesterone and androgen receptors, suggest that norgestrel inhibits the growth of these cells via an interaction of androgen and progesterone receptor-mediated mechanisms in the presence of oestrogens. In oestrogen-free medium, however, norgestrel stimulated the growth of these cells, an effect that was counteracted by the anti-oestrogen EM-139 (Poulin et al., 1990).

Norgestrel increased the secretion of vascular endothelial growth factor by the human breast cancer cell line T47D to an extent (two- to threefold over basal levels) similar to progesterone. This effect, which was progestogen-specific and did not occur in MCF-7, ZR-75 or MDA-MB-231 cells, suggests an angiogenic response of T47D cells to norgestrel (Hyder *et al.*, 1998).

4.3   Genetic and related effects

Most, if not all, of the genetic and related effects associated with use of oral contraceptives can be explained by oestrogen and progestogen receptor mechanisms (King, 1991), but non-receptor processes may also exist (Duval *et al.*, 1983; Yager & Liehr, 1996). The following descriptions indicate how the doses of hormone used relate to receptor and non-receptor mechanisms and to the concentrations achieved *in vivo* in women who use oral contraceptives or post-menopausal hormonal therapy. The concentrations in such formulations are usually several micrograms per kilogram body weight per day, which generate plasma concentrations of nanograms per millilitre for progestogens and picograms per millilitre for oestrogens (Orme *et al.*, 1983; Barnes & Lobo, 1987). Those are the concentrations at which receptor-mediated events can be saturated *in vitro*. Appreciably higher concentrations were used in many of the studies listed in Tables 42–46. The significance of the presence and absence of effects at these concentrations is uncertain, as is the mode of action in the case of effects.

4.3.1   *Combined oral contraceptives*

Genetic changes in cells from women taking steroid hormones have been compared with those in cells from unexposed women in five studies, in all of which few details are given about the hormonal exposure; however, use of oral contraceptives predominated.

Two of three reports described the effects of steroids on lymphocytes. Ghosh and Ghosh (1988) noted an increased frequency of sister chromatid exchange in lymphocytes from 51 healthy, non-smoking Indian women (mean age, 34.5 years) exposed to ethinyloestradiol plus levonorgestrel [doses not given] for 4–28 months as compared with 38 unexposed referents (mean age, 35.6 years). The numbers of sister chromatid exchanges per cell were 5.56 ± 0.21 for the referents and 8.63 ± 0.29 for women taking oral contraceptives ($p < 0.001$).

In contrast, a study in Denmark showed no effect on the sister chromatid exchange frequency in lymphocytes of exposure to oestrogen and progestogen [types and doses not stated] for a minimum of two months (Husum *et al.*, 1982). There were 25 non-smoking, healthy women aged 15–42 years in the referent group, who had 8.42 ± 0.21 sister chromatid exchanges per cell and 15 women with otherwise similar characteristics who used oral contraceptives and had 8.54 ± 0.24 sister chromatid exchanges per cell. Smoking of > 20 cigarettes per day produced the expected increase in sister chromatid exchange frequency, but no significant difference was observed between oral contraceptive users who smoked this number of cigarettes and comparable controls: 9.52 ± 0.30 sister chromatid exchanges per cell in 13 referents and 10.36 ± 0.75 sister chromatid exchanges per cell in six oral contraceptive users.

Chromosomal abnormalities were quantified in lymphocytes from 88 women aged 16–35 years in South Africa, equally divided into controls who had never used hormonal contraception and women who had used oral contraceptives [types and doses not stated] for 7–98 months. The groups were pair-matched for race, age, parity and condition of offspring, occupation, medication, X-irradiation and smoking habits (Pinto, 1986). Abnormal chromosomes were found in 31% (410/1286) of lymphocytes from oral contraceptive users and 18% (233/1255) of control cells ($p < 0.0001$). The abnormalities were sub-classified into those possibly caused by technical handling (0.29 ± 0.13 and 0.19 ± 0.07 abnormalities per cell in oral contraceptive users and controls, respectively ($p < 0.0001$)) and those not likely to be generated in this way (0.105 ± 0.077 and 0.018 ± 0.029 abnormalities per cell in oral contraceptive users and controls, respectively ($p < 0.0001$)).

Indications of hormone-related genetic damage in lymphocytes in two of the three well-conducted studies raised questions about the potential genotoxicity of steroid hormones in humans. As the relevance of effects in blood lymphocytes to mechanisms of carcinogenesis in tissues such as breast epithelium is unclear, two good analyses of the effects of oral contraceptives on subsequent changes in breast cancer DNA are noteworthy. The two studies were based on the same library of stored breast cancer tissues from women in Sweden whose previous exposure to oral contraceptives was known. At the time of first diagnosis of the cancer, pre-menopausal women were questioned about their earlier life style, including the age at which they had started using oral contraceptives. Tumours removed from these women were stored and subsequently used to analyse ploidy, aneuploidy and cell proliferative activity by flow cytometry (Olsson et al., 1991b) and oncogene amplification (Olsson et al., 1991c).

In the study of ploidy (Olsson et al., 1991b), 175 breast tumours from pre-meno-pausal women aged 26–52 years were used. Of the tumours from women who had started using oral contraceptives before 20 years of age, 81% ($n = 27$) were aneuploid, whereas only 53% ($n = 59$) of those from women who had never used oral contraceptives were aneuploid ($p < 0.04$). Tumours from women who had started using oral contraceptives at ages 20 to ≥ 24 years had intermediate percentages of aneuploid cells. There was a highly significant ($p = 0.0001$) correlation between early oral contraceptive use and age at diagnosis and other parameters such as proliferative activity, measured as the fraction of cells in S-phase. The statistical significance of the association between early oral contraceptive use and biological effects on the cancer cells was maintained when multivariate analysis was performed.

In the study of oncogenes (Olsson et al., 1991c), erbb2 (HER/neu) and int2 gene amplifications were assessed in 72 tumours from 28–50-year-old women. More cancers from women who had started using oral contraceptives before the age of 20 had erbb2 amplifications (11/19 or 58% of cancers) than those from women who started after that age (11/53 or 21% of cancers). The odds ratio for this difference was significant in both univariate (odds ratio, 5.3; 95% CI, 1.6–17) and multivariate (odds ratio, 6.8; 95% CI, 1.3–35) analyses. No link was seen between early oral contraceptive use and int2 amplification, but this effect was positively associated with any use of progestogens (multivariate odds ratio, 17; 95% CI, 1.8–170); amplification of *erbb2* was not related to progestogen use. Other variables considered were age at abortion and first full-term pregnancy, parity, age at diagnosis and tumour stage. The authors recognized the problems associated with interpreting data from such analyses in terms of cause and effect and correctly concluded that they should not be ignored.

4.3.2   *Ethinyloestradiol and some derivatives alone and in combination with progestogens* (Table 42)

No gene mutation was induced in *S. typhimurium* after treatment with ethinyloestradiol. In single studies, small increases in the frequency of unscheduled DNA synthesis were demonstrated in primary cultures of rat hepatocytes treated with ethinyloestradiol, particularly in cells from male rats, and cell transformation was demonstrated *in vitro* in BALB/c 3T3 mouse cells treated with ethinyloestradiol.

In vivo, covalent binding to DNA was demonstrated in the liver, pancreas and kidney of rats and in the kidneys of Syrian hamsters treated with ethinyloestradiol. Chromosomal aberrations were induced *in vivo* in kidney cells of exposed, castrated male Syrian hamsters and in bone-marrow cells of mice treated with high doses of ethinyloestradiol. Paradoxically, ethinyloestradiol at these high doses did not induce micronuclei in bone-marrow cells of mice.

Covalent binding to DNA was observed in the kidneys of Syrian hamsters treated with ethylethinyloestradiol and in those of animals that had received an implant of methylethinyloestradiol. Methoxyethinyloestradiol (Moxestrol) did not induce cell transformation in BALB/c 3T3 mouse cells *in vitro*, but it bound to DNA in the kidneys of Syrian hamsters that had received a Moxestrol implant.

Combinations of ethinyloestradiol and gestodene did not induce gene mutation in various *S. typhimurium* strains. Chromosomal aberrations were induced in the bone marrow of male mice treated *in vivo* with combinations of ethinyloestradiol and norethisterone acetate. In a single study, micronuclei were not induced in female mice exposed *in vivo* to ethinyloestradiol and norethisterone acetate. Primary cultures of baby rat kidney cells were transformed to anchorage-independent growth, and these cells induced tumour formation in syngeneic animals infected with HPV-16 DNA and Ha-*ras*-1 and exposed to an ethanolic extract of oral contraceptive tablets containing ethinyloestradiol and levonorgestrel.

DNA covalent binding was demonstrated in the liver, pancreas and kidney of male rats treated with ethinyloestradiol and tamoxifen.

4.3.3   *Mestranol alone and in combination with progestogens* (Table 43)

Gene mutations were not induced in *S. typhimurium* after treatment with mestranol itself or with ethanolic extracts of Ovulen 21 tablets, containing mestranol, or Enovid tablets, containing mestranol and norethynodrel. Also, gene mutations were not induced in *S. typhimurium* in a host-mediated assay in which the bacteria were recovered from the livers of mice. It has been reported, however, that mestranol and extracts of Ovulen 21 and

Table 42. Genetic and related effects of ethinyloestradiol and its derivatives

Test system	Result[a] Without exogenous metabolic system	Result[a] With exogenous metabolic system	Dose[b] (LED or HID)	Reference
Ethinyloestradiol				
Escherichia coli rec strains, differential toxicity	NT	–	1000 µg/plate	Mamber et al. (1983)
Bacillus subtilis rec strains, differential toxicity	–	NT	5000 µg/plate	Tanooka (1977)
Salmonella typhimurium TA100, TA1535, TA1537, TA1538, TA98, reverse mutation	–	–	2500 µg/plate	Lang & Redmann (1979)
Salmonella typhimurium TA100, TA1537, TA1538, TA98, reverse mutation	–	–	1000 µg/plate	Dayan et al. (1980)
Salmonella typhimurium TA100, TA1535, TA1537, TA1538, TA98, reverse mutation	–	–	500 µg/plate[c]	Lang & Reimann (1993)
Aneuploidy, male Chinese hamster DON cells *in vitro*	+	NT	22.2	Wheeler et al. (1986)
Gene mutation, Chinese hamster lung V79 cells, *hprt* locus *in vitro*	–	–	29.6	Drevon et al. (1981)
Gene mutation, Chinese hamster lung V79 cells, ouabain resistance *in vitro*	–	NT	29.6	Drevon et al. (1981)
Chromosomal aberrations, Chinese hamster ovary cells *in vitro*	–	NT	4	Ishidate et al. (1978)
Cell transformation, BALB/c 3T3 mouse cells	–	NT	5.0	Dunkel et al. (1981)
Cell transformation, BALB/c 3T3 mouse cells	+	NT	3.0	Liehr et al. (1987a)
Cell transformation, Syrian hamster embryo cells, clonal assay	–	NT	50	Dunkel et al. (1981)
Cell transformation, RMuLV/Fischer rat embryo cells	+	NT	10.7	Dunkel et al. (1981)
Chromosomal aberrations, human lymphocytes *in vitro*	–	NT	100	Stenchever et al. (1969)
Micronucleus induction, mice *in vivo*	–		0.2 po × 15	Shyama & Rahiman (1996)
Chromosomal aberrations, male Syrian hamster kidney cells *in vivo*	+		185 µg/d imp.; 5 mo	Banerjee et al. (1994)
Chromosomal aberrations, mouse bone-marrow cells *in vivo*	+		0.12 po × 15	Shyama & Rahiman (1996)
Binding (covalent) to DNA, female rat liver, pancreas, kidney *in vivo*	+		75 µg/d po; 12 mo	Shimomura et al. (1992)
Binding (covalent) to DNA, Syrian hamster kidney *in vivo*	+		22 mg imp. × 2	Liehr et al. (1987b)
Inhibition of metabolic cooperation, Chinese hamster V79 cells *in vitro*	(+)	NT	0.74	Yager (1983)

Table 42 (contd)

Test system	Result[a] Without exogenous metabolic system	With exogenous metabolic system	Dose[b] (LED or HID)	Reference
Ethinyloestradiol + gestodene (1 part + 2.5 parts)				
Salmonella typhimurium TA100, TA1535, TA1537, TA1538, TA98, reverse mutation	−	−	2000 µg/plate[c,d]	Lang & Reimann (1993)
Ethinyloestradiol + norethisterone acetate				
Chromosomal aberrations, female Swiss mouse bone-marrow cells *in vivo*	+		0.8 po × 15[d]	Shyama *et al.* (1991)
Micronucleus formation, female Swiss mouse bone-marrow cells *in vivo*	−		8.0 po × 15[d]	Shyama *et al.* (1991)
Ethinyloestradiol + (l)-norgestrel				
Cell transformation, primary baby rat kidney+ HPV-16 + H-*ras*-1	+	NT	0.3 (ethanol extract)[d]	Pater *et al.* (1990)
Ethinyloestradiol + tamoxifen				
Binding (covalent) to DNA, female rat liver, pancreas, kidney *in vivo*	+		75 µg + 500 µg/d po, 12 mo	Shimomura *et al.* (1992)
Ethylethinyloestradiol				
Binding (covalent) to DNA, Syrian hamster kidney *in vivo*	+		25 mg imp. × 2	Liehr *et al.* (1987b)
Methoxyethinyloestradiol (Moxestrol)				
Cell transformation, BALB/c 3T3 mouse cells *in vitro*	−	NT	16.3	Liehr *et al.* (1987a)
Binding (covalent) to DNA, Syrian hamster kidney *in vivo*	+		25 mg imp. × 2	Liehr *et al.* (1986)
Methylethinyloestradiol				
Binding (covalent) to DNA, Syrian hamster kidney *in vivo*	+		25 mg imp. × 2	Liehr *et al.* (1986, 1987b)

[a] +, positive; (+), weak positive; −, negative; NT, not tested; ?, inconclusive
[b] LED, lowest effective dose; HID, highest ineffective dose; in-vitro tests, µg/mL; in-vivo tests, mg/kg bw per day; po, oral; imp., implant; d, day; mo, month
[c] Toxicity was observed at higher dose(s) tested
[d] Total mixture

Table 43. Genetic and related effects of mestranol

Test system	Result[b] Without exogenous metabolic system	Result[b] With exogenous metabolic system	Dose[b] (LED or HID)	Reference
Mestranol				
Salmonella typhimurium TA100, TA1535, TA1537, TA1538, TA98, reverse mutation	–	–	12.5 µg/plate	Rao et al. (1983)
Salmonella typhimurium TA100, TA1535, TA97a, TA98, reverse mutation	–	–	1000 µg/plate[c]	Dhillon et al. (1994)
Drosophila melanogaster, sex-linked recessive lethal mutations	–	–	50000	Aguiar & Tordecilla (1984)
Sister chromatid exchange, human lymphocytes *in vitro*	+	NT	1	Dhillon et al. (1994)
Chromosomal aberrations, human lymphocytes *in vitro*	+	NT	10	Stenchever et al. (1969)
Chromosomal aberrations, human lymphocytes *in vitro*	+	NT	100	Dhillon et al. (1994)
DNA strand breaks, cross-links or related damage, Sprague-Dawley rats *in vivo*	–		250 ip × 1	Yager & Fifield (1982)
Chromosomal aberrations, mouse bone-marrow cells *in vivo*	–		100 po × 1	Ansari & Adhami (1977)
Chromosomal aberrations, mouse bone-marrow cells *in vivo*	+		0.01 ip × 1	Dhillon et al. (1994)
Micronucleus induction, mouse bone-marrow cells *in vivo*	+		1 ip × 1	Dhillon et al. (1994)
Sister chromatid exchange, mouse bone-marrow cells *in vivo*	+		0.1 ip × 1	Dhillon et al. (1994)
Host mediated assay (male Swiss albino mouse, intravenous inoculation), *S. typhimurium* TA100, TA1535, TA98, TA97a	–		100 ip × 1	Dhillon et al. (1994)
Inhibition of metabolic cooperation, Chinese hamster V79 cells *in vitro*	(+)	NT	0.78	Yager (1983)
Mestranol + 2-acetylaminofluorene (3 µg)				
Salmonella typhimurium TA100, TA98, reverse mutation	NT	+	0.62 µg/plate	Rao et al. (1983)
Mestranol + norethisterone				
Sister chromatid exchange, human lymphocytes *in vitro*	–	NT	0.0038 + 0.075	Dutkowski et al. (1983)
Micronucleus induction, human lymphocytes *in vitro*	–	NT	0.0038 + 0.075	Dutkowski et al. (1983)

Table 43 (contd)

Test system	Result[b] Without exogenous metabolic system	With exogenous metabolic system	Dose[b] (LED or HID)	Reference
Enovid extract (mestranol + norethynodrel)				
Salmonella typhimurium TA100, TA98, reverse mutation	–	–	625 µg/plate	Rao et al. (1983)
Enovid extract (mestranol + norethynodrel) + 2-acetylaminofluorene (3 µg)				
Salmonella typhimurium TA100, TA98, reverse mutation	–	+	31.3 µg/plate	Rao et al. (1983)
Enovid extract (mestranol + norethynodrel) + N-nitrosopiperidine (250 µg)				
Salmonella typhimurium TA100, reverse mutation	–	+	62.5 µg/plate	Rao et al. (1983)
Salmonella typhimurium TA1535, reverse mutation	–	+	31.3 µg/plate	Rao et al. (1983)
Ovulen 21 extract (mestranol)				
Salmonella typhimurium TA100, TA98, reverse mutation	–	–	50 µg/plate	Rao et al. (1983)
Ovulen 21 extract (mestranol) + 2-acetylaminofluorene (3 µg)				
Salmonella typhimurium TA98, reverse mutation	–	+	31.3 µg/plate	Rao et al. (1983)
Ovulen 21 extract (mestranol) + N-nitrosopiperidine (250 µg)				
Salmonella typhimurium TA1535, reverse mutation	–	+	31.3 µg/plate	Rao et al. (1983)

[a] +, positive; (+), weak positive; –, negative; NT, not tested

[b] LED, lowest effective dose; HID, highest ineffective dose; in-vitro tests, µg/mL; in-vivo tests, mg/kg bw per day; ip, intraperitoneal; po, oral

[c] Toxicity was observed at higher dose(s)

Enovid enhanced the mutation yield obtained with an ineffective dose of 2-acetyl-aminofluorene (3 µg/plate). The extracts also enhanced the mutation yield obtained with an ineffective dose of *N*-nitrosopiperidine (250 µg/plate).

In a single study, mestranol induced sister chromatid exchange and chromosomal aberrations in human lymphocytes *in vitro* and sister chromatid exchange, chromosomal aberrations and micronuclei in bone-marrow cells from mice treated *in vivo*.

Negative results were obtained with a combination of mestranol and norethisterone in a study of sister chromatid exchange and micronucleus formation in human lymphocyte cultures. The concentrations of the test material used in this study were in the nanogram per millilitre range, which are those that might be expected during human use.

4.3.4   *Cyproterone acetate, metabolites and derivatives* (Table 44)

Gene mutations were not induced in *Salmonella typhimurium* by cyproterone acetate or 6,7-epoxycyproterone acetate. Covalent binding to DNA was observed with cyproterone acetate in cultured rat liver cells, the binding being greater in cells from females than from males in all cases, according to one study. Cyproterone acetate also bound to DNA in human and porcine hepatocytes in culture, while a metabolite, 3-hydroxy-cyproterone acetate, and a derivative, 3-*O*-acetylcyproterone acetate, also bound to isolated calf thymus DNA. DNA strand breakage was induced in female rat hepatocytes *in vitro* in one study. No DNA breakage was observed in male human hepatocytes *in vitro*. DNA repair, including unscheduled DNA synthesis, of damage induced by cyproterone acetate appears to be sex specific, since these processes occur in cultured liver cells from female but not male rats. Gene mutations were not induced at the *hprt* locus of Chinese hamster V79 cells by cyproterone acetate in two studies; in one of the studies, the cells were co-cultured with rat hepatocytes. The frequency of chromosomal aberrations was not increased in a single study with cyproterone acetate in Chinese hamster V79 cells co-cultured with rat hepatocytes, whereas a study of the frequency of micronucleus formation *in vitro* in hepatocytes from female rats gave inconclusive results.

In vivo, covalent binding to DNA has been demonstrated in the livers of male and female rats and female mice (weak binding). No binding to male mouse liver DNA was observed. Unscheduled DNA synthesis was induced in one study in hepatocytes from rats exposed to cyproterone acetate. Also in single studies, this compound increased the frequency of micronucleus formation in hepatocytes from exposed female rats and induced γ-GT-positive foci in the livers of female rats. In one study, the frequency of mutation of the *Lac*I transgene was significantly increased in female BigBlue® transgenic Fischer 344 rats after exposure to 3-*O*-acetylcyproterone acetate. DNA adducts were quantified in the same experiment; the mutation frequency started to increase at doses at which the number of DNA adducts had already reached a plateau.

4.3.5   *Norethisterone alone and in combination with an oestrogen* (Table 45)

Gene mutation was not induced in *S. typhimurium* after treatment with norethisterone. Chromosomal aberrations were induced, but the frequency of micronucleus

Table 44. Genetic and related effects of cyproterone acetate and some derivatives

Test system	Result[a] Without exogenous metabolic system	Result[a] With exogenous metabolic system	Dose[b] (LED or HID)	Reference
Cyproterone acetate				
Salmonella typhimurium TA100, TA1535, TA1537, TA1538, TA98, reverse mutation	–	–	250 µg/plate[c]	Lang & Reimann (1993)
DNA strand breaks, alkaline elution assay, female rat hepatocytes in vitro	+	NT	20.85	Martelli et al. (1995)
DNA repair exclusive of unscheduled DNA synthesis, female rat hepatocytes in vitro	+	NT	0.83	Neumann et al. (1992)
DNA repair exclusive of unscheduled DNA synthesis, female rat hepatocytes in vitro	+	NT	0.83	Topinka et al. (1995)
DNA repair exclusive of unscheduled DNA synthesis, male rat hepatocytes in vitro	–	NT	20.9	Topinka et al. (1995)
Unscheduled DNA synthesis, female rat hepatocytes in vitro	+	NT	1.32	Kasper et al. (1995)
Unscheduled DNA synthesis, male rat hepatocytes in vitro	–	NT	20.85	Martelli et al. (1995)
Unscheduled DNA synthesis, female rat hepatocytes in vitro	+	NT	0.42	Martelli et al. (1995)
Unscheduled DNA synthesis, female rat hepatocytes in vitro	+	NT	0.84	Martelli et al. (1996a)
Gene mutation, Chinese hamster V79 cells, hprt locus in vitro	–	–	80[d]	Lang & Reimann (1993)
Gene mutation, Chinese hamster V79 cells, hprt locus in vitro (co-cultured with hepatocytes)	NT	–	41.7	Kasper et al. (1995)
Chromosomal aberrations, Chinese hamster V79 cells in vitro (co-cultured with hepatocytes)	NT	–	41.7	Kasper et al. (1995)
Micronucleus formation, female rat hepatocytes in vitro	(+)	NT	0.42	Kasper et al. (1995)
DNA strand breaks, alkaline elution assay, male human hepatocytes in vitro	–	NT	20.85 (1 sample)	Martelli et al. (1995)
DNA strand breaks, alkaline elution assay, female human hepatocytes in vitro	(+)	NT	20.8 (3/4 samples)	Martelli et al. (1995)
Unscheduled DNA synthesis, male and female human hepatocytes in vitro	+	NT	0.42	Martelli et al. (1995)
Unscheduled DNA synthesis, male and female human hepatocytes in vitro	+	NT	0.42	Martelli et al. (1996a)

Table 44 (contd)

Test system	Result[a] Without exogenous metabolic system	Result[a] With exogenous metabolic system	Dose[b] (LED or HID)	Reference
Cyproterone acetate (contd)				
Unscheduled DNA synthesis, female rat hepatocytes in vivo	+		100 po × 1	Kasper & Mueller (1996)
Gene mutation, female lacI transgenic rat (BigBlue®) in vivo	+		75 po × 1	Krebs et al. (1998)
Micronucleus formation, female rat hepatocytes in vivo	+		100 po × 1	Martelli et al. (1996b)
γ-Glutamyl transpeptidase-positive foci, female Sprague-Dawley rat liver in vivo	+		100 po × 6 (weekly)	Martelli et al. (1996b)
Binding (covalent) to DNA, female rat hepatocytes in vitro	+	NT	0.013	Topinka et al. (1993, 1995)
Binding (covalent) to DNA, male rat hepatocytes in vitro	+	NT	0.42	Topinka et al. (1993, 1995)
Binding (covalent) to DNA, human (male and female), rat (female) hepatocytes in vitro	+	NT	4.2	Werner et al. (1996)
Binding (covalent) to DNA, pig (male and female), rat (male) hepatocytes in vitro	(+)	NT	4.2	Werner et al. (1996)
Binding (covalent) to DNA, female rat liver in vivo	+		0.1 po × 1	Topinka et al. (1993)
Binding (covalent) to DNA, male rat liver in vivo	+		3 po × 1	Topinka et al. (1993)
Binding (covalent) to DNA, female rat liver in vivo	+		10 po × 1	Werner et al. (1995)
Binding (covalent) to DNA, male rat liver in vivo	+		100 po × 1	Werner et al. (1995)
Binding (covalent) to DNA, male rat liver in vivo	+		100 po × 1	Werner et al. (1996)
Binding (covalent) to DNA, male C57BL/6 mouse liver in vivo	–		35 po × 1	Werner et al. (1996)
Binding (covalent) to DNA, female rat liver in vivo	+		10 po × 1	Werner et al. (1996)
Binding (covalent) to DNA, female C57BL/6 mouse liver in vivo	(+)		35 po × 1	Werner et al. (1996)
Binding (covalent) to DNA, female rat liver in vivo	+		25 po × 1	Krebs et al. (1998)

Table 44 (contd)

Test system	Result[a]		Dose[b] (LED or HID)	Reference
	Without exogenous metabolic system	With exogenous metabolic system		
6,7-Epoxycyproterone acetate				
Salmonella typhimurium TA100, TA1535, TA1537, TA1538, TA98, reverse mutation	–	–	500 μg/plate[c]	Lang & Reimann (1993)
α-Hydroxycyproterone acetate				
Binding (covalent) to DNA, calf thymus *in vitro*	+	NT	1	Kerdar *et al.* (1995)
3-*O*-Acetyl cyproterone acetate (not a metabolite)				
Gene mutation, female *lacI* transgenic rat (BigBlue®) *in vivo*	+		75 po × 1	Krebs *et al.* (1998)
Binding (covalent) to DNA, calf thymus *in vitro*	+	NT	1	Kerdar *et al.* (1995)
Binding (covalent) to DNA, female rat liver *in vivo*	+		25 po × 1	Krebs *et al.* (1998)

[a] +, positive; (+), weak positive; –, negative; NT, not tested
[b] LED, lowest effective dose; HID, highest ineffective dose; in-vitro tests, μg/mL; in-vivo tests, mg/kg bw per day; po, oral
[c] Toxicity was observed at this dose in some or all strains
[d] Some toxicity was observed

Table 45. Genetic and related effects of norethisterone and its ester

Test system	Result[a]		Dose[b] (LED or HID)	Reference
	Without exogenous metabolic system	With exogenous metabolic system		
Norethisterone				
Salmonella typhimurium TA100, TA1535, TA1537, TA98, reverse mutation	–	–	1000 µg/plate	Peter et al. (1981)
Salmonella typhimurium TA100, TA1535, TA1537, TA1538, TA98, reverse mutation	–	–	750 µg/plate	Lang & Reimann (1993)
Unscheduled DNA synthesis, female rat hepatocytes in vitro	–	NT	150	Blakey & White (1985)
Unscheduled DNA synthesis, male rat hepatocytes in vitro	(+)	NT	15	Blakey & White (1985)
Micronucleus formation, female Swiss albino mouse bone-marrow cells in vivo	–		30 po × 15	Shyama & Rahiman (1993)
Chromosomal aberrations, female Swiss albino mouse bone-marrow cells in vivo	–		70 po × 1	Ansari & Adhami (1977)
Chromosomal aberrations, female Swiss albino mouse bone-marrow cells in vivo	+		3 po × 15	Shyama & Rahiman (1993)
Norethisterone acetate				
Salmonella typhimurium TA100, TA1535, TA1537, TA98, reverse mutation	–	–	2500 µg/plate	Lang & Redmann (1979)
Salmonella typhimurium TA100, TA1535, TA1537, TA1538, TA98, reverse mutation	–	–	1000 µg/plate	Dayan et al. (1980)
Salmonella typhimurium TA100, TA1535, TA1537, TA1538, TA98, reverse mutation	–	–	500 µg/plate[c]	Lang & Reimann (1993)
Salmonella typhimurium TA100, TA1535, TA97a, TA98, reverse mutation	–	–	1000 µg/plate[c]	Dhillon & Dhillon (1996)
Sister chromatid exchange, human male lymphocytes in vitro (24-h treatment)	+	NT	1	Dhillon & Dhillon (1996)
Sister chromatid exchange, human male lymphocytes in vitro (90-min treatment)	+	+	1	Dhillon & Dhillon (1996)
Chromosomal aberrations, human lymphocytes in vitro	–	NT	100	Stenchever et al. (1969)
Chromosomal aberrations, human male lymphocytes in vitro (72-h treatment)	+	NT	1	Dhillon & Dhillon (1996)
Chromosomal aberrations, human male lymphocytes in vitro (6-h treatment)	–	+	10	Dhillon & Dhillon (1996)
Host-mediated assay, male Swiss albino mouse (intravenous inoculation), S. typhimurium TA97a, TA98, TA100, TA1535	–		100 ip × 1	Dhillon & Dhillon (1996)
Sister chromatid exchange, Swiss albino mice bone-marrow cells in vivo	+		1 ip × 1	Dhillon & Dhillon (1996)
Micronucleus formation, male Swiss albino mouse bone-marrow cells in vivo	+		1 ip × 1	Dhillon & Dhillon (1996)
Dominant lethal mutation induction, C3H and NMRI mice in vivo	(+)		1 mg/animal po daily × 4 wk	Rohrborn & Hansmann (1974)
Aneuploidy, C3H mice in vivo	+		10 mg/animal po daily × 4 wk	Rohrborn & Hansmann (1974)

Table 45 (contd)

Test system	Result[a]		Dose[b] (LED or HID)	Reference
	Without exogenous metabolic system	With exogenous metabolic system		
Norethisterone + mestranol				
Sister chromatid exchange, human lymphocytes *in vitro*	–	NT	0.075 + 0.0038	Dutkowski *et al.* (1983)
Micronucleus formation, human lymphocytes *in vitro*	–	NT	0.075 + 0.0038	Dutkowski *et al.* (1983)
Norethisterone acetate + ethinyloestradiol				
Chromosomal aberrations, female Swiss albino mouse bone-marrow cells *in vivo*	+		0.79 + 0.01 po × 15	Shyama *et al.* (1991)
Micronucleus formation, female Swiss albino mouse bone-marrow cells *in vivo*	–		7.9 + 0.1 po × 15	Shyama *et al.* (1991)

[a] +, positive; (+), weak positive; –, negative; NT, not tested
[b] LED, lowest effective dose; HID, highest ineffective dose; in-vitro tests, μg/mL; in-vivo tests, mg/kg bw per day; po, oral; ip, intraperitoneal; wk, week
[c] Precipitation and/or toxicity was observed at higher dose(s).

formation was not increased in bone-marrow cells of female Swiss albino mice treated *in vivo* with norethisterone.

In a single study, the frequencies of sister chromatid exchange and micronuclei were not increased in cultured human lymphocytes treated with a combination of norethisterone and mestranol.

4.3.6 *Norethisterone acetate alone and in combination with an oestrogen* (Table 45)

Norethisterone acetate did not induce gene mutation in various strains of *S. typhimurium* with or without an exogenous metabolic activation system. In a single study, the frequencies of sister chromatid exchange and chromosomal aberrations were increased in human lymphocytes treated *in vitro* with norethisterone acetate. In the same study, sister chromatid exchange and micronucleus formation were induced in the bone-marrow cells of Swiss albino mice treated *in vivo* with norethisterone acetate, whereas gene mutations were not induced in *S. typhimurium* in a mouse host-mediated assay in which the bacteria were recovered from the livers of animals after treatment with norethisterone acetate.

The combination of norethisterone acetate plus ethinyloestradiol induced chromosomal aberrations in bone-marrow cells of female Swiss albino mice exposed *in vivo*, whereas micronuclei were not induced in the bone-marrow cells of these mice.

4.3.7 *Chlormadinone acetate* (Table 46)

After rat liver cells were incubated with chlormadinone acetate *in vitro*, covalent DNA binding was observed, particularly in cells from females. Unscheduled DNA synthesis was reported in female but not male rat hepatocytes *in vitro* and in male and female human hepatocytes *in vitro* after treatment with chlormadinone acetate. The BdUr density shift assay to determine DNA repair in female and male rat hepatocytes exposed to chlormadinone acetate *in vitro* gave negative results.

No DNA binding was observed in female rat liver *in vivo*, but micronuclei were induced in female rat hepatocytes *in vivo*.

4.3.8 *Gestodene* (Table 46)

Gene mutations were not induced in *S. typhimurium* by gestodene or combinations of gestodene and ethinyloestradiol.

4.3.9 *Megestrol acetate* (Table 46)

Low levels of covalent DNA binding were observed in rat liver cells treated with megestrol acetate *in vitro*, particularly in cells from females. Megestrol acetate induced unscheduled DNA synthesis in rat primary hepatocytes and gave rise to DNA repair in female and male rat liver cells and in human hepatocytes *in vitro*.

Weak covalent DNA binding was observed in female rat liver *in vivo*; however, micronucleus formation was not induced in female rat hepatocytes, and γ-GT-positive foci were not induced in rat liver *in vivo*.

Table 46. Genetic and related effects of other progestogens used in combined oral contraceptives

Test system	Result[a]		Dose[b] (LED or HID)	Reference
	Without exogenous metabolic system	With exogenous metabolic system		
Chlormadinone acetate				
Salmonella typhimurium TA100, TA1535, TA1537, TA1538, reverse mutation	–	–	1000 µg/plate	Dayan et al. (1980)
DNA repair exclusive of unscheduled DNA synthesis, female and male rat hepatocytes *in vitro*	–	NT	20.3	Topinka et al. (1995)
Unscheduled DNA synthesis, female rat hepatocytes *in vitro*	+	NT	0.81	Martelli et al. (1996a)
Unscheduled DNA synthesis, male rat hepatocytes *in vitro*	–	NT	8.1	Martelli et al. (1996a)
Cell transformation, rat liver cells treated *in vivo* scored *in vitro*	–		100 po × 6	Martelli et al. (1996b)
Unscheduled DNA synthesis, male and female human hepatocytes *in vitro*	+	NT	0.81	Martelli et al. (1996a)
Chromosomal aberrations, human lymphocytes *in vitro*	–	NT	100	Stenchever et al. (1969)
Micronucleus formation, female rat hepatocytes *in vivo*	+		100 po × 1	Martelli et al. (1996b)
Binding (covalent) to DNA, female rat hepatocytes *in vitro*	+	NT	1.2	Topinka et al. (1995)
Binding (covalent) to DNA, male rat hepatocytes *in vitro*	(+)	NT	1.2	Topinka et al. (1995)
Binding (covalent) to DNA, female rat liver *in vivo*	–		100 po × 1	Topinka et al. (1995)
Gestodene				
Salmonella typhimurium TA100, TA1535, TA1537, TA1538, TA98, reverse mutation	–	–	5 µg/plate	Lang & Reimann (1993)
Gestodene + ethinyloestradiol (2.5 parts + 1 part)				
Salmonella typhimurium TA100, TA1535, TA1537, TA1538, TA98, reverse mutation	–	–	200 µg/plate[c,d]	Lang & Reimann (1993)
Megestrol acetate				
DNA repair exclusive of unscheduled DNA synthesis, female and male rat hepatocytes *in vitro*	–	NT	19.3	Topinka et al. (1995)
Unscheduled DNA synthesis, female rat hepatocytes *in vitro*	+	NT	1.93	Martelli et al. (1996a)

Table 46 (contd)

Test system	Result[a]		Dose[b] (LED or HID)	Reference
	Without exogenous metabolic system	With exogenous metabolic system		
Megestrol acetate (contd)				
Unscheduled DNA synthesis, male rat hepatocytes *in vitro*	–	NT	19.3	Martelli *et al.* (1996a)
γ-Glutamyl transpeptidase-positive foci induction, female Sprague-Dawley rat liver *in vivo*	–		100 po × 6 (weekly)	Martelli *et al.* (1996b)
Unscheduled DNA synthesis, male and female human hepatocytes *in vitro*	+	NT	0.77	Martelli *et al.* (1996a)
Chromosomal aberrations, human lymphocytes *in vitro*	–	NT	10	Stenchever *et al.* (1969)
Micronucleus formation, female rat liver *in vivo*	–		100 po × 1	Martelli *et al.* (1996b)
Binding (covalent) to DNA, female rat hepatocytes *in vitro*	+	NT	1.2	Topinka *et al.* (1995)
Binding (covalent) to DNA, male rat hepatocytes *in vitro*	(+)	NT	1.2	Topinka *et al.* (1995)
Binding (covalent) to DNA, female rat liver *in vivo*	(+)	NT	10 po × 1	Topinka *et al.* (1995)
Norethynodrel				
Salmonella typhimurium TA100, TA1535, TA1537, TA1538, TA98, reverse mutation	–	–	1000 µg/plate	Lang & Redmann (1979)
Salmonella typhimurium TA100, TA1535, TA1537, TA1538, TA98, reverse mutation	–	–	250 µg/plate	Rao *et al.* (1983)
Salmonella typhimurium TA100, TA1535, TA1537, TA1538, TA98, reverse mutation	–	–	2000 µg/plate[d]	Lang & Reimann (1993)
Inhibition of metabolic cooperation, Chinese hamster V79 cells *in vitro*	(+)	NT	0.75	Yager (1983)
Norethynodrel + 2-acetylaminofluorene (3 µg)				
Salmonella typhimurium TA100, TA1535, TA98, reverse mutation	NT	–	150 µg/plate	Rao *et al.* (1983)

Table 46 (contd)

Test system	Result[a]		Dose[b] (LED or HID)	Reference
	Without exogenous metabolic system	With exogenous metabolic system		
Levonorgestrel				
Salmonella typhimurium TA100,TA1535, TA1537, TA1538, TA98, reverse mutation	–	–	2500 µg/plate	Lang & Redmann (1979)
Salmonella typhimurium TA100,TA1535, TA1537, TA1538, TA98, reverse mutation	–	–	1000 µg/plate	Dayan et al. (1980)
Salmonella typhimurium TA100,TA1535, TA1537, TA1538, TA98, reverse mutation	–	–	500 µg/plate	Lang & Reimann (1993)
Drosophila melanogaster, sex-linked recessive lethal mutations	–		3120	Parádi (1981)
Drosophila melanogaster, sex-linked recessive lethal mutations	(+)		5000	Aguiar & Tordecilla (1984)

[a] +, positive; (+), weak positive; –, negative; NT, not tested
[b] LED, lowest effective dose; HID, highest ineffective dose; in-vitro tests, µg/mL; in-vivo tests, mg/kg bw per day; po, oral; ip, intraperitoneal
[c] Total mixture
[d] Toxicity was observed at higher dose(s)

4.3.10   *Norethynodrel* (Table 46)

Gene mutations were not induced in *S. typhimurium* by norethynodrel, and it did not enhance the mutagenicity of a sub-threshold mutagenic dose of 2-acetylaminofluorene.

4.3.11   *Levonorgestrel* (Table 46)

Gene mutations were not induced in *S. typhimurium* by levonorgestrel. Ethanolic extracts of combinations of levonorgestrel and ethinyloestradiol induced cell transformation in baby rat kidney cells infected with HPV-16 and carrying the Ha-*ras*-1 oncogene (see Table 42).

4.4   Reproductive and prenatal effects

The literature up to 1979 on the developmental effects of sex hormones was reviewed in Volume 21 of the *IARC Monographs* (IARC, 1979). It has been shown in both humans and experimental animals that sex hormones can interfere with normal genital development. The effects observed with synthetic sex hormones are variable, and oestrogenic, androgenic and progestogenic effects may frequently be observed with one chemical, depending on the target tissues and the background levels of natural hormones acting at specific times. The effects on embryofetal development also depend on the relative importance of numerous conditioning factors and are not always easy to predict; however, masculinization of female fetuses and feminization of male fetuses are observed. Effects are found in many organ systems, and genital development, central nervous system development and sexual differentiation may be affected. The timing of exposure relative to embryofetal and postnatal development is critical in determining the type and site of the defect produced.

The literature on the effects of exposure to sex hormones during pregnancy on induction of other types of congenital malformation is much more controversial. Early case reports and epidemiological studies suggested that a wide variety of defects, affecting most organ systems, could be produced. Syndromes such as the VACTERL syndrome were reported, which involves malformations of one or more of the vertebral, anal, cardiac, tracheal, oesophageal, renal and limb systems. Numerous other studies failed to support the suggestion that these defects were related to hormonal treatment.

Three categories of exposure in pregnancy were considered. Accidental exposure to oral contraceptives comprised the major group, with the least convincing evidence for a connection with birth defects. The evidence related to use of hormonal pregnancy tests was a little stronger but still unsubstantiated; the use of such tests was discontinued many years ago. The third category is use of hormones to treat women with pregnancy problems, such as intermittent bleeding, repeated or threatened abortion and luteal failure. In those cases in which the pregnancy is maintained but the fetus has malformations, it is difficult to decide whether the cause was the hormonal treatment or the underlying disease.

Since the last IARC monograph on this subject (IARC, 1979), many papers have been published on the topic of exposure to hormones during pregnancy, and some have been reviewed. Schardein (1980b) reviewed the literature up to that time on the induction of genital and non-genital defects. He concluded that the commonest association for genital defects was masculinization of females, generally seen as clitoral hypertrophy, with exposure at around week 8–10 of pregnancy; the prevalence was low and the risk was estimated to be about 1% of exposed infants. The evidence for feminization of males was reported to be less convincing. Hypospadia has been the commonest defect reported, but recent analysis of more than 2000 cases of hypospadia has shown no association with maternal use of oral contraceptives (Källén et al., 1991). A meta-analysis of pregnancy outcomes after exposure to sex hormones during the first trimester showed no excess of genital malformations (Raman-Wilms et al., 1995).

The evidence accumulated since 1979 on the involvement of exposure to sex hormones in other non-genital malformations has been largely in favour of no association. In a short paper, Brent (1994) reviewed some of the reasons why false associations between congenital heart malformations and hormones may have been concluded in the past. These include the grouping of many different types of congenital heart disorder with different causes, inadequate knowledge about the critical times of exposure for specific defects, failure to differentiate between the actions of oestrogens and progestogens, and inclusion in some studies of syndromes with a known high incidence of heart defects. The paper lists 20 reviews on the subject of exposure to hormones and non-genital congenital malformations, none of which found a causal association. It can be concluded that most epidemiological studies do not indicate that progestogens are teratogenic for the cardio-vascular system; secular trend data do not support an association between exposure to sex hormones and cardiovascular disease; a very large number of experimental studies show no relationship between exposure to sex hormones and cardiac malformations; there are no sex hormone receptors in developing cardiac tissue; and no consistent syndrome of non-genital defects has been reported. In 1988, as a result of a meeting to review the evidence, the United States Food and Drug Administration removed the warning label on oral contraceptives which had previously stated that exposure during pregnancy could cause cardiac and limb defects (Brent, 1989).

Useful reviews of the data on congenital malformations have been published (Wilson & Brent, 1981; Polednak, 1985; Simpson, 1985; Bracken, 1990; Simpson & Phillips, 1990). Several case–control studies have been conducted that show little or usually no evidence of an association between birth defects and hormonal exposure (Lammer & Cordero, 1986; Hill et al., 1988; Ananijevic-Pandey et al., 1992; Pradat, 1992; Martínez-Frías et al., 1998). In a large cohort study in the United States (Harlap et al., 1985a), no increase in the incidence of malformations was found in relation to the use of oral or other methods of contraception. In a study of women in Thailand (Pardthaisong et al., 1988), no increase in the incidence of defects of the heart, central nervous system or limbs was found in the offspring of women using oral or injectable contraceptives, but an increased incidence of polysyndactyly and chromosomal anomalies was observed in women who had previously used medroxyprogesterone acetate (Depo Provera). The small numbers of affected children, the long interval between injection of medroxy-progesterone and the conception of the affected offspring and the unrelated nature of the effects led the authors to conclude that a causal relationship between treatment and effect was unlikely. Overall, the prevalence of major malformations was significantly lower in the oral contraceptive users than in the non-users.

A study of oral contraceptive use in 730 mothers of children with Down syndrome and 1035 mothers of children with other malformations (Lejeune & Prieur, 1979) showed that more of the mothers aged 30–38 years of children with Down syndrome had ceased contraceptive use within the six months prior to conception than in the other group. Three other studies, two of them prospective studies in which data on contraceptive use was obtained before the outcome of the pregnancy was known (Ericson *et al.*, 1983; Källén, 1989), and a smaller case–control study of contraceptive use in the mothers of Down cases and in mothers of normal children (Janerich *et al.*, 1976), found no association between use of oral contraceptives and the subsequent birth of a child with Down syndrome.

A study of chromosomal abnormalities in 33 551 births and abortions after 20 weeks was reported by Harlap *et al.* (1985b). No increased risk was found for women who used oral contraceptives prior to conception or who were still using contraceptives when they became pregnant.

4.4.1   *Ethinyloestradiol*

(*a*)   *Humans*

No data were available to the Working Group.

(*b*)   *Experimental systems*

A study was carried out with the inbred mouse strain 129SV-S1 C P, which is hetero-zygous for the *S1* gene shown to affect the development of primordial germ cells, and which has a 7% spontaneous incidence of testicular teratoma. Pregnant mice were injected subcutaneously with 0.02 or 0.2 mg/kg bw ethinyloestradiol in corn oil on days 11 and 12 of gestation (the day a vaginal plug was observed was considered to be day 0), which had been shown previously to be the critical period for induction of teratoma. The male pups were killed at 15 days of age and the testes examined for teratomas. A dose-related increase in the incidence of cryptorchid testes was found, with 4/107 in controls, 10/109 at the low dose and 23/115 at the high dose ($p < 0.0001$ for trend). A small increase was observed in the incidence of teratoma which was neither dose-related nor significant (odds ratio, 2.4; 95% CI, 0.7–9.1) for the pooled data. The authors suggested that different mechanisms are involved in the etiology of cryptorchidism and teratoma, although both may be induced by oestrogen stimulation (Walker *et al.*, 1990).

Oral administration of 0, 0.02, 0.2 or 2.0 mg/kg bw ethinyloestradiol in olive oil to pregnant Jcl:ICR mice (8–15 litters per group) on days 11–17 of gestation (the presence of a vaginal plug being considered day 0) resulted in a dose-dependent increase in the incidences of ovotestis and cryptorchidism in males, with persistent Müllerian and Wolffian ducts, when fetuses were examined on day 18 of gestation. Leydig-cell proli-feration was also seen at the two higher doses with alterations in cellular morphology suggestive of preneoplastic changes. Female fetuses showed ovarian hypoplasia, with decreased numbers of primordial follicles and increased follicular degeneration (Yasuda et al., 1985, 1986).

In a later study (Yasuda et al., 1988), pregnant ICR mice were given a daily dose of 0.02 or 0.2 mg/kg bw ethinyloestradiol in olive oil orally on days 11–17 of gestation. Dams at the low dose were allowed to deliver, and their male offspring were reared to maturity (20–22 months). The animals given the high dose had no live offspring. At day 18, male fetuses were recovered from mice at each dose, and the concentrations of testosterone and oestradiol were measured in testes. Ethinyloestradiol treatment significantly ($p < 0.001$) reduced the concentrations of testosterone in the testes of 18-day-old fetuses, from a mean of 5.21 ± 0.13 pg/testis in the controls ($n = 32$ testes) to 0.89 ± 0.11 pg/testis ($n = 30$) at the low dose and 0.40 ± 0.13 pg/testis ($n = 52$) at the high dose. Treatment at the high dose also reduced the oestradiol levels in the testis from 78.80 ± 0.49 pg/testis in controls to 42.25 ± 1.56 pg/testis ($p < 0.05$). The testosterone:oestradiol ratios were reduced from 1:15 in controls, to 1:77 at the low dose and 1:106 at the high dose. At 20–22 months, the offspring from the low-dose group were killed, and the testes and epididymides were removed, examined histologically and analysed for testosterone and oestradiol. There were significant ($p < 0.05$) increases in the frequency of testicular atrophy, Leydig-cell hyperplasia and absence of epididymal sperm in the treated compared with the control mice. The testosterone concentration was significantly decreased, from 84 to 28 ng/testis ($p < 0.01$), and the oestradiol level was increased, from 356 to 564 ng/testis ($p < 0.05$). The authors suggested that the dramatic fall in the testosterone:oestradiol ratio in the fetal testis results from greatly increased conversion of testosterone to oestradiol by the Leydig cells, so that insufficient amounts of testosterone are available for regulation of pro-spermatogenesis in the developing testis and spermatogenesis, eventually resulting in sterility.

4.4.2   Mestranol
(a)   Humans
No data were available to the Working Group.

(b)   Experimental systems
Daily oral administration of 0.05 or 0.2 mg/kg bw mestranol to female NMRI mice and $AFAF_1$ hybrid mice, on days 4–8 after mating, inhibited implantation and increased the number of resorptions. The fetuses of NMRI mice had accessory ribs. Treatment on days 7–11 with doses of 0.1–0.2 mg/kg bw induced abortions but had no teratogenic effects (Heinecke & Klaus, 1975).

In rats, subcutaneous injection of 0.002–0.02 mg/kg bw mestranol five days before and 30 days after mating prevented implantation in a dose-dependent manner. Subcutaneous injection of 0.02 mg/kg bw or oral administration of 0.1 mg/kg bw on days 2–4 of gestation terminated pregnancy (Saunders & Elton, 1967).

Charles River rats received daily oral doses of 0.05–0.2 mg/kg bw Enovid (2.5 mg norethynodrel, 0.1 mg mestranol) or 0.01–0.1 mg/kg bw mestranol throughout gestation and for 21 days after parturition. The highest dose of mestranol terminated a significant percentage of pregnancies. No genital defects were observed in surviving male offspring, but female offspring showed enlarged urethral papillae and prematurely opened vaginas, even at lower doses of mestranol. The fertility of female offspring of rats treated with 0.1 mg Enovid was impaired by 55%. Higher doses of Enovid or 0.02 mg mestranol induced complete sterility in female offspring; examination of the ovaries showed no corpora lutea and follicles of reduced size (Saunders, 1967).

Sixty female Wistar rats were given a daily dose of 1 mg/kg bw Enidrel (0.075 mg mestranol, 9.2 mg norethynodrel) intragastrically for two months, at which time they were mated. In 30 animals in which treatment was continued, complete fetal resorption occurred rapidly; however, after two weeks without treatment, the fertility rates and litter sizes were normal. In the 30 animals in which treatment was discontinued, the fertility and pre- and post-natal development of the offspring were also normal. No teratogenic effects were observed (Tuchmann-Duplessis & Mercier-Parot, 1972).

In rabbits, pregnancy was terminated by daily oral doses of > 0.02 mg/kg bw mestranol on days 0–28 or 0.05 mg/kg bw [lower doses not tested] on days 10–28 of gestation and by daily subcutaneous doses of 0.005 mg/kg bw on days 0–28 or > 0.002 mg/kg bw on days 10–28. Doses that did not terminate pregnancy had no effects on litter size or the weights of the offspring (Saunders & Elton, 1967).

In female Syrian golden hamsters that received a contraceptive steroid containing 18.7 μg mestranol and 0.6 mg lynoestrenol [route unspecified] daily for 4.5–8 months, fertility was found to be normal; no effects were seen on sexual behaviour or on the fecundity of the offspring of the following two generations (Cottinet et al., 1974).

When adult beagle bitches received 5 mg/kg bw mestranol orally on day 6 or 21 of gestation, the embryonic losses, based on corpora lutea counts, were 95.5% with early treatment and 67.3% with late mestranol treatment in comparison with 34.5% in controls. The surviving offspring appeared normal (Kennelly, 1969).

4.4.3   Chlormadinone acetate

(a)   Humans

No increase in the incidence of malformations was reported in 305 infants whose mothers had been exposed to chlormadinone and oestrogens during pregnancy (Goldzieher et al., 1968; Lepage & Gueguen, 1968; Larsson-Cohn, 1970).

(b)   Experimental systems

Groups of 8–12 male Sprague-Dawley Crl:CD(SD)Br rats were castrated and injected immediately thereafter twice daily for 14 days with one of a number of synthetic progestogens, including chlormadinone acetate, used in the treatment of prostate cancer. Controls received the vehicle, 1% gelatine in 0.9% saline. Dihydrotestosterone was injected at a dose of 150 μg twice daily for 14 days as a positive control. All animals were killed on the morning after the last day of treatment, and the ventral prostate and adrenals were removed and weighed; furthermore, the prostatic content of ornithine decarboxylase was measured, as it is considered to be a highly specific, sensitive marker of androgenic activity in the prostate. Dihydrotestosterone increased the ventral prostate weight to 43% above that of castrated controls. Chlormadinone acetate was less potent than dihydrotestosterone but caused significant increases in prostate weight, by about 22% at 3 mg and 36% at 10 mg per injection. Whereas dihydrotestosterone caused a 14-fold increase in ornithine decarboxylase activity in the prostate, chlormadinone acetate caused a 5.3-fold increase at 3 mg and an 11.8-fold increase at 10 mg. Chlormadinone acetate thus has weak but significant androgenic activity in the rat ventral prostate (Labrie *et al.*, 1987).

Pregnant Wistar rats were given 1, 5 or 10 mg chlormadinone acetate orally once a day for four days on days 17–20 of pregnancy, and the fetuses were removed on day 21. After fixation, histological sections of the pelvic region were examined and the uro-vaginal septum length measured. Masculinization of female fetuses was not observed, in the absence of change in the development of the urogenital septum (Kawashima *et al.*, 1977).

Chlormadinone acetate given orally at doses of 1–50 mg/kg bw on days 8–15 of pregnancy to Japanese ddS and CF1 mice caused a significant increase in the incidence of cleft palate. A dose of 10 mg/kg bw, but not of 1 or 3 mg/kg bw, given orally on days 8–20 of gestation to Japanese albino rabbits increased the incidence of cleft palate, abdominal wall defects and wrist contractures (Takano *et al.*, 1966).

4.4.4   *Cyproterone acetate*

(*a*)   *Humans*

Two men treated for prostatic carcinoma with high oral doses of cyproterone acetate (2×100 mg per day for seven months) had widespread testicular damage, with disappearance of Sertoli cells and spermatogonia and involution of Leydig cells (Re *et al.*, 1979). When cyproterone acetate was given at doses of 5–10 mg per day as a contraceptive in several other studies, decreased sperm concentration and motility and increased abnormal morphology, with—except in one study—decreased power to penetrate the mucus, were observed. Variable effects on plasma gonadotrophins and testosterone levels have been reported (Føgh *et al.*, 1979; Roy & Chatterjee, 1979; Moltz *et al.*, 1980; Wang & Yeung, 1980). Doses of 50–100 mg cyproterone acetate per day combined with testosterone induced azoospermia and decreased testis size in each of 10 subjects. All of the effects were reversible (Meriggiola *et al.*, 1996).

In women, ovulation is inhibited by 2 mg per day cyproterone acetate when given in combination with 35 μg ethinyloestradiol (Spona *et al.*, 1986). No controlled studies on developmental effects are available.

(*b*)   *Experimental systems*

Cyproterone acetate has been reported to have both androgenic and anti-androgenic activity in experimental animals (see also section 4.2.5).

Groups of 8–12 male Sprague-Dawley Crl:CD(SD)Br rats were castrated and then injected twice daily for 14 days with one of a number of synthetic progestogens, including cyproterone acetate. Treatment was begun one day after castration. Controls were injected with the vehicle, 1% gelatine in 0.9% saline. Dihydrotestosterone was injected twice daily at a dose of 125 µg for 14 days as a positive control. All animals were killed on the morning after the last day of treatment, and the ventral prostate and adrenals were removed and weighed. Dihydrotestosterone increased the ventral prostate weight to approximately five time that of castrated controls. Cyproterone acetate was less potent than dihydrotestosterone but caused a significant increase in prostate weight, by 60% at a dose of 5 mg per injection twice daily. Cyproterone acetate thus has weak but significant androgenic activity in the rat ventral prostate (Poyet & Labrie, 1985).

Anti-androgenic effects have also been reported. Groups of 10 albino Wistar mice were treated subcutaneously with vehicle alone or with 1 mg per animal per day of cyproterone acetate for seven days. The animals were killed on the eighth day and the testes removed for histological and morphometric examination. Treatment caused marked decreases in the volume, surface area and length of the seminiferous tubules, and it inhibited spermatogenesis (Umapathy & Rai, 1982).

The anti-androgenic activity of cyproterone and cyproterone acetate has been shown in mice (Umapathy & Rai, 1982; Homady *et al.*, 1986), rats (El Etreby *et al.* 1987), guinea-pigs (Tam *et al.*, 1985), ferrets (Kästner & Apfelbach, 1987), goats (Panda & Jindal, 1982; Kumar & Panda, 1983) and monkeys (Lohiya *et al.*, 1987; Kaur *et al.*, 1990, 1992). The effects observed include decreased sexual behaviour and inter-male aggression, reduced weights of testis and inhibition of spermatogenesis. Fertility can be reduced by low doses of cyproterone acetate even in the absence of reduced spermatogenesis (Rastogi *et al.*, 1980), which may be due to an effect on epididymal processing of sperm. In addition to reduced secretion of testosterone and luteinizing hormone (Clos *et al.*, 1988), there is also evidence that translocation of the testosterone receptor to the nucleus may be affected (Brinkmann *et al.*, 1983).

In rodents, cyproterone acetate has oestrogenic properties, increasing uterine weight and causing vaginal cornification in ovariectomized rats (Arya *et al.*, 1979). When the compound was administered to pregnant rats, feminization of male fetuses, including development of a vagina, has been reported (Neumann *et al.*, 1966; Forsberg & Jacobsohn, 1969).

Treatment of NMRI mice with doses of 5–900 mg/kg bw cyproterone acetate subcutaneously on day 2 of gestation (the day a vaginal plug was observed was considered to be day 0) or with 30 mg/kg bw on single days of pregnancy from day 1 to 12, resulted in a clear dose- and time-related increase in the incidences of cleft palate and of urinary tract and respiratory tract malformations, with up to 64% of fetuses affected after the single 900-mg/kg bw dose (Eibs *et al.*, 1982). Administration in late pregnancy or in the neonatal period can produce permanent changes in neuroendocrine and sexual function of rats. Groups of 15 male and 16 female offspring of rats treated subcutaneously with 1 mg cyproterone acetate on days 15–20 of gestation [strain and number of pregnant animals not specified] were studied when two to three months of age. The weight of the brain was reduced in animals of each sex and the weight of the testis in males. Cell density in the ventromedial nucleus of the hypothalamus was increased in males in comparison with females. The prolactin concentration in the pituitary was increased in animals of each sex (Rossi *et al.*, 1991). Groups of newborn male Swiss CD1 mice were injected with cyproterone acetate on days 1–10 (200 μg/day), 11–20 (400 μg), 21–30 (800 μg) or 31–40 (1 mg) of age. In all groups, there was an immediate reduction in the weights of the testis, epididymis, vas deferens, preputial gland and seminal vesicles relative to body weight. This reduction in the weight of the accessory sex organs was permanent in animals injected up to day 20 of age but was reversible in animals treated after day 20. In mice injected on days 1–10 of age, marked, permanent infertility was observed when they became adults, but spermatogenesis, the androgen concentration in plasma and sexual behaviour were not affected. The infertility appeared to be due to failure of sperm in the epididymis to mature (Jean-Faucher *et al.*, 1985).

4.4.5   *Levonorgestrel* (see also the monograph on 'Hormonal contraceptives, progestogens only', section 4.4.2)

(*a*)   *Humans*

No relevant data were available to the Working Group.

(*b*)   *Experimental systems*

Groups of six pregnant rats [strain not specified] were ovariectomized on day 8 of gestation and treated subcutaneously with doses of 0.01–0.3 mg levonorgestrel daily on days 8–21 of gestation; at the same time they received an injection of 1.0 μg oestrone. The rats were killed on day 22 to measure maintenance of pregnancy; satisfactory maintenance was achieved with 0.1 and 0.3 mg levonorgestrel. Immature castrated male rats [age not specified] were treated subcutaneously daily for 13 days with doses of 0.1–3 mg levonorgestrel and were killed the day after the last treatment; the weights of the prostate and seminal vesicles were measured. Levonorgestrel showed androgenic activity, as judged from the increased weight of both tissues (Kuhnz & Beier, 1994).

Groups of 10–12 Prob:WNZ New Zealand white rabbits were mated with Prob:KAL Californian rabbits, producing hybrid fetuses; the day of mating was called day 1. The animals were treated with 0.5 mg/kg bw levonorgestrel in sesame oil by gavage on days 5–25 of gestation and were killed on day 21. [The Working Group concluded that the animals must have been killed after day 25, but the fetal body weights were very low for full-term offspring.] The fetuses were examined macroscopically, and half of them were sliced for visceral examination and the other half examined for skeletal and cartilage malformations. No adverse effect of treatment on pregnancy rate, number of implantations, number of resorptions or number of live or dead fetuses was observed. The female fetal body weight at term was slightly but significantly reduced (15.2 ± 0.61 g versus 17.4 ± 0.74 g in the sesame oil control group). No malformations were observed (Heinecke & Kohler, 1983).

4.4.6   *Lynoestrenol*
(*a*)   *Humans*
No data were available to the Working Group.

(*b*)   *Experimental systems*
Groups of 14–20 inseminated belted Dutch rabbits were given lynoestrenol at a dose of 0, 0.1, 0.5 or 2.5 mg/kg bw orally on days 6–18 of gestation (the day of insemination being considered day 0). The does were killed on day 29 for examination of the fetuses. Increased post-implantation loss was observed at all doses: 1.3% in controls, 13.2% at the low dose, 17.1% at the intermediate dose and 90.9% at the high dose. A wide range of malformations of the brain and eye was observed in all groups, affecting 31–50% of fetuses and only 12% of controls. Cardiovascular malformations were observed in 2, 5 and 20% of fetuses, respectively, at the three doses. No masculinization of female fetuses was observed. In a second experiment with groups of five to six belted Dutch rabbits, lynoestrenol was administered at a dose of 0, 0.1 or 0.5 mg/kg bw on days 6–18 of gestation. The does were allowed to deliver naturally and raise their pups to four weeks of age. At the higher dose, the litter size was decreased and there was clear evidence of central nervous system abnormalities in surviving pups, with ataxia, disorientation, posterior paralysis and rotation of one or both hindlimbs. Anophthalmia and microphthalmia were seen in 3/10 pups at the high dose. Histological examination of the central nervous system revealed pathological changes in the ventral horns of the spinal cord, with a marked reduction in the number of neurons (Sannes *et al.*, 1983).

Pregnant Wistar rats were given 1 or 5 mg lynoestrenol orally once a day for four days on days 17–20 of gestation, and the fetuses were removed on day 21. After fixation, histological sections of the pelvic region were examined and the urovaginal septum length measured. Masculinization of female fetuses was seen at 5 mg, as evidenced by decreased development of the urogenital system (Kawashima *et al.*, 1977).

4.4.7   *Megestrol acetate*
(*a*)   *Humans*
No data were available to the Working Group.

(*b*)   *Experimental systems*
Megestrol acetate has some androgenic activity in rats (Poyet & Labrie, 1985; Labrie *et al.*, 1987). In the study of Labrie *et al.* (1987), described in section 4.4.3, the positive control dihydrotestosterone increased the ventral prostate weight to 43% above that of castrated controls. Megestrol acetate was less potent, but caused significant increases in prostate weight, by about 35% at 3 mg and 59% at 10 mg per injection. Whereas dihydrotestosterone caused a 14-fold increase in the activity of orthinine decarboxylase in the prostate, megestrol acetate caused an 11-fold increase at 3 mg and a 13-fold increase at 10 mg. Megestrol acetate thus has weak but significant androgenic activity in the rat ventral prostate.

In the study of Kawashima *et al*. (1977) described in section 4.4.3, megestrol acetate at a dose of 5 mg induced masculinization of female fetuses.

4.4.8   *Norethisterone*
(a)   Humans
No data were available to the Working Group.

(b)   Experimental systems
Ten groups of three timed-mated pregnant rhesus monkeys (*Macaca mulatta*) were treated with Norlestrin (norethisterone acetate, 2.5 mg and ethinyloestradiol, 0.05 mg per tablet) orally at a dose of 5, 10, 25 or 50 mg per monkey per day (on the basis of the norethisterone acetate content). [These doses are equivalent to 0.83, 1.67, 4.17 and 8.33 mg/kg bw daily on the basis of the information in the paper that the doses are equivalent to 20, 40, 100 and 200 times the human contraceptive dose.] The animals at the three lower doses were treated daily during early (days 21–35) or late (days 33–46) organogenesis or throughout (days 21–46) organogenesis and were allowed to deliver at term (165 days' gestation). Animals at 50 mg/day were dosed on days 21–35 only and delivered by caesarean section on day 50 of gestation for serial sectioning and histo-logical examination of the fetuses. Of 26 animals that were allowed to deliver at term, 16 delivered morphologically normal infants (nine male, seven female), eight aborted, and two had stillbirths, a rate of 7.4%, which was not different from that of controls. The overall pre-natal mortality rate was higher in the treated animals (10/26, 38.5%) than in the control colony (55/262, 21%). Two of nine animals at each of the 5- and 10-mg doses aborted, in comparison with 4/9 at 25 mg/day. Among those treated on days 21–35 or 21–46 of gestation, six (37.5%) aborted, in comparison with 2/9 (22.2%) of those treated later in organogenesis, on days 33–46. Only three aborted embryos were recovered, and all three were much smaller than expected for their gestational age; however, they were too severely autolysed for further examination. No morphological or histological abnormalities were detected in fetuses recovered on day 50 of gestation from females at 50 mg. The infants were followed up for a maximum of 2.5 years, and all three animals that died and the five that were sacrificed were necropsied and examined histopatho-logically. No malformations or significant lesions were found. Detailed physical exami-nation of the live infants showed no morphological changes, and the body weights and other measures were no different from those of controls. The serum oestrogen and progesterone concentrations of females treated with 25 mg on days 21–35 of gestation were measured daily on days 26–44 by immunoassay. The oestrogen concentrations were significantly lower ($p < 0.05$) than those of controls, but the progesterone levels were similar. As it has been shown in other studies that monkeys can be ovariectomized on day 23 of gestation without fetal loss, although the plasma oestrogen concentration falls almost to zero, the authors suggested that the reduction in oestrogen concentration was not the cause of the observed pre-natal deaths. They proposed that Norlestrin has a direct embryolethal effect. The normal progesterone concentrations indicate that

placental synthesis of progesterone is unaffected. The authors also pointed out that as the periods of treatment in this study did not extend into the early fetal period after day 46, when external genital development occurs in the rhesus monkey, genital malformations would not be expected to occur (Prahalada & Hendrickx, 1983).

Eight of the offspring in the study described above from females dosed with 5, 10 or 25 mg Norlestrin were subjected to limited behavioural examination up to 11 months of age. No serious deficiencies in the regulation of activity, motor maturity, manual dexterity or discrimination learning were observed at three to five months of age. Age-appropriate sex-differentiated behaviour was seen at five and 11 months of age. The authors noted, however, that Norlestrin was not given during the period of sexual differentiation of the brain in rhesus monkeys (Golub *et al.*, 1983).

In the study of Kawashima *et al.* (1977), described in section 4.4.3, norethisterone caused masculinization of female fetuses at doses of 5 or 10 mg but not at 1 mg.

4.4.9   *Norethynodrel*

(*a*)   *Humans*

No data were available to the Working Group.

(*b*)   *Experimental systems*

Mice given 10 mg/kg bw norethynodrel (with 2% mestranol) orally, daily on days 8–15 of gestation, had a very high rate of embryonic death (98.9%), but not when the dose was given on days 14–17 of gestation (Takano *et al.*, 1966).

In mice given 0.2–2.4 mg/kg bw norethynodrel or its 3-hydroxy metabolite as an oral or parenteral dose, either singly or on three consecutive days between days 6 and 16 of gestation, congenital anomalies were observed in near-term fetuses. A single dose of 1.2 mg/kg bw norethynodrel or its metabolite given between days 8 and 16 of gestation produced congenital abnormalities (retarded development, hydrocephalus, club-foot and minor skeletal anomalies) in 10–30% of offspring (Andrew *et al.*, 1972).

Mice that received a single subcutaneous injection of 0.1 mg/kg bw norethynodrel in combination with 1.5 µg/kg mestranol (Enovid) on day 7, 10, 12, 15 or 17 of gestation had normal fetuses, with no external or internal genital anomalies; however, treatment on day 10 of gestation led to a significant decrease in aggressive behaviour of male offspring later in life (Abbatiello & Scudder, 1970).

Oral administration of norethynodrel or its metabolites, 17α-ethynyl-oestr-5(10)-ene-3α,17β-diol and 17α-ethynyl-oestr-5(10)-ene-3β,17β-diol, at a daily dose of 0.15, 0.3 or 0.6 mg/kg bw on days 8–10 or 11–13 of gestation resulted in increased numbers of resorptions and intrauterine deaths on days 11–13. The teratogenic effects included exencephaly after treatment during days 8–10 and hydrocephalus and partial cryptorchidism after treatment on days 11–13. The most effective agent was 17α-ethynyl-oestr-5(10)-ene-3β,17β-diol (Gidley *et al.*, 1970).

Subcutaneous administration of 0.5 or 1 mg/kg bw norethynodrel to pregnant rats on days 2–4 of gestation terminated a significant number of pregnancies (Saunders, 1965).

Subcutaneous administration of 0.083–2.5 mg/kg bw per day norethynodrel to rats on days 10–17 of gestation induced 100% fetal resorptions, whereas a dose of 0.0083 mg/kg bw per day induced 42% resorptions; no virilizing effect was observed in females, but in males the weight of the testes was significantly lowered and the descent of testes was delayed in 35.5% of animals (Roy & Kar, 1967).

In the study of Tuchmann-Duplessis and Mercier-Parot (1972), described in section 4.4.2, complete fetal resorption occurred rapidly in 30 animals in which treatment with Enidrel (mestranol/norethynodrel) was continued for the first 15 days of gestation; however, after two weeks without treatment, the fertility rates and litter sizes were normal. In the 30 animals in which treatment was discontinued, the fertility and pre- and post-natal development of the offspring were normal. No teratogenic effects were observed.

Subcutaneous injection of 1 mg norethynodrel (Enovid) to guinea-pigs daily on days 18–60 of gestation prevented pregnancy (Foote *et al.*, 1968).

4.4.10   *Norgestimate*
   (*a*)   *Humans*
No data were available to the Working Group.

   (*b*)   *Experimental systems*
In the study of Kuhnz and Beier (1994), described in section 4.4.5, groups of rats were given doses of 0.03–1 mg/day norgestimate. Satisfactory maintenance of pregnancy was achieved with 0.3 and 1 mg. In immature male rats treated with 1–30 mg norgestimate, the weights of the prostate and seminal vesicles were increased, indicating androgenic activity, but norgestimate was less active than levonorgestrel. The blood concentrations of levonorgestrel were measured in animals treated with levonorgestrel or norgestimate, as levonorgestrel is the major metabolite of norgestimate. Both the pregnancy maintenance and the androgenic activity could be accounted for by the concentrations of levonorgestrel produced as a metabolite.

4.4.11   *Norgestrel*
   (*a*)   *Humans*
As the active isomer of norgestrel is levonorgestrel, the reader is referred to section 4.4.5 of this monograph.

   (*b*)   *Experimental systems*
Mature female B3C6F$_1$ mice were superovulated with serum gonadotropin from pregnant mares and 48 h later by human chorionic gonadotrophin; they were then mated overnight with males known to be fertile. The females were killed, and the fertilized pre-embryos were collected from the fallopian tubes 24 h (one-cell stage) or 48 h (2–4-cell stage) after the injection of human chorionic gonadotrophin. The pre-embryos were then cultured for up to 72 h in the absence or presence of 4 ng/mL (dl)-norgestrel, which is the peak plasma concentration of levonorgestrel found in women who use norgestrel as

a contraceptive. [It is unclear whether this dose refers to (dl)- or levonorgestrel.] After 24, 48 or 72 h of culture, the pre-embryos were examined microscopically, and the number of cells counted up to the morula and late blastocyst stages. A similar experiment was carried out in which one-cell pre-embryos were harvested 24 h after injection of human chorionic gonadotrophin and exposed in culture to norgestrel at a concentration of 8, 80 or 800 ng/mL for up to 72 h. In neither study was any difference found in the number of pre-embryos at various cell stages or in the number of degenerating or abnormal pre-embryos (Logan *et al.*, 1989).

5. Summary of Data Reported and Evaluation

5.1   Exposure

Oral contraceptives have been used since the early 1960s and are now used by about 90 million women worldwide. 'The pill' is given as a combination of an oestrogen and a progestogen or as sequential therapy. Since the 1970s, progestogen-only pills have been available. Continuous development of the formulas and the development of new progestogens have allowed for lower dosages with fewer acute side-effects, while offering effective, convenient contraception.

The oestrogen component of combined oral contraceptives is either ethinyloestradiol or mestranol, and the progestogens used are cyproterone acetate, desogestrel, ethynodiol diacetate, gestodene, levonorgestrel, lynoestrenol, megestrol, norethisterone, norethisterone acetate, norethynodrel, norgestimate and norgestrel. Currently, the most commonly used oestrogen is ethinyloestradiol, and commonly used progestogens are levonorgestrel and norethisterone.

Large differences exist in the worldwide use of oral contraceptives. These products were already being used extensively in the 1960s in northern Europe (e.g. the Netherlands, Sweden and the United Kingdom) and the United States. Extensive use of oral contraceptives by adolescents was documented in Sweden and the United Kingdom as early as 1964. Very little use of oral contraceptives is reported in Japan, the countries of the former Soviet Union and most developing countries. Contraceptive use also differs in relation to religion, ethnicity, educational level, use before or after marriage and use before or after first pregnancy.

The type of oral contraceptives prescribed differs between countries, and both the type of oral contraceptive and the doses of oestrogens and progestogens have changed between and within countries over time.

Oral contraceptives may be used for emergency post-coital contraception, and the components of oral contraceptives are used to treat peri- and post-menopausal symptoms and a number of other conditions.

It is important to stress that use of oral contraceptives is a recent human activity, and the health benefits and adverse effects in women have not yet been followed over a complete generation, even though they are some of the most widely used drugs in the world. Women who began using oral contraceptives before the age of 20 in the 1960s are only now reaching the ages (50–60 years) at which the incidences of most malignancies begin to increase.

Oestrogens and progestogens belonging to the same chemical groups may have different oestrogenic, androgenic and progestogenic effects. Little is known about the long-term health risks and potential protective effects of the individual components. The effects become increasingly complex as women grow older, as they may be exposed to different types and doses of hormones, starting with oral contraceptives and progressing to post-menopausal hormonal therapy.

5.2   Human carcinogenicity

Breast cancer

More than 10 cohort and 50 case–control studies have assessed the relationship between use of combined oral contraceptives and the risk for breast cancer. The studies included over 50 000 women with breast cancer. The weight of the evidence suggests a small increase in the relative risk for breast cancer among current and recent users, which is, however, unrelated to duration of use or type or dose of preparation. By 10 years after cessation of use, the risk of women who used oral contraceptives appears to be similar to that of women who never used them. Important known risk factors do not account for the association. The possibility that the association seen for current and recent users is due to detection bias has not been ruled out. Even if the association is causal, the excess risk for cancer associated with patterns of use that are typical today is very small.

Cervical cancer

Five cohort and 16 case–control studies of use of combined oral contraceptives and invasive cervical cancer have been published; these consistently show a small increase in relative risk associated with long duration of use. These associations were also seen in four studies in which some analyses were restricted to cases and controls who had human papillomavirus infections. Biases related to sexual behaviour, screening and other factors cannot be ruled out as possible explanations for the observed associations.

Endometrial cancer

Three cohort and 16 case–control studies addressed the relationship between use of combined oral contraceptives and the risk for endometrial cancer. The results of these studies consistently show that the risk for endometrial cancer of women who have taken these pills is approximately halved. The reduction in risk is generally stronger the longer the oral contraceptives are used and persists for at least 10 years after cessation of use. Few data are available on the more recent, low-dose formulations.

Use of sequential oral contraceptives which were removed from the consumer market in the 1970s was associated with an increased risk for endometrial cancer.

Ovarian cancer

Four cohort and 21 case–control studies addressed the relationship between ovarian cancer and use of combined oral contraceptives. Overall, these studies show a consistent reduction in the risk for ovarian cancer with increasing duration of use. The reduction is about 50% for women who have used the preparations for at least five years, and the reduction seems to persist for at least 10–15 years after use has ceased. Few data are available on the more recent, low-dose formulations. A reduction in risk for ovarian tumours of borderline malignancy is also observed.

Cancers of the liver and gall-bladder

Two case–control studies of benign hepatocellular tumours showed a strong relationship with duration of use of combined oral contraceptives. Three cohort studies showed no significant association between use of combined oral contraceptives and the incidence of or mortality from liver cancer, but the expected numbers of cases were very small, resulting in low statistical power. Long-term use of combined oral contraceptives was associated with an increase in risk for hepatocellular carcinoma in all nine case–control studies conducted in populations with low prevalences of hepatitis B and C viral infection and chronic liver disease, which are major causes of liver cancer, and in analyses in which women with these factors were excluded. Few data are available for the more recent, low-dose formulations. In the two case–control studies conducted in populations with a high prevalence of infection with hepatitis viruses, there was no increase in risk for hepatocellular carcinoma associated with use of combined oral contraceptives, but there was little information on long-term use.

Little information was available on the association between use of combined oral contraceptives and the risk for cholangiocarcinoma or cancer of the gall-bladder.

Colorectal cancer

Four cohort investigations and 10 case–control studies provided information on use of combined oral contraceptives and risk for colorectal cancer. None showed significantly elevated risks in women who used these preparations for any length of time. Relative risks lower than 1.0 were found in nine studies, and the risk was significantly reduced in two.

Cutaneous malignant melanoma

Four cohort investigations and 16 case–control studies provided information on use of combined oral contraceptives and the risk for cutaneous malignant melanoma. The relative risks were generally close to 1.0 and not related to duration of use.

Thyroid cancer

Ten case–control studies provided information on use of combined oral contraceptives and the risk for cancer of the thyroid gland. In general, there was no elevation in the risk associated with oral contraceptive use.

5.3   Carcinogenicity in experimental animals

Oestrogen–progestogen combinations

Several combinations of oral contraceptives have been tested alone and together with known carcinogens in mice, rats and monkeys. Consistent tumorigenic effects that are seen with various combinations which are important for classifying the degree of evidence for carcinogenicity of this class of compounds are as follows.

The incidences of pituitary adenoma in male and female mice were increased by administration of mestranol plus chlormadinone acetate, mestranol plus ethynodiol diacetate, ethinyloestradiol plus ethynodiol diacetate, mestranol plus norethisterone, ethinyloestradiol plus norethisterone (females only) and mestranol plus norethynodrel, which also increased the incidence of pituitary adenomas in female rats.

The incidence of benign mammary tumours was increased in mice by ethinyloestradiol plus chlormadinone acetate (in intact and castrated males) and by mestranol plus norethynodrel (only in castrated males). In rats, the incidence of benign mammary tumours was increased by administration of ethinyloestradiol plus norethisterone acetate. This combination did not cause tumour formation in any tissue in one study in monkeys.

The incidence of malignant mammary tumours was increased in male and female mice by ethinyloestradiol plus megestrol acetate and in rats by ethinyloestradiol plus ethynodiol diacetate (males and females), mestranol plus norethisterone (females) and mestranol plus norethynodrel (females).

In female mice, the incidence of malignant uterine tumours (non-epithelial) was increased by ethinyloestradiol plus ethynodiol diacetate and the incidence of vaginal or cervical tumours by norethynodrel plus mestranol. In mice treated with 3-methylcholanthrene to induce genital tumours, ethinyloestradiol plus lynoestrenol, ethinyloestradiol plus norgestrel and mestranol plus norethynodrel increased the incidence of uterine tumours; however, this occurred only at the highest doses of ethinyloestradiol plus lynoestrenol and ethinyloestradiol plus norgestrel that were tested. Lower doses inhibited tumorigenesis induced by 3-methylcholanthrene alone.

In rats, the incidence of benign liver tumours (adenomas) was increased by mestranol plus norethisterone (males) and by ethinyloestradiol plus norethisterone acetate (males); the latter combination also increased the incidence of hepatocellular carcinomas in females. Liver foci, which are putative preneoplastic lesions, were induced in rats by mestranol plus norethynodrel. In rats initiated for hepatocarcinogenesis with *N*-nitrosodiethylamine, mestranol plus norethynodrel increased the formation of altered hepatic foci.

Oestrogens

The synthetic oestrogens ethinyloestradiol and mestranol have been tested extensively alone and together with known carcinogens in mice, rats, hamsters, dogs and monkeys.

The incidence of pituitary adenomas was increased by ethinyloestradiol and mestranol in male and female mice and by ethinyloestradiol in female rats.

The incidences of malignant mammary tumours in male and female mice and female rats were increased by ethinyloestradiol and mestranol; however, mestranol did not increase the incidences of mammary tumours in dogs in a single study.

Ethinyloestradiol increased the incidence of cervical tumours in female mice.

In one mouse strain, ethinyloestradiol increased the incidences of hepatocellular adenomas. In female rats, ethinyloestradiol and mestranol increased the numbers of altered hepatic foci. Ethinyloestradiol increased the incidence of adenomas in males and females and of hepatocellular carcinomas in females, whereas mestranol increased the incidence of hepatic nodules and carcinomas combined in female rats.

The incidence of microscopic malignant kidney tumours was increased in hamsters exposed to ethinyloestradiol.

In mice initiated for liver carcinogenesis and exposed to unleaded gasoline, ethinyloestradiol increased the number of altered hepatic foci; however, when given alone after the liver carcinogen, it reduced the number of spontaneous foci.

In female rats initiated for liver carcinogenesis, ethinyloestradiol and mestranol increased the number of altered hepatic foci and the incidences of adenomas and carcinomas. Ethinyloestradiol also increased the incidences of kidney adenomas, renal-cell carcinomas and liver carcinomas in rats initiated with N-nitrosoethyl-N-hydroxyethylamine. In hamsters initiated with N-nitrosobis(2-oxopropyl)amine, ethinyloestradiol increased the incidence of renal tumours and the multiplicity of dysplasias.

Progestogens

Various progestogens have been tested alone and together with known carcinogens in mice, rats and dogs.

The incidence of pituitary adenomas was increased by norethisterone in female mice and by norethynodrel in male and female mice and male rats.

The incidence of malignant mammary tumours was increased in female mice by lynoestrenol, megestrol acetate and norethynodrel. In female rats, lynoestrenol and norethisterone slightly increased the incidence of malignant mammary tumours. Norethisterone also slightly increased the incidence of malignant mammary tumours in male rats, while norethynodrel increased the incidence of both benign and malignant mammary tumours in male rats. In dogs, chlormadinone acetate, lynoestrenol and megestrol acetate increased the incidence of benign and malignant mammary tumours; however, lynoestrenol had a protective effect at a low dose but enhanced tumour incidence at two higher doses. Levonorgestrel did not increase the incidence of mammary tumours in one study in dogs.

In female mice treated with 3-methylcholanthrene to induce uterine tumours, norethynodrel further increased the tumour incidence.

In male mice treated with chlormadinone acetate, ethynodiol diacetate, lynoestrenol, norethisterone or norethisterone acetate, the incidence of liver adenomas was increased. Megestrol acetate increased the incidence of adenomas in female mice. Cyproterone acetate increased the incidences of liver adenomas and hepatocellular carcinomas in male and female mice, but at doses exceeding the maximum tolerated dose. In rats, the incidence of liver adenomas was increased by norethisterone acetate (males and females), norethisterone (males), norethynodrel and cyproterone acetate (males and females). The numbers of altered hepatic foci in female rats were also increased by norethisterone acetate and cyproterone acetate. In rats treated with N-nitrosodiethylamine to initiate hepatocarcinogenesis, norethynodrel increased the number of altered hepatic foci. Norethynodrel alone was shown to increase the incidence of hepatocarcinomas in male rats.

Levonorgestrel in combination with N-nitrosobis(2-oxopropyl)amine did not enhance the incidence of renal dysplastic lesions or tumours in hamsters.

5.4   Other relevant data

After single or multiple doses, oestrogens and progestogens in combined oral contraceptives are rapidly absorbed and reach maximal serum levels quickly. The proportion of the absorbed hormone that becomes biologically available depends on the extent of enterohepatic circulation and metabolic transformation of pro-drugs. Interactions between some of these hormones affect their disposition and that of the oestrogen or progestogen with which they are combined. Several progestogens also exhibit some oestrogenic activity and can thus modify the effects of the oestrogens. In three studies, women taking oestrogen–progestogen combinations had increased epithelial cell proliferation in the breast, and in one of these studies the effect was related to the dose of oestrogen in the presence of progestogen. The constituents of combined oral contraceptives may stimulate rat hepatocyte cell proliferation *in vitro* and *in vivo*, and this growth potentiation may be selectively effective in preneoplastic hepatocytes. In addition to the major routes of metabolism, a minor proportion of oestrogen may be metabolized to catechol intermediates, with significant potential for formation of reactive intermediates and damage to DNA. Some of the constituents of combined oral contraceptives can cause changes in DNA at the nuclear level in some experimental systems. Most, but not all, human studies show effects of this type, which occur at conventional therapeutic doses of combined oral contraceptives. When given during pregnancy, combined oral contraceptives can cause developmental abnormalities of the genital tract of offspring. There is evidence for other malformations, but this is controversial and not considered proven.

5.5   Evaluation

There is *sufficient evidence* in humans for the carcinogenicity of combined oral contraceptives.

This classification is based on an increased risk for hepatocellular carcinoma in the absence of hepatitis viruses observed in studies of predominantly high-dose preparations.

There is *sufficient evidence* in experimental animals for the carcinogenicity of ethinyloestradiol plus ethynodiol diacetate and mestranol plus norethynodrel.

There is *limited evidence* in experimental animals for the carcinogenicity of ethinyloestradiol plus megestrol acetate, mestranol or ethinyloestradiol plus chlormadinone acetate, mestranol plus ethynodiol diacetate, mestranol plus lynoestrenol, mestranol or ethinyloestradiol plus norethisterone and ethinyloestradiol plus norgestrel.

There is *sufficient evidence* in experimental animals for the carcinogenicity of ethinyloestradiol and mestranol.

There is *sufficient evidence* in experimental animals for the carcinogenicity of norethynodrel and lynoestrenol.

There is *limited evidence* in experimental animals for the carcinogenicity of chlormadinone acetate, cyproterone acetate, ethynodiol diacetate, megestrol acetate, norethisterone acetate and norethisterone.

There is *inadequate evidence* in experimental animals for the carcinogenicity of levonorgestrel and norgestrel.

Overall evaluation

Combined oral contraceptives are *carcinogenic to humans (Group 1)*.

There is also conclusive evidence that these agents have a protective effect against cancers of the ovary and endometrium.

6.   References

Abbatiello, E. & Scudder, C.L. (1970) The effect of norethynodrel with mestranol treatment of pregnant mice on the isolation-induced aggression of their male offspring. *Int. J. Fertil.*, **15**, 182–189

Abdel-Aziz, M.T. & Williams, K.I.H. (1969) Metabolism of 17α-ethynylestradiol and its 3-methyl ether by the rabbit; an *in vivo* D-homoannulation. *Steroids*, **13**, 809–820

Adam, S.A., Sheaves, J.K., Wright, N.H., Mosser, G., Harris, R.W. & Vessey, M.P. (1981) A case–control study of the possible association between oral contraceptives and malignant melanoma. *Br. J. Cancer*, **44**, 45–50

Adami, H.O., Bergstrom, R., Persson, I. & Sparen, P. (1990) The incidence of ovarian cancer in Sweden, 1960–1984. *Am. J. Epidemiol.*, **132**, 446–452

Aguiar, M.L.J.B. & Tordecilla, J.M.C. (1984) Mutagenic effect of mestranol and norgestrel in *Drosophila melanogaster*. *Actual. biol.*, **13**, 43–47 (in Spanish)

Alton, K.B., Hetyei, N.S., Shaw, C. & Patrick, J.E. (1984) Biotransformation of norgestimate in women. *Contraception*, **29**, 19–29

Ananijevic-Pandey, J., Jarebinski, M., Kastratovic, B., Vlajinac, H., Radojkovic, Z. & Brankovic, D. (1992) Case–control study of congenital malformations. *Eur. J. Epidemiol.*, **8**, 871–874

Anderson, T.J., Ferguson, D.J.P. & Raab, G.M. (1982) Cell turnover in the 'resting' human breast: Influence of parity, contraceptive pill, age and laterality. *Br. J. Cancer*, **46**, 376–382

Anderson, T.J., Battersby, S., King, R.J.B., McPherson, K. & Going, J.J. (1989) Oral contraceptive use influences resting breast proliferation. *Hum. Pathol.*, **20**, 1139–1144

Andolsek, L., Kovacic, J., Kozuh, M. & Litt, B. (1983) Influence of oral contraceptives on the incidence of premalignant and malignant lesions of the cervix. *Contraception*, **28**, 505–519

Andrew, F.D., Williams, T.L., Gidley, J.T. & Wall, M.E. (1972) Teratogenicity of contraceptive steroids in mice (Abstract). *Teratology*, **5**, 249

Annapurna, V.V., Mukundan, M.A., Sesikeran, B. & Bamji, M.B. (1988) Long-term effects of female sex steroids on female rat liver in an initiator–promoter model of hepatocarcinogenesis. *Indian J. Biochem. Biophys.*, **25**, 708–713

Ansari, S.R. & Adhami, U.M. (1977) Effect of antifertility drugs (norethindrone and mestranol) on the bone marrow chromosomes of albino rat (*Rattus norvegicus*). *Indian J. Hered.*, **9**, 7–9

Ansari, G.A.S., Walker, R.D., Smart, V.B. & Smith, L.L. (1982) Further investigations of mutagenic cholesterol preparations. *Food chem. Toxicol.*, **20**, 35–41

Archer, D.F., Timmer, C.J. & Lammers, P. (1994) Pharmacokinetics of a triphasic oral contraceptive containing desogestrel and ethinyl estradiol. *Fertil. Steril.*, **61**, 645–651

Armstrong, B.K., Ray, R.M. & Thomas, D.B. (1988) Endometrial cancer and combined oral contraceptives. The WHO Collaborative Study of Neoplasia and Steroid Contraceptives. *Int. J. Epidemiol.*, **17**, 263–269

Arya, M., Gupta, S. & Dixit, V.P. (1979) Effect of cyproterone acetate on the reproductive system of the female rat. A histological review. *Acta anat. (Basel)*, **103**, 259–265

Aten, R.F. & Eisenfeld, A.J. (1982) Estradiol is less potent than ethinyl estradiol for *in vivo* translocation of the mammalian liver estrogen receptor to the nucleus. *Endocrinology*, **111**, 1292–1298

Augustsson, A., Stierner, U., Rosdahl, I. & Suurkula, M. (1991) Common and dysplastic naevi as risk factors for cutaneous malignant melanoma in a Swedish population. *Acta dermatol. venereol.*, **71**, 518–524

Bain, C., Hennekens, C.H., Speizer, F.E., Rosner, B., Willett, W. & Belanger, C. (1982) Oral contraceptive use and malignant melanoma. *J. natl Cancer Inst.*, **68**, 537–539

Ball, P., Gelbke, H.P., Haupt, O. & Knuppen, R. (1973) Metabolism of 17α-ethynyl-[4-^{14}C]-oestradiol and [4-^{14}C]mestranol in rat liver slices and interaction between 17α-ethynyl-2-hydroxyoestradiol and adrenalin. *Hoppe-Seyler's Z. physiol. Chem.*, **354**, 1567–1575

Banduhn, N. & Obe, G. (1985) Mutagenicity of methyl 2-benzimidazolecarbamate, diethylstilbestrol and estradiol: Structural chromosomal aberrations, sister-chromatid exchanges, C-mitoses, polyploidies and micronuclei. *Mutat. Res.*, **156**, 199–218

Banerjee, S.K., Banerjee, S., Li, S.A. & Li, J.J. (1994) Induction of chromosome aberrations in Syrian hamster renal cortical cells by various estrogens. *Mutat. Res.*, **311**, 191–197

Barnes, R.B. & Lobo, R.A. (1987) Pharmacology of estrogens. In: Mishell, D.R., Jr, ed., *Menopause: Physiology and Pharmacology*, Chicago, IL, Year Book Medical Publishers, pp. 301–315

Bauer, H.M., Hildesheim, A., Schiffman, M.H., Glass, A.G., Rush, B.B., Scott, D.R., Cadell, D.M., Kurman, R.J. & Manos, M.M. (1993) Determinants of genital human papillomavirus infection in low-risk women in Portland, Oregon. *Sex. transm. Dis.*, **20**, 274–278

Baumann, A., Kulmann, H., Gorkov, V., Mahler, M. & Kuhnz, W. (1996) Radioimmunological analysis of cyproterone acetate in human serum. *Arzneimittel-Forsch./Drug Res.*, **46**, 412–418

Becker, T.M., Wheeler, C.M., McGough, N., Stidley, C.A., Parmenter, C.A., Dorin, M.H. & Jordan, S.W. (1994) Contraceptive and reproductive risks for cervical dysplasia in southwestern Hispanic and non-Hispanic white women. *Int. J. Epidemiol.*, **23**, 913–922

Beral, V., Ramcharan, S. & Faris, R. (1977) Malignant melanoma and oral contraceptive use among women in California. *Br. J. Cancer*, **36**, 804–809

Beral, V., Evans, S., Shaw, H. & Milton, G. (1984) Oral contraceptive use and malignant melanoma in Australia. *Br. J. Cancer*, **50**, 681–685

Beral, V., Hannaford, P. & Kay, C. (1988) Oral contraceptive use and malignancies of the genital tract. Results of the Royal College of General Practitioners' Oral Contraception Study. *Lancet*, **ii**, 1331–1335

Beral, V., Hermon, C., Kay, C., Hannaford, P., Darby, S. & Reeves, G. (1999) Mortality in relation to oral contraceptive use: 25 year follow-up of women in the Royal College of General Practitioners Oral Contraception study. *Br. med. J.*, **318**, 96–100

Bergink, E.W., van Meel, F., Turpijn, W. & van der Vies, J. (1983) Binding of progestagens to receptor proteins in MCF-7 cells. *J. Steroid Biochem.*, **19**, 1563–1570

Bernstein, L., Pike, M.C., Krailo, M. & Henderson, B.E. (1990) Update of the Los Angeles study of oral contraceptives and breast cancer: 1981 and 1983. In: Mann, R.D., ed., *Oral Contraceptives and Breast Cancer*, Camforth, Publishing Group Limited, pp. 169–181

Blakey, D.C. & White, I.N.H. (1985) Unscheduled DNA synthesis caused by norethindrone and related contraceptive steroids in short-term male rat hepatocyte cultures. *Carcinogenesis*, **6**, 1201–1205

Blanzat-Reboud, S. & Russfield, A.B. (1969) Effect of parenteral steroids on induction of genital tumors in mice by 20-methylcholanthrene. *Am. J. Obstet. Gynecol.*, **103**, 96–101

Bokkenheuser, V.D., Winter, J., Mosenthal, A.C., Mosbach, E.H., McSherry, C.K., Ayengar, N.K.N., Andrews, A.W., Lebherz, W.B., III, Pienta, R.J. & Wallenstein, S. (1983) Fecal steroid 21-dehydroxylase, a potential marker for colorectal cancer. *Am. J. Gastroenterol.*, **78**, 469–475

Bolt, H.M. (1979) Metabolism of estrogens—natural and synthetic. *Pharmacol. Ther.*, **4**, 155–181

Bolt, H.M. & Bolt, W.H. (1974) Pharmacokinetics of mestranol in man in relation to its oestrogenic activity. *Eur. J. clin. Pharmacol.*, **7**, 295–305

Booth, M., Beral, V. & Smith, P. (1989) Risk factors for ovarian cancer: A case–control study. *Br. J. Cancer*, **60**, 592–598

Booth, M., Beral, V., Maconochie, N., Carpenter, L. & Scott, C. (1992) A case–control study of benign ovarian tumours. *J. Epidemiol. Community Health*, **46**, 528–531

Bosch, F.X., Muñoz, N., de Sanjosé, S., Izarzugaza, I., Gili, M., Viladiu, P., Tormo, M.J., Moreo, P., Ascunce, N., Gonzalez, L.C., Tafur, L., Kaldor, J.M., Guerrero, E., Aristizabal, N., Santamaria, M., de Ruiz, P.A. & Shah, K.V. (1992) Risk factors for cervical cancer in Colombia and Spain. *Int. J. Epidemiol.*, **52**, 750–758

Bosch, F.X., Muñoz, N., de Sanjosé, S., Eluf Neto, J., Orfila, J., Walboomers, J. & Shah, K. (1995) What is relevant in cervical carcinogenesis other than HPV? In: Monsonego, J., ed., *Challenges of Modern Medicine*, Vol. 9, *Papillomavirus in Human Pathology*, Paris, Ares-Serono Symposia Publications, pp. 173–181

Bostick, R.M., Potter, J.D., Kushi, L.H., Sellers, T.A., Steinmetz, K.A., McKenzie, D.R., Gapstur, S.M. & Folsom, A.R. (1994) Sugar, meat, and fat intake, and non-dietary risk factors for colon cancer incidence in Iowa women (United States). *Cancer Causes Control*, **5**, 38–52

Botella, J., Paris, J. & Lahlou, B. (1987) The cellular mechanism of the antiandrogenic action of nomegestrol acetate, a new 19-nor progestagen, on the rat prostate. *Acta endocrinol.*, **115**, 544–550

Botella, J., Duc, I., Delansorne, R., Paris, J. & Lahlou, B. (1990) Structure–activity and structure–affinity relationships of 19-nor-progesterone derivatives in rat uterus. *J. endocrinol. Invest.*, **13**, 905–910

Botella, J., Duranti, E., Duc, I., Cognet, A.M., Delansorne, R. & Paris, J.(1994) Inhibition by nomegestrol acetate and other synthetic progestins on proliferation and progesterone receptor content of T47-D human breast cancer cells. *J. Steroid Biochem. mol. Biol.*, **50**, 41–47

Botella, J., Duranti, E., Viader, V., Duc, I., Delansorne, R. & Paris, J. (1995) Lack of estrogenic potential of progesterone- or 19-nor-progesterone-derived progestins as opposed to testosterone or 19-nortestosterone derivatives on endometrial Ishikawa cells. *J. Steroid Biochem. mol. Biol.*, **55**, 77–84

Bracken, M.B. (1990) Oral contraception and congenital malformations in offspring: A review and meta-analysis of the prospective studies. *Obstet. Gynecol.*, **76**, 552–557

Breiner, M., Romalo, G. & Schweikert, H.-U. (1986) Inhibition of androgen receptor binding by natural and synthetic steroids in cultured human genital skin fibroblasts. *Klin. Wochenschr.*, **64**, 732–737

Brent, R.L. (1989) Kudos to the Food and Drug Administration: Reversal of the package insert warning for birth defects for oral contraceptives. *Teratology*, **39**, 93–94

Brent, R.L. (1994) Cardiovascular birth defects and prenatal exposure to female sex hormones: Importance of utilising proper epidemiological methods and teratologic principles. *Teratology*, **49**, 159–161

Brewster, D., Jones, R.S. & Symons, A.M. (1977) Effects of neomycin on the biliary excretion and enterohepatic circulation of mestranol and 17β-oestradiol. *Biochem. Pharmacol.*, **26**, 943–946

Briggs, M.H. (1975) Contraceptive steroid binding to the human uterine progesterone-receptor. *Curr. med. Res. Opin.*, **3**, 95–98

Brinkmann, A.O., Lindh, L.M., Breedveld, D.I., Mulder, E. & Van der Molen, H.J. (1983) Cyproterone acetate prevents translocation of the androgen receptor in the rat prostate. *Mol. cell. Endocrinol.*, **32**, 117–129

Brinton, L.A., Hoover, R., Szklo, M. & Fraumeni, F.J., Jr (1982) Oral contraceptives and breast cancer. *Int. J. Epidemiol.*, **11**, 316–322

Brinton, L.A., Huggins, G.R., Lehman, H.F., Mallin, K., Szvitz, D.A., Trapido, E., Rosenthal, J. & Hoover, R. (1986) Long-term use of oral contraceptives and risk of invasive cervical cancer. *Int. J. Cancer*, **38**, 339–344

Brinton, L.A., Tashima, K.T., Lehman, H.F., Levine, R.S., Mallin, K., Savitz, D.A., Stolley, P.D. & Fraumeni, J.F., Jr (1987) Epidemiology of cervical cancer by cell type. *Cancer Res.*, **47**, 1706–1711

Brinton, L.A., Reeves, W.C., Brenes, M.M., Herrero, R., De Britton, R.C., Gaitan, E., Tenorio, F., Garcia, M. & Rawls, W.E. (1990) Oral contraceptive use and risk of invasive cervical cancer. *Int. J. Epidemiol.*, **19**, 4–11

Brinton, L.A., Daling, J.A., Liff, J.M., Schoenberg, J.B., Malone, K.E., Stanford, J.L., Coates, R.J., Gammon, M.D., Hanson, L. & Hoover, R.N. (1995) Oral contraceptives and breast cancer risk among young women. *J. natl Cancer Inst.*, **87**, 827–835

British Medical Association (1997) *British National Formulary*, No. 34, London, Royal Pharmaceutical Society of Great Britain, pp. 345–349

Brock, K.E., Berry, G., Brinton, L.A., Kerr, C., MacLennan, R. & Mock, P.A. (1989) Sexual reproductive and contraceptive risk factors for carcinoma in situ of the uterine cervix in Sydney. *Med. J. Austr.*, **150**, 125–130

van der Burg, B., Kalkhoven, E., Isbrücker, L. & de Laat, S.W. (1992) Effects of progestins on the proliferation of estrogen-dependent human breast cancer cells under growth factor-defined conditions. *J. Steroid Biochem. mol. Biol.*, **42**, 457–465

Burk, R.D., Kelly, P., Feldman, J., Bromberg, J., Vermund, S.H., Dehovitz, J.A. & Landesman, S.H. (1996) Declining prevalence of cervicovaginal human papillomavirus infection with age is independent of other risk factors. *Sex. transm. Dis.*, **23**, 333–341

Bursch, W., Düsterberg, B. & Schulte-Hermann, R. (1986) Growth, regression and cell death in rat liver as related to tissue levels of the hepatomitogen cyproterone acetate. *Arch. Toxicol.*, **59**, 221–227

Bursch, W., Oberhammer, F., Jirtle, R.L., Askari, M., Sedivy, R., Grasl-Kraupp, B., Purchio, A.F. & Schulte-Hermann, R. (1993) Transforming growth factor-$\beta1$ as a signal for induction of cell death by apoptosis. *Br. J. Cancer*, **67**, 531–536

Burton, S. & Trachtenberg, J. (1986) Effectiveness of antiandrogens in the rat. *J. Urol.*, **136**, 932–935

Bustan, M.H., Coker, A.L., Addy, C.L., Macera, C.A., Greene, F. & Sampoerno, D. (1993) Oral contraceptive use and breast cancer in Indonesia. *Contraception*, **47**, 241–249

Campen, D., Maronpot, R. & Lucier, G. (1990) Dose–response relationships in promotion of rat hepatocarcinogenesis by 17β-ethinylestradiol. *J. Toxicol. environ. Health*, **29**, 257–268

Cancer and Steroid Hormone Study of the Centers for Disease Control and the National Institute of Child Health and Human Development (1986) Oral contraceptive use and the risk of breast cancer. *New Engl. J. Med.*, **315**, 405–411

Cancer and Steroid Hormone Study of the Centers for Disease Control and the National Institute of Child Health and Human Development (1987) The reduction in risk of ovarian cancer associated with oral contraceptive use. *New Engl. J. Med.*, **316**, 650–655

Carol, W., Klinger, G., Jäger, R., Kasch, R. & Brandstädt, A. (1992) Pharmacokinetics of ethinylestradiol and levonorgestrel after administration of two oral contraceptive preparations. *Exp. clin. Endocrinol.*, **99**, 12–17

Casagrande, J.T., Louie, E.W., Pike, M.C., Roy, S., Ross, R.K. & Henderson, B.E. (1979) Incessant ovulation and ovarian cancer. *Lancet*, **ii**, 170–173

Catherino, W.H. & Jordan, V.C. (1995) Nomegestrol acetate, a clinically useful 19-norprogesterone derivative which lacks estrogenic activity. *J. Steroid Biochem. mol. Biol.*, **55**, 239–246

Catherino, W.H., Jeng, M.H. & Jordan, V.C. (1993) Norgestrel and gestodene stimulate breast cancer cell growth through an oestrogen receptor mediated mechanism. *Br. J. Cancer*, **67**, 945–952

Cavalieri, E.L., Stack, D.E., Devanesan, P.D., Todorovic, R., Dwivedy, I., Higginbotham, S., Johansson, S.L., Patil, K.D., Gross, M.L., Gooden, J.K., Ramanathan, R., Cerny, R.L. & Rogan, E.G. (1997) Molecular origin of cancer: Catechol estrogen-3,4-quinones as endogenous tumor initiators. *Proc. natl Acad. Sci. USA*, **94**, 10937–10942

Caviezel, M., Lutz, W.K. & Minini, C. (1984) Interaction of estrone and estradiol with DNA and protein of liver and kidney in rat and hamster in vivo and in vitro. *Arch. Toxicol.*, **55**, 97–103

Celentano, D.D., Klassen, A.C., Weisman, C.S. & Rosenshein, N.B. (1987) The role of contraceptive use in cervical cancer: The Maryland cervical cancer case–control study. *Am. J. Epidemiol.*, **126**, 592–604

Centers for Disease Control and the National Institute of Child Health and Human Development, Cancer and Steroid Hormone Study (1987) Combination oral contraceptive use and the risk of endometrial cancer. *J. Am. med. Assoc.*, **257**, 796–800

Centers for Disease Control Cancer and Steroid Hormone Study (1983a) Long-term oral contraceptive use and the risk of breast cancer. *J. Am. med. Assoc.*, **249**, 1591–1595

Centers for Disease Control Cancer and Steroid Hormone Study (1983b) Oral contraceptive use and the risk of ovarian cancer. *J. Am. med. Assoc.*, **249**, 1596–1599

Cerbón, M.A., Pasapera, A.M., Gutiérrez-Sagal, R., García, G.A. & Pérez-Palacios, G. (1990) Variable expression of the uteroglobin gene following the administration of norethisterone and its A-ring reduced metabolites. *J. Steroid Biochem.*, **36**, 1–6

Chaouki, N., Bosch, F.X., Muñoz, N., Meijer, C.J.L.M., El Gueddari, B., El Ghazi, A., Deacon, J., Castellsagué, X. & Walboomers, J.M.M. (1998) The viral origin of cervical cancer in Rabat, Morocco. *Int. J. Cancer*, **75**, 546–554

Chhabra, S.K., Kaur, S. & Rao, A.R. (1995) Modulatory influence of the oral contraceptive pill, Ovral, on 3-methylcholanthrene-induced carcinogenesis in the uterus of mouse. *Oncology*, **52**, 32–34

Chilvers, C., Mant, D. & Pike, M.C. (1987) Cervical adenocarcinoma and oral contraceptives. *Br. med. J.*, **295**, 1446–1447

Chilvers, C.E.D., Smith, S.J. & Members of the UK National Case–Control Study Group (1994) The effect of patterns of oral contraceptive use on breast cancer risk in young women. *Br. J. Cancer*, **67**, 922–923

Chow, W.-H., McLaughlin, J.K., Mandel, J.S., Blot, W.J., Niwa, S. & Fraumeni, J.F., Jr (1995) Reproductive factors and the risk of renal cell cancer among women. *Int. J. Cancer*, **60**, 321–324

Chute, C.G., Willett, W.C., Colditz, G.A., Stampfer, M.J., Rosner, B. & Speizer, F.E. (1991) A prospective study of reproductive history and exogenous estrogens on the risk of colorectal cancer in women. *Epidemiology*, **2**, 201–207

Clarke, E.A., Hatcher, J., McKeown-Eyssen, G.E. & Lickrish, G.M. (1985) Cervical dysplasia: Association with sexual behavior, smoking, and oral contraceptive use? *Am. J. Obstet. Gynecol.*, **151**, 612–616

Clavel, F., Andrieu, N., Gairard, B., Brémand, A., Piana, L., Lansac, J., Bréart, G., Rumeau-Rouquette, C., Flamant, R. & Renaud, R. (1991) Oral contraceptives and breast cancer: A French case–control study. *Int. J. Epidemiol.*, **20**, 32–38

Clos, V., Esteve, A., Jane, F. & Salva, P. (1988) Microsomal effects of cyproterone acetate and flutamide in rat testis. *Gen. Pharmacol.*, **19**, 393–397

Coenen, C.M.H., Thomas, C.M.G., Borm, G.F., Hollanders, J.M.G. & Rolland, R. (1996) Changes in androgens during treatment with four low-dose contraceptives. *Contraception*, **53**, 171–176

Coezy, E., Auzan, C., Lonigro, A., Philippe, M., Menard, J. & Corvol, P. (1987) Effect of mestranol on cell proliferation and angiotensinogen production in HepG2 cells: Relation with the cell cycle and action of tamoxifen. *Endocrinology*, **120**, 133–141

Cohen, C.J. & Deppe, G. (1977) Endometrial carcinoma and oral contraceptive agents. *Obstet. Gynecol.*, **49**, 390–392

Coker, A.L., McCann, M.F., Hulka, B.S. & Walton, L.A. (1992) Oral contraceptive use and cervical intraepithelial neoplasia. *J. clin. Epidemiol.*, **45**, 1111–1118

Coldham, N.G. & James, V.H. (1990) A possible mechanism for increased breast cell proliferation by progestins through increased reductive 17β-hydroxysteroid dehydrogenase activity. *Int. J. Cancer*, **45**, 174–178

Colditz, G.A. for the Nurses' Health Study Research Group (1994) Oral contraceptive use and mortality during 12 years of follow-up: The Nurses' Health Study. *Ann. intern. Med.*, **120**, 821–826

Collaborative Group on Hormonal Factors in Breast Cancer (1996a) Breast cancer and hormonal contraceptives: Further results. *Contraception*, **54** (Suppl. 3), 1S–106S

Collaborative Group on Hormonal Factors in Breast Cancer (1996b) Breast cancer and hormonal contraceptives: Collaborative reanalysis of individual data on 53 297 women with breast cancer and 100 239 women without breast cancer from 54 epidemiological studies. *Lancet*, **347**, 1713–1727

Collaborative MILTS Project Team (1997) Oral contraceptives and liver cancer. *Contraception*, **56**, 275–284

Colletta, A.A., Howell, F.V. & Baum, M. (1989) A novel binding site for a synthetic progestagen in breast cancer cells. *J. Steroid Biochem.*, **33**, 1055–1061

Colletta, A.A., Wakefield, L.M., Howell, F.V., Danielpour, D., Baum, M. & Sporn, M.B. (1991) The growth inhibition of human breast cancer cells by a novel synthetic progestin involves the induction of transforming growth factor beta. *J. clin. Invest.*, **87**, 277–283

Committee on Safety of Medicines (1972) *Carcinogenicity Tests of Oral Contraceptives*, London, Her Majesty's Stationery Office

Coni, P., Simbula, G., DePrati, A.C., Menegazzi, M., Suzuki, H., Sarma, D.S.R., Ledda-Columbano, G.M. & Columbano, A. (1993) Differences in the steady-state levels of c-*fos*, c-*jun* and c-*myc* messenger RNA during mitogen-induced liver growth and compensatory regeneration. *Hepatology*, **17**, 1109–1116

Cooke, B.A. & Vallance, D.K. (1965) Metabolism of megestrol acetate and related progesterone analogues by liver preparations *in vitro*. *Biochem. J.*, **97**, 672–677

Cooper, J.M. & Kellie, A.E. (1968) The metabolism of megestrol acetate (17-alpha acetoxy-6-methylpregna-4,6-diene-3,20-dione) in women. *Steroids*, **11**, 133–149

Cottinet, D., Czyba, J.C., Dams, R. & Laurent, J.L. (1974) Effects of long-term administration of anti-ovulatory steroids on the fertility of female golden hamsters and their progeny. *C.R. Soc. Biol.*, **168**, 517–520 (in French)

Cramer, D.W., Hutchison, G.B., Welch, W.R., Scully, R.E. & Knapp, R.C. (1982) Factors affecting the association of oral contraceptives and ovarian cancer. *New Engl. J. Med.*, **307**, 1047–1051

Cuzick, J., Singer, A., De Stavola, B.L. & Chomet, J. (1990) Case–control study of risk factors for cervical intraepithelial neoplasia in young women. *Eur. J. Cancer*, **26**, 684–690

Daling, J.R., Madeleine, M.M., McKnight, B., Carter, J.J., Wipf, G.C., Ashley, R., Schwartz, S.M., Beckmann, A.M., Hagensee, M.E., Mandelson, M.T. & Galloway, D.A. (1996) The relationship of human papillomavirus-related cervical tumors to cigarette smoking, oral contraceptive use, and prior herpes simplex virus type 2 infection. *Cancer Epidemiol. Biomarkers Prev.*, **5**, 541–548

Darney, P.D. (1995) The androgenicity of progestins. *Am. J. Med.*, **98** (Suppl. 1A), 104S–110S

Dayan, J., Crajer, M.C., Bertozzi, S. & Lefrancois, S. (1980) Application of the *Salmonella typhimurium* microsome test to the study of 25 drugs belonging to 5 chemical series. *Mutat. Res.*, **77**, 301–306

Deml, E., Schwarz, L.R. & Oesterle, D. (1993) Initiation of enzyme-altered foci by the synthetic steroid cyproterone acetate in rat liver foci bioassay. *Carcinogenesis*, **14**, 1229–1231

De Vet, H.C.W., Knipschild, P.G. & Sturmans, F. (1993) The role of sexual factors in the aetiology of cervical dysplasia. *Int. J. Epidemiol.*, **22**, 798–803

Dhillon, V.S. & Dhillon, I.K. (1996) Genotoxicity evaluation of norethisterone acetate. *Mutat. Res.*, **367**, 1–10

Dhillon, V.S., Singh, J.S., Singh, H. & Kler, R.S. (1994) In vitro and in vivo genotoxicity evaluation of hormonal drugs. V. Mestranol. *Mutat. Res.*, **322**, 173–183

Di Carlo, F., Gallo, E., Conti, G. & Racca, S. (1983) Changes in the binding of oestradiol to uterine oestrogen receptors induced by some progesterone and 19-nor-testosterone derivatives. *J. Endocrinol.*, **98**, 385–389

Doll, R. (1985) Invasive cervical cancer and combined oral contraceptives (Letter to the Editor). *Br. med. J.*, **290**, 1210

Dragan, Y.P., Singh, J. & Pitot, H.C. (1996) Effect of the separate and combined administration of mestranol and phenobarbital on the development of altered hepatic foci expressing placental form of glutathione S-transferase in the rat. *Carcinogenesis*, **17**, 2043–2052

Drevon, C., Piccoli, C. & Montesano, R. (1981) Mutagenicity assays of estrogenic hormones in mammalian cells. *Mutat. Res.*, **89**, 83–90

Drill, V.A. (1966). *Oral Contraceptives*, New York, McGraw-Hill, pp. 6–7

Duc, I., Botella, J., Bonnet, P., Fraboul, F., Delansorne, R. & Paris, J. (1995) Antiandrogenic properties of nomegestrol acetate. *Arzneimittelforschung*, **45**, 70–74

Dugwekar, Y.G., Narula, R.K. & Laumas, K.R. (1973) Disappearance of 1α-^{3}H-chlormadinone acetate from the plasma of women. *Contraception*, **7**, 27–45

Duivenvoorden, W.C.M. & Maier, P. (1994) Nongenotoxic carcinogens shift cultured rat hepatocytes into G1 cell cycle phase: Influence of tissue oxygen tension on cells with different
ploidy. *Eur. J. Cell Biol.*, **64**, 368–375

Duivenvoorden, W.C.M., Schäfer, R., Pfeifer, A.M.A., Piquet, D. & Maier, P. (1995) Nuclear
matrix condensation and c-*myc* and c-*fos* expression are specifically altered in cultured rat
hepatocytes after exposure to cyproterone acetate and phenobarbital. *Biochem. biophys. Res.
Comm.*, **215**, 598–605

Dunkel, V.C., Pienta, R.J., Sivak, A. & Traul, K.A. (1981) Comparative neoplastic transformation
responses of Balb/3T3 cells, Syrian hamster embryo cells, and Rauscher murine leukemia
virus-infected Fischer 344 rat embryo cells to chemical carcinogens. *J. natl Cancer Inst.*, **67**,
1303–1315

Dunkel, V.C., Zeiger, E., Brusick, D., McCoy, E., McGregor, D., Mortelmans, K., Rosenkranz, H.S.
& Simmon, V.F. (1984) Reproducibility of microbial mutagenicity assays: I. Tests with
Salmonella typhimurium and *Escherichia coli* using a standardized protocol. *Environ. Mutag.*,
6 (Suppl. 2), 1–254

Dutkowski, R.T., Kevin, M.J. & Jenkins, E.C. (1983) The effect of oral contraceptives on sister
chromatid exchange, blast transformation, mitotic index and micronuclei formation. *Exp. Cell
Biol.*, **51**, 115–120

Duval, D., Durant, S. & Homo-Delarche, F. (1983) Non-genomic effects of steroids: Interactions of
steroid molecules with membrane structures and functions. *Biochim. biophys. Acta*, **737**,
409–442

Ebeling, K., Nischan, P. & Schindler, C. (1987) Use of oral contraceptives and risk of invasive
cervical cancer in previously screened women. *Int. J. Cancer*, **39**, 427–430

Ebeling, K., Ray, R., Nischan, P., Thomas, D.B., Kunde, D. & Stalsberg, H. (1991) Combined oral
contraceptives containing chlormadinone acetate and breast cancer: Results of a case–control
study. *Br. J. Cancer*, **63**, 804–808

Edmondson, H.A., Henderson, B. & Benton, B. (1976) Liver-cell adenomas associated with use of
oral contraceptives. *New Engl. J. Med.*, **294**, 470–472

Edwards, A.M. & Lucas, C.M. (1985) Induction of γ-glutamyl transpeptidase in primary cultures
of normal rat hepatocytes by liver tumor promoters and structurally related compounds.
Carcinogenesis, **6**, 733–739

Eibs, H.G., Spielmann, H. & Hägele, M. (1982) Teratogenic effects of cyproterone acetate and
medroxyprogesterone treatment during the pre- and postimplantation period of mouse
embryos.1. *Teratology*, **25**, 27–36

Eisenfeld, A.J., Aten, R.F. & Weinberger, M.J. (1978) Oral contraceptives—possible mediation of
side effects via an estrogen receptor in liver. *Biochem. Pharmacol.*, **27**, 2571–2575

El Etreby, M.F., Habenicht, U.-F., Louton, T., Nishino, Y. & Schröder, H.G. (1987) Effect of
cyproterone acetate in comparison to flutamide and megestrol acetate on the ventral prostate,
seminal vesicle and adrenal glands of adult male rats. *Prostate*, **11**, 361–375

Ellery, C., MacLennan, R., Berry, G. & Shearman, R.P. (1986) A case–control study of breast cancer
in relation to the use of steroid contraceptive agents. *Med. J. Aust.*, **144**, 173–176

Eluf-Neto, J., Booth, M., Muñoz, N., Bosch, F.X., Meijer, C.J.L.M. & Walboomers, J.M.M. (1994) Human papillomavirus and invasive cervical cancer in Brazil. *Br. J. Cancer*, **69**, 114–119

Epstein, S.S., Arnold, E., Andrea, J., Bass, W. & Bishop, Y. (1972) Detection of chemical mutagens by the dominant lethal assay in the mouse. *Toxicol. appl. Pharmacol.*, **23**, 288–325

Ericson, A., Källén, B. & Lindsten, J. (1983) Lack of correlation between contraceptive pills and Down's syndrome. *Acta obstet. gynecol. scand.*, **62**, 511–514

Ewertz, M. (1992) Oral contraceptives and breast cancer risk in Denmark. *Eur. J. Cancer*, **28A**, 1176–1181

Farley, T.M., Meirik, O., Poulter, N.R., Chang, C.L. & Marmot, M.G. (1996) Oral contraceptives and thrombotic diseases: Impact of new epidemiological studies. *Contraception*, **54**, 193–198

Fathalla, M.F. (1971) Incessant ovulation—a factor in ovarian neoplasia? (Letter to the Editor) *Lancet*, **ii**, 163

Fernandez, E., La Vecchia, C., D'Avanzo, B., Franceschi, S., Negri, E. & Parazzini, F. (1996) Oral contraceptives, hormone replacement therapy and the risk of colorectal cancer. *Br. J. Cancer*, **73**, 1431–1435

Fernandez, E., La Vecchia, C., Franceschi, S., Braga, C., Talamini, R., Negri, E. & Parazzini, F. (1998) Oral contraceptive use and risk of colorectal cancer. *Epidemiology*, **9**, 295–300

Fitzgerald, J., DeLaIglesia, F. & Goldenthal, E.I. (1982) Ten-year oral toxicity study with Norlestrin in rhesus monkey. *J. Toxicol. environ. Health*, **10**, 879–896

Føgh, M., Corker, C.S., Hunter, W.M., McLean, H., Philip, J., Schou, G. & Skakkebaek, N.E. (1979) The effects of low doses of cyproterone acetate on some functions of the reproductive systems in normal men. *Acta endocrinol.*, **91**, 545–552

Foote, W.D., Foote, W.C. & Foote, L.H. (1968) Influence of certain natural and synthetic steroids on genital development in guinea pigs. *Fertil. Steril.*, **19**, 606–615

Forman, D., Doll, R. & Peto, R. (1983) Trends in mortality from carcinoma of the liver and the use of oral contraceptives. *Br. J. Cancer*, **48**, 349–354

Forman, D., Vincent, T.J. & Doll, R. (1986) Cancer of the liver and the use of oral contraceptives. *Br. med. J.*, **292**, 1357–1361

Forsberg, J.-G. (1991) Estrogen effects on chromosome number and sister chromatid exchanges in uterine epithelial cells and kidney cells from neonatal mice. *Teratog. Carcinog. Mutag.*, **11**, 135–146

Forsberg, J.-G. & Jacobsohn, D. (1969) The reproductive tract of males delivered by rats given cyproterone acetate from days 7 to 21 of pregnancy. *J. Endocrinol.*, **44**, 461–462

Fotherby, K. (1995) Levonorgestrel: Clinical pharmacokinetics. *Clin. Pharmacokin.*, **28**, 203–215

Francavilla, A., Polimeno, L., DiLeo, A., Barone, M., Ove, P., Coetzee, M., Eagon, P., Makowka, L., Ambrosino, G., Mazzaferro, V. & Starzl, T.E. (1989) The effect of estrogen and tamoxifen on hepatocyte proliferation *in vivo* and *in vitro*. *Hepatology*, **9**, 614–620

Franceschi, S., La Vecchia, C., Helmrich, S.P., Mangioni, C. & Tognoni, G. (1982) Risk factors for epithelial ovarian cancer in Italy. *Am. J. Epidemiol.*, **115**, 714–719

Franceschi, S., Fassina, A., Talamini, R., Mazzolini, A., Vianello, S., Bidoli, E., Cizza, G. & La Vecchia, C. (1990) The influence of reproductive and hormonal factors on thyroid cancer in women. *Rev. Epidemiol. Santé publ.*, **38**, 27–34

Franceschi, S., Parazzini, F., Negri, E., Booth, M., La Vecchia, C., Beral, V., Tzonou, A. & Trichopoulos, D. (1991a) Pooled analysis of 3 European case–control studies of epithelial ovarian cancer. III. Oral contraceptive use. *Int. J. Cancer*, **49**, 61–65

Franceschi, S., Bidoli, E., Talamini, R., Barra, S. & La Vecchia, C. (1991b) Colorectal cancer in northeastern Italy: Reproductive, menstrual and female hormone-related factors. *Eur. J. Cancer*, **27**, 604–608

Fuhrmann, U., Bengtson, C., Repenthin, G. & Schillinger, E. (1992) Stable transfection of androgen receptor and MMTV-CAT into mammalian cells: Inhibition of CAT expression by anti-androgens. *J. Steroid Biochem. mol. Biol.*, **42**, 787–793

Fuhrmann, U., Slater, E.P. & Fritzemeier, K.-H. (1995) Characterization of the novel progestin gestodene by receptor binding studies and transactivation assays. *Contraception*, **51**, 45–52

Furner, S.E., Davis, F.G., Nelson, R.L. & Haenszel, W. (1989) A case–control study of large bowel cancer and hormone exposure in women. *Cancer Res.*, **49**, 4936–4940

Galanti, M.R., Hansson, L., Lund, E., Bergström, R., Grimelius, L., Stalsberg, H., Carlsen, E., Baron, J.A., Persson, I. & Ekbom, A. (1996) Reproductive history and cigarette smoking as risk factors for thyroid cancer in women: A population-based case–control study. *Cancer Epidemiol. Biomarkers Prev.*, **5**, 425–431

Gallagher, R.P., Elwood, J.M., Hill, G.B., Coldman, A.J., Threlfall, W.J. & Spinelli, J.J. (1985) Reproductive factors, oral contraceptives and risk of malignant melanoma: Western Canada melanoma study. *Br. J. Cancer*, **52**, 901–907

Gefeller, O., Hassan, K. & Wille, L. (1997) A meta-analysis on the relationship between oral contraceptives and melanoma: Results and methodological aspects. *J. Epidemiol. Biostat.*, **2**, 225–235

Ghia, M. & Mereto, E. (1989) Induction and promotion of γ-glutamyltranspeptidase-positive foci in the liver of female rats treated with ethinyl estradiol, clomiphene, tamoxifen and their associations. *Cancer Lett.*, **46**, 195–202

Ghosh, R. & Ghosh, P.K. (1988) Sister chromatid exchange in the lymphocytes of control women, pregnant women, and women taking oral contraceptives: Effects of cell culture temperature. *Environ. mol. Mutag.*, **12**, 179–183

Gidley, J.T., Christensen, H.D., Hall, I.H., Palmer, K.H. & Wall, M.E. (1970) Teratogenic and other effects produced in mice by norethynodrel and its 3-hydroxymetabolites. *Teratology*, **3**, 339–344

Giudice, L.C., Milkowski, D.A., Fielder, P.J. & Irwin, J.C. (1991) Characterization of the steroid-dependence of insulin-like growth factor-binding protein-2 synthesis and mRNA expression in cultured human endometrial stromal cells. *Hum. Reprod.*, **6**, 632–640

Going, J.J., Anderson, T.J., Battersby, S. & Macintyre, C.C.A. (1988) Proliferative and secretory activity in human breast during natural and artificial menstrual cycles. *Am. J. Pathol.*, **130**, 193–204

Goldzieher, J.W. & Brody, S.A. (1990) Pharmacokinetics of ethinyl estradiol and mestranol. *Am. J. Obstet. Gynecol.*, **163**, 2114–2119

Goldzieher, J.W., Maas, J.M. & Hines, D.C. (1968) Seven years of clinical experience with a sequential oral contraceptive. *Int. J. Fertil.*, **13**, 399–404

Golub, M.S., Hayes, L., Prahalada, S. & Hendrickx, A.G. (1983) Behavioral tests in monkey infants exposed embryonically to an oral contraceptive. *Neurobehav. Toxicol. Teratol.*, **5**, 301–304

Gomes, A.L.R.R., Guimarâes, M.D.C., Gomes, C.C., Chaves, I.G., Goff, H. & Camargos, A.F. (1995) A case–control study of risk factors for breast cancer in Brazil, 1978–87. *Int. J. Epidemiol.*, **24**, 292–299

Gram, I.T., Macaluso, M. & Stalsberg, H. (1992) Oral contraceptive use and the incidence of cervical intraepithelial neoplasia. *Am. J. Obstet. Gynecol.*, **167**, 40–44

Greb, R.R., Heikinheimo, O., Williams, R.F., Hodgem G.D. & Goodman, A.L. (1997) Vascular endothelial growth factor in primate endometrium is regulated by oestrogen-receptor and progesterone-receptor ligands *in vivo*. *Hum. Reprod.*, **12**, 1280–1292

Green, A. & Bain, C. (1985) Hormonal factors and melanoma in women. *Med. J. Austr.*, **142**, 446–448

Grill, H.J., Manz, B., Elger, W. & Pollow, K. (1985) 3H-Cyproterone acetate: Binding characteristics to human uterine progestagen receptors. *J. endocrinol. Invest.*, **8**, 135–141

Gross, T.P. & Schlesselman, J.J. (1994) The estimated effect of oral contraceptive use on the cumulative risk of epithelial ovarian cancer. *Obstet. Gynecol.*, **83**, 419–424

Gross, T.P., Schlesselman, J.J., Stadel, B.V., Yu, W. & Lee, N.C. (1992) The risk of epithelial ovarian cancer in short-term users of oral contraceptives. *Am. J. Epidemiol.*, **136**, 46–53

Guengerich, F.P. (1988) Oxidation of 17α-ethynylestradiol by human liver cytochrome P-450. *Mol. Pharmacol.*, **33**, 500–508

Hackenberg, R., Hofmann, J., Hölzel, F. & Schulz, K.-D. (1988) Stimulatory effects of androgen and antiandrogen on the in vitro proliferation of human mammary carcinoma cells. *J. Cancer Res. clin. Oncol.*, **114**, 593–601

Hajek, R.A., Van, N.T., Johnston, D.A. & Jones, L.A. (1993) In vivo induction of increased DNA ploidy of mouse cervicovaginal epithelium by neonatal estrogen treatment. *Biol. Reprod.*, **49**, 908–917

Hallquist, A., Hardell, L., Degerman, A. & Boquist, L. (1994) Thyroid cancer: Reproductive factors, previous diseases, drug intake, family history and diet. A case–control study. *Eur. J. Cancer Prev.*, **3**, 481–488

Hallstrom, I.P., Liao, D.-Z., Assefaw-Redda, Y., Ohlson, L.C., Sahlin, L., Eneroth, P., Eriksson, L.C., Gustafsson, J.-A. & Blanck, A. (1996) Role of the pituitary in tumor promotion with ethinyl estradiol in rat liver. *Hepatology*, **24**, 849–854

Han, X. & Liehr, J.G. (1994) DNA single-strand breaks in kidneys of Syrian hamsters treated with steroidal estrogens: Hormone-induced free radical damage preceding renal malignancy. *Carcinogenesis*, **15**, 997–1000

Han, X. & Liehr, J.G. (1995) Microsome-mediated 8-hydroxylation of guanine bases of DNA by steroid estrogens: Correlation of DNA damage by free radicals with metabolic activation to quinones. *Carcinogenesis*, **16**, 2571–2574

Han, X., Liehr, J.G. & Bosland, M.C. (1995) Induction of a DNA adduct detectable by ^{32}P-post-labelling in the dorsolateral prostate of NBL/Cr rats treated with estradiol-17β and testosterone. *Carcinogenesis*, **16**, 951–954

Handy, R.W., Palmer, K.H., Wall, M.E. & Piantadosi, C. (1974) The metabolism of antifertility steroids. The *in vitro* metabolism of chlormadinone acetate. *Drug Metab. Disposition*, **2**, 214–220

Hankinson, S.E., Colditz, G.A., Hunter, D.J., Willett, W.C., Stampfer, M.J., Rosner, B., Hennekens, C.H. & Speizer, F.E. (1995) A prospective study of reproductive factors and risk of epithelial ovarian cancer. *Cancer*, **76**, 284–290

Hannaford, P.C., Villard-Mackintosh, L., Vessey, M.P. & Kay, C.R. (1991) Oral contraceptives and malignant melanoma. *Br. J. Cancer*, **63**, 430–433

Hannaford, P.C., Kay, C.R., Vessey, M.P., Painter, R. & Mant, J. (1997) Combined oral contraceptives and liver disease. *Contraception*, **55**, 145–151

Harlap, S., Shiono, P.H. & Ramcharan, S. (1985a) Congenital abnormalities in the offspring of women who used oral and other contraceptives around the time of conception. *Int. J. Fertil.*, **30**, 39–47

Harlap, S., Shiono, P.H., Ramcharan, S., Golbus, M., Bachman, R., Mann, J. & Lewis, J.P. (1985b) Chromosomal abnormalities in the Kaiser-Permanente birth defects study, with special reference to contraceptive use around the time of conception. *Teratology*, **31**, 381–387

Harlow, B.L., Weiss, N.S., Roth, G.J., Chu, J. & Daling, J.R. (1988) Case–control study of borderline ovarian tumors: Reproductive history and exposure to exogenous female hormones. *Cancer Res.*, **48**, 5849–5852

Harris, R.W.C., Brinton, L.A., Cowdell, R.H., Skegg, D.C.G., Smith, P.G., Vessey, M.P. & Doll, R. (1980) Characteristics of women with dysplasia or carcinoma in situ of the cervix uteri. *Br. J. Cancer*, **42**, 359–369

Harris, N.V., Weiss, N.S., Francis, A.M. & Polissar, L.N. (1982) Breast cancer in relation to patterns of oral contraceptive use. *Am. J. Epidemiol.*, **116**, 643–651

Harris, R.E., Zang, E.A. & Wynder, E.L. (1990) Oral contraceptives and breast cancer risk: A case–control study. *Int. J. Epidemiol.*, **19**, 240–246

Harris, R., Whittemore, A.S., Itnyre, J. & the Collaborative Ovarian Cancer Group (1992) Characteristics relating to ovarian cancer risk: Collaborative analysis of 12 US case–control studies. III. Epithelial tumors of low malignant potential in white women. *Am. J. Epidemiol.*, **136**, 1204–1211

Hartge, P., Schiffman, M.H., Hoover, R., McGowan, L., Lesher, L. & Norris, H.J. (1989a) A case–control study of epithelial ovarian cancer. *Am. J. Obstet. Gynecol.*, **161**,10–16

Hartge, P., Tucker, M.A., Shields, J.A., Augsburger, J., Hoover, R.N. & Fraumeni, J.F., Jr (1989b) Case–control study of female hormones and eye melanoma. *Cancer Res.*, **49**, 4622–4625

Hatcher, R.A., Rinckart, W., Blackburn, R. & Geller, J.S. (1997) *The Essentials of Contraceptive Technology*, Baltimore, Population Information Program, Center for Communication Programs, The Johns Hopkins School of Public Health, pp. 5–23

Haukkamaa, M., Niemelä, A. & Tuohimaa, P. (1980) Progesterone-binding properties of the microsomal fraction from chick oviduct. *Mol. cell. Endocrinol.*, **19**, 123–130

Heinecke, H. & Klaus, S. (1975) Effect of mestranol on the gravidity of mice. *Pharmazie*, **30**, 53–56 (in German)

Heinecke, H. & Kohler, D. (1983) Prenatal toxic effects of STS557. II. Investigation in rabbits—preliminary results. *Exp. clin. Endocrinol.*, **81**, 206–209

Hellberg, D., Valentin, J. & Nilsson, S. (1985) Long-term use of oral contraceptives and cervical neoplasia: An association confounded by other risk factors? *Contraception*, **32**, 337–346

Helmrich, S.P., Rosenberg, L., Kaufman, D.W., Miller, D.R., Schottenfeld, D., Stolley, P.D. & Shapiro, S. (1984) Lack of an elevated risk of malignant melanoma in relation to oral contraceptive use. *J. natl Cancer Inst.*, **72**, 617–620

Henderson, B.E., Casagrande, J.T., Pike, M.C., Mack, T., Rosario, I. & Duke, A. (1983a) The epidemiology of endometrial cancer in young women. *Br. J. Cancer*, **47**, 749–756

Henderson, B., Preston-Martin, S., Edmonson, H.A., Peters, R.L. & Pike, M.C. (1983b) Hepatocellular carcinoma and oral contraceptives. *Br. J. Cancer*, **48**, 437–440

Hennekens, C.H., Speizer, F.E., Lipnick, R.J., Rosner, B., Bain, C., Belanger, C., Stampfer, M.J., Willett, W. & Peto, R. (1984) A case–control study of oral contraceptive use and breast cancer. *J. natl Cancer Inst.*, **72**, 39–42

Heuner, A., Kuhnz, W., Heger-Mahn, D., Richert, K. & Hümpel, M. (1995) A single-dose and 3-month clinical–pharmacokinetic study with a new combination oral contraceptive. *Adv. Contracept.*, **11**, 207–225

Hildesheim, A., Gravitt, P., Schiffman, M.H., Kurman, R.J., Barnes, W., Jones, S., Tchabo, J.-G., Brinton, L.A., Copeland, C., Epp, J. & Manos, M.M. (1993) Determinants of genital human papillomavirus infection in low-income women in Washington, DC. *Sex. transm. Dis.*, **20**, 279–285

Hildesheim, A., Schiffman, M.H., Gravitt, P.E., Glass, A.G., Greer, C.E., Zhang, T., Scott, D.R., Rush, B.B., Lawler, P., Sherman, M.E., Kurman, R.J. & Manos, M.M. (1994) Persistence of type-specific human papillomavirus infection among cytologically normal women. *J. infect. Dis.*, **169**, 235–240

Hildreth, N.G., Kelsey, J.L., LiVolsi, V.A., Fischer, D.B., Holford, T.R., Mostow, E.D., Schwartz, P.E. & White, C. (1981) An epidemiologic study of epithelial carcinoma of the ovary. *Am. J. Epidemiol.*, **114**, 398–405

Hill, A. & Wolff, S. (1983) Sister chromatid exchanges and cell division delays induced by diethylstilbestrol, estradiol, and estriol in human lymphocytes. *Cancer Res.*, **43**, 4114–4118

Hill, L., Murphy, M., McDowall, M. & Paul, A.H. (1988) Maternal drug histories and congenital malformations: Limb reduction defects and oral clefts. *J. Epidemiol. Community Health*, **42**, 1–7

Hillbertz-Nilsson, K. & Forsberg, J.-G. (1985) Estrogen effects on sister chromatid exchanges in mouse uterine cervical and kidney cells. *J. natl Cancer Inst.*, **75**, 575–580

Ho, G.Y.F., Burk, R.D., Klein, S., Kadish, A.S., Chang, C.J., Palan, P., Basu, J., Tachezy, R., Lewis, R. & Romney, S. (1995) Persistent genital human papillomavirus infection as a risk factor for persistent cervical dysplasia. *J. natl Cancer Inst.*, **87**, 1365–1371

Ho, G.Y.F., Bierman, R., Beardsley, L., Chang, C.J. & Burk, R.D. (1998) Natural history of cervicovaginal papillomavirus infection in young women. *New Engl. J. Med.*, **338**, 423–428

Hoffmann, H., Hillesheim, H.G., Güttner, J., Stade, K., Merbt, E.-M. & Holle, K. (1983) Long-term toxicological studies on the progestin STS 557. *Exp. clin. Endocrinol.*, **81**, 179–196

Holly, E.A., Weiss, N.S. & Liff, J.M. (1983) Cutaneous melanoma in relation to exogenous hormones and reproductive factors. *J. natl Cancer Inst.*, **70**, 827–831

Holly, E.A., Cress, R.D. & Ahn, D.K. (1994) Cutaneous melanoma in women: Ovulatory life, meno-pause, and use of exogenous oestrogens. *Cancer Epidemiol. Biomarkers Prev.*, **3**, 661–668

Holly, E.A., Cress, R.D. & Ahn, D.K. (1995) Cutaneous melanoma in women. III. Reproductive factors and oral contraceptive use. *Am. J. Epidemiol.*, **141**, 943–950

Holmberg, L., Lund, E., Bergström, R., Adami, H.-O. & Meirik, O. (1994) Oral contraceptives and prognosis in breast cancer: Effects of duration, latency, recency, age at first use and relation to parity and body mass index in young women with breast cancer. *Eur. J. Cancer*, **30A**, 351–354

Holtzman, S. (1988) Retinyl acetate inhibits estrogen-induced mammary carcinogenesis in female ACI rats. *Carcinogenesis*, **9**, 305–307

Homady, M.H., Al-Khayat, T.H.A. & Brain, P.F. (1986) Effects of different doses of cyproterone acetate (CA) on preputial gland structure and activity in intact male mice. *Comp. Biochem. Physiol.*, **85C**, 187–191

Honoré, L.H., Koch, M. & Brown, L.B. (1991) Comparison of oral contraceptive use in women with adenocarcinoma and squamous cell carcinoma of the uterine cervix. *Gynecol. obstet. Invest.*, **32**, 98–101

Hopkins, M.P. & Morley, G.W. (1991) A comparison of adenocarcinoma and squamous cell carci-noma of the cervix. *Obstet. Gynecol.*, **77**, 912–917

Horn-Ross, P.L., Whittemore, A.S., Harris, R., Itnyre, J. & the Collaborative Ovarian Cancer Group (1992) Characteristics relating to ovarian cancer risk: Collaborative analysis of 12 US case–control studies. VI. Nonepithelial cancers among adults. *Epidemiology*, **3**, 490–495

Hsing, A.W., Hoover, R.N., McLaughlin, J.K., Co-Chien, H.T., Wacholder, S., Blot, W.J. & Fraumeni, J.F. (1992) Oral contraceptives and primary liver cancer among young women. *Cancer Causes Control*, **3**, 43–48

Huber, J., Zeillinger, R., Schmidt, J., Täuber, U., Kuhnz, W. & Spona, J. (1988) Pharmacokinetics of cyproterone acetate and its main metabolite 15β-hydroxy-cyproterone acetate in young healthy women. *Int. J. clin. Pharmacol. Ther. Toxicol.*, **26**, 555–561

Hulka, B.S., Chambless, L.E., Kaufman, D.G., Fowler, W.C., Jr & Greenberg, B.G. (1982) Protec-tion against endometrial carcinoma by combination-product oral contraceptives. *J. Am. med. Assoc.*, **247**, 475–477

Hümpel, M., Täuber, U., Kuhnz, W., Pfeffer, M., Brill, K., Heithecker, R., Louton, T. & Steinberg, B. (1990) Comparison of serum ethinyl estradiol, sex-hormone-binding globulin, corticoid-binding globulin and cortisol levels in women using two low-dose combined oral contra-ceptives. *Hormone Res.*, **33**, 35–39

Hussain, S.P. & Rao, A.R. (1992) Modulatory influence of oral contraceptive pills Ovral and Nora-cycline on 3-methylcholanthrene-induced carcinogenesis in the uterine cervix of mouse. *Jpn. J. Cancer Res.*, **83**, 576–583

Hussain, S.P., Chhabra, S.K. & Rao, A.R. (1991) Effects of oral contraceptive pills on drug meta-bolizing enzymes and acid soluble sulfhydryl level in mouse liver. *Biochem. int.*, **25**, 973–984

Husum, B., Wulf, H.C. & Niebuhr, E. (1982) Normal sister-chromatid exchanges in oral contra-ceptive users. *Mutat. Res.*, **103**, 161–164

Hyder, S.M., Murthy, L. & Stancel, G.M. (1998) Progestin regulation of vascular endothelial growth factor in human breast cancer cells. *Cancer Res.*, **58**, 392–395

IARC (1974) *IARC Monographs on the Evaluation of Carcinogenic Risk of Chemicals to Man,* Vol. 6, *Sex Hormones,* Lyon

IARC (1979) *IARC Monographs on the Evaluation of the Carcinogenic Risk of Chemicals to Humans,* Vol. 21, *Sex Hormones (II),* Lyon, pp. 105–106

IARC (1987) *IARC Monographs on the Evaluation of the Carcinogenic Risks to Humans,* Suppl. 7, *Overall Evaluations of Carcinogenicity: An Updating of* IARC Monographs *Volumes 1–42,* pp. 272–310

IARC (1988) *IARC Monographs on the Evaluation of Carcinogenic Risks to Humans,* Vol. 44, *Alcohol Drinking,* Lyon

IARC (1994) *IARC Monographs on the Evaluation of Carcinogenic Risks to Humans,* Vol. 59, *Hepatitis Viruses,* Lyon

IARC (1995) *IARC Monographs on the Evaluation of Carcinogenic Risks to Humans,* Vol. 64, *Human Papillomaviruses,* Lyon

Ingerowski, G.H., Scheutwinkel-Reich, M. & Stan, H.-J. (1981) Mutagenicity studies on veterinary anabolic drugs with the *Salmonella*/microsome test. *Mutat. Res.,* **91**, 93–98

Iqbal, M.J. & Colletta, A.A. (1987) Characterisation of gestodene binding to the oestrogen receptor in human malignant breast tissue. *Anticancer Res.,* **7**, 45–48

Iqbal, M.J. & Valyani, S.H. (1988) Evidence for a novel binding site for the synthetic progestogen, gestodene on oestrogen receptor in human malignant tissue. *Anticancer Res.,* **8**, 351–354

Iqbal, M.J., Colletta, A.A., Houmayoun-Valyani, S.D. & Baum, M. (1986) Differences in oestrogen receptors in malignant and normal breast tissue as identified by the binding of a new synthetic progestogen. *Br. J. Cancer,* **54**, 447–452

Irwin, K.L., Rosero-Bixby, L., Oberle, M.W., Lee, N.C., Whatley, A.S., Fortney, J.A. & Bonhomme, M.G. (1988) Oral contraceptives and cervical cancer risk in Costa Rica. *J. Am. med. Assoc.,* **259**, 59–64

Ishidate, M., Jr, ed. (1983) *The Data Book of Chromosomal Aberration Tests in Vitro on 587 Chemical Substances using a Chinese Hamster Fibroblast Cell Line (CHL Cells),* Tokyo, Realize

Ishidate, M., Jr, Hayashi, M., Sawada, M., Matsuoka, A., Yoshikawa, K., Ono, M. & Nakadate, M. (1978) Cytotoxicity test on medical drugs—Chromosome aberration tests with Chinese hamster cells *in vitro*. *Eisei Shikenjo Hokoku,* **96**, 55–61 (in Japanese)

Jacobs, E.J., White, E. & Weiss, N.S. (1994) Exogenous hormones, reproductive history, and colon cancer (Seattle, Washington, United States). *Cancer Causes Control,* **5**, 359–366

Jacobson, J.S., Neugut, A.I., Garbowski, G.D., Ahsan, H., Waye, J.D., Treat, M.R. & Forde, K.A. (1995) Reproductive risk factors for colorectal adenomatous polyps (New York City, NY, United States). *Cancer Causes Control,* **6**, 513–518

Janerich, D.T., Flink, E.M. & Keogh, M.D. (1976) Down's syndrome and oral contraceptive usage. *Br. J. Obstet. Gynaecol.,* **83**, 617–620

Janerich, D.T., Polednak, A.P., Glebatis, D.M. & Lawrence, C.E. (1983) Breast cancer and oral contraceptive use: A case–control study. *J. chron. Dis.,* **36**, 639–646

Jean-Faucher, C., Berger, M., de Turckheim, M., Veyssiere, G. & Jean, C. (1985) Permanent changes in the functional development of accessory sex organs and in fertility in male mice after neonatal exposure to cyproterone acetate. *J. Endocrinol.,* **104**, 113–120

Jeng, M.-H. & Jordan, V.C. (1991) Growth stimulation and differential regulation of transforming growth factor-β1 (TGF β1), TGF β2, and TGF β3 messenger RNA levels by norethindrone in MCF-7 human breast cancer cells. *Mol. Endocrinol.*, **8**, 1120–1128

Jeng, M.-H., Parker, C.J. & Jordan, V.C. (1992) Estrogenic potential of progestins in oral contraceptives to stimulate human breast cancer cell proliferation. *Cancer Res.*, **52**, 6539–6546

Jiang, S.-Y., Shyu, R.-Y., Yeh, M.-Y. & Jordan, V.C. (1995) Tamoxifen inhibits hepatoma cell growth through an estrogen receptor independent mechanism. *J. Hepatol.*, **23**, 712–719

Jick, H., Walker, A.M., Watkins, R.N., Dewart, D.C., Hunter, J.R., Danford, A., Madsen, S., Dinan, B.J. & Rothman, K.J. (1980) Oral contraceptives and breast cancer. *Am. J. Epidemiol.*, **112**, 577–585

Jick, S.S., Walker, A.M., Stergachis, A. & Jick, H. (1989) Oral contraceptives and breast cancer. *Br. J. Cancer*, **59**, 618–621

Jick, S.S., Walker, A.M. & Jick, H. (1993) Oral contraceptives and endometrial cancer. *Obstet. Gynecol.*, **82**, 931–935

Jick, H., Jick, S.S., Gurewich, V., Myers, M.W. & Vasilakis, C. (1995) Risk of idiopathic cardiovascular death and non-fatal venous thromboembolism in women using oral contraceptives with differing progestagen components. *Lancet*, **346**, 1589–1593

John, E.M., Whittemore, A.S., Harris, R., Itnyre, J. & Collaborative Ovarian Cancer Group (1993) Characteristics relating to ovarian cancer risk: Collaborative analysis of seven US case–control studies. Epithelial ovarian cancer in black women. *J. natl Cancer Inst.*, **85**, 142–147

Jones, M.W. & Silverberg, S.G. (1989) Cervical adenocarcinoma in young women: Possible relationship to microglandular hyperplasia and use of oral contraceptives. *Obstet. Gynecol.*, **73**, 984–989

Jones, C.J., Brinton, L.A., Hamman, R.F., Stolley, P.D., Lehman, H.F., Levine, R.S. & Mallin, K. (1990) Risk factors for in situ cervical cancer: Results from a case–control study. *Cancer Res.*, **50**, 3657–3662

Juchem, M. & Pollow, K. (1990) Binding of oral contraceptive progestogens to serum proteins and cytoplasmic receptor. *Am. J. Obstet. Gynecol.*, **163**, 2171–2183

Juchem, M., Pollow, K., Elger, W., Hoffmann, G. & Möbus, V. (1993) Receptor binding of norgestimate—a new orally active synthetic progestational compound. *Contraception*, **47**, 283–294

Kalandidi, A., Tzonon, A., Lipworth, L., Garnatsi, L., Filippa, D. & Trichopoulos, D. (1996) A case–control study of endometrial cancers in relation to reproductive, somatometric and livestyle variables. *Oncology*, **53**, 354–359

Kalkhoven, E., Kwakkenbos-Isbrücker, L., de Laat, S.W., van der Saag, P.T. & van der Burg, B. (1994) Synthetic progestins induce proliferation of breast tumor cell lines via the progesterone or estrogen receptor. *Mol. cell. Endocrinol.*, **102**, 45–52

Kalkhoven, E., Beraldi, E., Panno, M.L., De Winter, J.P., Thijssen, J.H.H. & van der Burg, B. (1996) Growth inhibition by anti-estrogens and progestins in TGF-β-resistant and -sensitive breast-tumor cells. *Int. J. Cancer*, **65**, 682–687

Källén, B. (1989) Maternal use of contraceptives and Down syndrome. *Contraception*, **39**, 503–505

Källén, B., Mastroiacovo, P., Lancaster, P.A.L., Mutchinick, O., Kringelback, M., Martínez-Frías, M.L., Robert, E. & Castilla, E.E. (1991) Oral contraceptives in the etiology of isolated hypospadias. *Contraception*, **44**, 173–182

Kampman, E., Potter, J.D., Slattery, M.L., Caan, B.J. & Edward, S. (1997) Hormone replacement therapy, reproductive history, and colon cancer: A multicenter, case–control study in the United States. *Cancer Causes Control*, **8**, 146–158

Kappus, H., Bolt, H.M. & Remmer, H. (1973) Affinity of ethynyl-estradiol and mestranol for the uterine estrogen receptor and for the microsomal mixed function oxidase of the liver. *J. Steroid Biochem.*, **4**, 121–128

Kasid, A. & Laumas, K.R. (1981) Nuclear progestin receptors in human uterus. *Endocrinology*, **109**, 553–560

Kasper, P. & Mueller, L. (1996) Time-related induction of DNA repair synthesis in rat hepatocytes following *in vivo* treatment with cyproterone acetate. *Carcinogenesis*, **17**, 2271–2274

Kasper, P., Tegethoff, K. & Mueller, L. (1995) *In vitro* mutagenicity studies on cyproterone acetate using female rat hepatocytes for metabolic activation and as indicator cells. *Carcinogenesis*, **16**, 2309–2314

Kästner, D. & Apfelbach, R. (1987) Effects of cyproterone acetate on mating behaviour, testicular morphology, testosterone level, and body temperature in male ferrets in comparison with normal and castrated males. *Horm. Res.*, **25**, 178–184

Kaufman, R.H., Reeves, K.O. & Dougherty, C.M. (1976) Severe atypical endometrial changes and sequential contraceptive use. *J. Am. med. Assoc.*, **236**, 923–926

Kaufman, D.W., Shapiro, S., Slone, D., Rosenberg, L., Miettinen, O.S., Stolley, P.D., Knapp, R.C., Leavitt, T., Jr, Watring, W.G., Rosenshein, N.B., Lewis, J.L., Jr, Schottenfeld, D. & Engle, R.L., Jr (1980) Decreased risk of endometrial cancer among oral-contraceptive users. *New Engl. J. Med.*, **303**, 1045–1047

Kaur, J., Ramakrishnan, P.R. & Rajalakshmi, M. (1990) Inhibition of spermatazoa maturation in rhesus monkey by cyproterone acetate. *Contraception*, **42**, 349–359

Kaur, J., Ramakrishnan, P.R. & Rajalakshmi, M. (1992) Effect of cyproterone acetate on structure and function of rhesus monkey reproductive organs. *Anat. Rec.*, **234**, 62–72

Kawashima, K., Nakaura, S., Nagao, S., Tanaka, S., Kawamura, T. & Omori, Y. (1977) Virilizing activities of various steroids in female rat fetuses. *Endocrinol. Jpn.*, **24**, 77–81

Kay, C.R. (1981) Malignant melanoma and oral contraceptives (Letter to the Editor). *Br. J. Cancer*, **44**, 479

Kay, C.R. & Hannaford, P.C. (1988) Breast cancer and the pill—A further report from the Royal College of General Practitioners' oral contraceptive study. *Br. J. Cancer*, **58**, 675–680

Kelsey, J.L., Holford, T.R., White, C., Mayer, E.S., Kilty, S.E. & Acheson, R.M. (1978) Oral contraceptives and breast disease. An epidemiological study. *Am. J. Epidemiol.*, **107**, 236–244

Kelsey, J.L., LiVolsi, V.A., Holford, T.R., Fischer, D.B., Mostow, E.D., Schwartz, P.E., O'Connor, T. & White, C. (1982) A case–control study of cancer of the endometrium. *Am. J. Epidemiol.*, **116**, 333–342

Kennedy, A.R. & Weichselbaum, R.R. (1981) Effects of 17β-estradiol on radiation transformation in vitro; inhibition of effects by protease inhibitors. *Carcinogenesis*, **2**, 67–69

Kennelly, J.J. (1969) The effect of mestranol on canine reproduction. *Biol. Reprod.*, **1**, 282–288

Kerdar, R.S., Baumann, A., Brudny-Klöppel, M., Biere, H., Blode, H. & Kuhnz, W. (1995) Identification of 3α-hydroxy-cyproterone acetate as a metabolite of cyproterone acetate in the bile of female rats and the potential of this and other already known or putative metabolites to form DNA adducts *in vitro*. *Carcinogenesis*, **16**, 1835–1841

Kew, M.C., Song, E., Mohammed, A. & Hodkinson, J. (1990) Contraceptive steroids as a risk factor for hepatocellular carcinoma: A case–control study in South African black women. *Hepatology*, **11**, 298–302

Kiivet, R.A., Bergman, U., Rootslane, L., Rago, L. & Sjoqvist, F. (1998) Drug use in Estonia in 1994–1995: A follow-up from 1989 and comparison with two Nordic countries. *Eur. J. clin. Pharmacol.*, **54**, 119–124

Killinger, J., Hahn, D.W., Phillips, A., Hetyei, N.S. & McGuire, J.L. (1985) The affinity of norgestimate for uterine progestogen receptors and its direct action on the uterus. *Contraception*, **32**, 311–319

King, R.J.B. (1991) Biology of female sex hormone action in relation to contraceptive agents and neoplasia. *Contraception*, **43**, 527–542

Kjaer, S.K., Engholm, G., Dahl, C., Bock, J.E., Lynge, E. & Jensen, O.M. (1993) Case–control study of risk factors for cervical squamous-cell neoplasia in Denmark. III. Role of oral contraceptive use. *Cancer Causes Control*, **4**, 513–519

Kleinman, R.L. (1990) *Hormonal Contraception*, London, IPPF Medical Publications

Kleinman, R.L. (1996) *Directory of Hormonal Contraceptives*, London, IPPF Medical Publications

Kloosterboer, H.J., Vonk-Noordegraaf, C.A. & Turpijn, E.W. (1988) Selectivity in progesterone and androgen receptor binding of progestagens used in oral contraceptives. *Contraception*, **38**, 325–332

Kolonel, L.N., Hankin, J.H., Wilkens, L.R., Fukunaga, F.H. & Hinds, M.W. (1990) An epidemiologic study of thyroid cancer in Hawaii. *Cancer Causes Control*, **1**, 223–234

Kontula, K., Paavonen, T., Luukkainen, T. & Andersson, L.C. (1983) Binding of progestins to the glucocorticoid receptor. Correlation to their glucocorticoid-like effects on *in vitro* functions of human mononuclear leukocytes. *Biochem. Pharmacol.*, **32**, 1511–1518

Koper, N.P., Kiemeney, L.A.L.M., Massuger, L.F.A.G., Thomas, C.M.G., Schijf, C.P.T. & Verbeek, A.L.M. (1996) Ovarian cancer incidence (1989–1991) and mortality (1954–1993) in The Netherlands. *Obstet. Gynecol.*, **88**, 387–393

Kopera, H. (1985) Unintended effects of oral contraceptives. II. Progesterone-caused effects, interactions with drugs. *Wien med. Wochenschr.*, **17**, 415–419 (in German)

van Kordelaar, J.M.G., Vermorken, A.J.M., de Weerd, C.J.M. & van Rossum, J.M. (1975) Interaction of contraceptive progestins and related compounds with the oestrogen receptor. Part II: Effect on (3H)oestradiol binding to the rat uterine receptor *in vitro*. *Acta endocrinol.*, **78**, 165–179

Koumantaki, Y., Tzonou, A., Koumantakis, E., Kaklamani, E., Aravantinos, D. & Trichopoulos, D. (1989) A case–control study of cancer of endometrium in Athens. *Int. J. Cancer*, **43**, 795–799

Koutsky, L.A., Holmes, K.K., Critchlow, C.S., Stevens, C.E., Paavonen, J., Beckmann, A.M., DeRouen, T.A., Galloway, D.A., Vernon, D. & Kiviat, N.B. (1992) A cohort study of the risk of cervical intraepithelial neoplasia grade 2 or 3 in relation to papillomavirus infection. *New Engl. J. Med.*, **327**, 1272–1278

Krebs, O., Schäfer, B., Wolff, T., Oesterle, D., Deml, E., Sund, M. & Favor, J. (1998) The DNA damaging drug cyproterone acetate causes gene mutations and induces glutathione-S-transferase P in the liver of female Big Blue™ transgenic F344 rats. *Carcinogenesis*, **19**, 241–245

Kreitmann, B., Bugat, R. & Bayard, F. (1979) Estrogen and progestin regulation of the progesterone receptor concentration in human endometrium. *J. clin. Endocrinol. Metab.*, **49**, 926–929

Kuhl, H. (1990) Pharmacokinetics of oestrogens and progestogens. *Maturitas*, **12**, 171–197

Kuhl, H., Jung-Hoffmann, C. & Wiegratz, I. (1995) Gestodene-containing contraceptives. *Clin. Obstet. Gynecol.*, **38**, 829–840

Kuhnz, W. & Beier, S. (1994) Comparative progestational and androgenic activity of norgestimate and levonorgestrel in the rat. *Contraception*, **49**, 275–289

Kuhnz, W. & Löfberg, B. (1995) Urinary excretion of 6β-hydroxycortisol in women during treatment with different oral contraceptive formulations. *J. Steroid Biochem. mol. Biol.*, **55**, 129–133

Kuhnz, W., Hümpel, M., Schütt, B., Louton, T., Steinberg, B. & Gansau, C. (1990a) Relative bioavailability of ethinyl estradiol from two different oral contraceptive formulations after single oral administration to 18 women in an intraindividual cross-over design. *Hormone Res.*, **33**, 40–44

Kuhnz, W., Pfeffer, M. & Al-Yacoub, G. (1990b) Protein binding of the contraceptive steroids gestodene, 3-keto-desogestrel and ethinylestradiol in human serum. *J. Steroid Biochem.*, **35**, 313–318

Kuhnz, W., Sostarek, D., Gansau, C. & Louton, T. (1991) Single and multiple administration of a new triphasic oral contraceptive to women: Pharmacokinetics of ethinylestradiol and free and total testosterone levels in serum. *Am. J. Obstet. Gynecol.*, **165**, 596–602

Kuhnz, W., Al-Yacoub, G. & Fuhrmeister, A. (1992) Pharmacokinetics of levonorgestrel and ethinylestradiol in 9 women who received a low-dose oral contraceptive over a treatment period of 3 months and, after a wash-out phase, a single oral administration of the same contraceptive formulation. *Contraception*, **46**, 455–469

Kuhnz, W., Staks, T. & Jütting, G. (1993a) Pharmacokinetics of cyproterone acetate and ethinylestradiol in 15 women who received a combination oral contraceptive during three treatment cycles. *Contraception*, **48**, 557–575

Kuhnz, W., Baumann, A., Staks, T., Dibbelt, L., Knuppen, R. & Jütting, G. (1993b) Pharmacokinetics of gestodene and ethinylestradiol in 14 women during three months of treatment with a new tri-step combination oral contraceptive: Serum protein binding of gestodene and influence of treatment on free and total testosterone levels in the serum. *Contraception*, **48**, 303–322

Kuhnz, W., Staks, T. & Jütting, G. (1994a) Pharmacokinetics of levonorgestrel and ethinylestradiol in 14 women during three months of treatment with a tri-step combination oral contraceptive: Serum protein binding of levonorgestrel and influence of treatment on free and total testosterone levels in the serum. *Contraception*, **50**, 563–579

Kuhnz, W., Blode, H. & Mahler, M. (1994b) Systemic availability of levonorgestrel after single oral administration of a norgestimate-containing combination oral contraceptive to 12 young women. *Contraception*, **49**, 255–263

Kuhnz, W., Fritzemeier, K.H., Hegele-Hartung, C. & Krattenmacher, R. (1995) Comparative progestational activity of norgestimate, levonorgestrel-oxime and levonorgestrel in the rat and binding of these compounds to the progesterone receptor. *Contraception*, **51**, 131–139

Kumar, M.V. & Panda, J.N. (1983) Epididymal histoarchitecture of goats under chronic cyproterone acetate. *Andrologia*, **15**, 193–195

Kumasaka, T., Itoh, E., Watanabe, H., Hoshino, K., Yoshinaka, A. & Masawa, N. (1994) Effects of various forms of progestin on the endometrium of the estrogen-primed, ovariectomized rat. *Endocrine J.*, **41**, 161–169

Kune, G.A., Kune, S. & Watson, L.F. (1990) Oral contraceptive use does not protect against large bowel cancer. *Contraception*, **41**, 19–25

Kwapien, R.P., Giles, R.C., Geil, R.G. & Casey, H.W. (1980) Malignant mammary tumors in beagle dogs dosed with investigational oral contraceptive steroids. *J. natl Cancer Inst.*, **65**, 137–144

Labrie, C., Cusan, L., Plante, M., Lapointe, S. & Labrie, F. (1987) Analysis of the androgenic activity of synthetic 'progestins' currently used for the treatment of prostate cancer. *J. Steroid Biochem.*, **28**, 379–384

Lachnit-Fixson, U. (1996) The role of triphasic levonorgestrel in oral contraception: A review of metabolic and hemostatic effects. *Gynecol. Endocrinol.*, **10**, 207–218

Lammer, E.J. & Cordero, J.F. (1986) Exogenous sex hormone exposure and the risk of major malformations. *J. Am. med. Assoc.*, **255**, 3128–3132

Lande, R.E. (1995) New era for injectables. *Popul. Rep.*, **23**, 1–31

Landgren, B.M., Dada, O., Aedo, A.R., Johannisson, E. & Diczfalusy, E. (1990) Pituitary, ovarian and endometrial effects of 300 micrograms norethisterone and 30 micrograms levonorgestrel administered on cycle days 7 to 10. *Contraception*, **41**, 569–581

Lang, R. & Redmann, U. (1979) Non-mutagenicity of some sex hormones in the Ames *Salmonella/* microsome mutagenicity test. *Mutat. Res.*, **67**, 361–365

Lang, R. & Reimann, R. (1993) Studies for a genotoxic potential of some endogenous and exogenous sex steroids. *Environ. mol. Mutag.*, **21**, 272–304

Larsson-Cohn, U. (1970) Contraceptive treatment with low doses of gestagens. *Acta endocrinol.*, **144** (Suppl.), 7–46

La Vecchia, C., Decarli, A., Fasoli, M., Franceschi, S., Gentile, A., Negri, E., Parazzini, F. & Tognoni, G. (1986) Oral contraceptives and cancers of the breast and of the female genital tract. Interim results from a case–control study. *Br. J. Cancer*, **54**, 311–317

La Vecchia, C., Parazzini, F., Negri, E., Boyle, P., Gentile, A., Decarli, A. & Franceschi, S. (1989) Breast cancer and combined oral contraceptives: An Italian case–control study. *Eur. J. Cancer clin. Oncol.*, **25**, 1613–1618

La Vecchia, C., Lucchini, F., Negri, E., Boyle, P., Maisonneuve, P. & Levi, F. (1992) Trends of cancer mortality in Europe, 1955–1989: III. Breast and genital sites. *Eur. J. Cancer*, **28A**, 927–998

La Vecchia, C., D'Avanzo, B., Franceschi, S., Negri, E., Parazzini, F. & Decarli, A. (1994) Menstrual and reproductive factors and gastric-cancer risk in women. *Int. J. Cancer*, **59**, 761–764

La Vecchia, C., Negri, E., Franceschi, S., Talamini, R., Amadori, D., Filiberti, R., Conti, E., Montella, M., Veronesi, A., Parazzini, F., Ferraroni, M. & Decarli, A. (1995) Oral contraceptives and breast cancer: A cooperative Italian study. *Int. J. Cancer*, **60**, 163–167

La Vecchia, C., Tavani, A., Franceschi, S. & Parazzini, F. (1996) Oral contraceptives and cancer. *Drug Saf.*, **14**, 260–272

La Vecchia, C., Negri, E., Levi, F., Decarli, A. & Boyle, P. (1998) Cancer mortality in Europe: Effects of age, cohort of birth and period of death. *Eur. J. Cancer*, **34**, 118–141

Lax, E.R. (1987) Mechanisms of physiological and pharmacological sex hormone action on the mammalian liver. *J. Steroid Biochem.*, **27**, 1119–1128

Lax, E.R., Baumann, P. & Schriefers, H. (1984) Changes in the activities of microsomal enzymes involved in hepatic steroid metabolism in the rat after administration of androgenic, estrogenic, progestational, anabolic and catatoxic steroids. *Biochem. Pharmacol.*, **33**, 1235–1241

Lê, M.G., Cabanes, P.A., Desvignes, V., Chanteau, M.F., Mlika, N. & Avril, M.F. (1992) Oral contraceptive use and risk of cutaneous malignant melanoma in a case–control study of French women. *Cancer Causes Control*, **3**, 199–205

Lee, G.-H., Nomura, K. & Kitagawa, T. (1989) Comparative study of diethylnitrosamine-initiated two-stage hepatocarcinogenesis in C3H, C57BL and BALB mice promoted by various hepatopromoters. *Carcinogenesis*, **10**, 2227–2230

Lees, A.W., Burns, P.E. & Grace, M. (1978) Oral contraceptives and breast disease in premenopausal northern Albertan women. *Int. J. Cancer*, **22**, 700–707

Lejeune, J. & Prieur, M. (1979) Oral contraceptives and trisomy 21. A retrospective study of 730 cases. *Ann. Génét.*, **22**, 61–66 (in French)

Lemus, A.E., Vilchis, F., Damsky, R., Chavez, B.A., Garcia, G.A., Grillasca, I. & Perez-Palacios, G. (1992) Mechanism of action of levonorgestrel: In vitro metabolism and specific interactions with steroid receptors in target organs. *J. Steroid. Biochem. mol. Biol.*, **41**, 881–890

Lepage, F. & Gueguen, J. (1968) Results of a study on the possible teratogenic effects of chlormadinone and its possible action on the course of pregnancy. *Bull. Soc. fed. Gynecol. Obstet.*, **20** (Suppl.), 313–314 (in French)

Levi, F., Gutzwiller, F., Decarli, A. & La Vecchia, C. (1987) Oral contraceptive use and breast and ovarian cancer mortality in Switzerland. *J. Epidemiol. Community Health*, **41**, 267–268

Levi, F., La Vecchia, C., Gulie, C., Negri, E., Monnier, V., Franceschi, S., Delaloye, J.-F. & De Grandi, P. (1991) Oral contraceptives and the risk of endometrial cancer. *Cancer Causes Control*, **2**, 99–103

Levi, F., Franceschi, S., Gulie, C., Negri, E. & La Vecchia, C. (1993) Female thyroid cancer: The role of reproductive and hormonal factors in Switzerland. *Oncology*, **50**, 309–315

Levi, F., Lucchini, F., Pasche, C. & La Vecchia, C. (1996) Oral contraceptives, menopausal hormone replacement treatment and breast cancer risk. *Eur. J. Cancer Prev.*, **5**, 295–266

Lew, R.A., Sober, A.J., Cook, N., Marvell, R. & Fitzpatrick, T.B. (1983) Sun exposure habits in patients with cutaneous melanoma: A case–control study. *J. Dermatol. surg. Oncol.*, **9**, 981–986

Ley, C., Bauer, H.M., Reingold, A., Schiffman, M.H., Chamber, J.C., Tashiro, C.J. & Manos, M.M. (1991) Determinants of genital human papillomavirus infection in young women. *J. natl Cancer Inst.*, **83**, 997–1003

Li, J.J. & Li, S.A. (1984) Estrogen-induced tumorigenesis in hamsters: Roles for hormonal and carcinogenic activity. *Arch. Toxicol.*, **55**, 110–118

Li, J.J., Gonzalez, A., Banerjee, S., Banerjee, S.K. & Li, S.A. (1993) Estrogen carcinogenesis in the hamster kidney: Role of cytotoxicity and cell proliferation. *Environ. Health Perspectives*, **101** (Suppl, 5), 259–264

Liehr, J.G., Avitts, T.A., Randerath, E. & Randerath, K. (1986) Estrogen-induced endogenous DNA adduction: Possible mechanism of hormonal cancer. *Proc. natl Acad. Sci. USA*, **83**, 5301–5305

Liehr, J.G., Purdy, R.H., Baran, J.S., Nutting, E.F., Colton, F., Randerath, E. & Randerath, K. (1987a) Correlation of aromatic hydroxylation of 11β-substituted estrogens with morphological transformation *in vitro* but not with *in vivo* tumour induction by these hormones. *Cancer Res.*, **47**, 2583–2588

Liehr, J.G., Hall, E.R., Avitts, T.A., Randerath, E. & Randerath, K. (1987b) Localisation of estrogen-induced DNA adducts and cytochrome P-450 activity at the site of renal carcinogenesis in the hamster kidney. *Cancer Res.*, **47**, 2156–2159

Lindblad, P., Mellemgaard, A., Schlehofer, B., Adami, H.-O., McCredie, M., McLaughlin, J.K. & Mandel, J.S. (1995) International renal-cell cancer study. V. Reproductive factors, gynecologic operations and exogenous hormones. *Int. J. Cancer*, **61**, 192–198

Lipnick, R.J., Buring, J.E., Hennekens, C.H., Rosner, B., Willett, W., Bain, C., Stampfer, M.J., Colditz, G.A., Peto, R. & Speizer, F.E. (1986) Oral contraceptives and breast cancer. A prospective cohort study. *J. Am. med. Assoc.*, **255**, 58–61

Lippman, M., Bolan, G. & Huff, K. (1976) The effects of androgens and antiandrogens on hormone-responsive human breast cancer in long-term tissue culture. *Cancer Res.*, **36**, 4610–4618

Lipworth, L., Katsouyanni, K., Stuver, S., Samoli, E., Hankinson, S.E. & Trichopolous, D. (1995) Oral contraceptives, menopausal estrogens, and the risk of breast cancer: A case–control study in Greece. *Int. J. Cancer*, **62**, 548–551

Liu, T., Soong, S., Alvarez, R.D. & Butterworth, C.E., Jr (1995) A longitudinal analysis of human papillomavirus 16 infection, nutritional status, and cervical dysplasia progression. *Cancer Epidemiol. Biomarkers Prev.*, **4**, 373–380

Logan, J., Diamond, M.P., Lavy, G. & DeCherney, A.H. (1989) Effect of norgestrel on development of mouse pre-embryos. *Contraception*, **39**, 555–561

Lohiya, N.K. & Arya, M. (1981) Oestrogenic activity of cyproterone acetate in female mice. *Endokrinologie*, **78**, 21–27

Lohiya, N.K., Sharma, O.P., Sharma, R.C. & Sharma, R.S. (1987) Reversible sterility by cyproterone acetate plus testosterone enanthate in langur monkey with maintenance of libido. *Biomed. biochim. Acta*, **46**, 259–266

Lu, L.W., Liehr, J.G., Sirbasku, D.A., Randerath, E. & Randerath, K. (1988) Hypomethylation of DNA in estrogen-induced and -dependent hamster kidney tumours. *Carcinogenesis*, **9**, 925–929

Lubahn, D.B., McCarty, K.S., Jr & McCarty, K.S., Sr (1985) Electrophoretic characterization of purified bovine, porcine, murine, rat, and human uterine estrogen receptors. *J. biol. Chem.*, **260**, 2515–2526

Lumb, G., Mitchell, L. & DeLaIglesia, F.A. (1985) Regression of pathologic changes induced by the long-term administration of contraceptive steroids to rodents. *Toxicol. Pathol.*, **13**, 283–295

Lund, E., Meirik, O., Adami, H.-O., Bergström, R., Christoffersen, T. & Bergsjøss, P. (1989) Oral contraceptive use and premenopausal breast cancer in Sweden and Norway: Possible effects of different patterns of use. *Int. J. Epidemiol.*, **18**, 527–532

Lundgren, S., Lønning, P.E., Aakvaag, A. & Kvinnsland, S. (1990) Influence of aminoglutethimide on the metabolism of medroxyprogesterone acetate and megestrol acetate in postmenopausal patients with advanced breast cancer. *Cancer Chemother. Pharmacol.*, **27**, 101–105

Luthy, I.A., Begin, D.J. & Labrie, F. (1988) Androgenic activity of synthetic progestins and spironolactone in androgen-sensitive mouse mammary carcinoma (Shionogi) cells in culture. *J. Steroid Biochem.*, **31**, 845–852

Lyon, F.A. (1975) The development of adenocarcinoma of the endometrium in young women receiving long-term sequential oral contraception. *Am. J. Obstet. Gynecol.*, **123**, 299–301

Lyon, F.A. & Frisch, M.J. (1976) Endometrial abnormalities occurring in young women on long-term sequential oral contraceptives. *Obstet. Gynecol.*, **47**, 639–643

Madden, S. & Back, D.J. (1991) Metabolism of norgestimate by human gastrointestinal mucosa and liver microsomes *in vitro*. *J. Steroid Biochem. mol. Biol.*, **38**, 497–503

Madden, S., Back, D.J. & Orme, M.L'E. (1990) Metabolism of the contraceptive steroid desogestrel by human liver *in vitro*. *J. Steroid Biochem.*, **35**, 281–288

Málková, J., Michalová, K., Pribyl, T. & Schreiber, V. (1977) Chromosomal changes in rat pituitary and bone marrow induced by long-term estrogen administration. *Neoplasma*, **24**, 277–284

Malone, K.E. (1991) *Oral Contraceptives and Breast Cancer. A Review of the Epidemiological Evidence with an Emphasis on Younger Women*, Washington DC, National Academy Press, National Academy of Sciences

Malone, K.E., Daling, J.R. & Weiss, N.S. (1993) Oral contraceptives in relation to breast cancer. *Epidemiol. Rev.*, **15**, 80–97

Mamber, S.W., Bryson, V. & Katz, S.E. (1983) The *Escherichia coli* WP2/WP100 rec assay for detection of potential chemical carcinogens. *Mutat. Res.*, **119**, 135–144

Mant, J.W.F. & Vessey, M.P. (1995) Trends in mortality from primary liver cancer in England and Wales 1975–92: Influence of oral contraceptives. *Br. J. Cancer*, **72**, 800–803

Markiewicz, L. & Gurpide, E. (1994) Estrogenic and progestagenic activities coexisting in steroidal drugs: Quantitative evaluation by *in vitro* bioassays with human cells. *J. Steroid Biochem. mol. Biol.*, **48**, 89–94

Markiewicz, L., Hochberg, R.B. & Gurpide, E. (1992) Intrinsic estrogenicity of some progestagenic drugs. *J. Steroid Biochem. mol. Biol.*, **41**, 53–58

Marr, W., Elder, M.G. & Lim, L. (1980) The effects of oestrogens and progesterone on oestrogen receptors in female rat liver. *Biochem. J.*, **190**, 563–570

Martelli, A., Mattioli, F., Fazio, S., Andrae, U. & Brambilla, G. (1995) DNA repair synthesis and DNA fragmentation in primary cultures of human and rat hepatocytes exposed to cyproterone acetate. *Carcinogenesis*, **16**, 1265–1269

Martelli, A., Mattioli, F., Ghia, M., Mereto, E. & Brambilla, G. (1996a) Comparative study of DNA repair induced by cyproterone acetate, chlormadinone acetate, and megestrol acetate in primary cultures of human and rat hepatocytes. *Carcinogenesis*, **17**, 1153–1156

Martelli, A., Campart, G.B., Ghia, M., Allevena, A., Mereto, E. & Brambilla, G. (1996b) Induction of micronuclei and initiation of enzyme-altered foci in the liver of female rats treated with cyproterone acetate, chlormadinone acetate or megestrol acetate. *Carcinogenesis*, **17**, 551–554

Martinez, M.E., Grodstein, F., Giovannucci, E., Colditz, G.A., Speizer, F.E., Hennekens, C., Rosner, B., Willett, W.C. & Stampfer, M.J. (1997) A prospective study of reproductive factors, oral contraceptive use, and risk of colorectal cancer. *Cancer Epidemiol. Biomarkers Prev.*, **6**, 1–5

Martínez-Frías, M.-L., Rodríguez-Pinilla, E., Bermejo, E. & Prieto, L. (1998) Prenatal exposure to sex hormones: A case–control study. *Teratology*, **57**, 8–12

Maudelonde, T., Lavaud, P., Salazar, G., Laffargue, F. & Rochefort, H. (1991) Progestin treatment depresses estrogen receptor but not cathepsin D levels in needle aspirates of benign breast disease. *Breast Cancer Res. Treat.*, **19**, 95–102

Mayberry, R.M. & Stoddard-Wright, C. (1992) Breast cancer risk factors among black and white women: Similarities and differences. *Am. J. Epidemiol.*, **136**, 1445–1456

Mayol, X., Perez-Tomas, R., Cullere, X., Romero, A., Estadella, M.D. & Domingo, J. (1991) Cell proliferation and tumour promotion by ethinyl estradiol in rat hepatocarcinogenesis. *Carcinogenesis*, **12**, 1133–1136

McClamrock, H.D. & Adashi, E.Y. (1993) Pharmacokinetics of desogestrel. *Am. J. Obstet. Gynecol.*, **168**, 1021–1028

McGuire, J.L., Phillips, A., Hahn, D.W., Tolman, E.L., Flor, S. & Kafrissen, M.E. (1990) Pharmacologic and pharmacokinetic characteristics of norgestimate and its metabolites. *Am. J. Obstet. Gynecol.*, **163**, 2127–2131

McLaughlin, L. (1982) *The Pill, John Rock and the Church*, Toronto, Little, Brown & Co., pp. 138–145

McPherson, K., Vessey, M.P., Neil, A., Doll, R., Jones, L. & Roberts, M. (1987) Early oral contraceptive use and breast cancer: Results of another case–control study. *Br. J. Cancer*, **56**, 653–660

McTiernan, A.M., Weiss, N.S. & Daling, J.R. (1984) Incidence of thyroid cancer in women in relation to reproductive and hormonal factors. *Am. J. Epidemiol.*, **120**, 423–435

Meirik, O., Lund, E., Adami, H.-O., Bergström, R., Christoffersen, T. & Bergsjö, P. (1986) Oral contraceptive use and breast cancer in young women. A joint national case–control study in Sweden and Norway. *Lancet*, **ii**, 650–654

Meirik, O., Farley, T.M.M., Lund, E., Adami, H.-O., Christoffersen, T. & Bergsjö, P. (1989) Breast cancer and oral contraceptives: Patterns of risk among parous and nulliparous women—further analysis of the Swedish–Norwegian material. *Contraception*, **39**, 471–475

Menegazzi, M., Carcereri-De Prati, A., Suzuki, H., Shinozuka, H., Pibiri, M., Piga, R., Columbano, A. & Ledda-Columbano, G.M. (1997) Liver cell proliferation induced by nafenopin and cyproterone acetate is not associated with increases in activation of transcription factors NF-κB and AP-1 or with expression of tumor necrosis factor α. *Hepatology*, **25**, 585–592

Meriggiola, M.C., Bremner, W.J., Paulsen, C.A., Valdiserri, A., Incorvaia, L., Motta, R., Pavani, A., Capelli, M. & Flamigni, C. (1996) A combined regimen of cyproterone acetate and testosterone enanthate as a potentially highly effective male contraceptive. *J. clin. Endocrinol. Metab.*, **81**, 3018–3023

Miller, D.R., Rosenberg, L., Kaufman, D.W., Schottenfeld, D., Stolley, P.D. & Shapiro, S. (1986) Breast cancer risk in relation to early oral contraceptive use. *Obstet. Gynecol.*, **68**, 863–868

Miller, D.R., Rosenberg, L., Kaufman, D.W., Stolley, P., Warshauer, M.E. & Shapiro, S. (1989) Breast cancer before age 45 and oral contraceptive use: New findings. *Am. J. Epidemiol.*, **129**, 269–280

Mills, P.K., Beeson, L., Phillips, R.L. & Fraser, G.E. (1989) Prospective study of exogenous hormone use and breast cancer in Seventh-day Adventists. *Cancer*, **64**, 591–597

Misdorp, W. (1991) Progestagens and mammary tumors in dogs and cats. *Acta endocrinol.*, **125**, 27–31

Mitsumori, K., Furukawa, F., Sato, M., Yoshimura, H., Imazawa, T., Nishikawa, A. & Takahashi, M. (1994) Promoting effects of ethinyl estradiol on development of renal proliferative lesions induced by N-nitrosobis(2-oxopropyl)amine in female Syrian golden hamsters. *Cancer Res. clin. Oncol.*, **120**, 131–136

Molina, R., Thomas, D.B., Dabancens, A., Lopez, J., Ray, R.M., Martinez, L. & Salas, O. (1988) Oral contraceptives and cervical carcinoma in situ in Chile. *Cancer Res.*, **48**, 1011–1015

Moltz, L., Römmler, A., Post, K., Schwartz, U. & Hammerstein, J. (1980) Medium dose cyproterone acetate (CPA): Effects on hormone secretion and on spermatogenesis in men. *Contraception*, **21**, 393–413

Morabia, A., Szklo, M., Stewart, W., Schuman, L. & Thomas, D.B. (1993) Consistent lack of association between breast cancer and oral contraceptives using either hospital or neighborhood controls. *Prev. Med.*, **22**, 178–186

Mori, T., Cui, L., Satoru, K., Takahashi, S., Imaida, K., Iwasaki, S., Ito, N. & Shirai, T. (1996) Direct effects of testosterone, dihydrotosterone and estrogen on 3,2'-dimethyl-4-aminobiphenol-induced prostate carcinogenesis in castrated F344 rats. *Jpn. J. Cancer Res.*, **7**, 570–574

Moser, G.J., Wolf, D.C., Harden, R., Standeven, A.M., Mills, J., Jirtle, R.L. & Goldsworthy, T.L. (1996) Cell proliferation and regulation of negative growth factors in mouse liver foci. *Carcinogenesis*, **17**, 1835–1840

Muechler, E.K. & Kohler, D. (1980) Properties of the estrogen receptor in the human oviduct and its interaction with ethinylestradiol and mestranol *in vitro*. *J. clin. Endocrinol. Metab.*, **51**, 962–967

Muñoz, N., Bosch, F.X., de Sanjosé, S., Vergara, A., del Moral, A., Muñoz, M.T., Tafur, L., Gili, M., Izarzugaza, I., Viladiu, P., Navarro, C., de Ruiz, P.A., Aristizabal, N., Santamaria, M., Orfila, J., Daniel, R.W., Guerrero, E. & Shah, K.V. (1993) Risk factors for cervical intraepithelial neoplasia grade III/carcinoma in situ in Spain and Colombia. *Cancer Epidemiol. Biomarkers Prev.*, **2**, 423–431

Muñoz, N., Kato, I., Bosch, F.X., Eluf-Neto, J., de Sanjosé, S., Ascunce, N., Gili, M., Izarzugaza, I., Viladiu, P., Tormo, M.-J., Moreo, P., Gonzalez, L.C., Tafur, L., Walboomers, J.M.M. & Shah, K.V. (1996) Risk factors for HPV DNA detection in middle-aged women. *Sex. transm. Dis.*, **23**, 504–510

Narod, S.A., Risch, H., Moslehi, R., Dorum, A., Neuhausen, S., Olsson, H., Provencher, D., Radice, P., Evans, G., Bishop, S., Brunet, J.S. & Ponder, B.A. (1998) Oral contraceptives and the risk of hereditary ovarian cancer. Hereditary Ovarian Cancer Clinical Study Group. *New Engl. J. Med.*, **339**, 424–428

Negri, E., La Vecchia, C., Parazzini, F., Savoldelli, R., Gentile, A., D'Avanzo, B., Gramenzi, A. & Franceschi, S. (1989) Reproductive and menstrual factors and risk of colorectal cancer. *Cancer Res.*, **49**, 7158–7161

Negrini, B.P., Schiffman, M.H., Kurman, R.J., Barnes, W., Lannom, L., Malley, K., Brinton, L.A., Delgado, G., Jones, S., Tchabo, J.-G. & Lancaster, W.D. (1990) Oral contraceptive use, human papillomavirus infection, and risk of early cytological abnormalities of the cervix. *Cancer Res.*, **50**, 4670–4675

Neuberger, J., Forman, D., Doll, R. & Williams, R. (1986) Oral contraceptives and hepatocellular carcinoma. *Br. med. J.*, **292**, 1355–1357

Neumann, F., Elger, W. & Kramer, M. (1966) Development of a vagina in male rats by inhibiting androgen receptors through an antiandrogen during the critical phase of organogenesis. *Endocrinology*, **78**, 628–632

Neumann, I., Thierau, D., Andrae, U., Greim, H. & Schwartz, L.R. (1992) Cyproterone acetate induces DNA damage in cultured rat hepatocytes and preferentially stimulates DNA synthesis in γ-glutamyltranspeptidase-positive cells. *Carcinogenesis*, **13**, 373–378

Newcomb, P.A., Longnecker, M.P., Storer, B.E., Mittendorf, R., Baron, J., Clapp, R.W., Trentham-Dietz, A. & Willett, W.C. (1996) Recent oral contraceptive use and risk of breast cancer (United States). *Cancer Causes Control*, **7**, 525–532

New Zealand Contraception and Health Study Group (1994) Risk of cervical dysplasia in users of oral contraceptives, intrauterine devices or depot-medroxyprogesterone acetate. *Contraception*, **50**, 431–441

Ngelangel, C., Muñoz, N., Bosch, F.X., Limson, G.M., Festin, M.R., Deacon, J., Jacobs, M.V., Santamaria, M., Meijer, C.J.L.M. & Walboomers, J.M.M. (1998) Causes of cervical cancer in the Philippines: A case–control study. *J. natl Cancer Inst.*, **90**, 43–49

Ni, N. & Yager, J.D. (1994a) Comitogenic effects of estrogens on DNA synthesis induced by various growth factors in cultured female rat hepatocytes. *Hepatology*, **19**, 183–192

Ni, N. & Yager, J.D. (1994b) The co-mitogenic effects of various estrogens for TGF-α-induced DNA synthesis in cultured female rat hepatocytes. *Cancer Lett.*, **84**, 133–140

Nielsen, S.T., Conaty, J.M. & DiPasquale, G. (1987) Progesterone receptor of adult rabbit lung. *Pharmacology*, **35**, 217–226

Nilsson, B. & von Schoultz, B. (1989) Binding of levonorgestrel, norethisterone and desogestrel to human sex hormone binding globulin and influence on free testosterone levels. *Gynecol. obstet. Invest.*, **27**, 151–154

Nutter, L.M., Wu, Y., Ngo, E.O., Sierra, E.E., Gutierrez, P.L. & Abul-Hajj, Y.J. (1994) An o-quinone form of estrogen produces free radicals in human breast cancer cells: Correlation with DNA damage. *Chem. Res. Toxicol.*, **7**, 23–28

Oberhammer, F., Nagy, P., Tiefenbacher, R., Fröschl, G., Bouzahzah, B., Thorgeirsson, S.S. & Carr, B. (1996) The antiandrogen cyproterone acetate induces synthesis of transforming growth factor β1 in the parenchymal cells of the liver accompanied by an enhanced sensitivity to undergo apoptosis and necrosis without inflammation. *Hepatology*, **23**, 329–337

Ochs, H., Düsterberg, B., Günzel, P. & Schulte-Hermann, R. (1986) Effect of tumor promoting contraceptive steroids on growth and drug metabolizing enzymes in rat liver. *Cancer Res.*, **46**, 1224–1232

Odlind, V., Weiner, E., Victor, A. & Johansson, E.D.B. (1980) Effects on sex hormone binding globulin of different oral contraceptives containing norethisterone and lynestrenol. *Br. J. Obstet. Gynaecol.*, **87**, 416–421

Ogawa, T., Higashi, S., Kawarada, Y. & Mizumoto, R. (1995) Role of reactive oxygen in synthetic estrogen induction of hepatocellular carcinomas in rats and preventive effect of vitamins. *Carcinogenesis*, **16**, 831–836

Olsson, H. (1989) Oral contraceptives and breast cancer. A review. *Acta oncol.*, **6**, 849–863

Olsson, H., Möller, T.R. & Ranstam, J. (1989) Early oral contraceptive use and breast cancer among premenopausal women: Final report from a study in southern Sweden. *J. natl Cancer Inst.*, **81**, 1000–1004

Olsson, H., Borg, A., Fermö, M., Möller, T.R. & Ranstam, J. (1991a) Early oral contraceptive use and premenopausal breast cancer—a review of studies performed in southern Sweden. *Cancer Detect. Prev.*, **15**, 265–271

Olsson, H., Ranstam, J., Baldetorp, B., Ewers, S.-B., Fernö, M., Killander, D. & Sigurdsson, H. (1991b) Proliferation and DNA ploidy in malignant breast tumours in relation to early oral contraceptive use and early abortions. *Cancer*, **67**, 1285–1290

Olsson, H., Borg, A., Fernö, M., Ranstam, J. & Sigurdsson, H. (1991c) Her-2/neu and INT2 proto-oncogene amplification in malignant breast tumours in relation to reproductive factors and exposure to exogenous hormones. *J. natl Cancer Inst.*, **83**, 1483–1487

Olsson, H., Jernström, H., Alm, P., Kreipe, H., Ingvar, C., Jönsson, P.-E. & Rydén, S. (1996) Proliferation of the breast epithelium in relation to menstrual cycle phase, hormonal use and reproductive factors. *Breast Cancer Res. Treat.*, **40**, 187–196

Orme, M.L'E., Back, D.J. & Breckenridge, A.M. (1983) Clinical pharmacokinetics of oral contraceptive steroids. *Clin. Pharmacokin.*, **8**, 95–136

Ory, H., Cole, P., MacMahon, B. & Hoover, R. (1976) Oral contraceptives and reduced risk of benign breast diseases. *New Engl. J. Med.*, **294**, 419–422

Østerlind, A., Tucker, M.A., Stone, B.J. & Jensen, O.M. (1988) The Danish case–control study of cutaneous malignant melanoma. III. Hormonal and reproductive factors in women. *Int. J. Cancer*, **42**, 821–824

Paffenbarger, R.S., Jr, Fasal, E., Simmons, M.E. & Kampert, J.B. (1977) Cancer risk as related to use of oral contraceptives during fertile years. *Cancer*, **39**, 1887–1891

Palmer, J.R., Rosenberg, L., Kaufman, D.W., Warshauer, M.E., Stolley, P. & Shapiro, S. (1989) Oral contraceptive use and liver cancer. *Am. J. Epidemiol.*, **130**, 878–882

Palmer, J.R., Rosenberg, L., Strom, B.L., Harlap, S., Zauber, A.G., Warshauer, E.M. & Shapiro, S. (1992) Oral contraceptive use and risk of cutaneous malignant melanoma. *Cancer Causes Control*, **3**, 547–554

Palmer, J.R., Rosenberg, L., Rao, R.S., Strom, B.L., Warshauer, M.E., Harlap, S., Zauber, A. & Shapiro, S. (1995) Oral contraceptive use and breast cancer risk among African–American women. *Cancer Causes Control*, **6**, 321–331

Panda, J.N. & Jindal, S.K. (1982) Effect of chronic use of cyproterone acetate on the epididymis of goat. *Andrologia*, **14**, 397–402

Parádi, E. (1981) Mutagenicity of some contraceptive drugs in *Drosophila melanogaster*. *Mutat. Res.*, **88**, 175–178

Parazzini, F., La Vecchia, C., Negri, E., Fasoli, M. & Cecchetti, G. (1988) Risk factors for adenocarcinoma of the cervix: A case–control study. *Br. J. Cancer*, **57**, 201–204

Parazzini, F., La Vecchia, C., Franceschi, S., Negri, E. & Cecchetti, G. (1989) Risk factors for endometrioid, mucinous and serous benign ovarian cysts. *Int. J. Cancer*, **18**, 108–112

Parazzini, F., La Vecchia, C., Negri, E. & Maggi, R. (1990) Oral contraceptive use and invasive cervical cancer. *Int. J. Epidemiol.*, **19**, 259–263

Parazzini, F., La Vecchia, C., Negri, E., Bocciolone, L., Fedele, L. & Franceschi, S. (1991a) Oral contraceptives use and the risk of ovarian cancer: An Italian case–control study. *Eur. J. Cancer*, **27**, 594–598

Parazzini, F., Restelli, C., La Vecchia, C., Negri, E., Chiari, S., Maggi, R. & Mangioni, C. (1991b) Risk factors for epithelial ovarian tumours of borderline malignancy. *Int. J. Epidemiol.*, **20**, 871–877

Parazzini, F., Franceschi, S., La Vecchia, C. & Fasoli, M. (1991c) The epidemiology of ovarian cancer. *Gynecol. Oncol.*, **43**, 9–23

Parazzini, F., La Vecchia, C., Negri, E., Fedele, L., Franceschi, S. & Gallotta, L. (1992) Risk factors for cervical intraepithelial neoplasia. *Cancer*, **69**, 2276–2282

Parazzini, F., La Vecchia, C., Negri, E., Moroni, S. & Villa, A. (1995) Risk factors for benign ovarian teratomas. *Br. J. Cancer*, **71**, 644–646

Pardthaisong, T., Gray, R.H., McDaniel, E.B. & Chandacham, A. (1988) Steroid contraceptive use and pregnancy outcome. *Teratology*, **38**, 51–58

Parkin, D.M., Srivatanakul, P., Khlat, M., Chenvidhya, D., Chotiwan, P., Insiripong, S., L'Abbé, K.A. & Wild, C.P. (1991) Liver cancer in Thailand. I. A case–control study of cholangio-carcinoma. *Int. J. Cancer*, **48**, 323–328

Parzefall, W., Monschau, P. & Schulte-Hermann, R. (1989) Induction by cyproterone acetate of DNA synthesis and mitosis in primary cultures of adult rat hepatocytes in serum free medium. *Arch. Toxicol.*, **63**, 456–461

Parzefall, W., Erber, E., Sedivy, R. & Schulte-Hermann, R. (1991) Testing for induction of DNA synthesis in human hepatocyte primary cultures by rat liver tumor promoters. *Cancer Res.*, **51**, 1143–1147

Pasapera, A.M., Cerbón, M.A., Castro, I., Gutiérrez, R., Camacho-Arroyo, I., García, G.A. & Pérez-Palacios, G. (1995) Norethisterone metabolites modulate the uteroglobin and progesterone receptor gene expression in prepubertal rabbits. *Biol. Reprod.*, **52**, 426–432

Pater, A., Bayatpour, M. & Pater, M.M. (1990) Oncogenic transformation by human papilloma virus type 16 deoxyribonucleic acid in the presence of progesterone or progestins from oral contraceptives. *Am. J. Obstet. Gynecol.*, **162**, 1099–1103

Paul, C., Skegg, D.C.G., Spears, G.F.S. & Kaldor, J.M. (1986) Oral contraceptives and breast cancer: A national study. *Br. med. J.*, **293**, 723–726

Paul, C., Skegg, D.C.G. & Spears, G.F.S. (1990) Oral contraceptives and risk of breast cancer. *Int. J. Cancer*, **46**, 366–373

Paul, C., Skegg, D.C.G. & Spears, G.F.S. (1995) Oral contraceptive use and risk of breast cancer in older women (New Zealand). *Cancer Causes Control*, **6**, 485–491

Peek, M.J., Markham, R. & Fraser, I.S. (1995) The effects of natural and synthetic sex steroids on human decidual endothelial cell proliferation. *Hum. Reprod.*, **10**, 2238–2243

Peritz, E., Ramcharan, S., Frank, J., Brown, W.L., Huang, S. & Ray, R. (1977) The incidence of cervical cancer and duration of oral contraceptive use. *Am. J. Epidemiol.*, **106**, 462–469

Persson, E., Einhorn, N. & Pettersson, F. (1987) A case–control study of oral contraceptive use in women with adenocarcinoma of the uterine cervix. *Eur. J. Obstet. Gynecol. reprod. Biol.*, **26**, 85–90

Persson, I., Schmidt, M., Adami, H.O., Bergstrom, R., Pettersson, B. & Sparen, P. (1990) Trends in endometrial cancer incidence and mortality in Sweden, 1960–84. *Cancer Causes Control*, **1**, 201–208

Peter, H., Jung, R., Bolt, H.M. & Oesch, F. (1981) Norethisterone-4β,5-oxide and laevonorgestrel-4β,5-oxide: Formation in rat liver microsomal incubations and interference with microsomal epoxide hydrolase and cytoplasmic glutathione S-transferase. *J. Steroid Biochem.*, **14**, 83–90

Peters, R.K., Chao, A. Mack, T.M., Thomas, D., Bernstein, L. & Henderson, B.E. (1986a) Increased frequency of adenocarcinoma of the uterine cervix in young women in Los Angeles County. *J. natl Cancer Inst.*, **76**, 423–428

Peters, R.K., Thomas, D., Hagan, D.G., Mack, T.M. & Henderson, B.E. (1986b) Risk factors for invasive cervical cancer among Latinas and non-Latinas in Los Angeles County. *J. natl Cancer Inst.*, **77**, 1063–1077

Peters, R.K., Pike, M.C., Chang, W.W.L. & Mack, T.M. (1990) Reproductive factors and colon cancers. *Br. J. Cancer*, **61**, 741–748

Pettersson, B., Adami, H.O., Bergstrom, R. & Johansson, E.D. (1986) Menstruation span—A time-limited risk factor for endometrial carcinoma. *Acta obstet. gynecol. scand.*, **65**, 247–255

Phai, N.V., Knodel, J., Cam, M.V. & Xuyen, H. (1996) Fertility and family planning in Vietnam: Evidence from the 1994 inter-censal demographic survey. *Stud. Fam. Plann.*, **27**, 1–17

Phillips, A., Hahn, D.W., Klimek, S. & McGuire, J.L. (1987) A comparison of the potencies and activities of progestogens used in contraceptives. *Contraception*, **36**, 181–192

Phillips, A., Demarest, K., Hahn, D.W., Wong, F. & McGuire, J.L. (1990) Progestational and androgenic receptor binding affinities and *in vivo* activities of norgestimate and other progestins. *Contraception*, **41**, 399–410

Phillips, A., Hahn, D.W. & McGuire, J.L. (1992) Preclinical evaluation of norgestimate, a progestin with minimal androgenic activity. *Am. J. Obstet. Gynecol.*, **167**, 1191–1196

Pike, M.C., Henderson, B.E., Casagrande, J.T., Rosario, I. & Gray, G.E. (1981) Oral contraceptive use and early abortion as risk factors for breast cancer in young women. *Br. J. Cancer*, **43**, 72–76

Pike, M.C., Henderson, B.E., Krailo, M.D., Duke, A. & Roy, S. (1983) Breast cancer in young women and use of oral contraceptives: Possible modifying effect of formulations and age at use. *Lancet*, **ii**, 926–929

Pinto, M.R. (1986) Possible effects of hormonal contraceptives on human mitotic chromosomes. *Mutat. Res.*, **169**, 149-157

Piper, J.M. & Kennedy, D.L. (1987) Oral contraceptives in the United States: Trends in content and potency. *Int. J. Epidemiol.*, **16**, 215–221

Plante, M., Lapointe, S. & Labrie, F. (1988) Stimulatory effect of synthetic progestins currently used for the treatment of prostate cancer on growth of the androgen-sensitive Shionogi tumor in mice. *J. Steroid Biochem.*, **31**, 61–64

Polednak, A.P. (1985) Exogenous female sex hormones and birth defects. *Public Health Rev.*, **13**, 89–114

Pollow, K., Juchem, M., Grill, H.J., Elger, W., Beier, S., Schmidt-Gollwitzer, K. & Manz, B. (1990) Lack of binding of gestodene to estrogen receptor in human breast cancer tissue. *Eur. J. Cancer*, **26**, 608–610

Polychronopoulou, A., Tzonou, A., Hsieh, C., Kaprinis, G., Rebelakos, A., Toupadaki, N. & Trichopoulos, D. (1993) Reproductive variables, tobacco, ethanol, coffee and somatometry as risk factors for ovarian cancer. *Int. J. Cancer*, **55**, 402–407

Popov, A.A., Visser, A.P. & Ketting, E. (1993) Contraceptive knowledge, attitudes and practice in Russia during the 1980s. *Stud. Family Planning*, **24**, 227–235

Population Council (1994) Syria 1993: Results from the PAPCHILD Survey. *Stud. Fam. Plann.*, **25**, 248–252

Population Council (1995) Sudan 1992/93: Results from the PAPCHILD Health Survey. *Stud. Fam. Plann.*, **26**, 116–120

Population Council (1996a) Bolivia 1994: Results from the Demographic and Health Survey. *Stud. Fam. Plann.*, **27**, 172–176

Population Council (1996b) Morocco 1995: Results from the Demographic and Health Survey. *Stud. Fam. Plann.*, **27**, 344–348

Population Council (1997a) Uganda 1995: Results from the Demographic and Health Survey. *Stud. Fam. Plann.*, **28**, 156–160

Population Council (1997b) Egypt 1995: Results from the Demographic and Health Survey. *Stud. Fam. Plann.*, **28**, 251–255

Population Council (1997c) Guatemala 1995: Results from the Demographic and Health Survey. *Stud. Fam. Plann.*, **28**, 151–155

Population Council (1997d) Kazakstan 1995: Results from the Demographic and Health Survey. *Stud. Fam. Plann.*, **28**, 256–260

Population Council (1997e) Eritrea 1995: Results from the Demographic and Health Survey. *Stud. Fam. Plann.*, **28**, 336–340

Population Council (1997f) Mali 1995–96: Results from the Demographic and Health Survey. *Stud. Fam. Plann.*, **28**, 341–345

Population Council (1998a) Benin 1996: Results from the Demographic and Health Survey. *Stud. Fam. Plann.*, **29**, 83–87

Population Council (1998b) Brazil 1996: Results from the Demographic and Health Survey. *Stud. Fam. Plann.*, **29**, 88–92

Potter, J.D. & McMichael, A.J. (1983) Large bowel cancer in women in relation to reproductive and hormonal factors: A case–control study. *J. natl Cancer Inst.*, **71**, 703–709

Potter, J.D., Bostick, R.M., Grandits, G.A., Fosdick, L., Elmer, P., Wood, J., Grambsch, P. & Louis, T.A. (1996) Hormone replacement therapy is associated with lower risk of adenomatous polyps of the large bowel: The Minnesota Cancer Prevention Research Unit Case–Control Study. *Cancer Epidemiol. Biomarkers Prev.*, **5**, 779–784

Poulin, R., Baker, D., Poirier, D. & Labrie, F. (1990) Multiple actions of synthetic 'progestins' on the growth of ZR-75-1 human breast cancer cells: An *in vitro* model for the simultaneous assay of androgen, progestin, estrogen, and glucocorticoid agonistic and antagonistic activities of steroids. *Breast Cancer Res. Treat.*, **17**, 197–210

Powell-Jones, W., Thompson, C., Nayfeh, S.N. & Lucier, G.W. (1980) Sex differences in estrogen binding by cytosolic and nuclear components of rat liver. *J. Steroid Biochem.*, **13**, 219–229

Poyet, P. & Labrie, F. (1985) Comparison of the antiandrogenic/androgenic activities of flutamide, cyproterone acetate and megestrol acetate. *Mol. cell. Endocrinol.*, **42**, 283–288

Pradat, P. (1992) A case–control study of major congenital heart defects in Sweden—1981–1986. *Eur. J. Epidemiol.*, **8**, 789–796

Prahalada, S. & Hendrickx, A.G. (1983) Embryotoxicity of Norlestrin, a combined synthetic oral contraceptive, in rhesus macaques (*Macaca mulatta*). *Teratology*, **27**, 215–222

Prentice, R.L. & Thomas, D.B. (1987) On the epidemiology of oral contraceptives and breast disease. *Adv. Cancer Res.*, **49**, 284–401

Preston-Martin, S., Bernstein, L., Pike, M.C., Maldonado, A.A. & Henderson, B.E. (1987) Thyroid cancer among young women related to prior thyroid disease and pregnancy history. *Br. J. Cancer*, **55**, 191–195

Preston-Martin, S., Jin, F., Duda, M.J. & Mack, W.J. (1993) A case–control study of thyroid cancer in women under age 55 in Shanghai (People's Republic of China). *Cancer Causes Control*, **4**, 431–440

Primic-Žakelj, M., Evstifeeva, T., Ravnihar, B. & Boyle, P. (1995) Breast cancer risk and oral contraceptive use in Slovenia women aged 25 to 54. *Int. J. Cancer*, **62**, 414–420

Prost-Avallet, O., Oursin, J. & Adessi, G.L. (1991) *In vitro* effect of synthetic progestogens on estrone sulfatase activity in human breast carcinoma. *J. Steroid Biochem. mol. Biol.*, **39**, 967–973

Purdie, D., Green, A., Bain, C., Siskind, V., Ward, B., Hacker, N., Quinn, M., Wright, G., Russell, P. & Susil, B. for the Survey of Women's Health Group (1995) Reproductive and other factors and risk of epithelial ovarian cancer: An Australian case–control study. *Int. J. Cancer*, **62**, 678–684

Raman-Wilms, L., Tseng, A.L., Wighardt, S., Einarson, T.R. & Koren, G. (1995) Fetal genital effects of first-trimester sex hormone exposure: A meta-analysis. *Obstet. Gynecol.*, **85**, 141–149

Ramcharan, S., Pellegrin, F.A., Ray, R. & Hsu, J.P. (1981a) *The Walnut Creek Contraceptive Study. A Prospective Study of the Side Effects of Oral Contraceptives* (NIH Publ No. 81-564), Vol. III, Bethesda, MD, National Institutes of Health

Ramcharan, S., Pellegrin, F.A., Ray, R. & Hsu, J.-P. (1981b) *A Prospective Study of the Side Effects of Oral Contraceptives, Vol. III, An Interim Report. A Comparison of Disease Occurrence Leading to Hospitalization or Death in Users and Nonusers of Oral Contraceptives* (NIH Publication No. 81-564), Bethesda, MD, National Institutes of Health

Ranstam, J. & Olsson, H. (1993) Oral contraceptive use among young women in southern Sweden. *J. Epidemiol. Community Health*, **47**, 32–35

Rao, T.K., Allen, B.E., Cox, J.T. & Epler, J.L. (1983) Enhancement of mutagenic activity in *Salmonella* by contraceptive steroids. *Toxicol. appl. Pharmacol.*, **69**, 48–54

Rastogi, R.K., Milone, M. & Chieffi, G. (1980) A long-term study of the epididymal and fertility-suppressing effects of cyproterone acetate in the mouse. *Andrologia*, **12**, 476–481

Ravnihar, B., Siegel, D.G. & Lindtner, J. (1979) An epidemiologic study of breast cancer and benign breast neoplasia in relation to oral contraceptive and estrogen use. *Eur. J. Cancer*, **15**, 395–403

Ravnihar, B., Zakelj, P., Kosmelj, K. & Stare, J. (1988) A case–control study of breast cancer in relation to oral contraceptive use in Slovenia. *Neoplasma*, **35**, 109–121

Re, M., Micali, F., Santoro, L., Cuomo, M., Racheli, T., Scapellato, F. & Iannitelli, M. (1979) Histological characteristics of the human testis after long-term treatment with cyproterone acetate. *Arch. Androl.*, **3**, 263–268

Reboud, S. & Pageaut, G. (1977) Topographical response and epithelial abnormalities of the mouse cervix after parenteral administration of progestational compounds. *Contraception*, **16**, 357–366

Reel, J.R., Humphrey, R.R., Shih, Y.-H., Windsor, B.L., Sakowski, R., Creger, P.L. & Edgren, R.A. (1979) Competitive progesterone antagonists: Receptor binding and biological activity of testosterone and 19-nortestosterone derivatives. *Fertil. Steril.*, **31**, 552–561

Risch, H.A., Weiss, N.S., Lyon, J.L., Daling, J.R. & Liff, J.M. (1983) Events of reproductive life and the incidence of epithelial ovarian cancer. *Am. J. Epidemiol.*, **117**, 128–139

Risch, H.A., Marrett, L.D. & Howe, G.R. (1994) Parity, contraception, infertility, and the risk of epithelial ovarian cancer. *Am. J. Epidemiol.*, **140**, 585–597

Risch, H.A., Marrett, L.D., Jain, M. & Howe, G.R. (1996) Differences in risk factors for epithelial ovarian cancer by histologic type. Results of a case–control study. *Am. J. Epidemiol.*, **144**, 363–372

Roberts, R.A., Soames, A.R., Gill, J.H., James, N.H. & Wheeldon, E.B. (1995) Non-genotoxic hepatocarcinogens stimulate DNA synthesis and their withdrawal induces apoptosis, but in different hepatocyte populations. *Carcinogenesis*, **16**, 1693–1698

Rohan, T.E. & McMichael, A.J. (1988) Oral contraceptive agents and breast cancer: A population-based case–control study. *Med. J. Aust.*, **149**, 520–524

Röhrborn, G. & Hansmann, I. (1974) Oral contraceptives and chromosome segregation in oocytes of mice. *Mutat. Res.*, **26**, 535–544

Romieu, I., Willett, W.C., Colditz, G.A., Stampfer, M.J., Rosner, B., Hennekens, C.H. & Speizer, F.E. (1989) Prospective study of oral contraceptive use and risk of breast cancer in women. *J. natl Cancer Inst.*, **81**, 1313–1321

Romieu, I., Berlin, J.A. & Colditz, G. (1990) Oral contraceptives and breast cancer. Review and meta-analysis. *Cancer*, **66**, 2253–2263

Ron, E., Kleinerman, R.A., Boice, J.D., Jr, LiVolsi, V.A., Flannery, J.T. & Fraumeni, J.F., Jr (1987) A population-based case–control study of thyroid cancer. *J. natl Cancer Inst.*, **79**, 1–12

Rooks, J.B., Ory, H.W., Ishak, K.G., Strauss, L.T., Greenspan, J.R., Hill, A.P. & Tyler, C.W. (1979) Epidemiology of hepatocellular adenoma. The role of oral contraceptive use. *J. Am. med. Assoc.*, **242**, 644–648

Rookus, M.A., van Leeuwen, F.E., for The Netherlands Oral Contraceptives and Breast Cancer Study Group (1994) Oral contraceptives and risk of breast cancer in women aged 20–54 years. *Lancet*, **344**, 844–851

Rosenberg, L., Shapiro, S., Slone, D., Kaufman, D.W., Helmrich, S.P., Miettinen, P.S., Stolley, P.D., Rosenshein, N.B., Schottenfeld, D. & Engle, R.L., Jr (1982) Epithelial ovarian cancer and combination oral contraceptives. *J. Am. med. Assoc.*, **247**, 3210–3212

Rosenberg, L., Miller, D.R., Kaufman, D.W., Helmrich, S.P., Stolley, P.D., Shottenfeld, D. & Shapiro, S. (1984) Breast cancer and oral contraceptive use. *Am. J. Epidemiol.*, **119**, 167–176

Rosenberg, L., Palmer, J.P., Clarke, E.A. & Shapiro, S. (1992) A case–control study of the risk of breast cancer in relation to oral contraceptive use. *Am. J. Epidemiol.*, **136**, 1437–1444

Rosenberg, L., Palmer, J.R., Zauber, A.G., Warshauer, M.E., Lewis, J.L., Jr, Strom, B.L., Harlap, S. & Shapiro, S. (1994) A case–control study of oral contraceptive use and invasive epithelial ovarian cancer. *Am. J. Epidemiol.*, **139**, 654–661

Rosenberg, L., Palmer, J.R., Rao, R.S., Zauber, A.G., Strom, B.L., Warshauer, M.E., Harlap, S. & Shapiro, S. (1996) Case–control study of oral contraceptive use and risk of breast cancer. *Am. J. Epidemiol.*, **143**, 25–37

Rosenblatt, K.A., Thomas, D.B. & the WHO Collaborative Study of Neoplasia and Steroid Contraceptives (1991) Hormonal content of combined oral contraceptives in relation to the reduced risk of endometrial cancer. *Int. J. Cancer*, **49**, 870–874

Rosenblatt, K.A., Thomas, D.B., Noonan, E.A. & the WHO Collaborative Study of Neoplasia and Steroid Contraceptives (1992) High-dose and low-dose combined oral contraceptives: Protection against epithelial ovarian cancer and the length of the protective effect. *Eur. J. Cancer*, **28A**, 1872–1876

Rossi, G.L., Bestetti, G.E., Reymond, M.J. & Lemarchand-Béraud, T. (1991) Morphofunctional study of the effects of fetal exposure to cyproterone acetate on the hypothalamo-pituitary-gonadal axis of adult rats. *Exp. Brain Res.*, **83**, 349–356

Rossing, M.A., Stanford, J.L., Weiss, N.S. & Habel, L.A. (1996) Oral contraceptive use and risk of breast cancer in middle-aged women. *Am. J. Epidemiol.*, **144**, 161–164

Roy, S. & Chatterjee, S. (1979) The role of antiandrogenic action in cyproterone acetate-induced morphologic and biochemical changes in human semen. *Fertil. Steril.*, **32**, 93–95

Roy, S.K. & Kar, A.B. (1967) Foetal effect of norethynodrel in rats. *Indian J. exp. Biol.*, **5**, 14–16

Royal College of General Practitioners (1974) *Oral Contraceptives and Health*, London, Pitman Medical

Rudali, G. & Guggiari, M. (1974) Studies on the carcinogenic effect of two norgestrels on the mammary gland of the mouse. *C.R. Soc. Biol. Méd.*, **168**, 1190–1194 (in French)

Ruokonen, A. & Käär, K. (1985) Effects of desogestrel, levonorgestrel and lynestrenol on serum sex hormone binding globulin, cortisol binding globulin, ceruloplasmin and HDL-cholesterol. *Eur. J. Obstet. Gynecol. reprod. Biol.*, **20**, 13–18

Russell-Briefel, R., Ezzati, T. & Perlman, J. (1985) Prevalence and trends in oral contraceptive use in premenopausal females ages 12–54 years, United States, 1971–80. *Am. J. public Health*, **75**, 1173–1176

Russo, I.H. & Russo, J. (1991) Progestagens and mammary gland development: Differentiation versus carcinogenesis. *Acta endocrinol.*, **125**, 7–12

Russo, I.H., Frederick, J. & Russo, J. (1989) Hormone prevention of mammary carcinogenesis by norethynodrel–mestranol. *Breast Cancer Res. Treat.*, **14**, 43–56

Sannes, E., Lyngset, A. & Nafstad, I. (1983) Teratogenicity and embryotoxicity of orally administered lynestrenol in rabbits. *Arch. Toxicol.*, **52**, 23–33

dos Santos Silva, I. & Swerdlow, A.J. (1995) Recent trends in incidence of and mortality from breast, ovarian and endometrial cancers in England and Wales and their relation to changing fertility and oral contraceptive use. *Br. J. Cancer*, **72**, 485–492

Sartwell, P.E., Arthes, F.G. & Tonascia, J.A. (1977) Exogenous hormones, reproductive history, and breast cancer. *J. natl Cancer Inst.*, **59**, 1589–1592

Sasaki, M., Sugimura, K., Yoshida, M.A. & Abe, S. (1980) Cytogenetic effects of 60 chemicals on cultured human and Chinese hamster cells. *Kromosomo II*, **20**, 574–584

Saunders, F.J. (1965) Effects on the course of pregnancy of norethynodrel with mestranol (Enovid) administered to rats during early pregnancy. *Endocrinology*, **77**, 873–878

Saunders, F.J. (1967) Effects of norethynodrel combined with mestranol on the offspring when administered during pregnancy and lactation in rats. *Encocrinology*, **80**, 447–452

Saunders, F.J. & Elton, R.I. (1967) Effects of ethynodiol diacetate and mestranol in rats and rabbits, on conception, on the outcome of pregnancy and on the offspring. *Toxicol. appl. Pharmacol.*, **11**, 229–244

Schardein, J.L. (1980) Studies of the components of an oral contraceptive agent in albino rats. II. Progestogenic component and comparison of effects of the components and the combined agent. *J. Toxicol. environ. Health*, **6**, 895–906

Schauer, G., Blode, H. & Gunzel, P. (1996) Commentary on the publication: Tucker, M.J., Jones, D.V. Human and Exptl. Toxicol., 1996, **15**, 64-66 (Letter to the Editor). *Hum. exp. Toxicol.*, **15**, 597–598

Schiffman, M.H., Bauer, H.M., Hoover, R.N., Glass, A.G., Cadell, D.M., Rush, B.B., Scott, D.R., Sherman, M.E., Kurman, R.J., Wacholder, S., Stanton, C.K. & Manos, M.M. (1993) Epidemiologic evidence showing that human papillomavirus infection causes most cervical intraepithelial neoplasia. *J. natl Cancer Inst.*, **85**, 958–964

Schildkraut, J.M., Hulka, B.S. & Wilkinson, W.E. (1990) Oral contraceptives and breast cancer: A case–control study with hospital and community controls. *Obstet. Gynecol.*, **76**, 395–402

Schlesselman, J.J. (1995) Net effect of oral contraceptive use on the risk of cancer in women in the United States. *Obstet. Gynecol.*, **85**, 793–801

Schlesselman, J.J., Stadel, B.V., Murray, P. & Lai, S.-L. (1987) Breast cancer risk in relation to type of estrogen contained in oral contraceptives. *Contraception*, **3**, 595–613

Schlesselman, J.J., Stadel, B.V., Murray, P. & Lai, S. (1988) Breast cancer in relation to early use of oral contraceptives. No evidence of a latent effect. *J. Am. med. Assoc.*, **259**, 1828–1833

Schnitzler, R., Foth, J., Degen, G.H. & Metzler, M. (1994) Induction of micronuclei by stilbene-type and steroidal estrogens in Syrian hamster embryo & ovine seminal vesicle cells in vitro. *Mutat. Res.*, **311**, 85–93

Schoonen, W.G.E.J., Joosten, J.W.H. & Kloosterboer, H.J. (1995a) Effects of two classes of progestagens, pregnane and 19-nortestosterone derivatives, on cell growth of human breast tumor cells: I. MCF-7 cell lines. *J. Steroid Biochem. mol. Biol.*, **55**, 423–437

Schoonen, W.G.E.J., Joosten, J.W.H. & Kloosterboer, H.J. (1995b) Effects of two classes of progestagens, pregnane and 19-nortestosterone derivatives, on cell growth of human breast tumor cells: II. T47D cell lines. *J. Steroid Biochem. mol. Biol.*, **55**, 439–444

Schulte-Hermann, R., Hoffman, V., Parzefall, W., Kallenbach, M., Gerhardt, A. & Schuppler, J. (1980a) Adaptive responses of rat liver to the gestagen and anti-androgen cyproterone acetate and other inducers. II. Induction of growth. *Chem.–biol. Interactions*, **31**, 287–300

Schulte-Hermann, R., Hoffmann, V. & Landgraf, H. (1980b) Adaptive responses of rat liver to the gestagen and anti-androgen cyproterone acetate and other inducers. III. Cytological changes. *Chem.–biol. Interactions*, **31**, 301–311

Schulte-Hermann, R., Ochs, H., Bursch, W. & Parzefall, W. (1988) Quantitative structure–activity studies on effects of sixteen different steroids on growth and monooxygenases of rat liver. *Cancer Res.*, **48**, 2462–2468

Schuppler, J. & Gunzel, P. (1979) Liver tumors and steroid hormones in rats and mice. *Arch. Toxicol.*, **Suppl. 2**, 181–195

Schuppler, J., Gunzel, P. & El Etreby, M.F. (1977) Effect of progestogens on the liver: Comparative evaluation in rodents, dogs and monkeys in long-term toxicity studies. *J. Toxicol. environ. Health*, **3**, 370–371

Schuppler, J., Dammé, J. & Schulte-Hermann, R. (1983) Assay of some endogenous and synthetic sex steroids for tumor-initiating activity in rat liver using the Solt-Farber system. *Carcinogenesis*, **4**, 239–241

Schwartz, S.M. & Weiss, N.S. (1986) Increased incidence of adenocarcinoma of the cervix in young women in the United States. *Am. J. Epidemiol.*, **124**, 1045–1047

Shapiro, S.S., Dyer, R.D. & Colás, A.E. (1978) Synthetic progestins: In vitro potency on human endometrium and specific binding to cytosol receptor. *Am. J. Obstet. Gynecol.*, **132**, 549–554

Shenfield, G.M. & Griffin, J.M. (1991) Clinical pharmacokinetics of contraceptive steroids. An update. *Clin. Pharmacokinet.*, **20**, 15–37

Shi, Y.E. & Yager, J.D. (1989) Effects of the liver tumor promoter ethinyl estradiol on epidermal growth factor-induced DNA synthesis and epidermal growth factor receptor levels in cultured rat hepatocytes. *Cancer Res.*, **49**, 3574–3580

Shimomura, M., Higashi, S. & Mizumoto, R. (1992) ^{32}P-Postlabelling analysis of DNA adducts in rats during estrogen-induced hepatocarcinogenesis and effect of tamoxifen on DNA adduct level. *Jpn. J. Cancer Res.*, **83**, 438–444

Shirai, T., Fukushima, S., Ikawa, E., Tagawa, Y. & Ito, N. (1986) Induction of prostate carcinoma in situ at high incidence in F344 rats by a combination of 3,2'-dimethyl-4-aminobiphenyl and ethinyl estradiol. *Cancer Res.*, **46**, 6423–6426

Shirai, T., Tsuda, H., Ogiso, T., Hirose, M. & Ito, N. (1987) Organ specific modifying potential of ethinyl estradiol on carcinogenesis initiated with different carcinogens. *Carcinogenesis*, **8**, 115–119

Shirai, T., Nakamura, A., Fukushima, S., Yamamoto, A., Tada, A. & Ito, N. (1990) Different carcinogenic responses in a variety of organs, including the prostate, of five different rat strains given 3,2'-dimethyl-4-aminobiphenyl. *Carcinogenesis*, **11**, 793–797

Shoupe, D. (1994) New progestins—clinical experiences: Gestodene. *Am. J. Obstet. Gynecol.*, **170**, 1562–1568

Shu, X.O., Brinton, L.A., Gao, Y.T. & Yuan, J.M. (1989) Population-based case–control study of ovarian cancer in Shanghai. *Cancer Res.*, **49**, 3670–3674

Shu, X.-O., Brinton, L.A., Zheng, W., Gao, Y.T., Fan, J. & Fraumeni, J.F. (1991) A population-based case–control study of endometrial cancer in Shanghai, China. *Int. J. Cancer*, **49**, 38–43

Shyama, S.K. & Rahiman, M.A. (1993) Progestin (norethisterone)-induced genetic damage in mouse bone marrow. *Mutat. Res.*, **300**, 215–221

Shyama, S.K. & Rahiman, M.A. (1996) Genotoxicity of lynoral (ethinylestradiol, an estrogen) in mouse bone marrow cells, in vivo. *Mutat. Res.*, **370**, 175–180

Shyama, S.K., Rahiman, M.A. & Vijayalaxmi, K.K. (1991) Genotoxic effect of Anovlar 21, an oral contraceptive, on mouse bone marrow. *Mutat. Res.*, **260**, 47–53

Silverberg, S.G. & Makowski, E.L. (1975) Endometrial carcinoma in young women taking oral contraceptive agents. *Obstet. Gynecol.*, **46**, 503–506

Silverberg, S.G., Makowski, E.L. & Roche, W.D. (1977) Endometrial carcinoma in women under 40 years of age: Comparison of cases in oral contraceptive users and non-users. *Cancer*, **39**, 592–598

Simon, W.E., Albrecht, M., Hänsel, M., Dietel, M. & Hölzer, F. (1983) Cell lines derived from human ovarian carcinomas: Growth stimulation by gonadotropic and steroid hormones. *J. natl Cancer Inst.*, **70**, 839–845

Simpson, J.L. (1985) Relationship between congenital anomalies and contraception. *Adv. Contracept.*, **1**, 3–30

Simpson, J.L. & Phillips, O.P. (1990) Spermicides, hormonal contraception and congenital malformations. *Adv. Contracept.*, **6**, 141–167

Sina, J.F., Bean, C.L., Dysart, G.R., Taylor, V.I. & Bradley, M.O. (1983) Evaluation of the alkaline elution/rat hepatocyte assay as a predictor of carcinogenic/mutagenic potential. *Mutat. Res.*, **113**, 357–391

Singh, O.S. & Carr, D.H. (1970) A study of the effects of certain hormones on human cells in culture. *Can. med. Assoc. J.*, **103**, 349–350

Sisenwine, S.F., Kimmel, H.B., Liu, A.L. & Ruelius, H.W. (1975a) The presence of DL-, D-, and L-norgestrel and their metabolites in the plasma of women. *Contraception*, **12**, 339–353

Sisenwine, S.F., Kimmel, H.B., Liu, A.L. & Ruelius, H.W. (1975b) Excretion and stereoselective biotransformations of *dl*-, *d*- and *l*-norgestrel in women. *Drug. Metab. Disposition*, **3**, 180–188

Spona, J., Huber, J. & Schmidt, J.B. (1986) Inhibition of ovulation with 35 micrograms of ethinyl estradiol and 2 mg cyproterone acetate (Diane 35). *Geburtsh. Frauenheilk.*, **46**, 435–438 (in German)

Spritzer, P.M., Barbosa-Coutinho, L.M., Poy, M., Orsi, V., Dahlem, N. & Silva, I.S.B. (1995) Effects of norethisterone acetate and tamoxifen on serum prolactin levels, uterine growth and on the presence of uterine immunoreactive prolactin in estradiol-treated ovariectomized rats. *Braz. J. med. biol. Res.*, **28**, 125–130

Stadel, B.V., Rubin, G.L., Webster, L.A., Schlesselman, J.J., Wingo, P.A. for the Cancer and Steroid Hormone Group (1985) Oral contraceptives and breast cancer in young women. *Lancet*, **ii**, 970–973

Stadel, B.V., Lai, S., Schlesselman, S.S. & Murray, P. (1988) Oral contraceptives and premenopausal breast cancer in nulliparous women. *Contraception*, **38**, 287–299

Stanczyk, F.Z. & Roy, S. (1990) Metabolism of levonorgestrel, norethindrone, and structurally related contraceptive steroids. *Contraception*, **42**, 67–96

Standeven, A.M., Shi, Y.E., Sinclair, J.F., Sinclair, P.R. & Yager, J.D. (1990) Metabolism of the liver tumor promoter ethinyl estradiol by primary cultures of rat hepatocytes. *Toxicol. appl. Pharmacol.*, **102**, 486–496

Standeven, A.M., Wolf, D.C. & Goldsworthy, T.L. (1994) Interactive effects of unleaded gasoline and estrogen on liver tumor promotion in female B6C3F$_1$ mice. *Cancer Res.*, **54**, 1198–2104

Stanford, J.L., Brinton, L.A. & Hoover, R.N. (1989) Oral contraceptives and breast cancer: Results from an expanded case–control study. *Br. J. Cancer*, **60**, 375–378

Stanford, J.L., Brinton, L.A., Berman, M.L., Mortel, R., Twiggs, L.B., Barrett, R.J., Wilbanks, G.D. & Hoover, R.N. (1993) Oral contraceptives and endometrial cancer: Do other risk factors modify the association? *Int. J. Cancer*, **54**, 243–248

Stenchever, M.A., Jarvis, J.A. & Kreger, N.K. (1969) Effect of selected estrogens and progestins on human chromosomes in vitro. *Obstet. Gynecol.*, **34**, 249–252

Stone, S.C. (1995) Desogestrel. *Clin. Obstet. Gynecol.*, **38**, 821–828

Sutherland, R.L., Hall, R.E., Pang, G.Y.N., Musgrove, E.A. & Clarke, C.L. (1988) Effect of medroxyprogesterone acetate on proliferation and cell cycle kinetics of human mammary carcinoma cells. *Cancer Res.*, **48**, 5084–5091

Swenberg, J.A. (1981) Utilization of the alkaline elution assay as a short-term test for chemical carcinogens. In: Stich, H.F. & San, R.H.C., eds, *Short-term Tests for Chemical Carcinogens*, New York, Springer-Verlag, pp. 48–58

Takai, K., Kakizoe, T., Tanaka, Y., Tobisu, K.-I. & Aso, Y. (1991) Trial to induce prostatic cancer in ACI/Seg rats treated with a combination of 3,2′-dimethyl-4-aminobiphenyl and ethinyl estradiol. *Jpn. J. Cancer Res.*, **82**, 286–292

Takano, K., Yamamura, H., Suzuki, M. & Nishimura, H. (1966) Teratogenic effect of chlormadinone acetate in mice and rabbits. *Proc. Soc. exp. Biol. Med.*, **121**, 455–457

Talamini, K., La Vecchia, C., Franceschi, S., Colombo, F., Decarli, A., Grattoni, E., Grigoletto, E. & Tognoni, G. (1985) Reproductive and hormone factors and breast cancer in a northern Italian population. *Int. J. Epidemiol.*, **14**, 70–74

Talamini, R., Franceschi, S., Dal Maso, L., Negri, E., Conti, E., Filiberti, R., Montella, M., Nanni, O. & La Vecchia, C. (1998) The influence of reproductive and hormonal factors on the risk of colon and rectal cancer in women. *Eur. J. Cancer*, **34**, 1070–1076

Tam, C.C., Wong, Y.C. & Tang, F. (1985) Further regression of seminal vesicles of castrated guinea pig by administration of cyproterone acetate. *Acta anat.*, **124**, 65–73

Tamaya, T., Nioka, S., Furuta, N., Shimura, T., Takano, N. & Okada, H. (1977) Contribution of functional groups of 19-nor-progestogens to binding to progesterone and estradiol-17β receptors in rabbit uterus. *Endocrinology*, **100**, 1579–1584

Tanooka, H. (1977) Development and applications of *Bacillus subtilis* test systems for mutagens, involving DNA-repair deficiency and suppressible auxotrophic mutations. *Mutat. Res.*, **42**, 19–32

Täuber, U., Kuhnz, W. & Hümpel, M. (1990) Pharmacokinetics of gestodene and ethinyl estradiol after oral administration of a monophasic contraceptive. *Am. J. Obstet. Gynecol.*, **163**, 1414–1420

Tavani, A., Negri, E., Franceschi, S., Parazzini, F. & La Vecchia, C. (1993a) Oral contraceptives and breast cancer in Northern Italy. Final report from a case–control study. *Br. J. Cancer*, **68**, 568–571

Tavani, A., Negri, E., Parazzini, F., Franceschi, S. & La Vecchia, C. (1993b) Female hormone utilisation and risk of hepatocellular carcinoma. *Br. J. Cancer*, **67**, 635–637

Tavassoli, F.A., Casey, H.W. & Norris, H.J. (1988) The morphologic effects of synthetic reproductive steroids on the mammary gland of rhesus monkeys. Mestranol, ethynerone, mestranol–ethynerone, chloroethynyl norgestrel–mestranol, and anagestone acetate–mestranol combinations. *Am. J. Pathol.*, **131**, 213–234

Telang, N.T., Suto, A., Wong, G.Y., Osborne, M.P. & Bradlow, H.L. (1992) Induction by estrogen metabolite 16α-hydroxyestrone of genotoxic damage and aberrant proliferation in mouse mammary epithelial cells. *J. natl Cancer Inst.*, **84**, 634–638

Thomas, D.B. (1972) Relationship of oral contraceptives to cervical carcinogenesis. *Obstet. Gynecol.*, **40**, 508–518

Thomas, D.B. (1991a) Oral contraceptives and breast cancer: Review of the epidemiologic literature. *Contraception*, **43**, 597–642

Thomas, D.B. (1991b) The WHO Collaborative Study of Neoplasia and Steroid Contraceptives: The influence of combined oral contraceptives on risk of neoplasms in developing and developed countries. *Contraception*, **43**, 695–710

Thomas, D.B. & the WHO Collaborative Study of Neoplasia and Steroid Contraceptives (1991) The influence of combined oral contraceptives on risk of neoplasms in developing and developed countries. *Contraception*, **43**, 695–710

Thomas, D.B., Noonan, E.A. & the WHO Collaborative Study of Neoplasia and Steroid Contraceptives (1992) Breast cancer and specific types of combined oral contraceptives. *Br. J. Cancer*, **65**, 108–113

Thomas, E.J., Edridge, W., Weddell, A., McGill, A. & McGarrigle, H.H.G. (1993) The impact of cigarette smoking on the plasma concentrations of gonadotrophins, ovarian steroids and androgens and upon the metabolism of oestrogens in the human female. *Hum. Reprod.*, **8**, 1187–1193

Thomas, D.B., Noonan, E.A. & the WHO Collaborative Study of Neoplasia and Steroid Contraceptives (1994) Risk of breast cancer in relation to use of combined oral contraceptives near the age of menopause. *Cancer Causes Control*, **2**, 389–394

Thomas, D.B., Ray, R.M. & WHO Collaborative Study of Neoplasia and Steroid Contraceptives (1996) Oral contraceptives and invasive adenocarcinomas and adenosquamous carcinomas of the uterine cervix. *Am. J. Epidemiol.*, **144**, 281–289

Thorogood, M. & Villard-Mackintosh, L. (1993) Combined oral contraceptives: Risks and benefits. *Br. med. Bull.*, **49**, 124–139

Tomasson, H. & Tomasson, K. (1996) Oral contraceptives and risk of breast cancer. A historical prospective case–control study. *Acta obstet. gynaecol. scand.*, **75**, 157–161

Topham, J.C. (1980) Do induced sperm-head abnormalities in mice specifically identify mammalian mutagens rather than carcinogens? *Mutat. Res.*, **74**, 379–387

Topinka, J., Andrae, U., Schwartz, L.R. & Wolff, T. (1993) Cyproterone acetate generates DNA adducts in rat liver and in primary rat hepatocyte cultures. *Carcinogenesis*, **14**, 423–427

Topinka, J., Binkova, B., Zhu, H.K., Andrae, U., Neumann, I., Schwartz, L.R., Werner, S. & Wolff, T. (1995) DNA-damaging activity of the cyproterone acetate analogues chlormadinone acetate and megestrol acetate in rat liver. *Carcinogenesis*, **16**, 1483–1487

Trapido, E.J. (1983) A prospective cohort study of oral contraceptives and cancer of the endometrium. *Int. J. Epidemiol.*, **12**, 297–300

Tryggvadóttir, L., Tulinius, H. & Gudmundsdóttir, G.B. (1997) Oral contraceptive use at a young age and the risk of breast cancer: An Icelandic, population-based cohort study of the effect of birth year. *Br. J. Cancer*, **75**, 139–143

Tsutsui, T., Suzuki, N., Fukuda, S., Sato, M., Maizumi, H., McLacklan, J.A. & Barrett, J.C. (1987) 17β-Estradiol-induced cell transformation and aneuploidy of Syrian hamster embryo cells in culture. *Carcinogenesis*, **8**, 1715–1719

Tsutsui, T., Suzuki, N., Maizumi, H. & Barrett, J.C. (1990) Aneuploidy induction in human fibroblasts: Comparison with results in Syrian hamster fibroblasts. *Mutat. Res.*, **240**, 241–249

Tsutsui, T., Komine, A., Huff, J. & Barrett, J.C. (1995) Effects of testosterone, testosterone propionate, 17β-trenbolone and progesterone on cell transformation and mutagenesis in Syrian hamster embryo cells. *Carcinogenesis*, **16**, 1329–1333

Tsutsui, T., Taguchi, S., Tanaka, Y. & Barrett, C. (1997) 17β-Estradiol, diethylstilbestrol, tamoxifen, toremifene 7 ICI 164,384 induce morphological transformation and aneuploidy in cultured Syrian hamster embryo cells. *Int. J. Cancer*, **70**, 188–193

Tuchmann-Duplessis, H. & Mercier-Parot, L. (1972) Effect of a contraceptive steroid on offspring. *J. Gynécol. obstét. Biol. Reprod.*, **1**, 141–159 (in French)

Tucker, M.J. & Jones, D.V. (1996) Effects of cyproterone acetate in C57B1/10J mice. *Hum. exp. Toxicol.*, **15**, 64–66

Tucker, M.J., Kalinowski, A.E. & Orton, T.C. (1996) Carcinogenicity of cyproterone acetate in the mouse. *Carcinogenesis*, **17**, 1473–1476

Tzonou, A., Day, N.E., Trichopoulos, D., Walker, A., Saliaraki, M., Papapostolou, M. & Polychronopoulou, A. (1984) The epidemiology of ovarian cancer in Greece: A case–control study. *Eur. J. Cancer clin. Oncol.*, **20**, 1045–1052

UK National Case–Control Study Group (1989) Oral contraceptive use and breast cancer risk in young women. *Lancet*, **i**, 973–982

UK National Case–Control Study Group (1990) Oral contraceptive use and breast cancer risk in young women: Subgroup analyses. *Lancet*, **335**, 1507–1509

Umapathy, E. & Rai, U.C. (1982) Effect of antiandrogens and medroxyprogesterone acetate on testicular morphometry in mice. *Acta morphol. acad. sci. hung.*, **30**, 99–108

United Nations (1996) *Levels and Trends of Contraceptive Use as Assessed in 1994*, New York, Department for Economic and Social Information and Policy Analysis, Population Division

United States Census Bureau (1998) Int. Data Base http://www.census.gov/ipc/www/idbacc.html

Ursin, G., Aragaki, C.C., Paganini-Hill, A., Siemiatycki, J., Thompson, W.D. & Haile, R.W. (1992) Oral contraceptives and premenopausal bilateral breast cancer: A case–control study. *Epidemiology*, **3**, 414–419

Ursin, G., Peters, B.E., Henderson, B.E., d'Ablaing, G., III, Monroe, K.R. & Pike, M.C. (1994) Oral contraceptive use and adenocarcinoma of the cervix. *Lancet*, **344**, 1390–1394

Ursin, G., Hendersen, B.E., Haile, R.W., Pike, M.C., Zhou, N., Diep, A. & Bernstein, L. (1997) Does oral contraceptive use increase the risk of breast cancer in women with BrCA1/BrCA2 mutations more than in other women? *Cancer Res.*, **57**, 3678–3681

Vall Mayans, M., Calvet, X., Bruix, J., Bruguera, M., Costa, J., Estève, J., Bosch, F.X., Bru, C. & Rodés, J. (1990) Risk factors for hepatocellular carcinoma in Catalonia, Spain. *Int. J. Cancer*, **46**, 378–381

Vessey, M.P. & Painter, R. (1995) Endometrial and ovarian cancer and oral contraceptives—Findings in a large cohort study. *Br. J. Cancer*, **71**, 1340–1342

Vessey, M.P., Doll, R. & Sutton, P.M. (1972) Oral contraceptives and breast neoplasia: A retrospective study. *Br. med. J.*, **iii**, 719–724

Vessey, M.P., Doll, R. & Jones, K. (1975) Oral contraceptives and breast cancer. *Lancet*, **i**, 941–944

Vessey, M., Doll, R., Peto, R., Johnson, B. & Wiggins, P. (1976) A long-term follow-up study of women using different methods of contraception—An interim report. *J. biosoc. Sci.*, **8**, 373–427

Vessey, M.P., McPherson, K., Yeates, D. & Doll, R. (1982) Oral contraceptive use and abortion before first term pregnancy in relation to breast cancer risk. *Br. J. Cancer*, **45**, 327–331

Vessey, M., Buron, J., Doll, R., McPherson, K. & Yeates, D. (1983) Oral contraceptives and breast cancer: Final report of an epidemiologic study. *Br. J. Cancer*, **47**, 455–462

Vessey, M.P., McPherson, K., Villard-Mackintosh, L. & Yeates, D. (1989a) Oral contraceptives and breast cancer: Latest findings in a large cohort study. *Br. J. Cancer*, **59**, 613–617

Vessey, M.P., Villard-Mackintosh, L., McPherson, K. & Yeates, D. (1989b) Mortality among oral contraceptive users: 20 year follow up of women in a cohort study. *Br. med. J.*, **299**, 1487–1491

Vickers, A.E.M. & Lucier, G.W. (1991) Estrogen receptor, epidermal growth factor receptor and cellular ploidy in elutriated subpopulations of hepatocytes during liver tumor promotion by 17α-ethinylestradiol in rats. *Carcinogenesis*, **12**, 391–399

Vickers, A.E.M. & Lucier, G.W. (1996) Estrogen receptor levels and occupancy in hepatic sinusoidal endothelial and Kupffer cells are enhanced by initiation with diethylnitrosamine and promotion with 17α-ethinylestradiol in rats. *Carcinogenesis*, **17**, 1235–1242

Vickers, A.E.M., Nelson, K., McCoy, Z. & Lucier, G.W. (1989) Changes in estrogen receptor, DNA ploidy, and estrogen metabolism in rat hepatocytes during a two-stage model for hepato-carcinogenesis using 17α-ethinylestradiol as the promoting agent. *Cancer Res.*, **49**, 6512–6520

Villard-Mackintosh, L., Vessey, M.P. & Jones, L. (1989) The effects of oral contraceptives and parity on ovarian cancer trends in women under 55 years of age. *Br. J. Obstet. Gynaecol.*, **96**, 783–788

Vizcaino, A.P., Moreno, V., Bosch, F.X., Muñoz, N., Barros-Dios, X.M. & Parkin, D.M. (1998) International trends in the incidence of cervical cancer: I. Adenocarcinoma and adeno-squamous cell carcinomas. *Int. J. Cancer*, **75**, 536–545

Voigt, L.F., Deng, Q. & Weiss, N.S. (1994) Recency, duration, and progestin content of oral contra-ceptives in relation to the incidence of endometrial cancer (Washington, USA). *Cancer Causes Control*, **5**, 227–233

Waetjen, L.E. & Grimes, D.A. (1996) Oral contraceptives and primary liver cancer: Temporal trends in three countries. *Obstet. Gynecol.*, **88**, 945–949

Walker, A.H., Bernstein, L., Warren, D.W., Warner, N.E., Zheng, X. & Henderson, B.E. (1990) The effect of *in utero* ethinyl oestradiol exposure on the risk of cryptorchid testis and testicular teratoma in mice. *Br. J. Cancer*, **62**, 599–602

Walnut Creek Contraceptive Drug Study (1981) *A Prospective Study of the Side Effects of Oral Contraceptives*, Vol. 1, *Findings in Oral Contraceptive Users and Nonusers at Entry into the Study* (DHEW Publ. No. (NIH) 74-562), Bethesda, MD, National Institutes of Health

Wang, C. & Yeung, K.K. (1980) Use of low-dosage cyproterone acetate as a male contraceptive. *Contraception*, **21**, 245–272

Wanless, I.R. & Medline, A. (1982) Role of estrogens as promoters of hepatic neoplasia. *Lab. Invest.*, **46**, 313–320

Warriar, N., Pagé, N., Koutsilieris, M. & Govindan, M.V. (1993) Interaction of antiandrogen-androgen receptor complexes with DNA and transcription activation. *J. Steroid Biochem. mol. Biol.*, **46**, 699–711

Weinstein, A.L., Mahoney, M.C., Nasca, P.C., Leske, M.C. & Varma, A.O. (1991) Breast cancer risk and oral contraceptive use: Results from a large case–control study. *Epidemiology*, **2**, 353–358

Weiss, N.S. & Sayvetz, T.A. (1980) Incidence of endometrial cancer in relation to the use of oral contraceptives. *New Engl. J. Med.*, **302**, 551–554

Weiss, N.S., Lyon, J.L., Liff, J.M., Vollmer, W.M. & Daling, J.R. (1981a) Incidence of ovarian cancer in relation to the use of oral contraceptives. *Int. J. Cancer*, **28**, 669–671

Weiss, N.S., Daling, J.R. & Chow, W.H. (1981b) Incidence of cancer of the large bowel in women in relation to reproductive and hormonal factors. *J. natl Cancer Inst.*, **67**, 57–60

Werner, S., Topinka, J., Wolff, T. & Schwartz, L.R. (1995) Accumulation and persistence of DNA adducts of the synthetic steroid cyproterone acetate in rat liver. *Carcinogenesis*, **16**, 2369–2372

Werner, S., Topinka, J., Kunz, S., Beckurts, T., Heidecke, C.-D., Schwartz, L.R. & Wolff, T. (1996) Studies on the formation of hepatic DNA adducts by the antiandrogenic and gestagenic drug, cyproterone acetate. *Adv. exp. Med. Biol.*, **387**, 253–257

Westerdahl, J., Olsson, H., Måsbäck, A., Ingvar, C. & Jonsson, N. (1996) Risk of malignant melanoma in relation to drug intake, alcohol, smoking and hormonal factors. *Br. J. Cancer*, **73**,
1126–1131

Westhoff, C., Pike, M. & Vessey, M. (1988) Benign ovarian teratomas: A population-based case–
control study. *Br. J. Cancer*, **58**, 93–98

Wharton, C. & Blackburn, R. (1988) Lower dose pills. *Population Rep.*, **16**, 1–31

Wheeler, W.J., Cherry, L.M., Downs, T. & Hsu, T.C. (1986) Mitotic inhibition and aneuploidy
induction by naturally occuring synthetic estrogens in Chinese hamster cells in vitro. *Mutat.
Res.*, **171**, 31–41

Wheeler, C.M., Parmenter, C.A., Hung, W.C., Becker, T.M., Greer, C.E., Hildesheim, A. & Manos,
M.M. (1993) Determinants of genital human papillomavirus infection among cytologically
normal women attending the University of New Mexico Student Health Center. *Sex. transm.
Dis.*, **20**, 286–289

White, J.O., Moore, P.A., Marr, W., Elder, M.G. & Lim, L. (1982) Comparative effects of progesterone, norgestrel, norethisterone and tamoxifen on the abnormal uterus of the anovulatory rat.
Biochem. J., **208**, 199–204

White, E., Malone, K.E., Weiss, N.S. & Daling, J.R. (1994) Breast cancer among young US women
in relation to oral contraceptive use. *J. natl Cancer Inst.*, **86**, 505–514

Whittemore, A.S., Harris, R., Itnyre, J. & the Collaborative Ovarian Cancer Group (1992) Characteristics relating to ovarian cancer risk: Collaborative analysis of 12 US case–control studies.
II. Invasive epithelial ovarian cancers in white women. *Am. J. Epidemiol.*, **136**, 1184–1203

WHO (1992) *Oral Contraceptives and Neoplasia. Report of a WHO Scientific Group* (WHO Technical Report Series 817), Geneva, pp. 18–21

WHO Collaborative Study of Neoplasia and Steroid Contraceptives (1988) Endometrial cancer and
combined oral contraceptives. *Int. J. Epidemiol.*, **17**, 263–269

WHO Collaborative Study of Neoplasia and Steroid Contraceptives (1989a) Epithelial ovarian
cancer and combined oral contraceptives. *Int. J. Epidemiol.*, **18**, 538–545

WHO Collaborative Study of Neoplasia and Steroid Contraceptives (1989b) Combined oral contraceptives and liver cancer. *Int. J. Cancer*, **43**, 254–259

WHO Collaborative Study of Neoplasia and Steroid Contraceptives (1989c) Combined oral contraceptives and gallbladder cancer. *Int. J. Epidemiol.*, **18**, 309–314

WHO Collaborative Study of Neoplasia and Steroid Contraceptives (1990) Breast cancer and combined oral contraceptives: Results from multinational study. *Br. J. Cancer*, **61**, 110–119

WHO Collaborative Study of Neoplasia and Steroid Contraceptives (1993) Invasive squamous cell
cervical carcinoma and combined oral contraceptives: Results from a multinational study. *Int.
J. Epidemiol.*, **55**, 228–236

Wilde, M.I. & Balfour, J.A. (1995) Gestodene: A review of its pharmacology, efficacy and tolera-
bility in combined contraceptive preparations. *Drugs*, **50**, 365–395

Willett, W.C., Bain, C., Hennekens, C.H., Rosner, B. & Speizer, F.E. (1981) Oral contraceptives
and risk of ovarian cancer. *Cancer*, **48**, 1684–1687

Williams, C.L. & Stancel, G.M. (1996) Estrogens and progestins. In: Wonsiewicz, M.J. & McCurdy, P., eds, *Goodman & Gilman's The Pharmacological Basis of Therapeutics*, 9th Ed., New York, McGraw-Hill, pp. 1411–1440

Williams, G., Anderson, E., Howell, A., Watson, R., Coyne, J., Roberts, S.A. & Potten, C.S. (1991) Oral contraceptive (OCP) use increases proliferation and decreases oestrogen receptor content of epithelial cells in the normal human breast. *Int. J. Cancer*, **48**, 206–210

Wilson, J.G. & Brent, R.L. (1981) Are female sex hormones teratogenic? *Am. J. Obstet. Gynecol.*, **141**, 567–580

Wingo, P.A., Lee, N.C., Ory, H.W., Beral, V., Peterson, H.B. & Rhodes, P. (1991) Age-specific differences in relationship between oral contraceptive use and breast cancer. *Obstet. Gynecol.*, **78**, 161–170

Wingren, G., Hatschek, T. & Axelson, O. (1993) Determinants of papillary cancer of the thyroid. *Am. J. Epidemiol.*, **138**, 482–491

Worth, A.J. & Boyes, D.A. (1972) A case–control study into the possible effects of birth control pills on pre-clinical carcinoma of the cervix. *J. Obstet. Gynaecol. Br. Commonw.*, **79**, 673–679

Wu, M.L., Whittemore, A.S., Paffenbarger, R.S., Jr, Sarles, D.L., Kampert, J.B., Grosser, S., Jung, D.L., Ballon, S., Hendrickson, M. & Mohle-Boetani, J. (1988) Personal and environmental characteristics related to epithelial ovarian cancer. I. Reproductive and menstrual events and oral contraceptive use. *Am. J. Epidemiol.*, **128**, 1216–1227

Wu-Williams, A.H., Lee, M., Whittemore, A.S., Gallagher, R.P., Jiao, D., Zheng, S., Zhou, L., Wang, X., Chen, K., Jung, D., Teh, C.-Z., Ling, C., Xu, J.Y. & Paffenbarger, R.S., Jr (1991) Reproductive factors and colorectal cancer risk among Chinese females. *Cancer Res.*, **51**, 2307–2311

Yager, J.D., Jr (1983) Oral contraceptive steroids as promoters or complete carcinogens for liver in female Sprague-Dawley rats. *Environ. Health Perspectives*, **50**, 109–112

Yager, J.D., Jr & Fifield, D.S., Jr (1982) Lack of hepatogenotoxicity of oral contraceptive steroids. *Carcinogenesis*, **3**, 625–628

Yager, J.D. & Liehr, J.G. (1996) Molecular mechanisms of estrogen carcinogenesis. *Ann. Rev. Pharmacotoxicol.*, **36**, 203–232

Yager, J.D. & Yager, R. (1980) Oral contraceptive steroids as promoters of hepatocarcinogenesis in female Sprague-Dawley rats. *Cancer Res.*, **40**, 3680–3685

Yager, J.D., Campbell, H.A., Longnecker, D.S., Roebuck, B.D. & Benoit, M.C. (1984) Enhancement of hepatocarcinogenesis in female rats by ethinyl estradiol and mestranol, but not estradiol. *Cancer Res.*, **44**, 3862–3869

Yager, J.D., Roebuck, B.D., Paluszcyk, T.L. & Memoli, V.A. (1986) Effects of ethinyl estradiol and tamoxifen on liver DNA turnover and new synthesis and appearance of gamma glutamyl trans-peptidase-positive foci in female rats. *Carcinogenesis*, **7**, 2007–2014

Yager, J.D., Zurlo, J. & Ni, N. (1991) Sex hormones and tumor promotion in liver. *Proc. Soc. exp. Biol. Med.*, **198**, 667–674

Yager, J.D., Zurlo, J., Sewall, C.H., Lucier, G.E. & He, H. (1994) Growth stimulation followed by growth inhibition in livers of female rats treated with ethinyl estradiol. *Carcinogenesis*, **15**, 2117–2123

Yamafuji, K., Iiyama, S. & Shinohara, K. (1971) Mode of action of steroid hormones on deoxyribo-nucleic acid. *Enzymology*, **40**, 259–264

Yamagiwa, K., Higashi, S. & Mizumoto, R. (1991) Effect of alcohol ingestion on carcinogenesis by synthetic estrogen and progestin in the rat liver. *Jpn. J. Cancer Res.*, **82**, 771–778

Yamagiwa, K., Mizumoto, R., Higashi, S., Kato, H., Tomida, T., Uehara, S., Tanigawa, K., Tanaka, M. & Ishida, N. (1994) Alcohol ingestion enhances hepatocarcinogenesis induced by synthetic estrogen and progestin in the rat. *Cancer Detect. Prev.*, **18**, 103–114

Yamamoto, T., Terada, N., Nishizawa, Y. & Petrow, V. (1994) Angiostatic activities of medroxy-progesterone acetate and its analogues. *Int. J. Cancer*, **56**, 393–399

Yasuda, Y., Kihara, T., Tanimura, T. & Nishimura, H. (1985) Gonadal dysgenesis induced by pre-natal exposure to ethinyl estradiol in mice. *Teratology*, **32**, 219–227

Yasuda, Y., Konishi, H. & Tanimura, T. (1986) Leydig cell hyperplasia in fetal mice treated trans-placentally with ethinyl estradiol. *Teratology*, **33**, 281–288

Yasuda, Y., Ohara, I., Konishi, H. & Tanimura, T. (1988) Long-term effects on male reproductive organs of prenatal exposure to ethinyl estradiol. *Am. J. Obstet. Gynecol.*, **159**, 1246–1250

Ye, Z., Thomas, D.B., Ray, R.M. & WHO Collaborative Study of Neoplasia and Steroid Contra-ceptives (1995) Combined oral contraceptives and risk of cervical cancer in situ. *Int. J. Epi-demiol.*, **24**, 19–26

Yen, S., Hsieh, C.-C. & MacMahon, B. (1987) Extrahepatic bile duct cancer and smoking, beverage consumption, past medical history, and oral-contraceptive use. *Cancer*, **59**, 2112–2116

Yu, M.C., Tong, M.J., Govindarajan, S. & Henderson, B.E. (1991) Nonviral risk factors for hepato-cellular carcinoma in a low-risk population, the non-Asians of Los Angeles County, California. *J. natl Cancer Inst.*, **83**, 1820–1826

Yuan, J.-M., Yu, M.C., Ross, R.K., Gao, Y.-T. & Henderson, B.E. (1988) Risk factors for breast cancer in Chinese women in Shanghai. *Cancer Res.*, **48**, 1949–1953

Zanetti, R., Franceschi, S., Rosso, S., Bidoli, E. & Colonna, S. (1990) Cutaneous malignant mela-noma in females: The role of hormonal and reproductive factors. *Int. J. Epidemiol.*, **19**, 522–526

Zarghami, N., Grass, L. & Diamandis, E.P. (1997) Steroid hormone regulation of prostate-specific antigen gene expression in breast cancer. *Br. J. Cancer*, **75**, 579–588

Zaridze, D., Mukeria, A. & Duffy, S.W. (1992) Risk factors for skin melanoma in Moscow. *Int. J. Cancer*, **52**, 159–161

Zondervan, K.T., Carpenter, L.M., Painter, R. & Vessey, M.P. (1996) Oral contraceptives and cervical cancer—Further findings from the Oxford Family Planning contraceptive study. *Br. J. Cancer*, **73**, 1291–1297

HORMONAL CONTRACEPTIVES, PROGESTOGENS ONLY

1. Exposure

'Progestogen-only' contraceptives are available as injections, implants, oral preparations, hormone-releasing intrauterine devices and emergency contraceptives. These compounds can be used by women who are breast feeding or have other contra-indications to oestrogen therapy, such as immediately *post partum*, those with thalassaemia, sickle-cell disease, gall-bladder disease, past or present thrombo-embolic disorders, valvular heart disease, ischaemic heart disease, recent surgery, migraine or hypertension, and older women, particularly those over 35 who smoke (WHO Family Planning and Population Unit, 1996; see Annex 1 for guidelines for use). Parenteral methods of administration generally result in more effective contraception than oral routes, as they provide more constant concentrations of the hormone in the blood. Use of progestogen-only oral contraceptives leads to the peaks and troughs in concentration characteristic of oral medication but involves greater potential errors by the users, as placebo is given during seven days of the cycle.

The progestogens that are or have been used in 'progestogen-only' contraceptives are chlormadinone acetate, desogestrel, ethynodiol diacetate, levonorgestrel, lynoestrenol, medroxyprogesterone acetate, norethisterone, norethisterone acetate, norethisterone oenanthate, norgestrel, norgestrienone and progesterone. Of these, medroxyprogesterone acetate, norethisterone oenanthate and progesterone are used only in this way; the remaining progestogens are also used in combination with oestrogens. Thus, information on the progestogens used only in 'progestogen-only' hormonal contraceptives is given in this monograph, and studies on other progestogens are summarized in the monograph on 'Oral contraceptives, combined'.

1.1 Historical overview

The development of injectable progestogen-only contraceptives resulted from a growing understanding of steroid hormones and from the research that eventually led to the development of combined oral contraceptives. In 1953, Karl Junkman and colleagues synthesized the first injectable progestogens and then developed the first injectable contraceptive, norethisterone oenanthate, in 1957. This compound is now approved for contraceptive use in over 60 countries. Medroxyprogesterone acetate was synthesized in the late 1950s, and its depot form was subjected to clinical trials in 1963, before being released onto the international market. It has been approved for use as a contraceptive in a steadily increasing number of countries over the last 30 years and is now available in over 100 countries worldwide. Concern about an association with cancers of the breast, endometrium and cervix and other possible side-effects meant that depot medroxy-progesterone acetate was approved as a contraceptive in the United States only in 1992, some 25 years after the manufacturer's first application (Lande, 1995); however, it had already been approved for the treatment of conditions such as endometrial cancer, and legislation in the United States does not prohibit the use of approved drugs for non-approved indications. Nevertheless, there are still concerns in the international community about issues of informed consent for the use of these long-acting methods and the potential abuse of their administration to poorly educated groups (Kleinman, 1990).

Although the very first oral contraceptive, which was tested in Puerto Rico in 1955, contained only norethynodrel and was, technically speaking, a progestogen-only oral contraceptive (McLaughlin, 1982), it was superseded by the combination of mestranol and norethynodrel during development, as the combination was shown to prevent ovulation consistently. Progestogen-only oral contraceptives were developed in response to concern raised in the late 1960s about the side-effects of oestrogens in combined oral contraceptives. The prototype progestogen-only oral contraceptive contained chlormadinone acetate and was introduced in 1969. It was withdrawn in 1970 because of evidence that it induced breast nodules in laboratory animals. Other progestogen-only oral contraceptives were developed subsequently, containing progestogens of the norethisterone and levonorgestrel groups (Kleinman, 1990).

Subcutaneous progestogen implants were developed in the late 1960s and 1970s and were approved in Finland in 1983, in Sweden in 1985, the Dominican Republic, Ecuador, Indonesia and Thailand in 1986, China, Colombia, Peru and Venezuela in 1987, Chile and Sri Lanka in 1988 and the United States in 1990 (McCauley & Geller, 1992).

A device that releases progesterone into the uterus was developed in the early 1970s and has been available since 1976. This had the disadvantage of a high rate of hormone release, necessitating annual replacement (Kleinman, 1990; Treiman *et al.*, 1995). An intrauterine device that releases effective concentrations of levonorgestrel over a five-year period was approved in Finland in 1990 and in Sweden in 1992 (Chi, 1995); it has since been approved in Belgium, Denmark, France, Iceland, Norway, Singapore, Switzerland and the United Kingdom (Treiman *et al.*, 1995).

1.2   Injectable progestogens

Two progestogen-only injectable contraceptives are available worldwide, and their formulations have remained unchanged since their development in the late 1950s and early 1960s (Table 1).

Norethisterone oenanthate is a long-chain ester of norethisterone which is formulated in a solution of castor oil and benzyl benzoate and given intramuscularly into the gluteal or deltoid muscle. The ester is then distributed to adipose tissue throughout the body and is slowly released back into the bloodstream. It then undergoes hydrolysis in the liver to produce norethisterone, the active progestogen (Kleinman, 1990). It is most commonly

Table 1. Formulation and availability of injectable progestogen-only contraceptives

Brand name	Composition	Dose (mg) and schedule	No. of countries in which registered
Depo-Provera[a]	Medroxyprogesterone acetate	150, every 3 months	100
Dugen	Medroxyprogesterone acetate	150, every 3 months	100
Megestron	Medroxyprogesterone acetate	150, every 3 months	100
Noristerat, Norigest	Norethisterone oenanthate	200, every 2 months	60
Doryxus	Norethisterone oenanthate	200, every 2 months	60

From Kleinman (1990); Lande (1995)

[a] Other names include Depo-Cliovir, Depocon, Depo-Gestin, Depo-Geston, Depo-Prodasone, Depo-Progesta, Depo-Progestin, Depo-Progevera, Medroksiprogesteron

used as a 200-mg dose given every eight weeks or two months, although in some programmes it is given on a two-month schedule for the first six months and then every three months (Lande, 1995).

Depot medroxyprogesterone acetate is administered in an aqueous microcrystalline suspension by deep intramuscular injection into the gluteal or deltoid muscle. This depot results in a high plasma concentration of medroxyprogesterone acetate initially, which declines exponentially thereafter. It is given at a dose of 150 mg every 90 days or three months (Lande, 1995).

Menstrual disturbances are common in women using these compounds and may take the form of amenorrhoea or frequent and/or irregular bleeding. Weight gain is also a common side-effect.

1.2.1   Patterns of use

About 12 million women worldwide currently use injectable contraceptives, and the vast majority of these are progestogen-only preparations (Lande, 1995). Table 2 shows the percentage of married women or women in union, aged 15–49, currently using any method of contraception (including traditional methods) and the percentage currently using injectable contraceptives. The overall proportion of women using injectable contraceptives is low in most regions, except in Indonesia, Jamaica, Kenya, Namibia, New Zealand, Rwanda, South Africa and Thailand.

In a survey conducted in New Zealand between 1983 and 1987, 14% of women aged 25–54 reported ever having used depot medroxyprogesterone acetate; however, 26% of these had only ever received one injection (Paul *et al.*, 1997). In 1994, the Planned Parenthood Federation of America supplied depot medroxyprogesterone acetate to 141 000 women, representing around 7% of their clients (Lande, 1995).

Table 2. Use of injectable contraceptives by married women or women in union aged 15–49, by country

Country	Year	Any contraceptive (%)	Injectable contraceptives (%)
Africa			
Algeria	1992	51	0.1
Benin	1996	16	0.7
Botswana	1988	33	5.4
Burkina Faso	1993	8	0.1
Cameroon	1991	16	0.4
Côte d'Ivoire	1994	11	0.8
Egypt	1995	48	2.4
Eritrea	1995	8	0.8
Ghana	1993	20	1.6
Kenya	1993	33	7.2
Madagascar	1992	17	1.6
Malawi	1992	13	1.5
Mali	1995–96	7	0.2
Mauritius	1985	75	6
Morocco	1995	50	0.1
Namibia	1992	29	7.7
Niger	1992	4	0.5
Nigeria	1990	6	0.7
Rwanda	1992	21	8.4
Senegal	1992	7	0.2
South Africa	1987–89	50	23
Black		49	27
White		79	3
Sudan	1992–93	10	0.2
Swaziland	1988	20	4
Tunisia	1988	50	1
Uganda	1995	15	2.5
Zimbabwe	1994	48	3.2
Europe			
Austria	1981–82	71	0
Belgium	1982	81	0
Hungary	1986	73	0
Italy	1979	78	0
Portugal	1979–80	66	2
United Kingdom	1983	83	0
England	1995	Not reported	1.2
North America			
Canada	1984	73	0
United States	1988	74	0

Table 2 (contd)

Country	Year	Any contraceptive (%)	Injectable contraceptives (%)
Latin America and the Caribbean			
Bolivia	1994	45	0.8
Brazil	1996	77	1.2
Colombia	1995	72	2.5
Costa Rica	1981	65	2
Dominican Republic	1991	56	< 1
Ecuador	1987	44	< 1
El Salvador	1985	47	1
Guatemala	1995	31	2.5
Haiti	1994	18	2.7
Jamaica	1993	62	8
Mexico	1987	53	1
Nicaragua	1981	27	1
Panama	1984	58	1
Paraguay	1990	48	5.2
Peru	1996	64	8
Trinidad and Tobago	1987	53	0.8
Asia and Pacific			
Bangladesh	1993	45	4.5
China	1988	71	< 1
Hong Kong	1987	81	3
Indonesia	1994	55	15
Nepal	1991	25	2
Pakistan	1990–91	12	0.1
Philippines	1993	40	0.1
Sri Lanka	1987	62	3
Syria	1993	40	0
Thailand	1991	69	12
Turkey	1993	63	0.1
Yemen	1991–92	7	0.6

From Population Council (1994); Lande (1995); Population Council (1995, 1996a,b); Bost *et al.* (1997); Population Council (1997a,b,c,d,e,f, 1998a,b); United States Census Bureau (1998)

1.2.2   Action

Injectable progestogen-only contraceptives prevent ovulation (Lande, 1995) by inhibiting follicle-stimulating hormone and luteinizing hormone in a similar way to combined oral contraceptives. They also thicken the cervical mucus, making it relatively impenetrable to sperm, and make the endometrium less receptive to implantation (Kleinman, 1990). They are very effective contraceptives, with 0.3 pregnancies per 100 women per year for depot medroxyprogesterone acetate and 0.4 pregnancies per 100 women per year for norethisterone oenanthate, in the first year of use (Lande, 1995).

1.3   Progestogen implants

Subdermal implants release progestogen slowly over a long period and provide long-term, reversible contraception. The prototype is Norplant, which consists of six silicone rubber (Silastic) capsules 2.4 mm in diameter and 3.4 cm long which are inserted under the skin of the forearm or upper arm and provide contraception for five years. The capsules are each packed with 36 mg crystalline levonorgestrel, which is released at a rate of 85 μg/day initially, falling to 50 μg/day by nine months of use, to 35 μg/day by 18 months and then 30 μg/day during the third, fourth and fifth year of use (McCauley & Geller, 1992). They are non-biodegradable and must be removed in a minor surgical procedure. Implants consisting of two Silastic rods with similar release rates are effective for three years (Reynolds, 1996), and biodegradable implants that do not require removal are being developed.

Like the injectable progestogen-only contraceptives, progestogen implants cause amenorrhoea or frequent or irregular bleeding in most users. Implants are also more costly than many other methods (McCauley & Geller, 1992).

1.3.1   *Patterns of use*

Although implants are approved as a contraceptive in many countries, their use is not widespread. The country with the largest number of users is Indonesia, where over 1 million women had used them by 1992, and in 1994 they were currently being used by around 5% of married women aged 15–49 (United States Census Bureau, 1998). In the two years after their approval by the United States Food and Drug Administration in 1990, about 500 000 women in the United States obtained implants (McCauley & Geller, 1992). By mid-1992, 150 000 women in Thailand had used Norplant; in a survey in 1994, 1.2% of married women or women in union aged 15–49 in Haiti were reported to be currently using it (McCauley & Geller, 1992; United States Census Bureau, 1998).

1.3.2   *Action*

Implants suppress ovulation in up to 50% of women and have progestogenic effects on the cervical mucus and the endometrium (Kleinman, 1990; McCauley & Geller, 1992). The pregnancy rate is less than one per 100 women per year, averaged over five years of use (McCauley & Geller, 1992).

1.4   Progestogen-only oral contraceptives

Progestogen-only oral contraceptives generally contain a progestogen of the norethisterone or levonorgestrel group, given at a constant dose, to be taken at the same time every day, without a break. They are also called 'mini-pills'. Annex 2 (Table 2) lists the common brand names of progestogen-only oral contraceptives with their compositions. Typical pills contain 0.3–0.35 mg norethisterone or 30–37.5 μg levonorgestrel (Kleinman, 1996).

1.4.1   *Patterns of use*

Few systematic data are available on the prevalence of use of progestogen-only oral contraceptives worldwide, as in most surveys women are asked about their use of 'oral contraceptive pills' with no distinction between combined and progestogen-only oral contraceptive pills. Use is probably more common in Australia–New Zealand, Scandinavia and the United Kingdom than it is in the United States and other parts of Europe, but use has been increasing over the last 20 years. In the United Kingdom, progestogen-only oral contraceptives represented 0.9% of all oral contraceptives used in 1973 and 8.8% in 1987 (Thorogood & Villard-Mackintosh, 1993). The *Health Survey for England 1995* showed that 4% of English women aged 16–54 were currently using progestogen-only oral contraceptives and 19% were using combined oral contraceptives; in the age group 35–44 years, 4% of women were using progestogen-only oral contraceptives and 9% were using combined oral contraceptives (Bost *et al.*, 1997). In the United States, progestogen-only oral contraceptives accounted for less than 1% of oral contraceptive sales in 1984 (Piper & Kennedy, 1987). Table 3 indicates the percentages of women among the population-based controls in studies of oral contraceptives and breast cancer in Denmark, New Zealand, Sweden and the United Kingdom who reported any use of progestogen-only oral contraceptives (Collaborative Group on Hormonal Factors in Breast Cancer, 1996). In 1987, about 2% of oral contraceptives bought by pharmacies in 'developed' countries were progesterone-only pills, while they accounted for less than 1% of such sales in 'developing' countries (Wharton & Blackburn, 1988) .

Table 3. Percentages of women reporting any use of progestogen-only oral contraceptives in selected studies

Country	Study	Any use of progestogen-only oral contraceptives (%)
Denmark	Ewertz (1992)	5
Sweden	Meirik *et al.* (1986)	13
New Zealand	Paul *et al.* (1990)	9
United Kingdom	UK National Case–Control Study Group (1989)	15

From Collaborative Group on Hormonal Factors in Breast Cancer (1996)

1.4.2   *Action*

Progestogen-only oral contraceptives have variable effects on ovulation, suppressing it in about 40% of users. Their main contraceptive action is through a progestogenic effect on cervical mucus and, to a lesser extent, the endometrium. As the effect on cervical mucus lessens 20–22 h after administration of a pill, the user must be careful to take it regularly at a time that maximizes its effectiveness. The pregnancy rate is 0.3–5 per 100 women per year of use, with lower failure rates among older women, probably because of their lower overall fertility (Kleinman, 1990).

1.5   Other sources of exposure to progestogen-only contraceptives

The hormone-releasing intrauterine device 'Progestasert' contains 38 mg proges-terone, which is released at a rate of 65 µg/day for one year, after which time it should be replaced (Treiman *et al.*, 1995). The more recently developed LNG-20 intrauterine device contains 52 mg levonorgestrel which is released at a rate of 20–30 µg/day and lasts for at least five years (Treiman *et al.*, 1995; Kleinman, 1996). The progestogen enhances the contraceptive efficacy of the intrauterine device and also reduces menstrual loss. Although worldwide use of intrauterine devices is high, with at least 72 million users in China alone (Treiman *et al.*, 1995), only a small proportion of these contain pro-gestogen. Hormone-impregnated contraceptive vaginal rings which release levo-norgestrel into the systemic circulation have been developed but are not widely used (Kleinman, 1990).

Progestogen-only emergency contraception involves the administration of two doses of 750 µg levonorgestrel orally 12 h apart within 48 h of unprotected intercourse (Cullins & Garcia, 1997).

2.   Studies of Cancer in Humans

2.1   Breast cancer

2.1.1   *Results of published studies*

Eight studies have been published on the relationship between the incidence of breast cancer and use of progestogen-only hormonal contraceptives, i.e. progestogen-only pills or injectable progestogen (depot medroxyprogesterone acetate). They are described in Table 4. The studies were similar in that all were case–control studies of breast cancer in relation to oral contraceptive use; information was obtained on contraceptive use and other factors through interviews, with the exception of the study of Ewertz (1992), in which self-administered questionnaires were used; they confirmed the cancer diagnosis through medical records or cancer registry data; and important risk factors for breast cancer were controlled for in the analyses.

(a)   *Mini-pills*

A case–control study in the United Kingdom (Vessey *et al.*, 1983), in which 1176 cases and 1176 controls aged 16–50 years in 1968–80 were enrolled, showed no asso-ciation between the risk for breast cancer and use of progestogen-only pills. Such use was reported by 2.8% of the cases and 2.5% of the controls; the relative risk estimate was not given.

A population-based study (Cancer and Steroid Hormone Study of the Centers for Disease Control and the National Institute of Child Health and Human Development,

Table 4. Case–control studies of use of progestogen-only contraceptives and breast cancer

Reference	Country	Years of case diagnosis	Age (years)	No. of cases	No. of controls	Participation rates (%) (cases/ controls)	Type of progestogen assessed	Any use of progestogen-only contraceptives (%) (cases/ controls)	RR (95% CI) for any versus no use
Vessey et al. (1983)	United Kingdom	1968–80	16–50	1 176 Hospital-based	1 176	Not given	Pill	2.8/2.5	Not given
Cancer and Steroid Hormone Study (1986)	United States	1980–82	20–54	4 711 Population-based	4 676 Random digit-dialling	80/83	Pill	Not given	1.3 (CI not given)
Paul et al. (1989) (New Zealand National Study)	New Zealand	1983–87	25–54	891 Population-based	1 864 Electoral rolls	79/82	Injectable (DMPA)	12/14	1.0 (0.8–1.3)
UK National Case–Control Study Group (1989)	United Kingdom	1982–85	<36	755 Population-based	755 General practice	72/89	Pill	16/15	0.85 (per year of use)
Clavel et al. (1991)	France	1983–87	25–56	464 Hospital-based	542	99/99	Pill	1.9/1.9	1.1 (0.4–2.7)
WHO Collaborative Study (1991a)	Kenya, Mexico, Thailand	1979–88	<65	869 Hospital-based	11 890	97/98	Injectable (DMPA)	13/12	1.2 (0.96–1.5)
Ewertz (1992)	Denmark	1983–84	<40 40–59	203 856 Population-based	212 778	90/88 89/80	Pill	Not given	0.99 (0.57–1.7)
Skegg et al. (1996) (New Zealand National Study)	New Zealand	1983–87	25–54	891 Population-based	1 864 Electoral rolls	79/82	Pill	5.6/8.7	1.1 (0.73–1.5)

RR, relative risk; CI, confidence interval; DMPA, depot medroxyprogesterone acetate

1986), conducted between 1980 and 1982 in the United States, involved 4711 cases and 4676 controls 20–54 years of age. The investigators reported a relative risk estimate of 1.3 for use of progestogen-only pills; the confidence interval and numbers of case and control women who had used the formulations were not given.

In a multicentre study in the United Kingdom (UK National Case–Control Study Group, 1989), cases in women under the age of 36 years in 1982–85 were ascertained and matched to a control from the general practice in which the case was treated. Replies about contraceptive use obtained at interview were supplemented by the general practitioner for 90% of the 755 pairs. Progestogen-only pills had been used in 16% of cases and 15% of controls, but only 2.9% of the controls had used them for more than eight years. The relative risk estimate for use of progestogen-only pills was 1.35 for less than four years of use (90 cases and 67 controls), 0.73 for > 4–8 years of use (19 cases and 27 controls) and 0.59 for > 8 years of use (14 cases and 22 controls). The trend for the relative risk to decrease with increasing duration of use was of borderline statistical significance ($p = 0.05$).

Clavel et al. (1991) carried out a hospital-based case–control study in France between 1983 and 1987. Among 464 cases and 542 controls aged 25–56 years, nine cases (1.9%) and 10 controls (1.9%) had use of progestogen-only pills, yielding a multivariate relative risk estimate of 1.1 (95% confidence interval [CI], 0.4–2.7).

Ewertz (1992) carried out a population-based case–control study in Denmark of cases notified in 1983–84 and obtained data on contraceptive use from self-administered questionnaires. A total of 1059 cases and 990 controls were included. Among the 377 cases and 364 controls for which data on the type of preparation used were available, 28 cases and 29 controls had used a progestogen-only pill, yielding a relative risk estimate of 0.99 (95% CI, 0.57–1.71). For five or more years' use of progestogen-only pills, the estimate was 0.65 (95% CI, 0.28–1.5), based on nine case and 14 control users.

Skegg et al. (1996) assessed use of progestogen-only pills in data from the New Zealand National Study. On the basis of 50 cases (5.6%) and 163 controls (8.7%) with use of progestogen-only pills, the relative risk estimate for breast cancer was 1.1 (95% CI, 0.73–1.5) after adjustment for a number of factors, including age. There was a statistically significant increased risk (2.3; 95% CI, 1.2–4.3) among women aged 25–34, on the basis of 18 case and 70 control users. The corresponding estimates were 0.97 (95% CI, 0.6–1.6) for women aged 35–44, on the basis of 28 case and 80 control users, and 0.37 (95% CI, 0.12–1.2) for women aged 45–54, on the basis of four case and 13 control users; neither estimate was statistically significant. Virtually all of the women had used the preparations for fewer than six years; the estimates for fewer than two and two to five years of use were similar. In further analyses of women of all ages together, the relative risk estimate was increased for use that had begun in the previous 10 years (1.6; 95% CI, 1.0–2.4; 40 case and 111 control users) and reduced for use that had begun 10 or more years previously (0.44; 95% CI, 0.22–0.90; 10 case and 52 control users). When time since last use was assessed, the relative risk estimate was 1.4 (95% CI, 0.86–2.2) for last use fewer than five years previously (29 case and 91 control users), 1.0 (95% CI, 0.56–1.9) for use that had ceased five to nine years previously (16 case and 48 case users) and 0.44 (95% CI, 0.16–1.2) for use that had ceased at least 10 years previously (five case and 24 control users). There was no clear evidence of an effect of the age at which use began or the timing with respect to the first pregnancy.

(b) Depot medroxyprogesterone acetate

Paul *et al.* (1989) reported on the use of the injectable progestogen, depot medroxyprogesterone acetate, in a population-based case–control study of women aged 25–54 conducted in New Zealand between 1983 and 1987. A total of 110 (12%) of 891 cases and 252 (14%) of 1864 controls had used this preparation. There was no increase in risk overall (relative risk, 1.0; 95% CI, 0.8–1.3), but the relative risk estimate was increased among women aged 25–34 (2.0; 95% CI, 1.0–3.8; 16 case and 55 control users). The estimate was not increased in women aged 35–44 (0.94; 95% CI, 0.45–3.3; 48 case and 133 control users) or 45–54 (0.95; 95% CI, 0.63–1.4; 46 case and 64 control users). There was no trend in the overall data for an increase in risk with increasing duration of use, but only 1.5% of controls had used depot medroxyprogesterone acetate for six years or more. The relative risk estimates, although based on small numbers, were higher for women with two to five years of use before the age of 25 or before the first pregnancy than among women with less than two years of use. The relative risk estimate tended to be increased for recent users: it was 1.7 (95% CI, 0.88–3.4) for women who had begun use in the previous five years (16 case and 24 control users) and declined to 1.2 (95% CI, 0.76–1.9) five to nine years after first use, 0.92 (95% CI, 0.64–1.3) 10–14 years after first use and 0.73 (95% CI, 0.39–1.4) 15 or more years after first use; none of these estimates was statistically significant. A similar trend was seen with time since last use: the relative risk was 1.6 (95% CI, 1.0–2.5) for use within the previous five years, 0.99 (95% CI, 0.65–1.5) five to nine years after last use and 0.78 (95% CI, 0.53–1.2) 10 years or more after last use.

The WHO Collaborative Study of Neoplasia and Steroid Contraceptives (1991a) assessed use of depot medroxyprogesterone acetate in centres in Kenya, Mexico and Thailand in a hospital-based study conducted between 1979 and 1988 among women under 65 years of age. Among the 869 cases of breast cancer and 11 890 controls, 109 cases (13%) and 1452 controls (12%) reported use of depot medroxyprogesterone acetate, yielding an overall multivariate relative risk estimate of 1.2 (95% CI, 0.96–1.5). The relative risk estimate was 1.4 (95% CI, 0.88–2.2) for breast cancer at age < 35, 1.1 (95% CI, 0.75–1.55) at age 35–44 and 1.0 (95% CI, 0.68–1.5) at age 45 or older; none of these estimates was statistically significant. There was no trend for the risk to increase with duration of use; indeed, the largest relative risk estimate was for the shortest duration of use; however, only 3.6% of controls had been exposed for more than three years. The relative risk estimates tended to be highest among recent users: 2.0 (95% CI, 1.4–3.0) for women whose use had begun in the previous two years (31 case and 342 control users) and 1.6 (95% CI, 1.1–2.5) for current users (27 case and 291 control users).

2.1.2   *Pooled analysis of individual data*

The Collaborative Group on Hormonal Factors in Breast Cancer (1996) carried out a combined analysis of data on use of progestrogen-only oral contraceptives from 27 studies that provided information on these preparations to the investigators in 1995. On the basis of 725 of 27 054 cases and 528 of 25 551 controls with any use of these preparations, the relative risk estimate was 1.1 (95% CI, 0.99–1.2) (Figure 1). There was no significant trend with duration of use, time since first use or time since last use (Figures 2–4), although there was some suggestion that the risk was slightly elevated in current and recent users (1.2; 95% CI, 1.0–1.3) (Figure 4).

Skegg *et al.* (1995) published the results of a pooled analysis of individual data from two studies (Paul *et al.*, 1989; WHO Collaborative Study of Neoplasia and Steroid Contraceptives, 1991a) on depot medroxyprogesterone acetate. As had been observed in the separate studies, there was no association between use and overall risk, but an increased risk (not statistically significant) was found for women under 35 years of age and an increased risk (statistically significant) for women who had last used the preparation during the previous five years. The age-specific results for time since first use suggested an increased risk for use begun in the previous year in each age group: 2.0 (95% CI, 1.2–3.3) for < 35 years of age, 1.5 (95% CI, 0.9–2.4) for 35–44 years of age and 1.8 (95% CI, 0.81–4.0) for 45 years of age and older, although only the estimate for women < 35 years of age was statistically significant.

The Collaborative Group on Hormonal Factors in Breast Cancer (1996) also carried out a combined analysis of use of injectable progestogens. On the basis of any use in 339 of 17 639 cases and 1935 of 38 248 controls, the relative risk estimate was 1.0 (95% CI, 0.89–1.2) (Figure 5). There was no significant trend with duration of use (Figure 6). There was some evidence of an increased risk for users of depot progestogens (Figures 7 and 8), with a significant trend of decreasing risk with time since first use (Figure 7).

2.2   Endometrial cancer

2.2.1   *Cohort studies*

In a study at a family planning clinic in Atlanta, United States, one case of uterine cancer was found among 5000 African–American women aged 50 in 1967–76 who were receiving injections of depot medroxyprogesterone acetate, with 0.83 expected (relative risk, 1.2; 95% CI, 0.1–6.7) on the basis of the rates from the national Surveillance, Epidemiology and End Results programme (Liang *et al.*, 1983).

2.2.2   *Case–control studies* (Table 5)

In a multi-centre case–control study among women under 55 years of age in the United States, only one of the 433 women with endometrial cancer and six of the 3191 control women reported use of a progestogen-only oral contraceptive (odds ratio, 0.6; 95% CI, 0.1–5.0) in personal interviews (Centers for Disease Control and the National Institute of Child Health and Human Development, Cancer and Steroid Hormone Study, 1987).

Figure 1. Relative risks for breast cancer among women with any versus no use of progestogen-only oral contraceptives

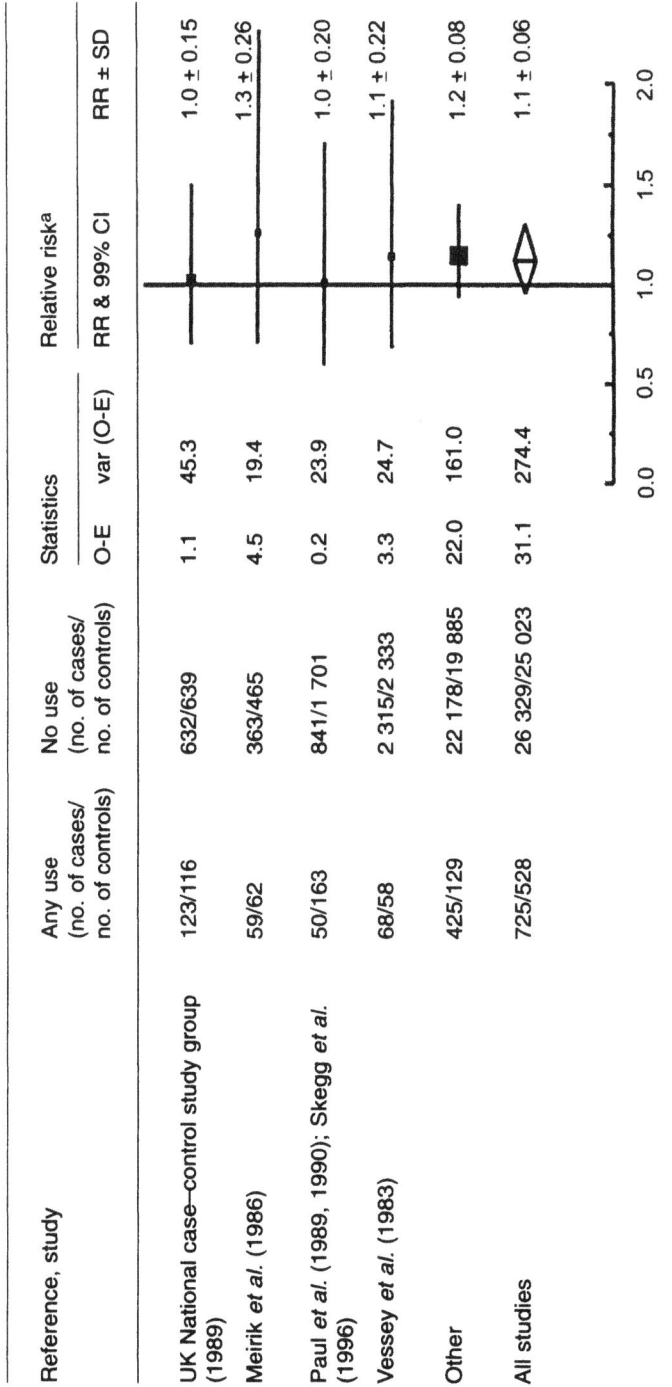

Reference, study	Any use (no. of cases/ no. of controls)	No use (no. of cases/ no. of controls)	Statistics		Relative risk[a]	
			O-E	var (O-E)	RR & 99% CI	RR ± SD
UK National case–control study group (1989)	123/116	632/639	1.1	45.3		1.0 ± 0.15
Meirik et al. (1986)	59/62	363/465	4.5	19.4		1.3 ± 0.26
Paul et al. (1989, 1990); Skegg et al. (1996)	50/163	841/1 701	0.2	23.9		1.0 ± 0.20
Vessey et al. (1983)	68/58	2 315/2 333	3.3	24.7		1.1 ± 0.22
Other	425/129	22 178/19 885	22.0	161.0		1.2 ± 0.08
All studies	725/528	26 329/25 023	31.1	274.4		1.1 ± 0.06

Test for heterogeneity between studies: χ^2 (4 d.f.) = 1.0; NS

Adapted from Collaborative Group on Hormonal Factors in Breast Cancer (1996)

O, observed; E, expected; RR, relative risk; CI, confidence interval; SD, standard deviation; d.f., degrees of freedom; NS, not significant

[a] Relative to no use, stratified by study, age at diagnosis, parity, age at first birth and age at which risk of conception ceased

Figure 2. Relative risk for breast cancer by duration of use of progestogen-only oral contraceptives

Duration of use (years)	No. of cases/ no. of controls	Statistics		Relative risk[a]	
		lnRR	1	RR (99% CI)	RR ± SD
		var(lnRR)	var(lnRR)		
Never	29 625/50 515	0.0	2469.0		1.0 ± 0.02
< 2	467/641	16.8	199.1		1.1 ± 0.07
2–3	120/150	7.6	52.2		1.2 ± 0.15
≥ 4	125/145	8.8	50.8		1.2 ± 0.15

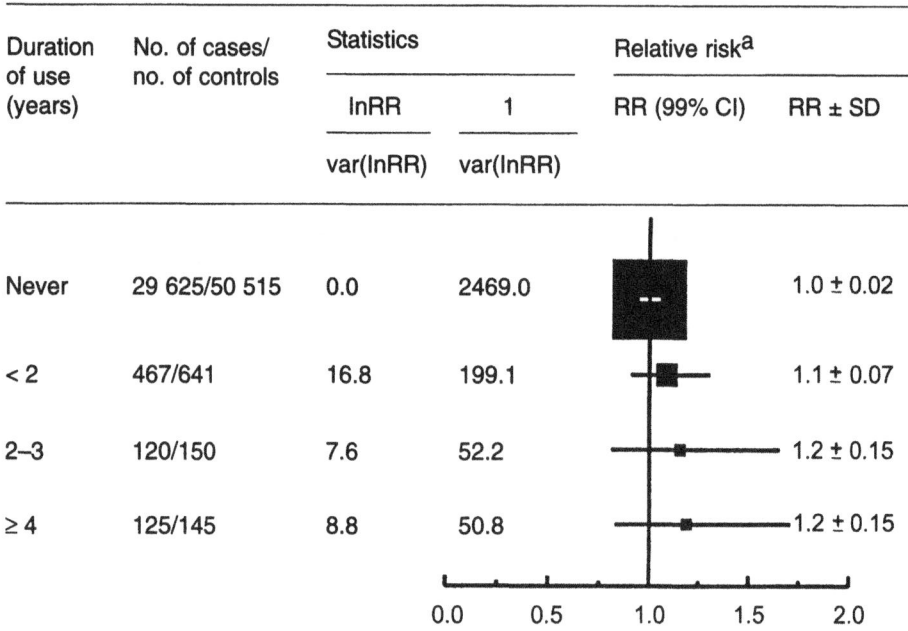

0.0   0.5   1.0   1.5   2.0

Adapted from Collaborative Group on Hormonal Factors in Breast Cancer (1996)
Test for trend with duration of use χ^2 (1 d.f.) = 0.4; NS
RR, relative risk; CI, confidence interval; SD, standard deviation; d.f., degree of freedom; NS, not significant
[a] Relative to no use, stratified by study, age at diagnosis, parity, age at first birth and age at which risk for conception ceased

A study in Bangkok and Chiang Mai, Thailand, found that the incidence of endometrial cancer was approximately 80% lower (odds ratio, 0.2; 95% CI, 0.1–0.8) among women (three cases and 84 controls) who reported using depot medroxyprogesterone acetate than among those who reported no use (119 cases and 855 controls) in personal interviews (WHO Collaborative Study of Neoplasia and Steroid Contraceptives, 1991b). All three case women who had used this preparation had also used pre-menopausal oestrogens.

2.3   Cervical cancer

2.3.1   *Methodological considerations*

The same methodological issues as are described in section 2.3 of the monograph on 'Oral contraceptives, combined' must be considered when assessing associations between use of injectable contraceptives and cervical carcinoma.

Figure 3. Relative risk for breast cancer by time since first use of progestogen-only oral contraceptives

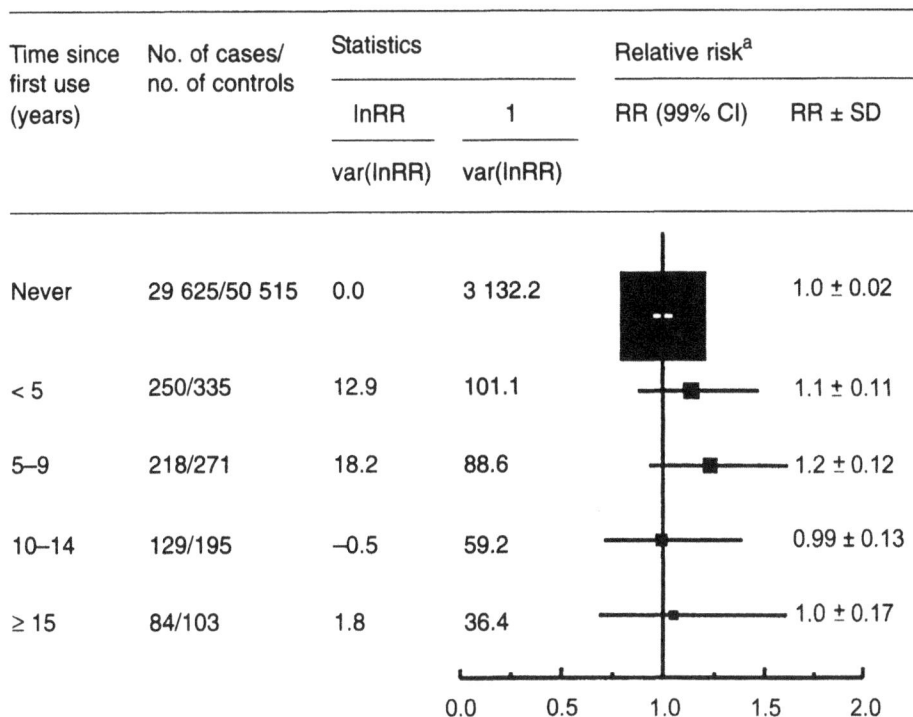

Time since first use (years)	No. of cases/ no. of controls	Statistics		Relative risk[a]	
		$\frac{\ln RR}{var(\ln RR)}$	$\frac{1}{var(\ln RR)}$	RR (99% CI)	RR ± SD
Never	29 625/50 515	0.0	3 132.2		1.0 ± 0.02
< 5	250/335	12.9	101.1		1.1 ± 0.11
5–9	218/271	18.2	88.6		1.2 ± 0.12
10–14	129/195	−0.5	59.2		0.99 ± 0.13
≥ 15	84/103	1.8	36.4		1.0 ± 0.17

Adapted from Collaborative Group on Hormonal Factors in Breast Cancer (1996)

Test for trend with time since first use: χ^2 (1 d.f.) = 0.6; NS

RR, relative risk; CI, confidence interval; SD, standard deviation; d.f., degree of freedom; NS, not significant

[a] Relative to no use, stratified by study, age at diagnosis, parity, age at first birth and age at which risk for conception ceased

2.3.2   *Cervical dysplasia and carcinoma* in situ

The New Zealand Contraception and Health Study Group (1994) followed a cohort of 7199 women for about five years. All of the women had two normal cervical smears at entry into the cohort and were using either oral contraceptives, an intrauterine device or depot medroxyprogesterone acetate as their method of contraception. The risk for dysplasia per 1000 women was 58.7 for the users of depot medroxyprogesterone acetate and 44.4 for those with an intrauterine device. This difference was not statistically significant. The incidence rate of more severe dysplasia or carcinoma *in situ* was 0.9/1000 in both groups. After control for multiple confounding factors, including the number of sexual partners, the risk of the progestogen users relative to that of women with an intrauterine device was 1.2.

From data on women included in the WHO Collaborative Study of Neoplasia and Steroid Contraceptives in Mexico and Thailand, Thomas *et al.* (1995a) estimated that the

Figure 4. Relative risk for breast cancer by time since last use of progestogen-only oral contraceptives

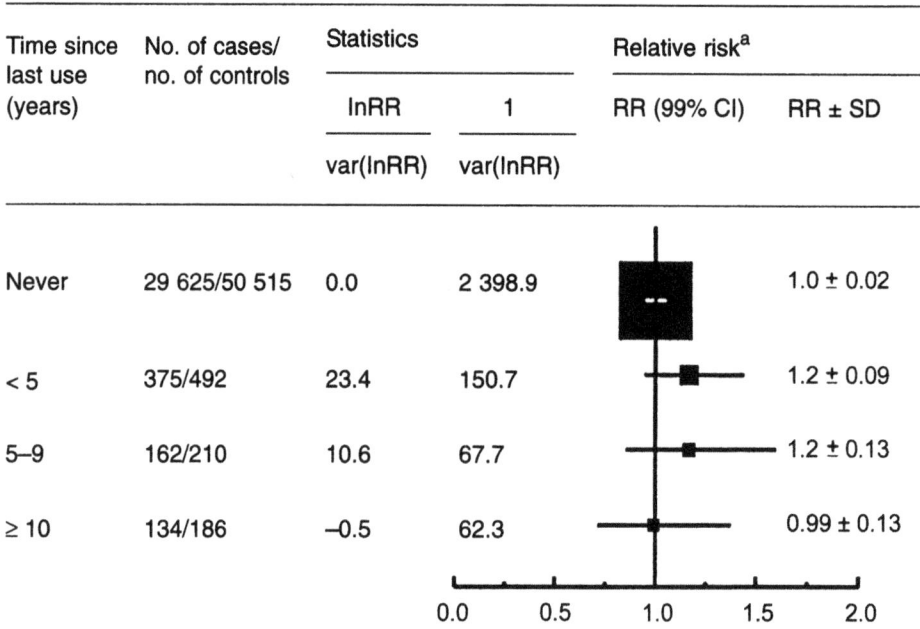

Time since last use (years)	No. of cases/ no. of controls	Statistics		Relative risk[a]	
		$\dfrac{\ln RR}{var(\ln RR)}$	$\dfrac{1}{var(\ln RR)}$	RR (99% CI)	RR ± SD
Never	29 625/50 515	0.0	2 398.9		1.0 ± 0.02
< 5	375/492	23.4	150.7		1.2 ± 0.09
5–9	162/210	10.6	67.7		1.2 ± 0.13
≥ 10	134/186	−0.5	62.3		0.99 ± 0.13

```
        0.0      0.5      1.0      1.5      2.0
```

Adapted from Collaborative Group on Hormonal Factors in Breast Cancer (1996)

Test for trend with time since last use: χ^2 (1 d.f.) = 1.0; NS

RR, relative risk; CI, confidence interval; SD, standard deviation; d.f., degree of freedom; NS, not significant

[a] Relative to no use, stratified by study, age at diagnosis, parity, age at first birth and age at which risk for conception ceased

relative risk for cervical carcinoma *in situ* of women who had ever used depot medroxyprogesterone acetate was 1.4 (95% CI, 1.2–1.7); however, when the analyses were restricted to women with symptoms of vaginal bleeding or discharge, to minimize the possibility of bias due to selective screening of women on this preparation, the relative risk estimate was 1.2 (95% CI, 1.0–1.5). Nonetheless, women with symptoms had a significant trend ($p = 0.017$) in risk with duration of use: women who had used depot medroxyprogesterone acetate for more than five years had a relative risk of 1.8 (95% CI, 1.2–2.6). There was no trend in risk with time since first or last use. When considering women who had used this preparation for more than five years, the risk was increased for those who had last used it within the previous 10 years but not for those who had used it before that time.

2.3.3   *Invasive cervical carcinoma*

Two case–control studies have been conducted of the risk for invasive cervical cancer and use of injectable contraceptives. Herrero *et al.* (1990) recruited cases from six hospitals in Colombia, Costa Rica, Mexico and Panama. Controls were selected from the

Figure 5. Relative risk for breast cancer among women with any use of depot progestogens versus those who had never used them

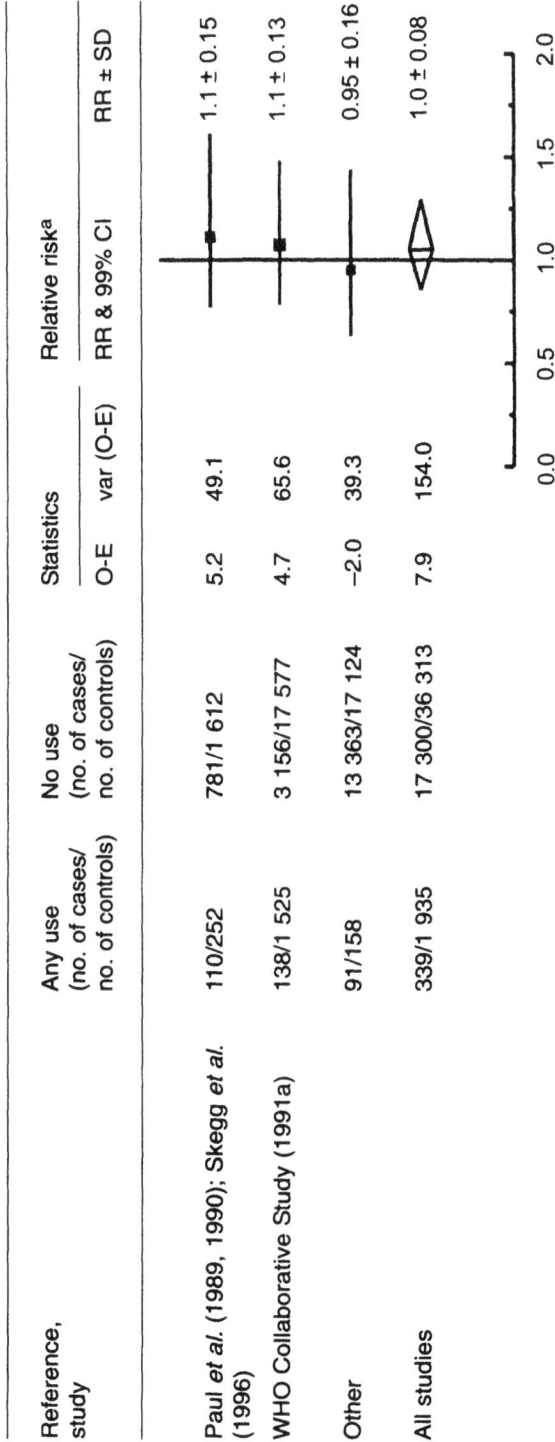

Reference, study	Any use (no. of cases/ no. of controls)	No use (no. of cases/ no. of controls)	Statistics		Relative risk[a]	
			O-E	var (O-E)	RR & 99% CI	RR ± SD
Paul et al. (1989, 1990); Skegg et al. (1996)	110/252	781/1 612	5.2	49.1		1.1 ± 0.15
WHO Collaborative Study (1991a)	138/1 525	3 156/17 577	4.7	65.6		1.1 ± 0.13
Other	91/158	13 363/17 124	-2.0	39.3		0.95 ± 0.16
All studies	339/1 935	17 300/36 313	7.9	154.0		1.0 ± 0.08

Adapted from Collaborative Group on Hormonal Factors in Breast Cancer (1996)
Test for heterogeneity between studies: χ^2 (2 d.f.) = 0.6; NS

O, observed; E, expected; RR, relative risk; CI, confidence interval; SD, standard deviation; d.f., degree of freedom; NS, not significant
[a] Relative to no use, stratified by study, age at diagnosis, parity, age at first birth and age at which risk for conception ceased

Figure 6. Relative risk for breast cancer by duration of use of depot progestogens

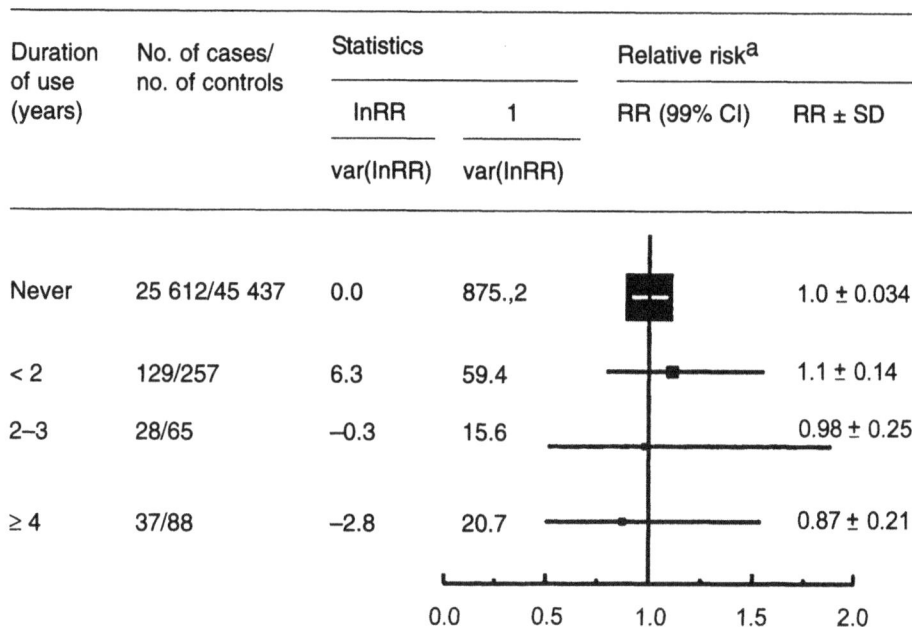

Duration of use (years)	No. of cases/ no. of controls	Statistics		Relative risk[a]	
		lnRR	1	RR (99% CI)	RR ± SD
		var(lnRR)	var(lnRR)		
Never	25 612/45 437	0.0	875.,2		1.0 ± 0.034
< 2	129/257	6.3	59.4		1.1 ± 0.14
2–3	28/65	–0.3	15.6		0.98 ± 0.25
≥ 4	37/88	–2.8	20.7		0.87 ± 0.21

0.0   0.5   1.0   1.5   2.0

Adapted from Collaborative Group on Hormonal Factors in Breast Cancer (1996)
Test for trend with duration of use χ^2 (1 d.f.) = 0.4; NS
RR, relative risk; CI, confidence interval; SD, standard deviation; d.f., degree of freedom; NS, not significant
[a] Relative to no use, stratified by study, age at diagnosis, parity, age at first birth and age at which risk for conception ceased

same hospitals from which the cases were recruited; in Costa Rica and Panama, community controls were also selected. The results were reported for use of all injectable contraceptives combined and not separately for specific agents. Of the users, 55% reported using injectable contraceptives monthly and 45% reported using them every three months. The preparation used more frequently than every three months was probably norethisterone oenanthate and that used every three months was probably depot medroxyprogesterone acetate. Cervical swabs were taken from the study subjects and tested for type-specific human papillomavirus DNA by filter in-situ hybridization. After control for age, age at first intercourse, number of sexual partners, number of pregnancies, detected presence of human papillomavirus type-16/-18 DNA, interval since last Papanicolaou (Pap) smear and socioeconomic status, the risk of women who had ever used injectable contraceptives for six or more months, relative to non-users, was estimated to be 0.8 (95% CI, 0.5–1.2). The risk was not increased for women who had used these products for fewer than five years (0.5; 95% CI, 0.3–0.9) but was 2.4 (95% CI, 1.0–5.7) for women who had used them for five or more years. There were no significant trends in risk with time since first or last use;

Figure 7. Relative risk for breast cancer by time since first use of depot progestogens

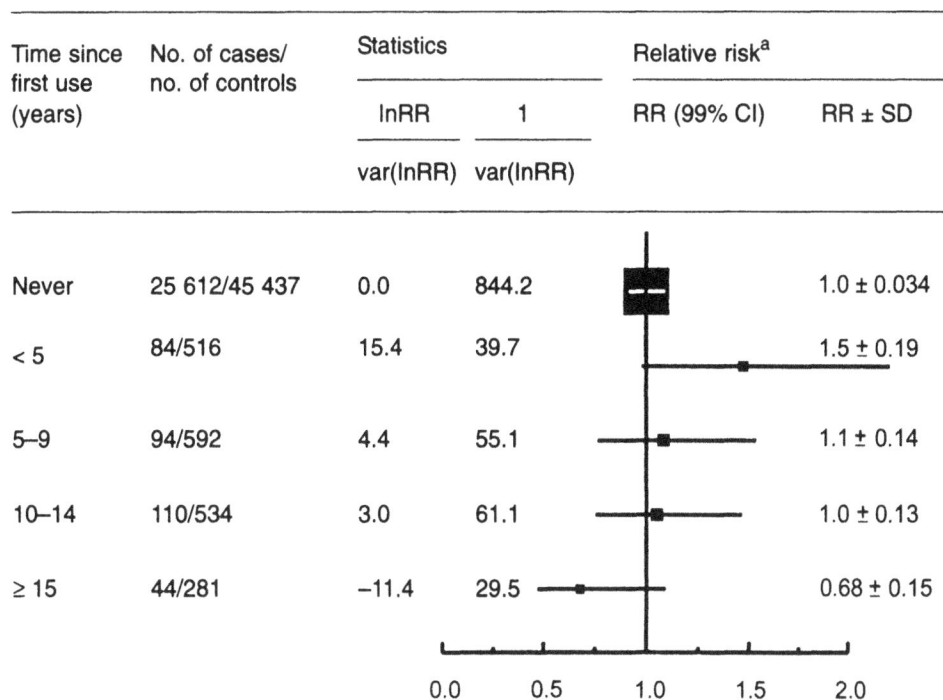

Time since first use (years)	No. of cases/ no. of controls	Statistics		Relative risk[a]	
		lnRR	1	RR (99% CI)	RR ± SD
		var(lnRR)	var(lnRR)		
Never	25 612/45 437	0.0	844.2		1.0 ± 0.034
< 5	84/516	15.4	39.7		1.5 ± 0.19
5–9	94/592	4.4	55.1		1.1 ± 0.14
10–14	110/534	3.0	61.1		1.0 ± 0.13
≥ 15	44/281	−11.4	29.5		0.68 ± 0.15

```
        0.0      0.5      1.0     1.5      2.0
```

Adapted from Collaborative Group on Hormonal Factors in Breast Cancer (1996)
Test for trend with duration of use χ^2 (1 d.f.) = 8.8; p = 0.003
RR, relative risk; CI, confidence interval; SD, standard deviation; d.f., degree of freedom
[a] Relative to no use, stratified by study, age at diagnosis, parity, age at first birth and age at which risk for conception ceased

however, the highest relative risks were observed for women who had used these products for more than five years and who had first used them more than 10 years previously (relative risk, 3.4; 95% CI, 1.1–25) and for women who had used the products for more than five years and who had last used them more than five years previously (relative risk, 5.3; 95% CI, 1.1–10). These increased risks must be interpreted with caution, however, because significantly reduced risks were observed for women who had used the products for fewer than five years and had used them for the first time within the past 10 years (relative risk, 0.4; 95% CI, 0.2–0.8) or within the past five years (relative risk, 0.4; 95% CI, 0.2–0.8). The reduced risks in relatively recent users could be due to more intensive screening in women receiving depot medroxyprogesterone acetate, so that earlier stages of disease are detected before progression to invasive disease.

In the WHO Collaborative Study of Neoplasia and Steroid Contraceptives (1992), described in section 2.1.1(b), 2009 women with invasive cervical cancer were compared

Figure 8. Relative risk for breast cancer by time since last use of depot pro-gestogens

Time since last use (years)	No. of cases/ no. of controls	Statistics		Relative risk[a]	
		$\frac{\text{lnRR}}{\text{var(lnRR)}}$	$\frac{1}{\text{var(lnRR)}}$	RR (99% CI)	RR ± SD
Never	25 612/45 437	0.0	809.0		1.0 ± 0.035
< 5	137/921	11.4	71.5		1.2 ± 0.13
5–9	82/514	−0.9	51.1		0.98 ± 0.14
≥ 10	101/467	−3.3	55.5		0.94 ± 0.13

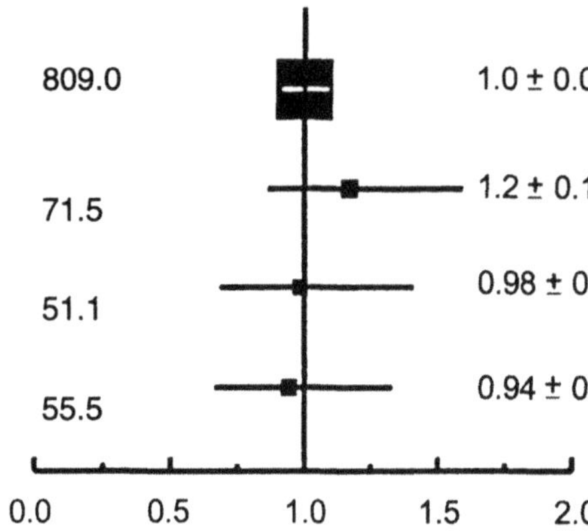

```
        0.0    0.5    1.0    1.5    2.0
```

Adapted from Collaborative Group on Hormonal Factors in Breast Cancer (1996)

Test for trend with duration of use χ^2 (1 d.f.) = 1.6; NS

RR, relative risk; CI, confidence interval; SD, standard deviation; d.f., degree of freedom; NS, not significant

[a] Relative to no use, stratified by study, age at diagnosis, parity, age at first birth and age at which risk for conception ceased

with 9583 hospital controls. After taking into consideration age, total number of pregnancies, number of prior Pap smears, use of oral contraceptives and centre, the relative risk for women who had ever used depot medroxyprogesterone acetate was estimated to be 1.1 (95% CI, 1.0–1.3).

Using data from this study, Thomas *et al.* (1995b) also assessed risks for adenocarcinoma and adenosquamous carcinoma in relation to use of depot medroxyprogesterone acetate. On the basis of 239 women with adenocarcinoma and 85 with adenosquamous carcinoma, the risks of women who had ever used this preparation relative to 2534 age-matched hospital controls were estimated to be 0.8 (95% CI, 0.5–1.3) for adenocarcinomas and 0.7 (95% CI, 0.3–1.7) for adenosquamous carcinoma. All of the relative risks in this study were assessed for possible confounding by variables including numbers of pregnancies, live births and sexual partners, history of abortion and stillbirths, age at first live birth, age at first sexual intercourse, marital status, history of a variety of sexually transmitted diseases, serological evidence of herpes simplex virus infection, prior Pap smears, level of education and use of other methods of contraception. Because the relative

Table 5. Case–control studies of use of progestogen-only contraceptives and endometrial cancer

Reference	Location/period/ ages	Source of controls	Ascertain- ment	Participation (%)		Type/measure of therapy	No. of subjects		OR (95% CI)
				Cases	Controls		Cases	Controls	
Centers for Disease Control (1987)	Eight US SEER areas/Dec. 1980– Dec. 1982/ 20–54 years	General population	Personal interviews	73	84	Never used POC Any use of POC	250 1	1 147 6	Referent 0.6 (0.1–5.0)
WHO Collaborative Study (1991b)	Bangkok, Chiang Mai, Thailand/ Jan. 1979–Feb. 1986/< 60 years	Hospital patients	Personal interviews	98	96	Never used DMPA Ever used DMPA	119 3	855 85	Referent 0.2 (0.1–0.81)

OR, odds ratio; CI, confidence interval; POC, progestogen-only contraceptives; DMPA, depot medroxyprogesterone acetate

risk estimates for the two histological types were similar, the data for the two types were combined, giving a relative risk of 0.8 (95% CI, 0.5–1.1) for women who had ever used depot medroxyprogesterone acetate. No trends in relative risk with length of use or time since first or last use were observed. The relative risk of women who had used the product for more than four years was estimated to be 0.7 (95% CI, 0.4–1.4).

2.4   Ovarian cancer

2.4.1   *Cohort studies*
In the study of Liang *et al.* (1983) described in section 2.2, one case of ovarian cancer was observed with 1.2 expected, corresponding to a relative risk of 0.8 (95% CI, 0.1–4.6).

2.4.2   *Case–control studies*
Within the framework of the WHO Collaborative Study of Neoplasia and Steroid Contraceptives (1991c), hospital-based data from Mexico and Thailand were analysed with reference to use of depot medroxyprogesterone acetate and the risk for epithelial ovarian cancer. A total of 224 cases and 1781 hospital controls were collected between 1979 and 1988. The multivariate relative risk for any use was 1.1 (95% CI, 0.6–1.8) in the absence of any duration–risk relationship (relative risk, 1.1 for ≥ 5 years of use; 95% CI, 0.4–3.2).

Little information is available on progestogen-only oral contraceptives. In a hospital-based case–control study of 441 cases and 2065 controls recruited between 1977 and 1991 from various areas of the United States (Rosenberg *et al.*, 1994), 1% of cases and 3% of controls had ever used such preparations. [The unadjusted odds ratio was 0.3.]

2.5   Liver cancer

The WHO Collaborative Study of Neoplasia and Steroid Contraceptives (1991d) also addressed the association between use of depot medroxyprogesterone acetate and the risk for cancer of the liver. Cases were women diagnosed with cancer in three centres in Thailand in 1979–88 and one centre in Kenya in 1979–86. Of the 94 eligible cases, 71 (75.5%) were interviewed. About two controls were identified for each case, chosen from the same hospital but not otherwise matched; women were not eligible as potential controls if they had been admitted to the hospital for conditions that might have altered their use of steroid contraceptives. Of 10 796 eligible controls that were identified, 10 382 (96.2%) were interviewed. Eight controls per case of liver cancer were randomly selected from the pool, resulting in the inclusion of 530 controls, matched on hospital, age and date of diagnosis. Information on smoking was not collected. As alcohol intake was not associated with the risk for liver cancer in these women, the relative risks were not adjusted for alcohol intake. Subjects were not tested for evidence of infection with hepatitis B virus, but both countries are endemic for this infection. The relative risks were adjusted for age, centre, date of diagnosis and number of live births and were presented separately for Kenya and Thailand. In Kenya, four out of 22 cases (18.2%) had used depot medroxyprogesterone acetate; the relative risks were 1.6 (95% CI, 0.4–6.6) for any use, 0.7 (95% CI, 0.1–6.8) for use for 1–26 months and 2.9 (95% CI, 0.5–15.2) for use for more than 26 months. Fifteen of the 22 cases in Kenya were diagnosed only on clinical grounds. In Thailand, four out of 49 cases (8.2%) had used depot medroxy-progesterone acetate; the relative risks were 0.3 (95% CI, 0.1–1.0) for any use, 0.2 (95% CI, 0.0–1.2) for use for 1–26 months, 0.3 (95% CI, 0.0–2.5) for 27–58 months and 0.7 (95% CI, 0.2–3.2) for more than 58 months.

Kew *et al.* (1990) conducted a hospital-based case–control study in Johannesburg, South Africa. The cases were those of patients with histologically confirmed hepato-cellular carcinoma which had been diagnosed when they were aged 19–54. Two controls per case were selected, matched on age, race, tribe, rural or urban birth, hospital and ward; patients with diseases in which contraceptive steroids might be causally implicated were not eligible as controls. The response rates were not given. Smoking and alcohol intake were associated with the risk for liver cancer, but inclusion of these variables in the analysis did not alter the results. Five of 46 cases (11%) and 21 of 92 controls (23%) had used injectable progestogens, giving an overall relative risk of 0.4 (95% CI, 0.1–1.2). Nineteen of the 46 cases had antibodies to hepatitis B surface antigen, 25 had evidence of past infection with hepatitis B virus, and two had no evidence of infection.

2.6   Malignant melanoma

One Danish case–control study of malignant melanoma (Østerlind *et al.*, 1988), described in detail in the monograph on 'Post-menopausal oestrogen therapy', provided data on the use of progestogens alone. These preparations were used as oral contraceptives by 14 cases and 23 controls (relative risk, 1.2; 95% CI, 0.6–2.6) and as post-menopausal therapy by three cases and four controls (crude relative risk, 1.5; 95% CI, 0.3–8.1).

3.   Studies of Cancer in Experimental Animals

In the only study evaluated previously (IARC, 1979) on the carcinogenicity of pro-gestogen-only contraceptives in experimental animals, medroxyprogesterone acetate, tested by intramuscular injection in dogs, produced malignant mammary tumours. No information was available at that time on levonorgestrel. The results of relevant studies published since that time are described below. Except where indicated, tumour deve-lopment in tissues other than those mentioned was not reported.

3.1   Medroxyprogesterone acetate

3.1.1   *Subcutaneous implantation*

(*a*)   *Mouse*

A group of virgin female BALB/c mice, eight weeks of age, was divided into three subgroups: 44 received 60 mg progesterone, as 40 mg in a Silastic pellet implanted sub-cutaneously initially and 20 mg six months later; 45 received 60 mg medroxyprogesterone acetate, as a 40-mg pellet initially and 20 mg six months later; and 47 received 160 mg of the progestogen, 40 mg subcutaneously every three months for one year, representing the protocol used in the development of this model (Lanari *et al.*, 1986). The incidence of mammary adenocarcinoma and the numbers and latency of the tumours are shown in Table 6. The carcinomas induced by medroxyprogesterone acetate were predominantly ductal but included some lobular carcinomas. The incidence of mammary carcinomas in untreated controls was reported previously by Lanari *et al.* (1986) to be 0/42 at 80–90 weeks of age (Kordon *et al.*, 1993).

Table 6. Mammary tumour incidence, number and latency in BALB/c mice treated with medroxyprogesterone acetate (MPA)

Treatment	Dose (mg)	Mammary tumour incidence		No. of tumours	Latency (weeks)
		No.	%		
Progesterone	60	9/44	28	10	46.2
MPA	60	18/45	58[a]	30	51.3
MPA	160	34/38	98[b]	38	50.1

From Kordon *et al.* (1993)
[a] Significantly greater than with progesterone ($p < 0.05$)
[b] Significantly greater than with 60 mg MPA ($p < 0.0001$)

Female BALB/c mice, two months of age, were either left intact or sialoadenectomized. One month after sialoadenectomy, all mice were injected subcutaneously with 40 mg depot medroxyprogesterone acetate, and the same treatment was given every three months for one year. The incidence of ductal and lobular mammary adenocarcinomas in the intact mice was 34/47, and that in the sialoadenectomized group was significantly less (11/48; $p < 0.001$). The tumour latency was similar: 52.5 ± 3.8 and 50.1 ± 2.1 weeks, respectively (Kordon *et al.*, 1994).

(b)   Dog

Groups of 20 virgin beagle bitches were hysterectomized at four to six months of age and given medroxyprogesterone acetate intramuscularly as an aqueous suspension, at a dose of 0 (control), 30, 180 or 690 mg every three months for 48 months, corresponding to one, six and 23 times the human contraceptive dose. As shown in Table 7, the incidence of mammary tumour nodules was increased in treated animals. Histopathological examination of the nodules revealed the presence of hyperplasia, including 13 animals at the high dose with complex lobular hyperplasias. At that dose, the tumour type was predominantly (12/14) complex adenoma. No carcinomas were detected (Frank *et al.*, 1979).

Table 7. Mammary tumour nodules in beagle bitches treated with medroxyprogesterone acetate (MPA)

Dose of MPA (mg/kg bw)	No. of surviving bitches	No. of bitches with nodules	No. of nodules
0 (vehicle)	17	2	2
3	19	13	29
30	18	15	93
75	14	12	105

From Frank *et al.* (1979)

Data on mammary tumour incidence in dogs treated therapeutically with medroxy-progesterone acetate for the prevention of oestrus were obtained from 10 veterinary practices in the Netherlands (van Os *et al.*, 1981) for 341 bitches; 339 untreated bitches were included as controls. The minimum age was two years, but most were older. The practitioners had used the recommended dose, which was 50–100 mg per bitch, with an interval of six months between doses, except at the start when dosing was more frequent. Putative mammary tumours were generally not examined histologically and are thus referred to as 'nodules', which were classed by size as < 1, 1–< 2, 2–< 3 and ≥ 3 cm. The first two sizes were combined and referred to as 'small' nodules and the last two were combined and referred to as 'large' nodules. The appearance of nodules was reported as a function of age, and the data were stratified in ranges of 2–< 4, 4–< 6, 6–< 9 and ≥ 9 years. Table 8 shows the incidence of mammary nodules by age in the treated and untreated groups. Treatment with medroxyprogesterone acetate increased the incidence of mammary nodules of all sizes in comparison with controls, and the tumour incidence increased with time, although treatment caused a significant increase even when given for less than four years.

Table 8. Mammary nodules in bitches treated with medroxy-progesterone acetate (MPA)

Age (years)	Controls (% with nodules)		MPA (% with nodules)	
	All sizes	2–≥ 3 cm	All sizes	2–≥ 3 cm
2–< 4	0	0	5	2
4–< 6	5	5	19[a]	14[a]
6–< 9	21	13	50[a]	39[a]
≥ 9	53	43	71[a]	56[a]

From van Os *et al.* (1981)
[a] Significantly greater than untreated controls by χ^2 test

Beagle bitches, one to six years of age, were used to determine the effect of medroxy-progesterone acetate on mammary tumour development. In one study, the progestogen was given as a single intramuscular injection into alternate rear legs every three months at a dose of 2 or 10 mg/kg bw, measured at the start of the experiment. Half of the animals in each group received seven injections and were killed at 20–22 months; the other half received six injections and were then maintained for 19 months without further treatment. In the second study, the protocol was similar except that the amount of progestogen administered was based on body weight at the time of treatment. The doses injected were 0.2, 0.8 and 1.2 mg/kg bw, made by diluting Depo-Provera in vehicle. A total dose of 75 mg/kg bw was given at two to three intramuscular sites in the hind legs. Controls received the vehicle alone. The incidences of gross mammary gland nodules observed at necropsy in bitches treated with medroxyprogesterone acetate are shown in Table 9. The nodular lesions consisted of simple or complex lobular hyperplasia, simple adenomas, complex adenomas and benign mixed tumours; no malignant tumours were observed. In similar groups of bitches given 75 mg/kg bw medroxyprogesterone acetate, prior ovari-ectomy did not significantly affect the induced mammary gland enlargement or nodule development, and prior hypophysectomy did not affect the induced mammary gland enlargement but significantly reduced the incidence of nodules (Concannon *et al.*, 1981).

Data were collected from eight veterinary practices around Amsterdam, the Netherlands, on 2031 bitches, comprising 576 with mammary tumours and 1455 control animals. Of the animals studied, 441 had been ovariectomized (most were ovariohyste-rectomized); 350 of these were controls. Medroxyprogesterone acetate was used in seven practices and proligestone in one [the data were not stratified for progestogen type]. Three groups were formed: animals in which tumours were diagnosed in 1976–79, animals in which tumours were diagnosed in 1980 and a control group formed in 1980. The groups were subdivided into age strata of 0–3, 4–5, 6–7, 8–9, 10–11 and 12 years and older. A

Table 9. Mammary gland nodules in beagle bitches treated with medroxyprogesterone acetate (MPA)

Dose of MPA (mg/kg bw)	No. of animals	Bitches with nodules (%)		
		5–9 mm	10–14 mm	≥ 15 mm
0	24	25	4	0
1.2[a,b]	6	7	0	0
2[b]	6	0	0	0
10[b]	7	57	14	14
75[a,c]	12	92	58	75

From Concannon et al. (1981)
[a] Data from second study
[b] Killed at 20–22 months
[c] Combination of animals killed at 20–22 months and 24 months

comparison of the two tumour groups with the controls showed that the progestogen-treated bitches had a somewhat greater risk for developing benign and malignant mammary tumours combined. The calculated relative risks for the most recent tumour group were 1.5 ($p < 0.05$) for regular progestogen treatment and 1.3 ($p < 0.05$) for irregular treatment. The proportions of malignant mammary tumours were similar after regular and irregular treatment; however, the author reported that progestogen treatment caused an earlier appearance of both benign and malignant mammary tumours (Misdorp, 1988, 1991).

Two groups of seven elderly beagle bitches weighing 10–15 kg (median ages, 7 and 6.8 years) that had not previously been treated with progestogens were subjected to surgical ovariohysterectomy to eliminate endogenous progesterone. Four to six weeks later, depot medroxyprogesterone acetate (10 mg/kg bw) or proligestone (50 mg/kg bw) was administered subcutaneously at three-week intervals for a total of eight injections. Four to eight weeks after the last injection, three dogs per group were killed for analysis of tissues, and the remaining four per group were maintained for six months without additional progestogen treatment. After this time, treatment was resumed at the same intervals, for a total of five more injections. The dogs were killed five to eight weeks later. Four dogs served as untreated controls; no abnormalities were found in any organ. The most frequent changes in the progestogen-treated dogs were adrenal atrophy (6/7 receiving medroxyprogesterone acetate and 7/7 receiving proligestone) and benign mammary tumours (5/7 receiving medroxyprogesterone acetate and 5/7 receiving proligestone). Some hepatic and pancreatic toxicity was also observed (Selman *et al.*, 1995).

(c)   Cat

Misdorp (1991) obtained data on 735 cats from the same veterinary practices as those from which data were obtained on dogs; 154 of the cats had mammary carcinomas, 35 had benign tumours, and 546 were used as controls. Medroxyprogesterone acetate was the commonest progestogen used, but some cats had been treated with megestrol acetate and some with proligestone. The type of progestogen was not taken into account in the analysis. Regular progestogen treatment was associated with a significantly increased relative risk (2.8; $p < 0.001$) for developing mammary carcinoma and a significantly increased risk (5.3; $p < 0.001$) for developing benign mammary tumours. Irregular treatment was not associated with an increased risk.

(d)   Monkey

[The Working Group was aware of an unpublished study on female rhesus monkeys reviewed by Jordan (1994). In this 10-year study, treatment with doses 50 times the human contraceptive dose of depot medroxyprogesterone acetate increased the incidence of endometrial carcinomas, two tumours appearing in the treated monkeys and none in controls.]

3.1.2   *Administration with known carcinogens*
    (*a*)   *Mouse*

Two groups of 20 female BALB/c mice, two to three months of age, received medroxy-progesterone acetate as a subcutaneous implant of 40-mg Silastic pellets followed after four months with 20 mg, and a further group received pellets without medroxyprogesterone acetate. One week later, mice in one of the treated groups and the controls were injected intraperitoneally three times at monthly intervals with 50 mg/kg bw N-methyl-N-nitroso-urea (MNU). The mammary tumour incidences and latencies were increased in the group given the combined treatment (Table 10) after seven months, before mammary tumours induced by medroxyprogesterone acetate would have appeared. The differences in tumour incidence and latency between the groups receiving MNU and without the progestogen were significant ($p < 0.01$ and $p < 0.05$, respectively) (Pazos *et al.*, 1991).

Table 10. Mammary tumour incidence and latency in BALB/c mice treated with medroxyprogesterone acetate (MPA) followed by N-methyl-N-nitrosourea (MNU)

Treatment	Tumour incidence		Latency (days)
	No.	%	
MPA + MNU	15/19	79	154 ± 19
MNU	3/20	15	179 ± 7
MPA	0/20	0	> 180

From Pazos *et al.* (1991)

Adult virgin female Swiss albino mice, eight to nine weeks of age, were given about 300 μg 3-methylcholanthrene intracervically in beeswax-impregnated threads. Medroxy-progesterone acetate was given intramuscularly at a dose of 50 μg/mouse every fifth day for 30, 60 or 90 days, with or without 3-methylcholanthrene, and mice were killed after 30, 60 and 90 days and observed for cervical lesions. The incidences of cervical invasive squamous-cell carcinomas in mice given the carcinogen plus medroxyprogesterone acetate were 0/30 after 30 days, 4/30 after 60 days and 22/38 after 90 days ($p < 0.05$). 3-Methyl-cholanthrene alone caused small increases in tumour incidence after 60 days (2/20) and 90 days (8/26) in comparison with the wax thread alone. Cervical dysplasia, but no cervical tumours, was observed in mice receiving medroxyprogesterone acetate alone (Hussain & Rao, 1991).

Groups of 35, 30 and 30 female ICR mice, 10 weeks of age, were treated with 10 mg/kg bw MNU after laparotomy by injection into the left uterine tube; the right uterine tube received saline. A group of 20 mice did not receive MNU. Two of the groups receiving MNU were fed a diet containing 5 ppm oestradiol and the other group and those not receiving MNU were fed basal diet. One group given both MNU and oestradiol and those not given MNU received subcutaneous injections of 2 mg/mouse medroxyprogesterone acetate every four weeks from week 7 after MNU or no treatment. The duration of the experiment was 30 weeks. As shown in Table 11, adenocarcinomas and preneoplastic lesions developed in the uteri of mice in all groups treated with MNU. Medroxyprogesterone acetate significantly decreased the incidence of endometrial adenocarcinomas. In addition, while it caused a reduction in uterine weight, it had no effect on body weight. Medroxyprogesterone acetate alone did not induce either uterine or mammary tumours (Niwa *et al.*, 1995).

Table 11. Uterine tumour incidence in ICR mice treated with *N*-methyl-*N*-nitrosourea (MNU) followed by medroxyprogesterone acetate (MPA), with or without oestradiol

Treatment	Atypical hyperplasia	Adenocarcinoma
MNU + oestradiol + MPA	4/30*	2/30**
MNU + oestradiol	16/24	8/24
MNU alone	7/26	3/26
MPA alone	0/20	0/20

From Niwa *et al.* (1993)
* Significantly less than with MNU plus oestradiol ($p < 0.001$)
**Significantly less than with MNU plus oestradiol ($p < 0.05$)

Four groups of 40 virgin female CD2F$_1$ (BALB/c × DBA/2) mice, six weeks of age, received six doses of 1 mg 7,12-dimethylbenz[*a*]anthracene (DMBA) by gavage at 6, 9, 10, 11, 12 and 13 weeks; four doses of DMBA at 9, 10, 12 and 13 weeks; a subcutaneous implant of a 20-mg pellet of medroxyprogesterone acetate at six weeks plus DMBA at 9 and 10 weeks; or an implant of medroxyprogesterone acetate at six weeks plus DMBA at 9, 10, 12 and 13 weeks. A control group of 20 mice received a subcutaneous implant of medroxyprogesterone acetate at six weeks. The experiment was terminated at 56 weeks. The incidences of mammary adencarcinoma and the latencies are shown in Table 12 (Aldaz *et al.*, 1996). Medroxyprogesterone acetate shortened the latency and enhanced the incidences of mammary adenocarcinomas. [The Working Group noted that it is not possible to assess whether medroxyprogesterone acetate alone produces mammary adeno-carcinomas in this strain of mice, since the latency for mammary tumour induction in BALB/c mice by this compound alone is > 50 weeks (Lanari *et al.*, 1986).]

Virgin female BALB/c mice, two months of age, were injected subcutaneously with 40 mg depot medroxyprogesterone acetate once or twice at three-month intervals with and without one dose of 50 mg/kg bw MNU administered either one week before or one week after the first injection of medroxyprogesterone acetate. The experiment was terminated at nine months to avoid detection of tumours induced by medroxyprogesterone acetate alone, which have a latency of 52 weeks (Lanari *et al.*, 1986). No mammary tumours developed in 43 mice given MNU only or in the 22 given the progestogen only.

Table 12. Incidence, number and latency of mammary tumours in CD2F₁ mice treated with 7,12-dimethylbenz[a]anthracene (DMBA) with and without medroxyprogesterone acetate (MPA)

Treatment	No. of mice	Mammary adenocarcinoma incidence	Total no. of mammary tumours	Latency (days)
DMBA × 6	32	5/32	8	152 ± 75
DMBA × 4	35	15/35	24	218 ± 72
MPA + DMBA × 2	36	21/36	28	210 ± 65
MPA + DMBA × 4	30	21/30	35	99 ± 51[a]
MPA	20	0/20	0	–

From Aldaz et al. (1996)
[a] Significantly less than the other groups ($p < 0.0001$)

A significant increase in the incidence of lobular adenocarcinomas was observed in the groups treated with MNU plus two injections of medroxyprogesterone acetate. When the first of the two progestogen treatments preceded MNU by one week, the incidence was 16/44 with a latency of 223 ± 34 days; a total of 23 tumours developed. When the first of the two progestogen treatments followed MNU by one week, the incidence was 9/43 with a latency of 211 ± 38 days; a total of 10 tumours was observed. The difference in the number of tumours between these two groups was significant ($p < 0.01$), but the difference in tumour incidence was not. When medroxyprogesterone acetate was given once one week after MNU and then withdrawn two months later, the tumour incidence was significantly ($p < 0.01$) reduced to 3/42 (Pazos et al., 1998).

(b)   Rat

Groups of 75 female Sprague-Dawley rats, 45, 55, 65 and 75 days of age at the start of treatment, respectively, were further subdivided into three groups of 25 rats each: one control and the two others implanted with a 21-day time-release pellet that contained 0.5 or 5 mg medroxyprogesterone acetate. The low dose corresponded to doses of 3.1, 2.8, 2.7 and 2.5 mg/kg bw, respectively, estimated to be equivalent to the amount of hormone administered to women weighing 50–60 kg and receiving an injection of 140 mg Depo-Provera every 90 days. At the end of 21 days, the remains of the pellets were removed. After a further 21 days, 20 rats per group were treated with 8 mg/kg bw DMBA by gavage. Mammary tumour development was monitored twice a week, and all animals were killed after 24 weeks. DMBA induced mammary tumours, including adenocarcinomas, in both control and progestogen-treated rats. The results are summarized in Table 13. Susceptibility to DMBA-induced mammary carcinogenesis declined and the latency increased with increasing age at the start of treatment. The low dose of medroxyprogesterone acetate did not alter the probability of mammary tumour development in younger rats; however, both

Table 13. Mammary tumour formation in Sprague-Dawley rats treated with medroxyprogesterone acetate (MPA) followed by 7,12-dimethylbenz-[a]anthracene (DMBA)

Treatment	No. of rats evaluated for tumours	Rats with tumours		Rats with adenocarcinomas		No. of tumours/ rat	Latency (days)
		No.	%	No.	%		
45 days							
Control[a]	12	9	75	5	42	1.8	82
MPA, low dose	11	9	82	5	46	1.6	115
MPA, high dose	8	7	88	4	50	1.8	116
55 days							
Control[a]	15	7	47	6	40	1.3	121
MPA, low dose	18	5	28	1	6	0.5	73
MPA, high dose	17	12	71	6	35	2.9	41
65 days							
Control[a]	12	6	50	5	42	1.6	110
MPA, low dose	15	7	47	4	27	0.6	60
MPA, high dose	16	10	63	6	38	1	90
75 days							
Control[a]	18	8	44	4	22	1.2	177
MPA, low dose	16	10	63	7	44	1.9	95
MPA, high dose	16	11	69	7	44	2.3	120

From Russo *et al.* (1989a)

[a] Controls received 8 mg/kg bw DMBA and cholesterol pellets

the low and the high dose caused a twofold increase in the incidence of adenocarcinoma in older animals over that with DMBA alone (Russo *et al.*, 1989a). [The Working Group noted that statistical analysis of the data did not allow an evaluation of the effects of medroxyprogesterone acetate on DMBA-induced mammary tumorigenesis.]

3.2   Levonorgestrel

Rabbit: One hundred and fourteen does, approximately 2.5 years old, were subjected to laparotomy and cross-sectional endomyometrial biopsy. Randomly selected rabbits then received a levonorgestrel-containing or an inert intrauterine implant in the right uterine horn. The implants consisted of a 0.3 × 2 cm core of either polydimethylsiloxane or 50% polydimethylsiloxane and 50% levonorgestrel. The rabbits then underwent a second cross-sectional endomometrial biopsy at six, 12 and 24 months. Of the 55 rabbits that received levonorgestrel and the 53 rabbits that received inert implants, 29 given levonorgestrel and 33 given inert implants survived 24 months. After 24 months, the incidence of endometrial carcinomas in rabbits receiving levonorgestrel (17%) was significantly lower ($p < 0.05$)

than that developing spontaneously in rabbits receiving the inert implant (42%) (Nisker *et al.*, 1988).

Hamster: Groups of 30 Syrian golden hamsters, five weeks of age, received four weekly subcutaneous injections of *N*-nitrosobis(2-oxypropyl)amine (NBOPA) at a dose of 10 mg/kg bw to initiate renal tumorigenesis and then received either control diet or a diet containing 10 mg/kg diet (ppm) levonorgestrel for 27 weeks. A third group of animals was not treated with the nitrosamine but was fed the diet containing levonorgestrel. Levonorgestrel alone did not cause renal tumours or dysplasia. Initiation with NBOPA caused nephroblastoma in 1/21 animals and 469 dysplastic tubules. Levonorgestrel did not significantly enhance the incidence of renal tumours in initiated animals (2/27 nephroblastomas and 2/27 renal adenomas) or increase the total number of dysplastic tubules (747) (Mitsumori *et al.*, 1994).

4. Other Data Relevant to an Evaluation of Carcinogenicity and its Mechanisms

4.1   Absorption, distribution, metabolism and excretion

4.1.1   *Medroxyprogesterone acetate*

(*a*)   *Humans*

Three women received intramuscular injections of 150 mg medroxyprogesterone acetate, and blood was obtained several times on the first day after injection, then daily for two weeks, then less frequently. The serum concentration of medroxyprogesterone acetate was measured by a sensitive radioimmunoassay. The concentrations rose rapidly after injection, reaching 0.26–0.47 ng/mL within 0.5 h and increasing to 0.97–2.66 ng/mL by 24 h; the concentrations remained in the range of 1.0–1.5 ng/mL for the first two to three months (Ortiz *et al.*, 1977).

Depot medroxyprogesterone acetate was administered intramuscularly to four groups of five healthy ovulating women at a dose of 25, 50, 100 or 150 mg. Medroxyprogesterone acetate was measured by radioimmunoassay in serum samples obtained periodically over the course of six months. All four doses initially produced serum concentrations that were above the sensitivity limit of the assay, ranging from 0.1 to 0.3 ng/mL. The concentration decreased with time, and the two lower doses reached the sensitivity limit more rapidly than the higher doses (Bassol *et al.*, 1984).

Medroxyprogesterone acetate was administered orally at a daily dose of 5 or 10 mg to groups of five women, and blood samples were obtained several times on the first day of treatment and daily 12 h after intake of the tablets. The serum concentrations were measured by radioimmunoassay. The concentrations rose rapidly within 1–3 h to peak values of 1.2–5.3 nmol/L [0.46–2.05 ng/mL] after the first 5-mg dose and to about 4.2–6.7 nmol/L [1.62–0.84 ng/mL] after the 10-mg dose (Wikström *et al.*, 1984).

Twenty women were given 150 mg medroxyprogesterone acetate intramuscularly every 90 days for 12 months. They were subjected to an oral glucose tolerance test before and 3, 6 and 12 months after the start of treatment, and fasting and post-oral glucose load (2-h) measurements were made of glucose, insulin, growth hormone, glucagon, pyruvate and cortisol. Significant increases in mean blood glucose, blood pyruvate, serum insulin, growth hormone and serum glucagon concentrations were seen after three months, which progressed to their highest concentrations at 12 months (Fahmy *et al.*, 1991).

Groups of 22 women recruited in roughly equal proportions from medical centres in Hungary, Mexico and Thailand were treated with 12.5 or 25 mg medroxyprogesterone acetate by intramuscular injection at 28-day intervals for three consecutive months. Blood samples were obtained for measurement of serum medroxyprogesterone acetate, oestradiol and progesterone before treatment, three times per week after treatment and for two months after the end of the last treatment. Ovulation was inhibited in all women. Restoration of ovulation after cessation of treatment occurred more slowly in the group given the high dose. The pharmacokinetic profiles differed between the three medical centres: dose-dependent differences in the serum concentration of medroxyprogesterone acetate were observed in the Thai women but not in Mexican women (Garza-Flores *et al.*, 1987).

(*b*)   *Experimental systems*

No data were available to the Working Group.

4.1.2   *Levonorgestrel* (see also the monograph on 'Oral contraceptives, combined', section 4.1.7)

(*a*)   *Humans*

Ball *et al.* (1991) reported on 16 women who were treated with 30 µg/day levonorgestrel for six months. At the end of the treatment period, plasma cholesterol, lipoprotein, triglyceride and glucose concentrations, and fibrinogen, plasminogen, factor VII, factor X and antithrombin III activities were compared with pre-treatment values and with those of a group of 23 women treated with 350 µg/day norethisterone for six months. There were no significant differences between the two groups.

A group of 47 healthy women received subdermal implants in the arm of Norplant®, from which levonorgestrel alone is released at a rate of about 30 µg/day. The women were compared with two groups given combined oral contraceptives: 25 received 1 mg norethisterone plus 50 µg mestranol per day for 21 days of a 28-day cycle, and 30 women received 150 µg levonorgestrel plus 30 µg ethinyloestradiol in a similar regimen. Blood samples were taken at admission and after one, three and six months. Coagulation parameters were measured, including platelet count, prothrombin time, thrombin time, partial thromboplastin time with kaolin, clotting factors I, II, V, VII–XIII, plasminogen, antithrombin III, α_1-antitrypsin, α_2-macroglobulin and fibrinogen degradation products. In contrast to the group receiving combined oral contraceptives, the Norplant® users had little alteration in coagulation parameters; the only significant changes were an increase in factor VII and a decrease in antithrombin III six months after implantation (Shaaban *et al.*, 1984).

(b)   *Experimental systems*

See the monograph on 'Oral contraceptives, combined'.

4.1.3   *Norethisterone* (see also the monograph on 'Oral contraceptives, combined', section 4.1.9)

(a)   *Humans*

In the study of Ball *et al.* (1991) described in section 4.1.2, 23 women were treated with 350 µg/day norethisterone for six months. No significant differences in the end-points measured were seen in comparison with pre-treatment values or with those of 16 women treated with 30 µg/day levonorgestrel for six months.

In the study of Fahmy *et al.* (1991) described in section 4.1.1, 20 women were treated with 200 mg norethisterone oenanthate intramuscularly every 60 days for six months, then with 200 mg every 84 days for another six months. Significant increases in mean blood glucose, pyruvate, serum insulin, growth hormone and glucagon concentrations were seen after three months, which reached a peak at six months. The concentrations reverted to normal at 12 months after the frequency of treatments was reduced.

(b)   *Experimental systems*

Three adult female baboons were injected intramuscularly with conventional bio-degradable microspheres containing 75 mg norethisterone which was released conti-nuously, while three other baboons received 75 mg norethisterone in encapsulated micro-spheres. The animals with the encapsulated microspheres showed two peaks of the blood concentration of norethisterone, while those given conventional microspheres showed a single peak. In addition, norethisterone was released for about 40–50 days longer from the encapsulated microspheres (Cong & Beck, 1991).

4.2   Receptor-mediated effects

4.2.1   *Medroxyprogesterone acetate*

(a)   *Humans*

Zalanyi *et al.* (1986) gave groups of women 5 or 10 mg medroxyprogesterone acetate orally on days 7–10 of the menstrual cycle and took endometrial biopsy samples on the 11th day before treatment and on the 11th day after the last dose of medroxyprogesterone acetate. Medroxyprogesterone acetate reduced the numbers of glandular and stromal mitoses, reduced the epithelial height, increased glandular diameter and increased the numbers of vacuolated cells in the endometrium.

Tiltman (1985) examined archived specimens from hysterectomies and determined the number of mitotic figures in uterine fibromyomas from 61 women who had received unknown oral or subcutaneous doses of medroxyprogesterone acetate and 71 women who had not received any hormonal treatment. The mitotic activity was significantly higher in fibromyomas from the progestogen-exposed women than in the control samples or in 63 samples from women treated with a combined oestrogen–progestogen oral contraceptive.

(b)   *Experimental systems*

Medroxyprogesterone acetate bound with high affinity to the progesterone receptor of human endometrium (Briggs, 1975), human MCF-7 breast cancer cells (Schoonen *et al.*, 1995a) and canine uterus (Selman *et al.*, 1996), its relative binding affinity exceeding that of progesterone by 2.5-fold in uterine tissue (Shapiro *et al.*, 1978; Selman *et al.*, 1996) and 10-fold in MCF-7 cells (Schoonen *et al.*, 1995a). Medroxyprogesterone acetate down-regulated the mRNA and protein expression of both progesterone receptor-A and -B iso-forms in primary cultures of isolated human endometrial epithelial cells, but surprisingly up-regulated these two receptor isoforms in human endometrial stromal cells, an effect that was inhibited by the anti-progestogen RU486 (Tseng & Zhu, 1997).

Medroxyprogesterone acetate had clear progestational activity *in vivo*, as measured by inhibition of ovulation and endometrial stimulation in rabbits, indicating that its activity is similar to that of progesterone (Phillips *et al.*, 1987).

Progestogen-specific stimulation of alkaline phosphatase activity in T47D human breast cancer cells indicated that medroxyprogesterone acetate has agonist activity, which was equal to that of progesterone (Markiewicz & Gurpide, 1994). It was eightfold more potent than progesterone in increasing glycogen levels in human endometrial explant cultures (Shapiro *et al.*, 1978).

Medroxyprogesterone acetate bound with much lower affinity than the natural ligand to the oestrogen receptor in whole rat uterine homogenate (van Kordelaar *et al.*, 1975); no binding occurred in MCF-7 human breast cancer cells (Schoonen *et al.*, 1995a). It had no oestrogenic activity at concentrations of 10^{-7}–10^{-6} mol/L, as demonstrated by oestrogen-stimulated alkaline phosphatase activity in Ishikawa-Var I human endometrial cancer cells, which is an oestrogen-specific response inhibited by 4-hydroxytamoxifen (Markiewicz *et al.*, 1992; Markiewicz & Gurpide, 1994; Botella *et al.*, 1995); however, the binding of oestradiol to rat uterine cytoplasmic oestrogen receptor was reduced by medroxy-progesterone acetate both *in vivo* and *in vitro* (Di Carlo *et al.*, 1983). Medroxyprogesterone acetate also slightly reduced the hyperplastic response in the endometrium of oestrogen-primed ovariectomized rats treated with conjugated equine oestrogen; tamoxifen did not have a similar effect (Kumasaka *et al.*, 1994). In addition, medroxyprogesterone acetate inhibited the up-regulation of mRNA expression of fibroblast growth factors-1 and -2 by oestradiol in Ishikawa human endometrial cancer cells; the effect was similar to that of the anti-oestrogen tamoxifen (Fujimoto *et al.*, 1997).

Medroxyprogesterone acetate did not affect the growth of most oestrogen-sensitive human mammary cancer cell lines tested, at concentrations of 10^{-8}–10^{-6} mol/L (Jeng & Jordan, 1991; Jeng *et al.*, 1992; Catherino & Jordan, 1995; Schoonen *et al.*, 1995a,b). It stimulated cell proliferation only in two human breast cancer cell sub-lines (MCF-7 sub-line M and T47D sub-line A) at concentrations of 10^{-6} mol/L and 10^{-8}–10^{-6} mol/L, respec-tively (Schoonen *et al.*, 1995a,b). Cappelletti *et al.* (1995) also found stimulation of prolife-ration of an MCF-7 line by medroxyprogesterone acetate at concentrations of 10^{-7}–10^{-6} mol/L. The latter effects were not changed by addition of tamoxifen or RU486, but both anti-progestogens and anti-oestrogens by themselves strongly counteracted oestradiol-stimulated cell proliferation in T47D cells (Schoonen *et al.*, 1995a,b). All of these experiments were performed with breast cancer cell lines grown in phenol red-free medium which contained steroid-free (dextran-coated charcoal-stripped) fetal bovine serum (Jeng *et al.*, 1992; Cappelletti *et al.*, 1995; Schoonen *et al.*, 1995a,b). Sutherland *et al.* (1988) found a high degree of variability in the inhibitory effects of medroxyprogesterone acetate on various human breast cancer cell lines, with about 50% inhibition at concentrations of 10^{-10} mol/L in T47D cells and 10^{-6} mol/L in MCF-7 cells and no effect in ZR75-1 cells; these studies were performed in the presence of phenol red and serum. Musgrove *et al.* (1991) reported that progestogens, including medroxyprogesterone acetate at 10^{-9} mol/L, could both stimulate and inhibit the cell cycle progression of the same human breast cancer cell line; they demonstrated an initial growth acceleration, increasing the number of cells in S-phase, followed later by growth inhibition due to G_1 arrest. The discrepancies in the response of different breast cancer cell sub-lines to medroxyprogesterone acetate may be related to differences in the time course of the biphasic effect of progestogens on their growth.

Medroxyprogesterone acetate did not *trans*-activate oestradiol-responsive reporter constructs containing oestrogen response elements in oestrogen receptor-positive cells (Jeng *et al.*, 1992; Catherino & Jordan, 1995), and did not alter the mRNA expression of transforming growth factors (TGF)-$\beta1$, -$\beta2$ and -$\beta3$ (Jeng & Jordan, 1991).

Oestradiol at concentrations of 10^{-10}–10^{-8} mol/L strongly induced the growth of MCF-7 and T47D cell lines, regardless of the sub-line used (Cappelletti *et al.*, 1995; Schoonen *et al.*, 1995a,b). Medroxyprogesterone acetate did not affect the growth stimulation of MCF-7 sub-lines L and M or T47D sub-line A by oestrogen (at 10^{-10} mol/L), but it inhibited stimulation of the growth of sub-line B MCF-7 cells and sub-line S T47D cells in a dose-dependent fashion at concentrations of 10^{-11}–10^{-6} mol/L and 10^{-10}–10^{-6} mol/L, respectively. These inhibitory effects at 10^{-8} mol/L were not blocked by the anti-progestogen RU486 at a concentration of 10^{-6} mol/L (Schoonen *et al.*, 1995a,b). Cappelletti *et al.* (1995), Botella *et al.* (1994) and Sutherland *et al.* (1988) also reported inhibition of oestradiol stimulation of growth of MCF-7 and T47D cell sub-lines by medroxyprogesterone acetate at concentrations of 10^{-8}–10^{-6} mol/L. Cappelletti *et al.* (1995) found that medroxyprogesterone acetate inhibited stimulation of MCF-7 breast cancer cell growth by TGF-α, but not by insulin-like growth factor-I and -II.

Medroxyprogesterone acetate increased the reductive activity of 17β-hydroxysteroid dehydrogenase in an oestrogen- and progestogen-stimulated MCF-7 cell line in phenol red-free medium (Coldham & James, 1990), indicating a possible mechanism for its stimulating effects on the growth of breast cancer cells *in vivo*, by increasing the formation of oestradiol. Medroxyprogesterone acetate also inhibited the activity of microsomal oestrone sulfatase in human breast carcinoma tissue, however, suggesting that it could reduce the intracellular formation of biologically active oestrogen in human breast cancer cells via the sulfatase pathway (Prost-Avallet *et al.*, 1991).

Administration of medroxyprogesterone acetate to 50-day-old virgin female Sprague-Dawley rats at a dose of 0.5 or 5 mg/rat per day for 21 days reduced the tritiated thymidine labelling index (an indicator of cell proliferation) in the terminal ducts and alveolar buds, but not in the terminal end-buds (Russo & Russo, 1991). This effect protected against the induction of mammary cancer by DMBA in a similar study with a norethynodrel–mestranol combination (Russo *et al.*, 1989b).

Subcutaneous administration of medroxyprogesterone acetate at doses of 1–1.5 mg/rat twice daily for 18 days inhibited stimulation by oestrone (1 μg/rat subcutaneously twice daily) of the growth of mammary gland carcinomas induced by DMBA in female Sprague-Dawley rats which were ovariectomized after tumours had developed; the effect of medroxyprogesterone acetate and the tumour growth inhibition caused by treatment with the anti-oestrogens EM-219 and EM-800 were additive (Li *et al.*, 1995; Luo *et al.*, 1997). Uterine weight was increased by medroxyprogesterone acetate in ovariectomized animals, while adrenal weights were decreased; the anti-oestrogens EM-219 and EM-800 did not have similar effects and did not alter the effects of the medroxyprogesterone acetate. The reductive activity of 17β-hydroxysteroid dehydrogenase in mammary tumour tissue was altered by medroxyprogesterone acetate in such a way that the formation of oestradiol in tumours of the ovariectomized oestrone-treated animals was reduced by more than 50%, while anti-oestrogens had no significant effect. In the uterus, medroxyprogesterone acetate caused 48% inhibition of the stimulatory effect of oestrone on 17β-hydroxysteroid dehydrogenase activity in the ovariectomized animals, while the anti-oestrogens reduced this enzymic activity to the levels found in ovariectomized animals.

Detectable but variable levels of either oestrogen or progesterone receptors were found in four of seven mammary adenocarcinomas induced by medroxyprogesterone acetate in BALB/c mice, while only three tumours contained both receptor types (Molinolo *et al.*, 1987).

Medroxyprogesterone acetate bound to the glucocorticoid receptor in canine liver cytosol (Selman *et al.*, 1996) and human mononuclear leukocytes and induced glucocorticoid-like effects in these cells, including reduced proliferative responses to mitogenic stimuli (Kontula *et al.*, 1983).

In studies with ovariohysterectomized bitches, administration of depot medroxyprogesterone acetate at three-week intervals for a total of eight subcutaneous injections of 10 mg/kg bw increased the concentrations of circulating growth hormones. This effect was reversed within 2 h after surgical removal of all mammary tissue, which contained the highest levels of growth hormone; there was also a distinct arterio-venous gradient of growth hormone across the mammary glands. This study provides evidence for local production of growth hormone in the canine mammary gland in response to medroxyprogesterone acetate treatment (Selman *et al.*, 1994). Further evidence for local production came from the demonstration by reverse transcriptase polymerase chain reaction (Mol *et al.*, 1995a,b) of the induction of growth hormone mRNA in canine, feline and human tumours. As growth hormone has been shown to stimulate human breast cancer cells (Biswas & Vonderhaar, 1987; Bonneterre *et al.*, 1990), the induction of mammary growth hormone production may be a major mechanism for the development of proliferative lesions in canine and perhaps human mammary gland (Mol *et al.*, 1996). It should be noted, however, that medroxyprogesterone acetate did not increase circulating growth hormone levels in men and women given a dose of 150 mg per day for three weeks to six months (Dhall *et al.*, 1977; Meyer *et al.*, 1977).

Medroxyprogesterone acetate stimulated the growth of androgen-sensitive mouse mammary carcinoma Shionogi cells with a reduction in the doubling time of approximately 75% at a concentration of 10^{-6} mol/L. This effect could be counteracted by blocking the androgen receptor with 5×10^{-6} mol/L of the anti-androgen hydroxyflutamide, which itself did not stimulate the growth of these cells (Luthy *et al.*, 1988). Consistent with these obser-vations, medroxyprogesterone acetate weakly bound to the rat ventral prostate androgen receptor (Botella *et al.*, 1987); however, it has been shown to be a strong competitor for binding of 5α-dihydrotestosterone to the androgen receptor in human foreskin fibroblasts, with activity similar to that of testosterone (Breiner *et al.*, 1986). Medroxyprogesterone acetate inhibited the growth of an oestrogen and progesterone receptor-negative human breast cancer cell line (MFM-223), the growth of which is inhibited by androgens (Hackenberg & Schulz, 1996).

Subcutaneous injection of medroxyprogesterone acetate to castrated male rats at a dose of 0.15 mg/rat twice daily for 14 days increased the ventral prostate weight by about 50% and stimulated the activity of the cell proliferation-related enzyme ornithine decarboxylase in the ventral prostate by almost 20-fold. Effects of similar magnitude were found with a dose of 0.15 mg 5α-dihydrotestosterone twice daily. No evidence for any anti-androgenic activity of medroxyprogesterone acetate was detected in these studies (Labrie *et al.*, 1987). Phillips *et al.* (1987), however, found no androgenic activity of medroxyprogesterone acetate in immature, castrated rats. The compound also increased the activity of 5α-reductase and decreased the activity of hepatic 3α- and 3β-hydroxysteroid dehydrogenase in male and female rats, which could lead to increased circulating levels of 5α-reduced androgens. These effects were blocked by flutamide or oestradiol, suggesting that androgen receptor mediation was involved (Lax *et al.*, 1984).

In dogs, medroxyprogesterone acetate induced cystic endometrial hyperplasia when administered subcutaneously at 10 mg/kg bw 5–13 times at intervals of three weeks. Although the presence of growth hormone was demonstrated in glandular epithelial cells by immunohistochemistry, no evidence could be found for local production in this tissue (Kooistra *et al.* 1997), in contrast to the canine mammary gland (Mol *et al.*, 1995a). A role for the elevated levels of circulating growth hormone in medroxyprogesterone acetate-induced canine endometrial hyperplasia has not been determined.

In cultured human endometrial stromal cells, medroxyprogesterone acetate and pro-gesterone were equally effective in markedly stimulating protein and mRNA expression of insulin-like growth factor binding protein-2. This response was inhibited by RU486 (Giudice *et al.*, 1991).

Medroxyprogesterone acetate and progesterone increased secretion of vascular endo-thelial growth factor by the human breast cancer cell line T47D to a similar extent (three- to fourfold over basal levels). This effect, which was progestogen-specific and did not occur in MCF-7, ZR-75 or MDA-MB-231 cells, suggests an angiogenic response of this cell line to medroxyprogesterone acetate (Hyder *et al.*, 1998).

Treatment of isolated primary normal human endometrial cells with medroxy-progesterone acetate, oestradiol or their combination *in vitro* increased mRNA expression of vascular endothelial growth factor in the cells by 3.1-, 2.8- and 4.7-fold, respectively, over control values (Shifren *et al.*, 1996). Intramuscular injection of medroxyprogesterone acetate at 2 mg/mouse one to three times at weekly intervals did not alter the expression of vascular endothelial growth factor in the tumour tissue of oestradiol-treated ovariectomized nude mice carrying a human endometrial carcinoma xenograft line (Kim *et al.*, 1996).

Medroxyprogesterone acetate weakly inhibited induction of angiogenesis by basic fibroblast growth factor and TGF-α in rabbit cornea *in vitro*. This anti-angiogenic activity was not correlated with its binding to glucocorticoid, progesterone or androgen receptors (Yamamoto *et al.*, 1994).

Medroxyprogesterone acetate at concentrations of 0.5–5.0 ng/mL did not affect the growth of decidual endothelial cells derived from human endometrium, which was stimulated by exposure to 5 ng/mL oestradiol (Peek *et al.*, 1995).

Using migration and invasion assays which involve cell growth along a fibronectin gradient, Ueda *et al.* (1996) demonstrated the inhibitory activity of 10^{-7}–10^{-5} mol/L medroxyprogesterone acetate on endometrial adenocarcinoma SNG-M cells in both systems. At these concentrations, medroxyprogesterone acetate did not affect the growth of these cells but inhibited cell locomotion, as determined in a monolayer wounding model *in vitro*. The secretion by these cells of matrix metalloproteinases and stromelysin was not affected. Fujimoto *et al.* (1996a,b) demonstrated, however, that medroxyproges-terone acetate does not affect the migration of human endometrial cancer-derived cells (Ishikawa, HEC-1 or HHUA cell lines) through an artificial basement membrane or their expression of cell adhesion-related molecules such as E-cadherin and α- and β-catenins. Oestradiol increased the migration of these cells and their expression of the cell adhesion-related molecules.

Medroxyprogesterone acetate given to female Wistar rats at an oral dose of 15 mg/kg per day for seven days increased the liver weight and increased oxidation of aminopyrine and ethyl morphine but had no significant effect on the liver DNA content (Schulte-Hermann *et al.*, 1988). This perhaps reflects the hepatic enzyme-inducing activity of me-droxyprogesterone acetate (Lax *et al.*, 1984).

4.2.2 *Levonorgestrel*

(a) *Humans*

Anderson *et al.* (1989) obtained breast biopsy samples from 347 pre-menopausal women and determined the tritiated thymidine labelling index for epithelial cells. The 14 women in this group who used progestogen-only contraceptives [not specified] had a mean labelling index of 1.55% (95% CI, 0.87–2.75), whereas the labelling index in 83 unexposed women was 0.66% (95% CI, 0.52–0.85). This study indicates that progestogen-only contraceptive use is associated with increased epithelial breast cell proliferation.

The mRNA expression of progesterone receptor in endometrial biopsy samples from 39 women using Norplant® (subcutaneous implants of levonorgestrel) was examined by in-situ hybridization and compared with that in 53 unexposed women (Lau *et al.*, 1996a). Exposure to levonorgestrel resulted in a signal intensity in endometrial glands that was comparable with that observed in control women during the menstrual and early proliferative phase, which was lower than that found during the early to mid-proliferative and secretory phases. The expression of progesterone receptor in endometrial stromal cells of levonorgestrel-exposed women was reduced by approximately 20–25% as compared with control tissue. The expression of cathepsin D, an indirect marker of the functional status of progesterone receptors, was examined in 46 women using Norplant® and 45 unexposed women (Lau *et al.*, 1996b). No differences were detected between these two groups, and no differences were found between phases of the menstrual cycle.

The effects of levonorgestrel administered from an intrauterine device on the expression of insulin growth factor (IGF)-I and IGF-II and those of IGF-binding protein I in the human endometrium were examined by Pekonen *et al.* (1992) and Rutanen *et al.* (1997). Endometrial tissue was obtained from surgical hysterectomy specimens and uterine biopsies taken from women who had carried intrauterine devices releasing levonorgestrel at a rate of 20 µg/day for 6–36 months ($n = 60$) (Rutanen *et al.*, 1997) or four months to seven years ($n = 11$) (Pekonen *et al.*, 1992). Control tissue was taken from 49 women carrying copper-releasing intrauterine devices (Pekonen *et al.*, 1992) or 13 untreated women (Rutanen *et al.*, 1997). Levonorgestrel induced expression of endometrial IGF-binding protein I (detected by immunohistochemistry and western blot) in 58/60 women, whereas none of 49 control women had detectable expression of this protein (Pekonen *et al.*, 1992). This finding was confirmed at the mRNA level by northern hybridization and reverse transcriptase polymerase chain reaction (Rutanen *et al.*, 1997); no expression occurred in either normal proliferative or secretory-phase endometrium, except for a very low level in late secretory-phase endometrium. IGF-I and IGF-II transcripts were found in all endometria, but expression was markedly higher for IGF-I in proliferative-phase endometrium and for IGF-II in endometrium from levonorgestrel-exposed women. IGF-binding protein-I was also expressed consistently in the latter group. Pekonen *et al.* (1992) also studied a group of six women with subcutaneous Norplant® capsules releasing 30–70 µg/day levonorgestrel. This treatment, in contrast to the effect of local progestogen, induced IGF-binding protein-I expression in the endometrium of only one of the women. None of the treatments resulted in increased serum concentrations of IGF-binding protein-I.

Using a cell migration assay for endothelial cells taken from endometrial biopsy samples, Subakir *et al.* (1995, 1996) showed that levonorgestrel reduced the mobility of these cells. Migration of human umbilical vein endothelial cells towards endometrial explants occurred in only 16/46 (35%) explant samples taken from women using Norplant® but in 22/30 (73%) explant samples from unexposed women. Furthermore, the median migratory scores were higher in the latter group.

(b)   *Experimental systems*

See the monograph on 'Oral contraceptives, combined', section 4.2.9.

4.3   Genetic and related effects

4.3.1   *Humans*

See the monograph on 'Oral contraceptives, combined', section 4.3.1.

4.3.2   *Experimental systems*

Progesterone did not induce DNA repair in female rat liver cells *in vitro*. It induced cell transformation in Syrian hamster embryo cells *in vitro* at a dose that did not induce chromosomal aberrations. Progesterone also induced cell transformation in baby rat kidney cells infected with human papillomavirus-16 carrying the Ha-*ras*-1 oncogene (Table 14).

See also the monograph on 'Oral contraceptives, combined', section 4.3.2.

4.4   Reproductive and prenatal effects

4.4.1   *Medroxyprogesterone acetate*

   (a)   *Humans*

When used as a contraceptive agent, medroxyprogesterone acetate at intramuscular doses of 100–150 mg reaches serum concentrations of 0.1–1 ng/mL, which inhibit ovulation for several months (Ortiz *et al.*, 1977; Bassol *et al.*, 1984). Oral administration of 5–10 mg per day results in serum concentrations of 0.4–1.7 nmol/L [0.125–0.531 ng/mL] 12 h after dosing; this also inhibits ovulation but less reliably (Wikström *et al.*, 1984). The steroid hormone profiles in early pregnancy are not affected by large doses of medroxyprogesterone given for the treatment of threatened abortion, although increased plasma concentrations of progesterone and decreased plasma concentrations of oestrogen were observed after the 20th week of gestation (Willcox *et al.*, 1985; Yovich *et al.*, 1985).

A number of early studies reported associations between the use of medroxyprogesterone acetate during pregnancy and the induction of a variety of congenital malformations in offspring (reviewed by Schardein, 1980). It was concluded that the evidence for malformations, such as cardiac, limb or central nervous system defects, was unconvincing. In a well-controlled study of 1608 infants born to women treated for genital bleeding during the first trimester of pregnancy with medroxyprogesterone acetate or other progestogens and 1147 infants born to women who had no treatment, the prevalence of congenital malformations, including genital malformations, was similar in the two groups (Katz *et al.*, 1985). A group of 449 subfertile pregnant women with high rates of recurrent abortion or who suffered a threatened abortion were treated with medroxyprogesterone (80–120 mg per day orally) from week 5 after the last menstrual period until at least the 18th week of pregnancy and were compared with a matched group of 464 women from the same clinic who were untreated. No difference was found in the prevalence of congenital malformations between the two groups: there were 15/366 (4.1%) infants with malformations in the treated group and 15/428 (3.5%) in the control group. In particular,

Table 14. Genetic and related effects of progesterone

Test system	Result[a] Without exogenous metabolic system	Result[a] With exogenous metabolic system	Dose[b] (LED or HID)	Reference
Salmonella typhimurium TA100, TA1535, TA1537, TA1538, TA98, reverse mutation	–	NT	40000 µg/plate	Ansari et al. (1982)
Salmonella typhimurium TA100, TA98, reverse mutation	–	–	500 µg/plate	Bokkenheuser et al. (1983)
Salmonella typhimurium TA100, TA1535, TA1537, TA1538, TA98, reverse mutation	–	–	333 µg/plate	Dunkel et al. (1984)
Escherichia coli WP2 *uvrA*, reverse mutation	–	–	333 µg/plate	Dunkel et al. (1984)
DNA strand breaks, cross-links and related damage, Chinese hamster V79 cells	–	–	94.5	Swenberg (1981)
DNA repair exclusive of unscheduled DNA synthesis, female rat hepatocytes *in vitro*	–	NT	15.7	Neumann et al. (1992)
Chromosomal aberrations, Chinese hamster ovary cells *in vitro*	–	–	480	Ishidate (1983)
Chromosomal aberrations, Syrian hamster embryo cells *in vitro*	–	NT	30	Tsutsui et al. (1995)
Cell transformation, BALB/3T3 mouse cells	(+)	NT	0.08	Dunkel et al. (1981)
Cell transformation, Syrian hamster embryo cells, clonal assay	+	NT	50	Dunkel et al. (1981)
Cell transformation, Syrian hamster embryo cells, clonal assay	+	NT	30	Tsutsui et al. (1995)
Cell transformation, RLV/Fischer rat embryo cells	+	NT	2.6	Dunkel et al. (1981)
Cell transformation, primary baby rat kidney + HPV16 + H-*ras*	+	NT	0.31	Pater et al. (1990)
Sister chromatid exchange, HE2144 human fibroblasts *in vitro*	–	NT	15.7	Sasaki et al. (1980)
Chromosomal aberrations, human lymphocytes *in vitro*	–	NT	100	Stenchever et al. (1969)
Chromosomal aberrations, HE2144 human fibroblasts *in vitro*	–	NT	31.4	Sasaki et al. (1980)
Dominant lethal mutation, mice *in vivo*	–		167 ip × 1	Epstein et al. (1972)
Sperm morphology, mice *in vivo*	–		500 ip × 5	Topham (1980)

[a] +, positive; (+), weak positive; –, negative; NT, not tested
[b] LED, lowest effective dose; HID, highest ineffective dose; in-vitro tests, µg/mL; in-vivo tests, mg/kg bw per day; ip, intraperitoneal

there was no suggestion of an increase in the incidence of cardiac or limb defects (Yovich *et al.*, 1988).

Long-term follow-up studies have been reported on more than 2000 people exposed to medroxyprogesterone acetate prenatally; most have shown no treatment-related effects on health or development (Jaffe *et al.*, 1990; Gray & Pardthaisong, 1991a; Pardthaisong & Gray, 1991; Pardthaisong *et al.*, 1992). In a large study in Thailand of 1431 children of mothers who had used depot medroxyprogesterone acetate as a contraceptive (Pardthaisong & Gray, 1991), a small but significant increase in the prevalence of low-birth-weight infants was found, accompanied by an increase in perinatal and infant mortality (Gray & Pardthaisong, 1991a). The treated and control groups in this study were not well matched, as the women taking medroxyprogesterone acetate had a higher incidence of pregnancy risk factors, and the conclusions of the study have been debated (Gray & Pardthaisong, 1991b; Hogue, 1991).

As treatment of men with medroxyprogesterone acetate can reduce their testosterone levels and sperm counts, it has been tested as a male contraceptive. Testosterone must be given at the same time to counter the decreased testosterone effects (Melo & Coutinho, 1977; Soufir *et al.*, 1983). In a study of 25 healthy men, who had each fathered at least two children, monthly injections of 100 mg medroxyprogesterone acetate and 250 mg testosterone oenanthate were given for 4–16 months. In 24 of the men, a marked drop in sperm count was observed one to three months after the first injection. By nine months, 11/14 men were azoospermic or had marked oligospermia (< 1 million sperm per millilitre). One subject was unresponsive, but no reason could be found (Melo & Coutinho, 1977).

Six men were given a daily oral dose of 20 mg medroxyprogesterone acetate in combination with 50 or 100 mg testosterone for one year. From the third month, the sperm count was $< 10^6$/mL. The sperm count returned to normal levels ($> 20 \times 10^6$/mL) three to six months after cessation of treatment (Soufir *et al.*, 1983).

(b) *Experimental systems*

Groups of 8–12 male Sprague-Dawley Crl:CD(SD)Br rats were castrated and injected immediately thereafter twice daily for 14 days with one of a number of synthetic progestogens, including medroxyprogesterone acetate, used in the treatment of prostate cancer. Controls were injected with the vehicle, 1% gelatine, in 0.9% saline. Dihydrotestosterone was injected at a dose of 150 µg twice daily for 14 days as a positive control. All of the animals were killed on the morning after the last day of treatment, and the ventral prostate and adrenals were removed and weighed; furthermore, the prostatic content of ornithine decarboxylase was measured, as it is considered to be a highly specific, sensitive marker of androgenic activity in the prostate. Dihydrotestosterone increased the ventral prostate weight to 43% above that of castrated controls. Medroxyprogesterone acetate was equipotent with dihydrotestosterone and caused significant increases in prostate weight, by about 49% at 150 µg and 162% at a dose of 500 µg per injection. Whereas dihydrotestosterone caused a 14-fold increase in ornithine decarboxylase activity in the prostate, medroxyprogesterone acetate caused a 20-fold increase at the same dose. Medroxyprogesterone acetate thus has very powerful androgenic activity in the rat ventral prostate, equal to that of the potent natural androgen dihydrotestosterone (Labrie *et al.*, 1987).

Pregnant Wistar rats were given 1 or 5 mg medroxyprogesterone acetate orally for four days on days 17–20 of pregnancy, and the fetuses were removed on day 21. After fixation, histological sections of the pelvic region were examined and the urovaginal septum length measured. Very marked masculinization of female fetuses was detected, as evidenced by decreased development of the urogenital septum at both doses (Kawashima *et al.*, 1977).

In a study in which Silastic intrauterine devices containing medroxyprogesterone acetate were implanted between fetal implantation sites on day 9 in groups of 16 pregnant Wistar rats, masculinization of female fetuses and feminization of males occurred, as judged from changes in anogenital distance and the morphology of the genital papilla (Barlow & Knight, 1983).

Anti-androgenic effects have also been reported. Groups of 10 albino Wistar mice were treated subcutaneously with vehicle alone or with 1.0 mg per animal per day of medroxyprogesterone acetate for seven days. The mice were killed on the eighth day and the testes removed for histological and morphometric examination. Treatment inhibited spermatogenesis and caused marked decreases in the volume, surface area and length of the seminiferous tubules (Umapathy & Rai, 1982).

In the previous monograph (IARC, 1979), it was reported that medroxyprogesterone acetate caused facial clefts in rabbits but not in rats or mice. A low incidence of facial clefts and malformations of the respiratory tract and renal system was reported in NMRI mice by Eibs *et al.* (1982) after subcutaneous injection of 30 mg/kg bw medroxyprogesterone acetate. Injection of doses up to 900 mg/kg on day 2 of gestation also increased the incidence of facial clefts and reduced fetal weight, but the effects were not dose-related. Genital anomalies, masculinization of females and feminization of males have been reported in rats (Lerner *et al.*, 1962; Barlow & Knight, 1983) and non-human primates. Time-mated cynomolgus monkeys were injected once intramuscularly with 25 (11 animals) or 100 (4 animals) mg/kg bw medroxyprogesterone acetate on day 27 (± 2) of gestation (10 and 40 times the human dose). All of the fetuses were affected: the female offspring had labial fusion, clitoral hypertrophy and penile urethra, while the male offspring had short penis, reduced scrotal swelling and hypospadia. The adrenal weight was markedly reduced in animals at the high dose, but no other malformation was observed, and no genital effects were seen in animals treated with 2.5 mg/kg bw, which is equivalent to the human dose (Prahalada *et al.*, 1985). Similar effects were reported in baboons at three to four times the human dose (8–10 mg/kg bw on day 30) (Tarara, 1984).

4.4.2   *Levonorgestrel*

(a)   *Humans*

The primary contraceptive mechanism of action of levonorgestrel is inhibition of ovulation, although effects on cervical mucus and on maturation of oocytes are also involved.

In a study of 32 women using Norplant® implants, daily blood samples were obtained for hormone analysis throughout most of one menstrual cycle. Half of the women had anovulatory cycles, and the others had abnormal concentrations of hormones in comparison with women not taking contraceptives. Reduced progesterone concentrations and short luteal phases were seen. None of the women using Norplant® had increased concentrations of human chorionic gonadotrophin, indicating that early abortion is not the mechanism of contraceptive action (Faundes *et al.*, 1991; Segal *et al.*, 1991). In a study of 178 women who had requested removal of their Norplant® implant for a planned pregnancy and 91 women who had requested removal of intrauterine devices containing Norplant®, fertility was unimpaired after cessation of use. Most of the women had used their contraceptive method for two to four years (Silvin *et al.*, 1992).

(*b*) *Experimental systems*
See the monograph on 'Oral contraceptives, combined', section 4.4.5.

5. Summary of Data Reported and Evaluation

5.1 Exposure

Progestogen-only contraceptives have been available worldwide for over 40 years. Intramuscular depot injections and subcutaneous implants are the most common routes of administration in developing countries, where there is the widest use. Oral progestogen-only 'mini pills' are used primarily in Europe and North America, but fewer women use these preparations than parenterally administered progestogens and combined oral contraceptives.

5.2 Human carcinogenicity

Breast cancer

Data on injectable progestogen-only contraceptives were available from two case–control studies and a pooled analysis of original data, overall including about 350 women with breast cancer who had used these drugs. Data on oral progestogen-only contraceptives were available from a pooled analysis of original data on 725 women with breast cancer who had used these drugs. Overall, there is no evidence of an increased risk for breast cancer.

Endometrial cancer

One case–control study addressed the relationship between use of oral progestogen-only contraceptives and risk for endometrial cancer; less than 2% of the control women had used these preparations. Women with endometrial cancer were less likely to have used oral progestogen-only contraceptives than control women but not significantly so.

The effects of use of depot medroxyprogesterone acetate on the risk for endometrial cancer have been evaluated in one cohort and one case–control study. No reduction in risk was seen in the cohort study, whereas a strong reduction was observed in the case–control study. Although the evidence is based on small numbers of women, the results of these studies suggest that women who use progestogen-only contraceptives have a reduced risk for endometrial cancer.

Cervical cancer

There is little evidence that use of depot medroxyprogesterone acetate or other pro-gestational injectable contraceptives alters the risk for either squamous-cell carcinoma or adenocarcinoma of the uterine cervix.

Ovarian cancer

One case–control study addressed use of progestogen-only oral contraceptives, and one case–control study specifically addressed any use of depot medroxyprogesterone acetate. Neither showed any alteration in risk, either overall or in relation to duration of use.

Liver cancer

Two case–control studies have addressed the association between risk for liver cancer and use of injectable progestogen-only contraceptives. In neither study did the risk for liver cancer differ significantly between women who had ever or never used these contra-ceptives. Both studies were conducted in areas endemic for hepatitis viruses.

Cutaneous malignant melanoma

One case–control study of cutaneous malignant melanoma showed no increase in risk among users of progestogen-only contraceptives.

5.3   Carcinogenicity in experimental animals

Medroxyprogesterone acetate has been tested for carcinogenicity in mice by sub-cutaneous implantation of pellets or injection and in dogs by subcutaneous or intra-muscular administration. In mice, it induced mammary adenocarcinomas; in dogs, it induced mammary hyperplasia, nodules and benign mammary tumours. Tumour deve-lopment in other organs and tissues of these animals was not reported.

Medroxyprogesterone acetate was tested in combination with some known carci-nogens. With 7,12-dimethylbenz[*a*]anthracene or *N*-methyl-*N*-nitrosourea, it increased the incidence of mammary adenocarcinomas in mice and shortened the latency to tumour appearance. Medroxyprogesterone acetate enhanced the incidence of cervical invasive squamous-cell carcinomas in mice treated with 3-methylcholanthrene. It decreased the incidence of endometrial adenocarcinoma in mice previously treated with *N*-methyl-*N*-nitrosourea plus oestradiol.

Two studies in dogs and one study in cats treated by veterinarians for suppression of oestrus and compared with untreated animals indicated that medroxyprogesterone acetate increases the risk for developing benign and malignant mammary tumours in both species.

Levonorgestrel was tested by implantation into the uterus of rabbits, with no indication of carcinogenicity. In combination with *N*-nitrosobis(2-oxopropyl)amine, levonorgestrel did not enhance the incidence of renal dysplastic lesions or tumours in hamsters.

5.4   Other relevant data

Use of depot injections of progestogens or subcutaneous implants of controlled-release devices results in sustained levels of hormone release over long periods. Progestogens used in this way vary in their spectrum of hormonal activities. In addition to progestational activity, levonorgestrel has some oestrogenic activity. In contrast, medroxyprogesterone acetate has no marked oestrogenic activity but has some androgenic activity. Both compounds can modify oestrogenic effects. Progestogen-only contraceptives have growth potentiating effects in the human mammary gland, as indicated by elevated rates of cell proliferation. No data were available on the genetic activity of these progestogens in humans, but norethisterone induced some changes in DNA and chromosomes in experimental systems. Progesterone induced cell transformation in mammalian cells *in vitro*. Early studies on use of depot medroxyprogesterone acetate during pregnancy suggested that genital malformations were induced in the fetus, but the results of later studies provided no support for that suggestion. Medroxyprogesterone acetate administered to men can reduce testosterone levels and semen production.

5.5   Evaluation

There is *inadequate evidence* in humans for the carcinogenicity of progestogen-only contraceptives.

There is *sufficient evidence* in experimental animals for the carcinogenicity of medroxyprogesterone acetate.

Overall evaluation

Progestogen-only contraceptives are *possibly carcinogenic to humans (Group 2B)*.

6.   References

Aldaz, C.M., Liao, Q.Y., LaBate, M. & Johnston, D.A. (1996) Medroxyprogesterone acetate accelerates the development and increases the incidence of mouse mammary tumors induced by dimethylbenzanthracene. *Carcinogenesis*, **17**, 2069–2072

Anderson, T.J., Battersby, S., King, R.J.B., McPherson, K. & Going, J.J. (1989) Oral contraceptive use influences resting breast proliferation. *Hum. Pathol.*, **20**, 1139–1144

Ansari, G.A.S., Walker, R.D., Smart, V.B. & Smith, L.L. (1982) Further investigations of mutagenic cholesterol preparations. *Food chem. Toxicol.*, **20**, 35–41

Ball, M.J., Ashwell, E. & Gillmer, M.D.G. (1991) Progestagen-only oral contraceptives: Comparison of the metabolic effects of levonorgestrel and norethisterone. *Contraception*, **44**, 223–233

Barlow, S.M. & Knight, A.F. (1983) Teratogenic effects of Silastic intrauterine devices in the rat with or without added medroxyprogesterone acetate. *Fertil. Steril.*, **39**, 224–230

Bassol, S., Garza-Flores, J., Cravioto, M.C., Diaz-Sanchez, V., Fotherby, K., Lichtenberg, R. & Perez-Palacios, G. (1984) Ovarian function following a single administration of depo-medroxy-progesterone acetate (DMPA) at different doses. *Fertil. Steril.*, **42**, 216–222

Biswas, R. & Vonderhaar, B.K. (1987) Role of serum in the prolactin responsiveness of MCF-7 human breast cancer cells in long-term tissue culture. *Cancer Res.*, **47**, 3509–3514

Bokkenheuser, B.D., Winter, J., Mosenthal, A.C., Mosbach, E.H., McSherry, C.K., Ayengar, N.K.N., Andrews, A.W., Lebherz, W.B., III, Pienta, R.J. & Wallstein, S. (1983) Fecal steroid 21-dehydroxylase, a potential marker for colorectal cancer. *Am. J. Gastroenterol.*, **78**, 469–475

Bonneterre, J., Peyrat, J.P., Beuscart, R. & Demaille, A. (1990) Biological and clinical aspects of prolactin receptors (PRL-R) in human breast cancer. *J. Steroid Biochem. mol. Biol.*, **37**, 977–981

Bost, L., Dong, W., Hedges, B., Primatesta, P., Prior, G., Purdon, S. & di Salvo, P. (1997) *Health Survey for England 1995*, Vol. I, *Findings*, London, The Stationery Office, p. 254

Botella, J., Paris, J. & Lahlou, B. (1987) The cellular mechanism of the antiandrogenic action of nomegestrol acetate, a new 19-nor progestagen, on the rat prostate. *Acta endocrinol.*, **115**, 544–550

Botella, J., Duranti, E., Duc, I., Cognet, A.M., Delansorne, R. & Paris, J. (1994) Inhibition by nomegestrol acetate and other synthetic progestins on proliferation and progesterone receptor content of T47-D human breast cancer cells. *J. Steroid Biochem. mol. Biol.*, **50**, 41–47

Botella, J., Duranti, E., Viader, V., Duc, I., Delansorne, R. & Paris, J. (1995) Lack of estrogenic potential of progesterone- or 19-nor-progesterone-derived progestins as opposed to testosterone or 19-nortestosterone derivatives on endometrial Ishikawa cells. *J. Steroid Biochem. mol. Biol.*, **55**, 77–84

Breiner, M., Romalo, G. & Schweikert, H.U. (1986) Inhibition of androgen receptor binding by natural and synthetic steroids in cultured human genital skin fibroblasts. *Klin. Wochenschr.*, **64**, 732–737

Briggs, M.H. (1975) Contraceptive steroid binding to the human uterine progesterone-receptor. *Curr. med. Res. Opin.*, **3**, 95–98

Cancer and Steroid Hormone Study of the Centers for Disease Control and the National Institute of Child Health and Human Development (1986) Oral contraceptive use and the risk of breast cancer. *New Engl. J. Med.*, **315**, 405–411

Cappelletti, V., Miodini, P., Fioravanti, L. & DiFronzo, G. (1995) Effect of progestin treatment on estradiol- and growth factor-stimulated breast cancer cell lines. *Anticancer Res.*, **15**, 2551–2555

Catherino, W.H. & Jordan, V.C. (1995) Nomegestrol acetate, a clinically useful 19-norprogesterone derivative which lacks estrogenic activity. *J. Steroid Biochem. mol. Biol.*, **55**, 239–246

Centers for Disease Control and the National Institute of Child Health and Human Development, Cancer and Steroid Hormone Study (1987) Combination oral contraceptive use and the risk of endometrial cancer. *J. Am. med. Assoc.*, **257**, 796–800

Chi, I.-C. (1995) The progestin-only pills and the levonorgestrel-releasing IUD: Two progestin-only contraceptives. *Clin. Obstet. Gynecol.*, **38**, 872–889

Clavel, F., Andrieu, N., Gairard, B., Brémand, A., Piana, L., Lansac, J., Bréart, G., Rumeau-Rouquette, C., Flamant, R. & Renaud, R. (1991) Oral contraceptives and breast cancer: A French case–control study. *Int. J. Epidemiol.*, **20**, 32–38

Coezy, E., Auzan, C., Lonigro, A., Philippe, M., Menard, J. & Corvol, P. (1987) Effect of mestranol on cell proliferation and angiotensinogen production in HepG2 cells: Relation with the cell cycle and action of tamoxifen. *Endocrinology*, **120**, 133–141

Coldham, N.G. & James, V.H.T. (1990) A possible mechanism for increased breast cell proliferation by progestins through increased reductive 17β-hydroxysteroid dehydrogenase activity. *Int. J. Cancer*, **45**, 174–178

Collaborative Group on Hormonal Factors in Breast Cancer (1996) Breast cancer and hormonal contraceptives: Further results. *Contraception*, **54** (Suppl. 3), 1S–106S

Concannon, P.W., Spraker, T.R., Casey, H.W. & Hansel, W. (1981) Gross and histopathologic effects of medroxyprogesterone acetate and progesterone on the mammary glands of adult beagle bitches. *Fertil. Steril.*, **36**, 373–387

Cong, H. & Beck, L.R. (1991) Preparation and pharmacokinetic evaluation of a modified long-acting injectable norethisterone microsphere. *Adv. Contracep.*, **7**, 251–256

Cullins, V.E. & Garcia, F.A.R. (1997) Implantable hormonal and emergency contraception. *Curr. Opin. Obstet. Gynecol.*, **9**, 169–174

Dhall, K., Kumar, M., Rastogi, G.K. & Devi, P.K. (1977) Short-term effects of norethisterone oenanthate and medroxyprogesterone acetate on glucose, insulin, growth hormone, and lipids. *Fertil. Steril.*, **28**, 154–158

Di Carlo, F., Gallo, E., Conti, G. & Racca, S. (1983) Changes in the binding of oestradiol to uterine oestrogen receptors induced by some progesterone and 19-nor-testosterone derivatives. *J. Endocrinol.*, **98**, 385–389

Dunkel, V.C., Pienta, R.J., Sivak, A. & Traul, K.A. (1981) Comparative neoplastic transformation responses of Balb/3T3 cells, Syrian hamster embryo cells, and Rauscher murine leukemia virus-infected Fischer 344 rat embryo cells to chemical carcinogens. *J. natl Cancer Inst.*, **67**, 1303–1315

Dunkel, V.C., Zeiger, E., Brusick, D., McCoy, E., McGregor, D., Mortelmans, K., Rosenkranz, H.S. & Simmon, V.F. (1984) Reproducibility of microbial mutagenicity assays: I. Tests with *Salmonella typhimurium* and *Escherichia coli* using a standardized protocol. *Environ. Mutag.*, **6** (Suppl. 2), 1–254

Eibs, H.G., Spielmann, H. and Hagele, M. (1982) Teratogenic effects of cyproterone acetate and medroxyprogesterone treatment during the pre- and postimplantation period of mouse embryos. 1. *Teratology*, **25**, 27–36

Englund, D.E. & Johansson, E.D. (1980) Endometrial effect of oral estriol treatment in post-menopausal women. *Acta obstet. gynecol. scand.*, **59**, 449–451

Epstein, S.S., Arnold, E., Andrea, J., Bass, W. & Bishop, Y. (1972) Detection of chemical mutagens by the dominant lethal assay in the mouse. *Toxicol. appl. Pharmacol.*, **23**, 288–325

Ewertz, M. (1992) Oral contraceptives and breast cancer risk in Denmark. *Eur. J. Cancer*, **28A**, 1176–1181

Fahmy, K., Abdel-Razik, M., Shaaraway, M., Al-Kholy, G., Saad, S., Wagdi, A. & Al-Azzony, M. (1991) Effect of long-acting progestagen-only injectable contraceptives on carbohydrate metabolism and its hormonal profile. *Contraception*, **44**, 419–430

Faundes, A. Brache, V., Tejada, A.S., Cochon, L. & Alvarez-Sanchez, F. (1991) Ovulatory dysfunction during continuous administration of low-dose levonorgestrel by subdermal implants. *Fertil. Steril.*, **56**, 27–31

Frank, D.W., Kirton, K.T., Murchison, T.E., Quinlan, W.J., Coleman, M.E., Gilbertson, T.J., Feenstra, E.S. & Kimball, F.A. (1979) Mammary tumors and serum hormones in the bitch treated with medroxyprogesterone acetate or progesterone for four years. *Fertil. Steril.*, **31**, 340–346

Fujimoto, J., Hori, M., Ichigo, S., Morishita, S. & Tamaya, T. (1996a) Estrogen activates migration potential of endometrial cancer cells through basement membrane. *Tumour Biol.* **17**, 48–57

Fujimoto, J., Ichigo, S., Hori, M., Morishita, S. & Tamaya, T. (1996b) Progestins and danazol effect on cell-to-cell adhesion, and E-cadherin and alpha- and beta-catenin mRNA expressions. *J. Steroid Biochem. med. Biol.*, **57**, 275–282

Fujimoto, J., Hori, M., Ichigo, S. & Tamaya, T. (1997) Antiestrogenic compounds inhibit estrogen-induced expression of fibroblast growth factor family (FGF-1,2, and 4) mRNA in well-differentiated endometrial cancer cells. *Eur. J. Gynaecol. Oncol.*, **18**, 497–501

Garza-Flores, J., Rodriguez, V., Perez-Palacios, G., Virutamasen, P., Tang-Keow, P., Konsayreepong, R., Kovacs, L., Koloszar, S. & Hall, P.E. (1987) A multicentered pharmacokinetic, pharmacodynamic study of once-a-month injectable contraceptives. I. Different doses of HRP112 and of Depoprovera (Task Force of WHO). *Contraception*, **36**, 441–457

Giudice, L.C., Milkowski, D.A., Fielder, P.J. & Irwin, J.C. (1991) Characterization of the steroid-dependence of insulin-like growth factor-binding protein-2 synthesis and mRNA expression in cultured human endometrial stromal cells. *Hum. Reprod.*, **5**, 632–640

Gray, R.H. & Pardthaisong, T. (1991a) In utero exposure to steroid contraceptives and survival during infancy. *Am. J. Epidemiol.*, **134**, 804–811

Gray, R.H. & Pardthaisong, T. (1991b) The authors' response to Hogue. *Am. J. Epidemiol.*, **134**, 816–817

Hackenberg, R. & Schultz, K.D. (1996) Androgen receptor mediated growth control of breast cancer and endometrial cancer modulated by antiandrogen- and androgen-like steroids. *J. Steroid Biochem. mol. Biol.*, **56**, 113–117

Herrero, R., Brinton, L.A., Reeves, W.C., Brenes, M.M., de Britton, R.C., Tenorio, F. & Gaitan, E. (1990) Injectable contraceptives and risk of invasive cervical cancer: Evidence of an association. *Int. J. Cancer*, **46**, 5–7

Hogue, C.J. (1991) Invited commentary: The contraceptive technology tightrope. *Am. J. Epidemiol.*, **134**, 812–817

Hussain, S.P. & Rao, A.R. (1991) Modulatory influence of injectable contraceptive steroid medroxyprogesterone acetate on methylcholanthrene-induced carcinogenesis in the uterine cervix of mouse. *Cancer Lett.*, **61**, 187–193

Hyder, S.M., Murthy, L. & Stancel, G.M. (1998) Progestin regulation of vascular endothelial growth factor in human breast cancer cells. *Cancer Res.*, **58**, 392–395

IARC (1979) *IARC Monographs on the Evaluation of the Carcinogenic Risk of Chemicals to Humans*, Vol. 21, *Sex Hormones (II)*, Lyon

Ishidate, M., Jr, ed. (1983) *The Data Book of Chromosomal Aberration Tests in Vitro on 587 Chemical Substances using a Chinese Hamster Fibroblast Cell Line (CHL Cells)*, Tokyo, Realize

Jaffe, B., Shye, D., Harlap, S., Baras, M., Belmaker, E., Gordon, L., Magidor, S. & Fortney, J. (1990) Health, growth and sexual development of teenagers exposed in utero to medroxy-progesterone acetate. *Paediatr. perinat. Epidemiol.*, **4**, 184–195

Jeng, M.H. & Jordan, V.C. (1991) Growth stimulation and differential regulation of transforming growth factor-β1 (TGF β1), TGF β2, and TGF β3 messenger RNA levels by norethindrone in MCF-7 human breast cancer cells. *Mol. Endocrinol.*, **8**, 1120–1128

Jeng, M.H., Parker, C.J. & Jordan, V.C. (1992) Estrogenic potential of progestins in oral contra-ceptives to stimulate human breast cancer cell proliferation. *Cancer Res.* **52**, 6539–6546

Jordan, A. (1994) Toxicology of depot medroxyprogesterone acetate. *Contraception*, **49**, 189–201

Katz, Z., Lancet, M., Skornik, J., Chemke, J., Mogilner, B.M. & Klinberg, M. (1985) Terato-genicity of progestogens given during the first trimester of pregnancy. *Obstet. Gynecol.*, **65**, 775–780

Kawashima, K., Nakaura, S., Nagao, S., Tanaka, S., Kuwamura, T. & Omori, Y. (1977) Virilizing activities of various steroids in female rat fetuses. *Endocrinol. Jpn.*, **24**, 77–81

Kew, M.C., Song, E., Mohammed, A. & Hodkinson, J. (1990) Contraceptive steroids as a risk factor for hepatocellular carcinoma: A case–control study in South African black women. *Hepatology*, **11**, 298–302

Kim, Y.B., Berek, J.S., Martinez-Maza, O. & Satyaswaroop, P.G. (1996) Vascular endothelial growth factor expression is not regulated by estradiol or medroxyprogesterone acetone in endometrial carcinoma. *Gynecol. Oncol.*, **61**, 97–100

Kleinman, R.L. (1990) *Hormonal Contraception*, London, IPPF Medical Publications

Kleinman, R.L. (1996) *Directory of Hormonal Contraceptives*, London, IPPF Medical Publications

Kontula, K., Paavonen, T., Luukkainen, T. & Andersson, L.C. (1983) Binding of progestins to the glucocorticoid receptor. Correlation to their glucocorticoid-like effects on *in vitro* functions of human mononuclear leukocytes. *Biochem. Pharmacol.*, **32**, 1511–1518

Kooistra, H.S., Okkens, A.C., Mol, J.A., van Garderen, E., Kirpensteijn, J. & Rijnberk, A. (1997) Lack of association of progestin-induced cystic endometrial hyperplasia with GH gene expression in the canine uterus. *J. Reprod. Fertil.*, **Suppl. 51**, 355–361

van Kordelaar, J.M.G., Vermorken, A.J.M., de Weerd, C.J.M. & van Rossum, J.M. (1975) Inter-action of contraceptive progestins and related compounds with the oestrogen receptor. Part II: Effect on [³H]oestradiol binding to the rat uterine receptor in vitro. *Acta endocrinol.*, **78**, 165–179

Kordon, E.C., Molinolo, A.A., Pasqualini, C.D., Pazos, P., Dran, G. & Lanari, C. (1993) Proges-terone induction of mammary carcinomas in female BALB/c mice. *Breast Cancer Res. Treat.*, **28**, 29–39

Kordon, E.C., Guerra, F., Molinolo, A.A., Elizalde, P., Charreau, E.H., Pasqualini, C.D., Montecchia, F., Pazos, P., Dran, G. & Lanari, C. (1994) Effect of sialoadenectomy on medoxyprogesterone-acetate-induced mammary carcinogenesis in BALB/c mice. Correlation between histology and epidermal-growth-factor receptor content. *Int. J. Cancer*, **59**, 196–203

Kumasaka, T., Itoh, E., Watanabe, H., Hoshino, K., Yoshinaka, A. & Masawa, N. (1994) Effects of various forms of progestin on the endometrium of the estrogen-primed, ovariectomized rat. *Endocrine J.*, **41**, 161–169

Labrie, C., Cusan, L., Plante, M., Lapointe, S. & Labrie, F. (1987) Analysis of the androgenic activity of synthetic 'progestins' currently used for the treatment of prostate cancer. *J. Steroid Biochem.*, **28**, 379–384

Lanari, C., Molinolo, A.A. & Pasqualini, C.D. (1986) Induction of mammary adenocarcinomas by medroxyprogesterone acetate in BALB/c female mice. *Cancer Lett.*, **33**, 215–233

Lande, R.E (1995) New era for injectables. *Popul. Rep.*, **23**, 1–31

Lau, T.M., Witjaksono, J., Affandi, B. & Rogers, P.A.W. (1996a) Expression of progesterone receptor mRNA in the endometrium during the normal menstrual cycle and in Norplant users. *Hum. Reprod.*, **12**, 2629–2634

Lau, T.M., Affandi, B. & Rogers, P.A.W. (1996b) Immunohistochemical detection of cathepsin D in endometrium from long-term subdermal levonorgestrel users and during the normal menstrual cycle. *Mol. hum. Reprod.*, **4**, 233–237

Lax, E.R., Baumann, P. & Schriefers, H. (1984) Changes in the activities of microsomal enzymes involved in hepatic steroid metabolism in the rat after administration of androgenic, estrogenic, progestational, anabolic and catatoxic steroids. *Biochem. Pharmacol.*, **33**, 1235–1241

Lerner, L.J., dePhillipo, M., Yiacas, E., Brennan, D. & Borman, A. (1962) Comparison of the acetophenone derivative of 16α,17α-dihydroprogesterone with other progestational steroids for masculinisation of the rat fetus. *Endocrinology*, **71**, 448–451

Li, S., Lévesque, C., Geng, C.-S., Yan, X. & Labrie, F. (1995) Inhibitory effects of medroxyprogesterone acetate (MPA) and the pure antiestrogen EM-219 on estrone (E_1)-stimulated growth of dimethylbenz(a)anthracene (DMBA)-induced mammary carcinoma in the rat. *Breast Cancer Res. Treat.*, **34**, 147–159

Liang, A.P., Levenson, A.G., Layde, P.M., Shelton, J.D., Hatcher, R.A., Potts, M. & Michelson, M.J. (1983) Risk of breast, uterine corpus, and ovarian cancer in women receiving medroxyprogesterone injection. *J. Am. med. Assoc.*, **249**, 2909–2912

Luo, S., Stojanovic, M., Labrie, C. & Labrie, F. (1997) Inhibitory effect of the novel anti-estrogen EM-800 and medroxyprogesterone acetate on estrone-stimulated growth of dimethylbenz[a]anthracene-induced mammary carcinoma in rats. *Int. J. Cancer*, **73**, 580–586

Luthy, I.A., Begin, D.J. & Labrie, F. (1988) Androgenic activity of synthetic progestins and spironolactone in androgen-sensitive mouse mammary carcinoma (Shionogi) cells in culture. *J. Steroid Biochem.*, **31**, 845–852

Markiewicz, L. & Gurpide, E. (1994) Estrogenic and progestagenic activities coexisting in steroidal drugs: Quantitative evaluation by *in vitro* bioassays with human cells. *J. Steroid Biochem. mol. Biol.*, **48**, 89–94

Markiewicz, L., Hochberg, R.B. & Gurpide, E. (1992) Intrinsic estrogenicity of some progestagenic drugs. *J. Steroid Biochem. mol. Biol.*, **41**, 53–58

Maudelonde, T., Lavaud, P., Salazar, G., Laffargue, F. & Rochefort, H. (1991) Progestin treatment depresses estrogen receptor but not cathepsin D levels in needle aspirates of benign breast disease. *Breast Cancer Res. Treat.*, **19**, 95–102

McCauley, A. & Geller, J. (1992) Decisions for Norplant programs. *Popul. Rep.*, **24**, 1–31

McLaughlin, L. (1982) *The Pill, John Rock and the Church*, Toronto, Little, Brown & Co., pp. 138–145

Meirik, O., Lund, E., Adami, H.O., Bergstrom, R., Christoffersen, T. & Bergsjo, P. (1986) Oral contraceptive use and breast cancer in young women. *Lancet*, **ii**, 650–654

Melo J.F. & Coutinho, E.M. (1977) Inhibition of spermatogenesis in men with monthly injections of medroxyprogesterone acetate and testosterone enanthate. *Contraception*, **15**, 627–633

Meyer, W.J., Walker, P.A., Wideking, C., Money, J., Kowarski, A.A., Migeon, C.J. & Borgaonkar, D.S. (1977) Pituitary function in adult males receiving medroxyprogesterone acetate. *Fertil. Steril.*, **28**, 1072–1076

Misdorp, W. (1988) Canine mammary tumours: Protective effect of late ovariectomy and stimulating effect of progestins. *Vet. Q.*, **10**, 26–33

Misdorp, W. (1991) Progestagens and mammary tumors in dogs and cats. *Acta endocrinol.*, **125**, 27–31

Mitsumori, K., Furukawa, F., Sato, M., Yoshimura, H., Imazawa, T., Nishikawa, A. & Takahashi, M. (1994) Promoting effects of ethinyl estradiol on development of renal proliferative lesions induced by *N*-nitrosobis(2-oxopropyl)amine in female Syrian golden hamsters. *Cancer Res. clin. Oncol.*, **120**, 131–136

Mol, J.A., Henzen-Logmans, S.C., Hageman, P., Misdorp, W., Blankenstein, M.A. & Rijnberk, A. (1995a) Expression of the gene encoding growth hormone in the human mammary gland. *J. clin. Endocrinol. Metab.*, **80**, 3094–3096

Mol, J.A., van Darderen, E., Selman, P.J., Wolfswinkel, J., Rijnberk, A. & Rutteman, G.R. (1995b) Growth hormone mRNA in mammary gland tumors of dogs and cats. *J. clin. Invest.*, **95**, 2028–2034

Mol, J.A., van Garderen, E., Rutteman, G.R. & Rijnberk, A. (1996) New insights in the molecular mechanism of progestin-induced proliferation of mammary epithelium: induction of the local biosynthesis of growth hormone (GH) in the mammary gland of dogs, cats and humans. *J. Steroid Biochem. mol. Biol.*, **57**, 67–71

Molinolo, A.A., Lanari, C., Charreau, E.H., Sanjuan, N. & Dosne Pasqualini, C. (1987) Mouse mammary tumors induced by medroxyprogesterone acetate: Immunohistochemistry and hormonal receptors. *J. natl Cancer Inst.*, **79**, 1341–1350

Musgrove, E.A., Lee, C.S.L. & Sutherland, R.L. (1991) Progestins both stimulate and inhibit breast cancer cell cycle progression while increasing expression of transforming growth factor α, epidermal growth factor receptor, c-*fos*, and c-*myc* genes. *Mol. cell. Biol.*, **11**, 5032–5043

Neumann, I., Thierau, D., Andrae, U., Greim, H. & Schwartz, L.R. (1992) Cyproterone acetate induces DNA damage in cultured rat hepatocytes and preferentially stimulates DNA synthesis in γ-glutamyltranspeptidase-positive cells. *Carcinogenesis*, **13**, 373–378

New Zealand Contraception and Health Study Group (1994) Risk of cervical dysplasia in users of oral contraceptives, intrauterine devices, or depot-medroxyprogesterone acetate. *Contraception*, **50**, 431–441

Nisker, J.A., Kirk, M.E. & Nunez-Troconis, J.T. (1988) Reduced incidence of rabbit endometrial neoplasia with levonorgestrel implant. *Am. J. Obstet. Gynecol.*, **158**, 300–303

Niwa, K., Morishita, S., Murase, T., Itoh, N., Tanaka, T., Mori, H. & Tamaya, T. (1995) Inhibitory effects of medroxyprogesterone acetate on mouse endometrial carcinogenesis. *Jpn. J. Cancer Res.*, **86**, 724–729

Odlind, V., Weiner, E., Victor, A. & Johansson, E.D. (1980) Effects of sex hormone binding globulin of different oral contraceptives containing norethisterone and lynestrenol. *Br. J. Obstet. Gynaecol.*, **87**, 416–421

Ortiz, A., Hiroi, M., Stanczyk, F.Z., Goebelsmann, U. & Mishell, D.R., Jr (1977) Serum medroxyprogesterone acetate (MPA) concentrations and ovarian function following intramuscular injections of Depo-MPA. *J. clin. Endocrinol. Metab.*, **44**, 32–38

van Os, J.L., van Laar, P.H., Oldenkamp, E.P. & Verschoor, J.S. (1981) Oestrus control and the incidence of mammary nodules in bitches, a clinical study with two progestogens. *Vet. Q.*, **3**, 46–56

Østerlind, A., Tucker, M.A., Stone, B.J. & Jensen, O.M. (1988) The Danish case–control study of cutaneous malignant melanoma. III. Hormonal and reproductive factors in women. *Int. J. Cancer*, **42**, 821–824

Pardthaisong, T. & Gray, R.H. (1991) In utero exposure to steroid contraceptives and outcome of pregnancy. *Am. J. Epidemiol.*, **134**, 795–803

Pardthaisong, T., Yenchit, C. & Gray, R.H. (1992) The long-term growth and development of children exposed to Depo-Provera during pregnancy or lactation. *Contraception*, **45**, 313–324

Parzefall, W., Monschau, P. & Schulte-Hermann, R. (1989) Induction by cyproterone acetate of DNA synthesis and mitosis in primary cultures of adult rat hepatocytes in serum free medium. *Arch. Toxicol.*, **63**, 456–461

Pater, A., Bayatpour, M. & Pater, M.M. (1990) Oncogenic transformation by human papilloma virus type 16 deoxyribonucleic acid in the presence of progesterone or progestins from oral contraceptives. *Am. J. Obstet. Gynecol.*, **162**, 1099-1103

Paul, C., Skegg, D.C.G. & Spears, G.F.S. (1989) Depot medroxyprogesterone (Depo-Provera) and risk of breast cancer. *Br. med. J.*, **299**, 759–762

Paul, C., Skegg, D.C.G. & Spears, G.F.S. (1990) Oral contraceptives and risk of breast cancer. *Int. J. Cancer*, **46**, 366–373

Paul, C., Skegg, D.C.G. & Williams, S. (1997) Depot medroxyprogesterone acetate: Patterns of use and reasons for discontinuation. *Contraception*, **56**, 209–214

Pazos, P., Lanari, C., Meiss, R., Charreau, E.H. & Pasqualini, C.D. (1991) Mammary carcinogenesis induced by N-methyl-N-nitrosourea (MNU) and medroxyprogesterone acetate (MPA) in BALB/c mice. *Breast Cancer Res. Treat.*, **20**, 133–138

Pazos, P., Lanari, C., Eizalde, P., Montecchia, F., Charreau, E.H. & Molinolo, A.A. (1998) Promoter effect of medroxyprogesterone acetate (MPA) in N-methyl-N-nitrosourea (MNU) induced mammary tumors in BALB/c mice. *Carcinogenesis*, **19**, 529–531

Peek, M.J., Markham, R. & Fraser, I.S. (1995) The effects of natural and synthetic sex steroids on human decidual endothelial cell proliferation. *Hum. Reprod.*, **10**, 2238–2243

Pekonen, F., Nyman, T. & Rutanen, E.M. (1994) Differential expression of mRNAs for endothelin-related proteins in human endometrium, mymetrium and leiomyoma. *Mol. cell. Endocrinol.*, **103**, 165–170

Phillips, A., Hahn, D.W., Klimek, S. & McGuire, J.L. (1987) A comparison of the potencies and activities of progestogens used in contraceptives. *Contraception*, **36**, 181–192

Piper, J.M. & Kennedy, D.L. (1987) Oral contraceptives in the United States: Trends in content and potency. *Int. J. Epidemiol.*, **16**, 215–221

Population Council (1994) Syria 1993: Results from the PAPCHILD Survey. *Stud. Fam. Plann.*, **25**, 248–252

Population Council (1995) Sudan 1992/93: Results from the PAPCHILD Health Survey. *Stud. Fam. Plann.*, **26**, 116–120

Population Council (1996a) Bolivia 1994: Results from the Demographic and Health Survey. *Stud. Fam. Plann.*, **27**, 172–176

Population Council (1996b) Morocco 1995: Results from the Demographic and Health Survey. *Stud. Fam. Plann.*, **27**, 344–348

Population Council (1997a) Uganda 1995: Results from the Demographic and Health Survey. *Stud. Fam. Plann.*, **28**, 156–160

Population Council (1997b) Egypt 1995: Results from the Demographic and Health Survey. *Stud. Fam. Plann.*, **28**, 251–255

Population Council (1997c) Guatemala 1995: Results from the Demographic and Health Survey. *Stud. Fam. Plann.*, **28**, 151–155

Population Council (1997d) Kazakstan 1995: Results from the Demographic and Health Survey. *Stud. Fam. Plann.*, **28**, 256–260

Population Council (1997e) Eritrea 1995: Results from the Demographic and Health Survey. *Stud. Fam. Plann.*, **28**, 336–340

Population Council (1997f) Mali 1995–96: Results from the Demographic and Health Survey. *Stud. Fam. Plann.*, **28**, 341–345

Population Council (1998a) Benin 1996: Results from the Demographic and Health Survey. *Stud. Fam. Plann.*, **29**, 83–87

Population Council (1998b) Brazil 1996: Results from the Demographic and Health Survey. *Stud. Fam. Plann.*, **29**, 88–92

Prahalada, S., Carroad, E., Cukierski, M. & Hendrickx, A.G. (1985) Embryotoxicity of a single dose of medroxyprogesterone acetate (MPA) and maternal serum MPA concentrations in cynomolgus monkey (*Macaca fascicularis*). *Teratology*, **32**, 421–432

Prost-Avallet, O., Oursin, J. & Adessi, G. (1991) *In vitro* effect of synthetic progestogens on estrone sulfatase activity in human breast carcinoma. *J. Steroid Biochem. mol. Biol.*, **39**, 967–973

Reynolds, J.E.F., ed. (1996) *Martindale: The Extra Pharmacopoeia*, 31st Ed., London, The Pharmaceutical Press, pp. 1495–1496, 1500–1501

Rosenberg, L., Palmer, J.R., Zauber, A.G., Warshauer, M.E., Lewis, J.L., Jr, Strom, B.L., Harlap, S. & Shapiro, S. (1994) A case–control study of oral contraceptive use and invasive epithelial ovarian cancer. *Am. J. Epidemiol.*, **139**, 654–661

Russo, I.H. & Russo, J. (1991) Progestagens and mammary gland development: Differentiation versus carcinogenesis. *Acta endocrinol.*, **125**, 7–12

Russo, I.H., Gimotty, P., Dupuis, M. & Russo, J. (1989a) Effect of medroxyprogesterone acetate on the response of the rat mammary gland to carcinogenesis. *Br. J. Cancer*, **59**, 210–216

Russo, I.H., Frederick, J. & Russo, J. (1989b) Hormone prevention of mammary carcinogenesis by norethynodrel-mestranol. *Breast Cancer Res. Treat.*, **14**, 43–56

Rutanen, E.M., Salmi, A. & Nyman, T. (1997) mRNA expression of insulin-like growth factor-I (IGF-I) is suppressed and those of IGF-II and IGF-binding protein-1 are constantly expressed in the endometrium during use of an intrauterine levonorgestrel system. *Mol. hum. Reprod.*, **9**, 749–754

Sasaki, M., Sugimura, K., Yoshida, M.A. & Aber, S. (1980) Cytogenetic effects of 60 chemicals on cultured human and Chinese hamster cells. *Kromosomo*, **20**, 574–584

Schardein, J.L. (1980) Congenital abnormalities and hormones during pregnancy: A clinical review. *Teratology*, **22**, 251–270

Schoonen, W.G.E.J., Joosten, J.W.H. & Kloosterboer, H.J. (1995a) Effects of two classes of progestagens, pregnane and 19-nortestosterone derivatives, on cell growth of human breast tumor cells: I. MCF-7 cell lines. *J. Steroid Biochem. mol. Biol.*, **55**, 423–437

Schoonen, W.G.E.J., Joosten, J.W.H. & Kloosterboer, H.J. (1995b) Effects of two classes of progestagens, pregnane and 19-nortestosterone derivatives, on cell growth of human breast tumor cells: II. T47D cell lines. *J. Steroid Biochem. mol. Biol.*, **55**, 439–444

Schulte-Hermann, R., Ochs, H., Bursch, W. & Parzefall, W. (1988) Quantitative structure–activity studies on effects of sixteen different steroids on growth and monooxygenases of rat liver. *Cancer Res.*, **48**, 2462–2468

Segal, S.J., Alvarez-Sanchez, F., Brache, V., Faundes, A., Vilja, P. & Tuohimaa, P. (1991) Norplant® implants: The mechanism of contraceptive action. *Fertil. Steril.*, **56**, 273–277

Selman, P.J., Mol, J.A., Rutteman, G.R., van Garderen, E. & Rijnberk, A.D. (1994) Progestin-induced growth hormone excess in the dog originates in the mammary gland. *Endocrinology*, **134**, 287–292

Selman, P.J., van Garderen, E., Mol, J.A. & van den Ingh, T.S. (1995) Comparison of the histological changes in the dog after treatment with the progestins medroxyprogesterone acetate and proligestone. *Veter. Q.*, **17**, 128–133

Selman, P.J., Wolfswinkel, J. & Mol, J.A. (1996) Binding specificity of medroxyprogesterone acetate and proligestone for the progesterone and glucocorticoid receptor in the dog. *Steroids*, **61**, 133–137

Shaaban, M.M., Elwan, S.I., El-Kabsh, M.Y., Farghaly, S.A. & Thabet, N. (1984) Effect of levonorgestrel contraceptive implants, Norplant®, on blood coagulation. *Contraception*, **30**, 421–450

Shapiro, S.S., Dyer, R.D. & Colas, A.E. (1978) Synthetic progestins: In vitro potency on human endometrium and specific binding to cytosol receptor. *Am. J. Obstet. Gynecol.*, **132**, 549–554

Shifren, J.L., Tseng, J.F., Zaloudek, C.J., Ryan, I.P., Meng, Y.G., Ferrara, N., Jaffe, R.B. & Taylor, R.N. (1996) Ovarian steroid regulation of vascular endothelial growth factor in the human endometrium: Implications for angiogenesis during the menstrual cycle and in the pathogenesis of endometriosis. *J. clin. Endocrinol. Metab.*, **8**, 3112–3118

Silvin, I., Stern, J., Diaz, S., Pavéz, M., Alvarez-Sanchez, F., Brache, V., Mishell, D.R., Macarra, M., McCarthy, T., Holma, P., Darney, P., Klaisle, C., Olsson, S.E. & Odlind, V. (1992) Rates and outcomes of planned pregnancy after use of Norplant capsules, Norplant II rods, or levonorgestrel-releasing or copper TCu 380Ag intrauterine contraceptive devices. *Am. J. Obstet. Gynecol.*, **166**, 1208–1213

Skegg, D.C., Noonan, E.A., Paul, C., Spears, G.F.S., Meirik, O. & Thomas, D.B. (1995) Depot medroxyprogesterone acetate and breast cancer. A pooled analysis of the World Health Organization and New Zealand studies. *J. Am. med. Assoc.*, **273**, 799–804

Skegg, D.C., Paul, C., Spears, G.F.S. & Williams, S.M. (1996) Progestogen-only oral contraceptives and risk of breast cancer in New Zealand. *Cancer Causes Control*, **7**, 513–519

Soufir, J.-C., Jouannet, P., Marson, J. & Soumah, A. (1983) Reversible inhibition of sperm production and gonadotrophin secretion in men following combined oral medroxyprogesterone acetate and percutanoeus testosterone treatment. *Endocrinologia*, **102**, 625–632

Stenchever, M.A., Jarvis, J.A. & Kreger, N.K. (1969) Effect of selected estrogens and progestins on human chromosomes in vitro. *Obstet. Gynecol.*, **34**, 249–252

Subakir, S.B., Hadisaputra, W., Siregar, B., Irawati, D., Santoso, D.I., Cornain, S. & Affandi, B. (1995) Reduced endothelial cell migratory signal production by endometrial explants from women using Norplant contraception. *Hum. Reprod.*, **10**, 2579–2583

Subakir, S.B., Hadisaputra, W., Handoyo, A.E. & Affandi, B. (1996) Endometrial angiogenic response in Norplant users. *Hum. Reprod.*, **11**, 51–55

Sutherland, R.L., Hall, R.E., Pang, G., Sutherland, R.L., Hall, R.E., Pang, G.Y., Musgrove, E.A. & Clarke, C.L. (1988) Effect of medroxyprogesterone acetate on proliferation and cell cycle kinetics of human mammary carcinoma cells. *Cancer Res.*, **48**, 5084–5091

Swenberg, J.A. (1981) Utilization of the alkaline elution assay as a short-term test for chemical carcinogens. In: Stich, H.F. & San, R.H.C., eds, *Short-term Tests for Chemical Carcinogens*, New York, Springer-Verlag, pp. 48–58

Tarara, R. (1984) The effect of medroxyprogesterone acetate (Depo-provera) on prenatal development in the baboon (*Papio anubis*): A preliminary study. *Teratology*, **30**, 181–185

Thomas, D.B., Ye, Z., Ray, R.M. & the WHO Collaborative Study of Neoplasia and Steroid Contraceptives (1995a) Cervical carcinoma in situ and use of depot-medroxyprogesterone acetate (DMPA). *Contraception*, **51**, 25–31

Thomas, D.B., Ray, R.M. & the WHO Collaborative Study of Neoplasia and Steroid Contraceptives (1995b) Depot-medroxyprogesterone acetate (DMPA) and risk of invasive adenocarcinomas and adenosquamous carcinomas of the uterine cervix. *Contraception*, **52**, 307–312

Thorogood, M. & Villard-Mackintosh, L. (1993) Combined oral contraceptives: Risks and benefits. *Br. med. Bull.*, **49**, 124–139

Tiltman, A.J. (1985) The effect of progestins on the mitotic activity of uterine fibromyomas. *Int. J. Gynecol. Pathol.*, **4**, 89–96

Topham, J.C. (1980) Do induced sperm-head abnormalities in mice specifically identify mammalian mutagens rather than carcinogens? *Mutat. Res.*, **74**, 379–387

Treiman, K., Liskin, L., Kols, A. & Ward, R. (1995) IUDs—An update. *Popul. Rep.*, **23**, 1–35

Tseng, L. & Zhu, H.H. (1997) Regulation of progesterone receptor messenger ribonucleic acid by progestin in human endometrial stromal cells. *Biol. Reprod.*, **57**, 1360–1366

Tsutsui, T., Komine, A., Huff, J. & Barrett, J.D. (1995) Effects of testosterone, testosterone propionate, 17β-trenbolone and progesterone on cell formation and mutagenesis in Syrian hamster embryo cells. *Carcinogenesis*, **16**, 1329–1333

Ueda, M., Fujii, H., Yoshizawa, K., Abe, F. & Ueki, M. (1996) Effects of sex steroids and growth factors on migration and invasion of endometrial adenocarcinoma SNG-M cells *in vitro*. *Jpn. J. Cancer Res.*, **87**, 524–533

UK National Case–Control Study Group (1989) Oral contraceptive use and breast cancer risk in young women. *Lancet*, **i**, 973–982

Umapathy, E. & Rai, U.C. (1982) Effect of antiandrogens and medroxyprogesterone acetate on testicular morphometry in mice. *Acta morphol. acad. sci. hung.*, **30**, 99–108

United States Census Bureau (1998) Int. Data Base http://www.census.gov/ipc/www/idbacc.html.

Vanderboom, R.J. & Sheffield, L.G. (1993) Estrogen enhances epidermal growth factor-induced DNA synthesis in mammary epithelial cells. *J. Cell Physiol.*, **156**, 367–372

Vessey, M., Buron, J., Doll, R., McPherson, K. & Yeates, D. (1983) Oral contraceptives and breast cancer: Final report of an epidemiologic study. *Br. J. Cancer*, **47**, 455–462

Wharton, C. & Blackburn, R. (1988) Lower dose pills. *Popul. Rep.*, **16**, 1–31

WHO Collaborative Study of Neoplasia and Steroid Contraceptives (1991a) Breast cancer and depot medroxyprogesterone acetate: A national study. *Lancet*, **338**, 833–838

WHO Collaborative Study of Neoplasia and Steroid Contraceptives (1991b) Depot medroxyprogesterone acetate (DMPA) and risk of endometrial cancer. *Int. J. Cancer*, **49**, 186–190

WHO Collaborative Study of Neoplasia and Steroid Contraceptives (1991c) Depot-medroxyprogesterone acetate (DMPA) and risk of epithelial ovarian cancer. *Int. J. Cancer*, **49**, 191–195

WHO Collaborative Study of Neoplasia and Steroid Contraceptives (1991d) Depot-medroxyprogesterone acetate (DMPA) and risk of liver cancer. *Int. J. Cancer*, **49**, 182–185

WHO Collaborative Study of Neoplasia and Steroid Contraceptives (1992) Depot-medroxyprogesterone acetate (DMPA) and risk of invasive squamous cell cervical cancer. *Contraception*, **45**, 299–312

WHO Family Planning and Population Unit (1996) Family planning methods: New guidance. *Popul. Rep.*, **24**, 1–48

Wikström, A., Green, B. & Johansson, E.D.B. (1984) The plasma concentration of medroxyprogesterone acetate and ovarian function during treatment with medroxyprogesterone acetate in 5 and 10 mg doses. *Acta obstet. gynecol. scand.*, **63**, 163–168

Willcox, D.L., Yovich, J.L., McColm, S.C. & Schmitt, L.H. (1985) Changes in total and free concentrations of steroid hormones in the plasma of women throughout pregnancy: Effects of medroxyprogesterone acetate in the first trimester. *J. Endocrinol.*, **107**, 293–300

Yamamoto, T., Terada, N., Nishizawa, Y. & Petrow, V. (1994) Angiostatic activities of medroxyprogesterone acetate and its analogues. *Int. J. Cancer*, **56**, 393–399

Yovich, J.L., Willcox, D.L., Wilkinson, S.P., Poletti, V.M. & Hähnel, R. (1985) Medroxy-progesterone acetate does not perturb the profile of steroid metabolites in urine during pregnancy. *J. Endocrinol.*, **104**, 453–459

Yovich, J.L., Turner, S.R. & Draper, R. (1988) Medroxyprogesterone acetate therapy in early pregnancy has no apparent fetal effects. *Teratology*, **38**, 135–144

Zalanyi, S., Jr, Aedo, A.R., Johannisson, E., Landgren, B.M. & Diczfalusy, E. (1986) Pituitary, ovarian and endometrial effects of graded doses of medroxyprogesterone acetate admi-nistered on cycle days 7 to 10. *Contraception*, **33**, 567–578

POST-MENOPAUSAL OESTROGEN THERAPY

1. Exposure

'Post-menopausal oestrogen therapy' refers to the use of oestrogen without progestogen for women in the period around the menopause, primarily for the treatment of menopausal symptoms but increasingly for the prevention of conditions that become more common in the post-menopausal period, such as osteoporosis and ischaemic heart disease. Currently, it is mainly given to women who have had a hysterectomy, as treatment with oestrogen alone in women with a uterus increases the risk for endometrial cancer. In the past, women with a uterus were often prescribed post-menopausal oestrogen therapy, although predominantly in the United States. Post-menopausal therapy with combined oestrogen and progestogen is discussed in another monograph in this volume.

Post-menopausal oestrogen therapy can be administered orally, transdermally (by patch or gel), by injection or by implant. Local, topical preparations are also available for relief of urogenital symptoms. Annex 2 (Table 3) gives a list of common brands of post-menopausal oestrogen therapy, with their constituents and doses and examples of countries in which they are available. Post-menopausal oestrogen therapy can also be administered in combination with an androgen or with an anxiolytic, and examples of such brands and formulations are given in Annex 2 (Table 4).

1.1 Historical overview

Whether menopause is natural or induced surgically, women in this condition have long been known to suffer from problems such as hot flushes (or 'flashes') and urogenital atrophy and to have increased rates of fracture and cardiovascular disease, in comparison with pre-menopausal women. These problems are particularly severe in women who have a premature menopause. In 1895, Marie Bra suggested that ovarian secretions could be used to treat ovarian failure (Bush & Barrett-Connor, 1985), and the first therapeutic investigations of the administration of ovarian tissue for the relief of climacteric symptoms were reported in 1896. Subsequently, researchers and clinicians investigated the use of various ovarian, placental and urine extracts, implantation of ovarian tissue and oral administration of dried ovarian tissue (Kopera & van Keep, 1991).

The identification of the ovarian hormones allowed a more specific understanding of the factors that might be responsible for climacteric symptoms. Oestrone, oestriol and progesterone were identified in 1929, and oestradiol was identified in 1936 (IARC, 1979). The first synthetic oestrogens, diethylstilboestrol and ethinyloestradiol, were isolated in 1938 (Bush & Barrett-Connor, 1985).

Clinical use of oestrogen for women with premature surgical or natural menopause began in the 1930s (Stadel & Weiss, 1975; Kopera & van Keep, 1991). Campbell and Collip (1930) demonstrated the clinical efficacy of extracts of human placenta in relieving menopausal symptoms and deviations from the normal menstrual cycle, like dysmenorrhoea. Although a product containing these extracts was introduced onto the market, it was impractical to produce on a large scale (Stern, 1982); most oestrogen was therefore administered by injection or subcutaneous implant. The earliest use of an implant was reported by Bishop (1938), who administered oestrogen to women after oophorectomy.

Clinical trials of conjugated equine oestrogens from the urine of pregnant mares were initiated in 1941 (Stern, 1982). In 1943, these preparations became available in the United States for use as oral post-menopausal oestrogen therapy and were introduced onto the market in the United Kingdom in 1956 (Godfree, 1994). Over the following years, post-menopausal oestrogen therapy began to be used less for women who had had a premature menopause than for women who had had menopause at a normal age, although women who had undergone a hysterectomy or an oophorectomy have been consistently more likely to receive post-menopausal oestrogen therapy than women who have had a natural menopause (Brett & Madans, 1997). The indications for use also widened, from short-term treatment for menopausal symptoms to longer-term treatment for the prevention of osteoporosis and cardiovascular disease; some clinicians advocated near-universal prescription for women after the menopause (Schleyer-Saunders, 1973).

Use of post-menopausal oestrogen therapy became widespread in the United States in the 1960s: the number of women using it was estimated to have increased by 240% between 1962 and 1967 (Bush & Barrett-Connor, 1985), such that approximately 13% of women in the United States aged 45–64 used post-menopausal oestrogen therapy (Stadel & Weiss, 1975). Figure 1 gives the estimated numbers of prescriptions for non-contraceptive oestrogens and progestogens from the National Prescription Audit in the United States (Kennedy et al., 1985; Wysowski et al., 1995) between 1966 and 1992. The dose of oral oestrogen prescribed decreased over the period 1975–83, as did the use of injectable post-menopausal oestrogen therapy (Kennedy et al., 1985). By 1992, transdermal oestradiol accounted for 15% of post-menopausal oestrogen therapy prescriptions in the United States (Jewelewicz, 1997).

In the United Kingdom, around 2% of English women aged 40–64 were using post-menopausal hormonal therapy during the period 1980–87, the prevalence rising rapidly to reach 22% by 1994. The majority of these prescriptions were for combined oestrogen–progestogen therapy (Townsend, 1998).

The fall in the number of prescriptions of oestrogen in the United States corresponded to scientific reports and growing public awareness of the elevated risks for endometrial cancer of women using post-menopausal oestrogen therapy who had not had a hysterectomy (Smith et al., 1975; Ziel & Finkle, 1975). Thereafter, the prescription rates for such therapy in the United States began to rise but more frequently in combination with a progestogen (Hemminki et al., 1988; see the monograph on 'Post-menopausal oestrogen–progestogen therapy'). Administration of unopposed therapy to women with a uterus

Figure 1. Estimated numbers of dispensed prescriptions (in millions) of non-contraceptive oestrogens and progestogens in the United States, 1966–92

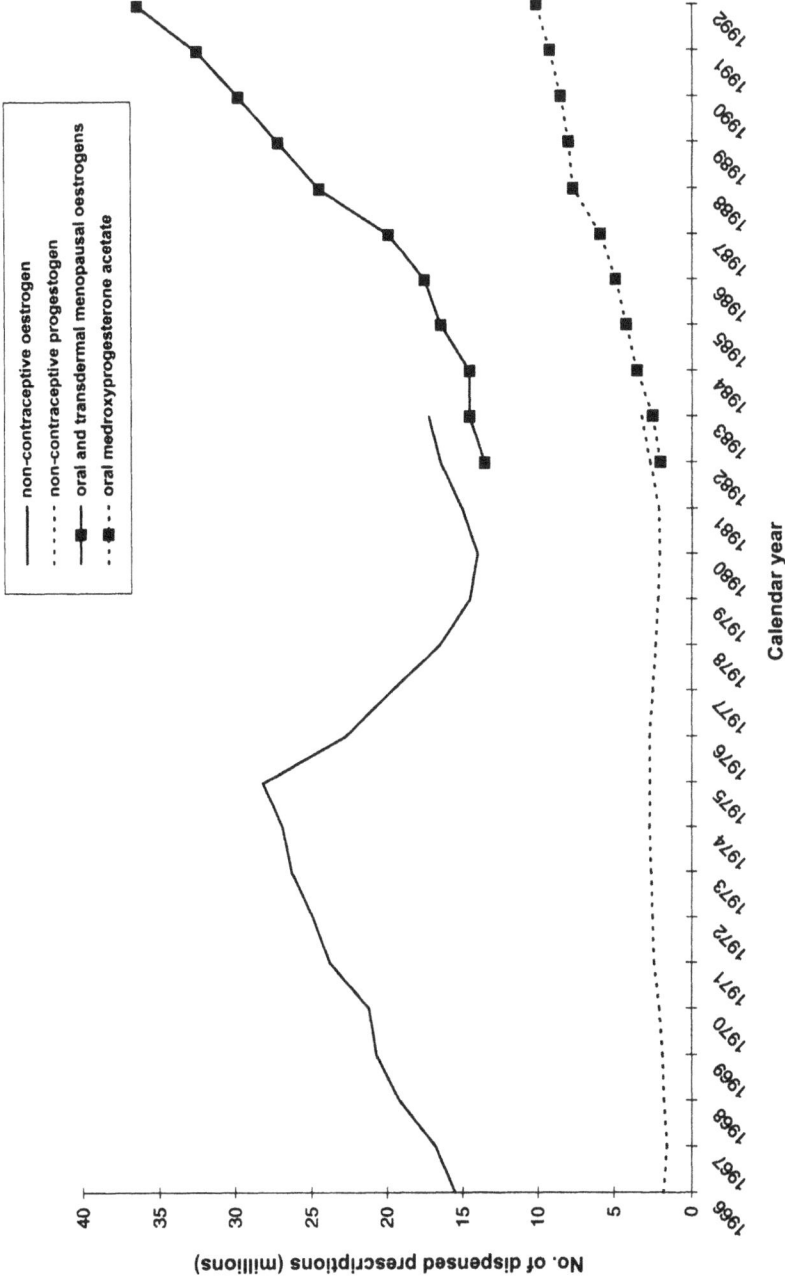

Adapted from Kennedy *et al.* (1985) and Wysowski *et al.* (1995)
The estimates for 1966–83 are for prescribed oestrogens and progestogens other than those that are part of an oral contraceptive, and the estimates for 1982–92 are for the more specific categories of oral and transdermal menopausal oestrogens and oral medroxyprogesterone acetate (the most commonly prescribed menopausal progestogen in the United States).

continued, predominantly in the United States, with the recommendation that the endometrium be monitored (e.g. American College of Physicians, 1992). A more substantial shift in consciousness in the United States occurred in 1995, with the publication of the results of a trial that showed the occurrence of adenomatous or atypical endometrial hyperplasia in 34% of women receiving 0.625 mg of unopposed conjugated equine oestrogens daily (Writing Group for the PEPI Trial, 1995). Subsequently, the protocol of the nationwide Women's Health Initiative trial of post-menopausal hormonal therapy was amended so that women with a uterus could be randomized to receive only combined oestrogen–progestogen therapy or placebo (Finnegan et al., 1995).

Oestrogen–androgen combinations accounted for an estimated 14% of non-contraceptive oestrogen prescriptions in the United States in 1966, but this had fallen to less than 2% in 1983 (Kennedy et al., 1985). The number of oestrogen–androgen prescriptions then began to increase again, from 0.1 million in 1982 to 0.8 million in 1992 (Wysowski et al., 1995). Oestrogen in combination with a tranquillizer represented an estimated 3% of non-contraceptive oestrogen prescriptions in the United States in 1975, falling to less than 1% of prescriptions in 1983 (Kennedy et al., 1985).

Outside the United States, use of post-menopausal oestrogen therapy was generally uncommon until the late 1970s and 1980s and was prescribed mainly to women who had had a hysterectomy (although very few data are available about international use before the 1980s). In Europe, women with an intact uterus have been treated with combined oestrogen–progestogen therapy since the early 1970s (Maddison, 1973).

Transdermal post-menopausal oestrogen therapy became available in the mid-1980s.

1.2   Post-menopausal oestrogen therapy preparations

The main oestrogens used in oral post-menopausal oestrogen therapy are conjugated equine oestrogens, oestradiol and oestradiol valerate, although esterified oestrogens, mestranol, oestriol and oestropipate, are also used. Oestriol is more commonly used in Scandinavia (Persson et al., 1983; Stadberg et al., 1997). The appropriate dose of oestrogen varies with the indication for therapy; for menopausal symptoms, it can be raised until a minimum effective dose is found. The usual oral dose of conjugated equine oestrogens is 0.625–1.25 mg daily, and the usual oral dose of oestradiol is 0.5–4.0 mg daily (British Medical Association, 1997). For prevention of osteoporosis, the United Kingdom guidelines stipulate minimal doses of 0.625 mg/day oral conjugated equine oestrogens, 2 mg/day oral oestradiol or 0.050 mg/day oestradiol by patch, and not all types of oestradiol patches are specifically licensed for this indication (Anon., 1996).

Oestradiol can also be administered transdermally via a gel or patch, which avoids the first-pass effect of the liver, where a substantial proportion of orally administered oestrogen is deactivated, thus providing more constant blood hormone concentrations than oral preparations. In addition, because it does not cause the peaks and troughs in hormone concentration characteristic of oral medication, a lower overall dose of oestrogen can be given by transdermal administration (Williams & Stancel, 1996). Transdermal doses of oestradiol range from 0.025 mg to 0.1 mg per 24 h (British Medical Association, 1997).

The patches available initially consisted of a central oestradiol reservoir and an external adhesive ring, while in those developed more recently oestradiol is distributed throughout the adherent part of the patch (Anon., 1996). The patches are applied to a clean, non-hairy area of the skin, generally below the waist, and are reapplied every three to four days at a different site.

The available implants consist of crystalline pellets of oestradiol which are inserted subcutaneously under local anaesthesia and provide continuous oestrogen therapy for several months (Anon., 1996). Implants containing 50 mg oestradiol provide effective concentrations for approximately six months, and those containing 100 mg may last for up to nine months (Studd, 1976).

Oestrogen combined with androgen is usually taken orally but can also be given by implant. The usual indication for this type of therapy is menopausal symptoms accompanied by loss of libido (British Medical Association, 1997; Reynolds, 1998). A combination of esterified oestrogen and the anxiolytic chlordiazepoxide (given as 5–10 mg daily) is available in the United States for menopausal symptoms accompanied by anxiety (Reynolds, 1998).

Local topical preparations are available in the form of creams, pessaries and vaginal tablets containing oestriol, oestradiol, conjugated oestrogens, dienoestrol or other oestrogens. They generally have low systemic absorption and are given for urogenital symptoms when systemic therapy is not required. They are not discussed further in this monograph.

1.2.1 *Patterns of use*

Menses cease normally around the age of 50, often preceded and accompanied by climacteric symptoms. Women who have had a hysterectomy often have earlier onset of symptoms, and those who have had pre-menopausal oophorectomy often develop symptoms soon after their operation. Treatment of climacteric symptoms with post-menopausal oestrogen therapy is generally begun around or before the age of menopause and continued until withdrawal of treatment does not lead to a return of the symptoms. Symptomatic treatment generally lasts for less than five years and often for one to two years. Longer-term treatment for the prevention of osteoporosis and other conditions may continue for 10 years or more.

Table 1 shows the prevalence of use of post-menopausal oestrogen therapy in selected international population-based studies. These studies are difficult to interpret and compare as they tended to involve regions within a country that are not necessarily representative of the nation as a whole, include different age groups and usually do not allow a distinction between post-menopausal oestrogen therapy and oestrogen–progestogen therapy. Use of post-menopausal oestrogen therapy varies enormously from country to country and may also show substantial variation within a particular country (Keating *et al.*, 1997). This regional variation is particularly marked in the United States. No figures on prevalence of use are available for many countries. Use is generally considered to be low in most of Africa and Asia.

Table 1. Prevalence of use of post-menopausal hormonal therapy (HT) in selected studies, 1975–97

Country	Reference	Year(s)	Age group (years)	Current use (%)			Any use (%)		
				HT	Oestrogen alone	Oestrogen–progestogen	HT	Oestrogen alone	Oestrogen–progestogen
Australia	MacLennan et al. (1993)	1991	>40	14			25		
Denmark	Pedersen & Jeune (1988)	1983	40–59	16			33	16	12
	Køster (1990)	1987	51	22			37	10	17[a]
	Oddens & Boulet (1997)	1994	45–65	18			31		
Finland	Topo et al. (1995)	1989	45–64	22					
France	Ringa et al. (1992)	1986–87	45–55[b]	8	3	3[a]			
Norway	Topo et al. (1995)	1981	45–55	9					
Sweden	Persson et al. (1983)	1980	50–54	9					
			55–59	6					
	Lindgren et al. (1993)	1988	55, 57, 59 and 65	10			20		
	Stadberg et al. (1997)	1992	46, 50, 54, 58 and 62	21			41		
	Hammar et al. (1996)	1995	55–56	35[c]			40[c]		
United Kingdom	Spector (1989)	Late 1980s	45–65	10					
	Sinclair et al. (1993)	1991	33–69[b]	9			16		
	Griffiths & Jones (1995)	1993	45–65	20			33		
	Lancaster et al. (1995)	1993	45–64	15					
	Banks et al. (1996)	1994–95	50–64	30			43		
	Porter et al. (1996)	NR	45–54	19					
	Kuh et al. (1997)	1993	47	18			25		
	Townsend (1998)	1987	40–64	3					

Table 1 (contd)

Country	Reference	Year(s)	Age group (years)	Current use (%)			Any use (%)		
				HT	Oestrogen alone	Oestrogen–progestogen	HT	Oestrogen alone	Oestrogen–progestogen
United States	Stadel & Weiss (1975)	1973–74	>18[b]				51		
	Barrett-Connor et al. (1979)	1973–75	55–74	39					
	Egeland et al. (1988)	1983–84	40–52	6	4	1			
	Barrett-Connor et al. (1989)	1984–87	50–79	31					
	Harris et al. (1990)	1986–87	NR	32	26	6			
	Cauley et al. (1990)	1986–88	>65	18	15	3			
	Derby et al. (1993)	1981–82	40–64	5					
	Derby et al. (1993)	1989–90	40–64	11					
	Nabulsi et al. (1993)	1986–89	45–64						
	Black			17	16	1	33		
	White			22	17	5	39		
	Johannes et al. (1994)	1981–87	45–61	12[d]					
	Handa et al. (1996)	1986–87	>65	6			25		
	Salamone et al. (1996)	1991		17			45		
	Brett & Madans (1997)	1982–92	25–74[b]				45	31	14
	Keating et al. (1997)	1995	45–74[b]	38					

NR, not reported

[a] 2% progestogen only

[b] Post-menopausal women only

[c] Oestriol users excluded

[d] Any use during study period

In the United States, the sales of non-contraceptive oestrogens increased from around 16 million per year in 1966 to around 36 million in 1992 (Kennedy *et al.*, 1985; Wysowski *et al.*, 1995). Use of post-menopausal hormonal therapy is more common in southern and western United States than in other regions (Keating *et al.*, 1997). In England, a 10-fold increase in the estimated proportion of women using post-menopausal oestrogen therapy was seen in the period 1987–94, with less than 1% of women using oestradiol or conjugated oestrogens in 1987 and 10% in 1994 (Townsend, 1998). Table 1 shows that the prevalence of post-menopausal hormonal therapy in the mid-1990s was about 20% in the age group 45–64. In Scandinavia, use of post-menopausal hormonal therapy increased throughout the 1980s and early 1990s, Norway appearing to have consistently lower rates of use than Sweden, Finland and Denmark (Topo *et al.*, 1995). Sales of post-menopausal hormones (mainly oestradiol compounds cyclically or continuously combined with progestogens) have risen in Sweden since the 1970s, with a clear acceleration and doubling of use rates since the beginning of the 1990s (National Corporation of Pharmacies, 1997). Use of post-menopausal hormonal therapy in general appears to be also relatively common in Australia (MacLennan *et al.*, 1993).

Estimates based on sales data for 1991–92 show that enough post-menopausal hormonal therapy was sold to supply 20% of 45–70-year-old women in the United States (assuming only long-term use), 9–16% of women in Scandinavia and the United Kingdom, 7% in France, 5% in Belgium, 4% in the Netherlands, 3% in Austria and less than 1% of women in this age group in Italy and Spain (Jolleys & Olesen, 1996). Use of post-menopausal hormonal therapy is low in Japan (Nagata *et al.*, 1996).

The post-menopausal oestrogen therapy used in the United States is predominantly conjugated equine oestrogens, Premarin® being the single most commonly prescribed proprietary medicine overall in 1995 (Reynolds, 1998). The oestrogen composition of Premarin® is shown in Table 2. In Scandinavia and the United Kingdom, oestradiol is the oestrogen therapy most commonly prescribed for the menopause (Persson *et al.*, 1997a; Townsend, 1998). Studies from Sweden show that 15–20% of current users of post-menopausal hormonal therapy take oestriol (Persson *et al.*, 1983; Stadberg *et al.*, 1997).

Women taking post-menopausal oestrogen therapy differ from women who do not take it in a number of ways; most notably, they are more likely to have had a hysterectomy and/or oophorectomy (Cauley *et al.*, 1990; Derby *et al.*, 1993; MacLennan *et al.*, 1993; Brett & Madans, 1997). Hysterectomy not only increases the likelihood that a woman will take post-menopausal hormonal therapy in general but also affects the type of therapy taken. Lancaster *et al.* (1995) reported from their general practice-based study in the United Kingdom that, of women taking post-menopausal hormonal therapy, 96% of those with a hysterectomy were taking oestrogen alone and 96% of women without a hysterectomy were taking combined oestrogen and progestogen. As post-menopausal oestrogen therapy is increasingly reserved for women who have had a hysterectomy, the relative use of oestrogen and combined oestrogen and progestogen therapy increasingly reflects the prevalence of hysterectomy in a population. Several studies have shown that, in comparison with non-users, post-menopausal oestrogen therapy users are more likely to have

Table 2. Oestrogen composition (as sulfates) of Premarin®

Oestrogen	% of total
Oestrone sulfate	42
8-Dehydrooestrone sulfate	18
Equilin sulfate	17
17α-Dehydroequilenin sulfate	10
Equilenin sulfate	4.3
17α-Dehydroequilin sulfate	3.4
17α-Oestradiol sulfate	2.4
17β-Oestradiol sulfate	1.5
17β-Dehydroequilin sulfate	0.7
17β-Dehydroequilenin sulfate	0.7

From Li *et al.* (1995)

taken the oral contraceptive pill in the past and to suffer from more severe menopausal symptoms (Sinclair *et al.*, 1993; Handa *et al.*, 1996; Persson *et al.*, 1997a). The relationship between post-menopausal oestrogen therapy and factors such as education, alcohol consumption, smoking and parity is not consistent from study to study.

2. Studies of Cancer in Humans

The use of oestrogen by post-menopausal women is referred to in the following text as 'oestrogen therapy' when oestrogen alone is specified or assumed and as 'oestrogen plus progestogen therapy' when the combination has been specified. The term 'hormone replacement therapy' is not used because none of the currently prescribed regimens offers physiological hormone replacement.

2.1 Breast cancer

Most of the established risk factors for breast cancer seem to operate through hormonal pathways. The fundamental importance of ovarian hormones in the etiology of breast cancer is evident from the established associations with early age at menarche, late age at first full-time pregnancy and late age at menopause (Kelsey *et al.*, 1993). Of particular relevance for the assessment of risk after hormonal therapy is the effect of age when menopause or oestrogen deficiency occurs. Re-analyses of individual data from 51 epidemiological studies on breast cancer showed that the risk for breast cancer increased by about 3% per year the later a woman began menopause in the absence of hormonal therapy (Collaborative Group on Hormonal Factors in Breast Cancer, 1997). Because the serum concentrations of hormones among post-menopausal women taking oestrogen therapy are increased to those of pre-menopausal women, it is reasonable to hypothesize *a priori* that such treatment can cause a similar increase in risk as delay of natural menopause (Colditz, 1996).

2.1.1   Descriptive studies

The sales of orally administered non-contraceptive hormones have surged during recent years in the United States (see section 1.2.1), and analyses of age-adjusted trends in breast cancer incidence in some areas of the United States (Devesa et al., 1987) have revealed an increase that might be compatible with increasing exposure to hormonal therapy. The trends in incidence, which were related mainly to birth cohorts (Holford et al., 1991), could, however, have other explanations, such as increasing intensity of mammography screening, changes in reproductive behaviour and life-style factors.

With the increased use of hormonal therapy in Sweden (see section 1.2.1), the nation-wide age-standardized incidence of breast cancer has increased linearly, by an average of 1.3% since the 1960s up through the mid-1980s (Persson et al., 1993). Thereafter, transient, period-related increases were seen in women aged 50–69 years, which are probably associated with the implementation of population-based mammography screening in Sweden from the late 1980s (Persson et al., 1998). These ecological relationships between use of hormonal therapy and breast cancer incidence are, however, difficult to interpret.

2.1.2   Analytical cohort and case–control studies

Owing to concern in the 1970s that oestrogen therapy might increase the risk for breast cancer, numerous epidemiological studies have been conducted to evaluate possible relationships. Most explored the risk associated with intake of conjugated oestrogens, as predominantly practised in the United States; a few late studies also addressed the risk associated with oestradiol compounds, mainly prescribed in Europe. These studies are summarized in Tables 3a and 3b.

The Collaborative Group on Hormonal Factors in Breast Cancer (1997) reanalysed the original data from 51 out of 61 epidemiological studies with relevant data. Tables 3a and 3b give the relative risks found in those studies and those derived in this reanalysis. The study covered a total of 52 705 cases of breast cancer and 108 411 control subjects. The key results showed that use of hormonal therapy at the time the breast cancer was diagnosed or that had ceased within five years of the diagnosis was associated with a 2.3% (95% confidence interval [CI], 1.1–3.6%) increase in the relative risk for breast cancer for each year of intake (Figure 2). The relative risk reached 1.3 (95% CI, 1.2–1.5) after five to nine years and 1.6 (95% CI, 1.3–1.8) after 15 years of intake for current or recent users. No excess risk was seen five years after discontinuation of treatment. Further, the effect of current or recent long-term treatment was greater in lean than in overweight women (Figure 3) and seen chiefly for clinically less advanced tumours.

The results of selected, large, published studies are reviewed in more detail, and abstracted information from these 15 cohort and 23 case–control studies is given in Tables 4 and 5, respectively. The risk relationships with regard to any use, duration, recency, latency, dose, type of oestrogen, regimens and route of administration are reviewed for

Table 3a. Prospective studies of post-menopausal oestrogen therapy and breast cancer

Reference, country	Original data or reanalysis[a]	No. of cases	Any use	
			Relative risk	95% CI
Hoover et al. (1976), USA	Original	49	1.3	1.0–1.7
Hunt et al. (1987), UK	Original	50	1.6	1.2–2.1
Miller et al. (1992), Canada	Reanalysis	448	1.0	[0.78–1.2]
Schairer et al. (1994), USA	Original	1 185	1.0	0.9–1.2
Risch & Howe (1994), Canada	Original	742	NR	
Colditz et al. (1995), USA	Original	1 935	1.3	1.1–1.5
Schuurman et al. (1995), Netherlands	Original	471	0.99	0.68–1.4
Folsom et al. (1995), USA	Reanalysis	468	1.2	[0.94–1.5]
Thomas et al. (1982), USA; Hiatt et al. (1984), USA; Alexander et al. (1987), UK; Wang et al. (1987), UK; Kay & Hannaford (1988), UK; Bergkvist et al. (1989), Sweden; Mills et al. (1989), USA; Vessey et al. (1989), UK; Willis et al. (1996), USA; Goodman et al. (1997a), Japan	Grouped reanalysis	667	0.62	[0.24–1.0]
Persson et al. (1997b), Sweden	Original	435	1.1	0.8–1.4

[a] Reanalyses by the Collaborative Group on Hormonal Factors in Breast Cancer (1997)
NR, not reported

cohort and case–control studies together. Some comments on methods are given in the tables.

(a) Use of any type of oestrogen for any length of time

Most studies give risk estimates reflecting 'ever use', i.e. use of any type of compound for any amount of time. Most of the relative risks are close to 1.0, and only a few significantly exceed that value (La Vecchia et al., 1986; Hunt et al., 1987; Mills et al., 1989; Colditz et al., 1995; Lipworth et al., 1995). Comparisons of any use of hormones with no use are not, however, very informative, since most use has been short.

(b) Duration of intake

Long-term use was linked to an increased incidence of breast cancer in seven cohort studies and six case–control studies (Ross et al., 1980; Hoover et al., 1981; Brinton et al., 1986; La Vecchia et al., 1986; Hunt et al., 1987; Ewertz, 1988; Bergkvist et al., 1989;

Table 3b. Case–control studies of post-menopausal oestrogen therapy and breast cancer

Reference, country	Original data or reanalysis[a]	No. of cases/ no. of controls	Any use	
			Relative risk	95% CI
Hoover et al. (1981), USA	Original	345/611	1.4	1.0–2.0
Kaufman et al. (1984), USA and Canada	Original	1 610/1 606	1.0	0.8–1.2
Brinton et al. (1986), USA	Original	1 960/2 258	1.0	0.9–1.2
Wingo et al. (1987), USA	Original	1 369/1 645	1.0	0.9–1.2
Hislop et al. (1986), Canada	Reanalysis	361/366	1.2	[0.67–1.6]
Siskind et al. (1989), Australia	Reanalysis	265/544	1.3	[0.64–2.0]
Ewertz (1988), Denmark	Original	1 486/1 336	1.3	0.96–1.7
Kaufman et al. (1991), USA	Original	1 686/2 077	1.2	1.0–1.6
Harris et al. (1992a), USA	Original	604/520	NR	
Weinstein et al. (1993), USA	Original	1 436/1 419	1.1	0.86–1.4
Newcomb et al. (1995), USA	Original	3 130/3 698	1.1	0.9–1.2
Yang et al. (1992), Canada	Original	699/685	1.0	0.8–1.3
Stanford et al. (1995), USA	Original	537/492	0.9	0.6–1.1
Ross et al. (1980), USA; Nomura et al. (1986), USA; Lee et al. (1987), Costa Rica; Rohan & McMichael (1988), Australia; Paul et al. (1990), New Zealand; Palmer et al. (1991), Canada; Ursin et al. (1992), USA; Rookus et al. (1994), Netherlands; White et al. (1994), USA; Brinton et al. (1995), USA	Grouped reanalysis	1 080/1 640 (with population controls)	0.96	[0.66–1.3]
Morabia et al. (1993), USA	Reanalysis	184/322	1.4	[0.67–2.2]
Vessey et al. (1983); McPherson et al. (1987), UK	Original	416/462	1.2	[0.53–1.9]
La Vecchia et al. (1992a), Italy	Reanalysis	1 615/1 450	1.7	[1.2–2.2]
Lipworth et al. (1995), Greece	Reanalysis	446/840	1.2	[0.55–1.8]
La Vecchia et al. (1995), Italy	Original	2 569/2 588	1.2	0.9–1.5
Talamini et al. (1985), Italy; Marubini et al. (1988), Italy; Ravnihar et al. (1988), Slovenia; Hulka et al. (1982), USA; WHO Collaborative Study (1990) (multinational); Ngelangel et al. (1994), Philippines; Levi et al. (1996), Italy	Grouped reanalysis	1 470/5 144 (with hospital controls)	1.0	[0.75–1.3]

[a] Reanalyses by the Collaborative Group on Hormonal Factors in Breast Cancer (1997)
NR, not reported

Figure 2. Relative risks (RR) for breast cancer by duration of use within categories of time since last use of post-menopausal hormonal therapy

Duration of use and time since last use	No. of cases/ no. of controls	RR (FSE)[a]	RR and 99% FCI[a]
No use	12 467/23 568	1.0 (0.021)	
Last use < 5 years before diagnosis (including current use)			
< 1 year	368/860	0.99 (0.085)	
1–4 years	891/2 037	1.1 (0.06)	
5–9 years	588/1 279	1.3 (0.079)	
10–14 years	304/633	1.26 (0.11)	
≥ 15 years	294/514	1.6 (0.13)	
Last use ≥ 5 years before diagnosis			
< 1 year	437/890	1.1 (0.079)	
1–4 years	566/1 256	1.1 (0.068)	
5–9 years	151/374	0.90 (0.12)	
≥ 10 years	93/233	0.95 (0.14)	

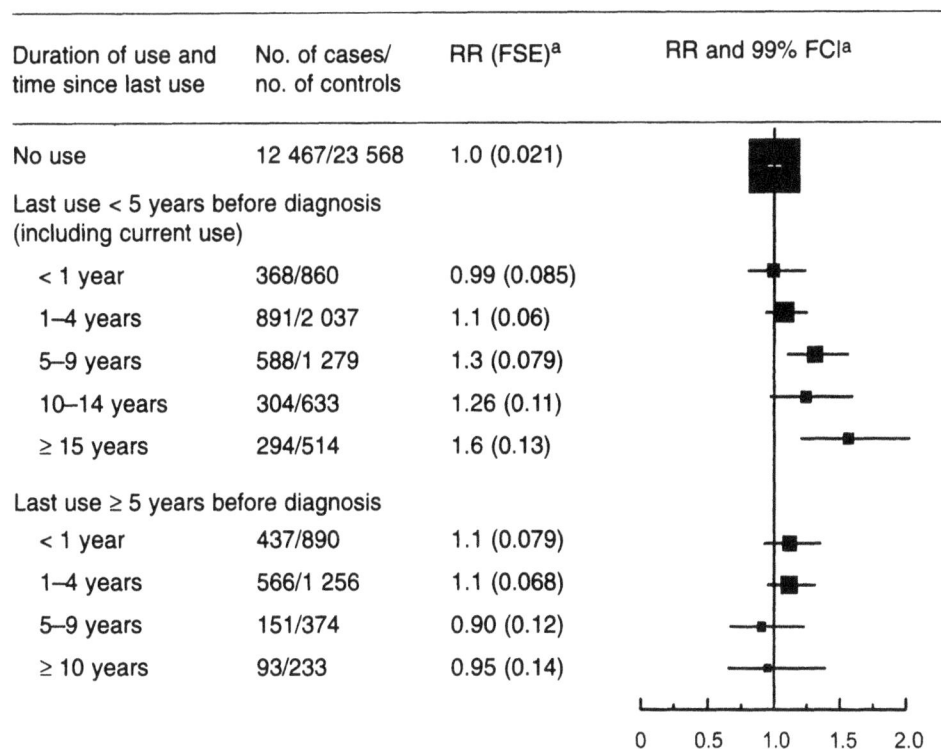

Adapted from Collaborative Group on Hormonal Factors in Breast Cancer (1997)

FSE, floated standard error; FCI, floated confidence interval

[a] Relative to no use, stratified by study, age at diagnosis, time since menopause, body-mass index, parity and age when first child was born

Mills *et al.*, 1989; Yang *et al.*, 1992; Risch & Howe, 1994; Schairer *et al.*, 1994; Colditz *et al.*, 1995; Persson *et al.*, 1997b). At least six case–control studies (Hulka *et al.*, 1982; Kaufman *et al.*, 1984; Wingo *et al.*, 1987; Kaufman *et al.*, 1991; Newcomb *et al.*, 1995; Stanford *et al.*, 1995) and one cohort study (Schuurman *et al.*, 1995) found no statistically significant association with years of oestrogen intake. In two European studies (Ewertz, 1988; Bergkvist *et al.*, 1989), the excess risks seemed to be higher with shorter periods of intake, the relative risk estimates exceeding 2.0 after six years of intake, than in studies in the United States (Brinton *et al.*, 1986; Colditz *et al.*, 1995). The American cohort studies gave increases in risk that are best explained by current intake rather than duration (Mills *et al.*, 1989; Colditz *et al.*, 1992, 1995), although there seemed to be duration-dependent effects in these data for current hormone takers (see Table 4).

Two recent, large population-based case–control studies in the United States (Newcomb *et al.*, 1995; Stanford *et al.*, 1995), the latter with considerable power to examine risk after long-term use, reported no effect of exposure of any duration.

Figure 3. Relative risks for breast cancer according to use of post-menopausal hormonal therapy by women with various characteristics

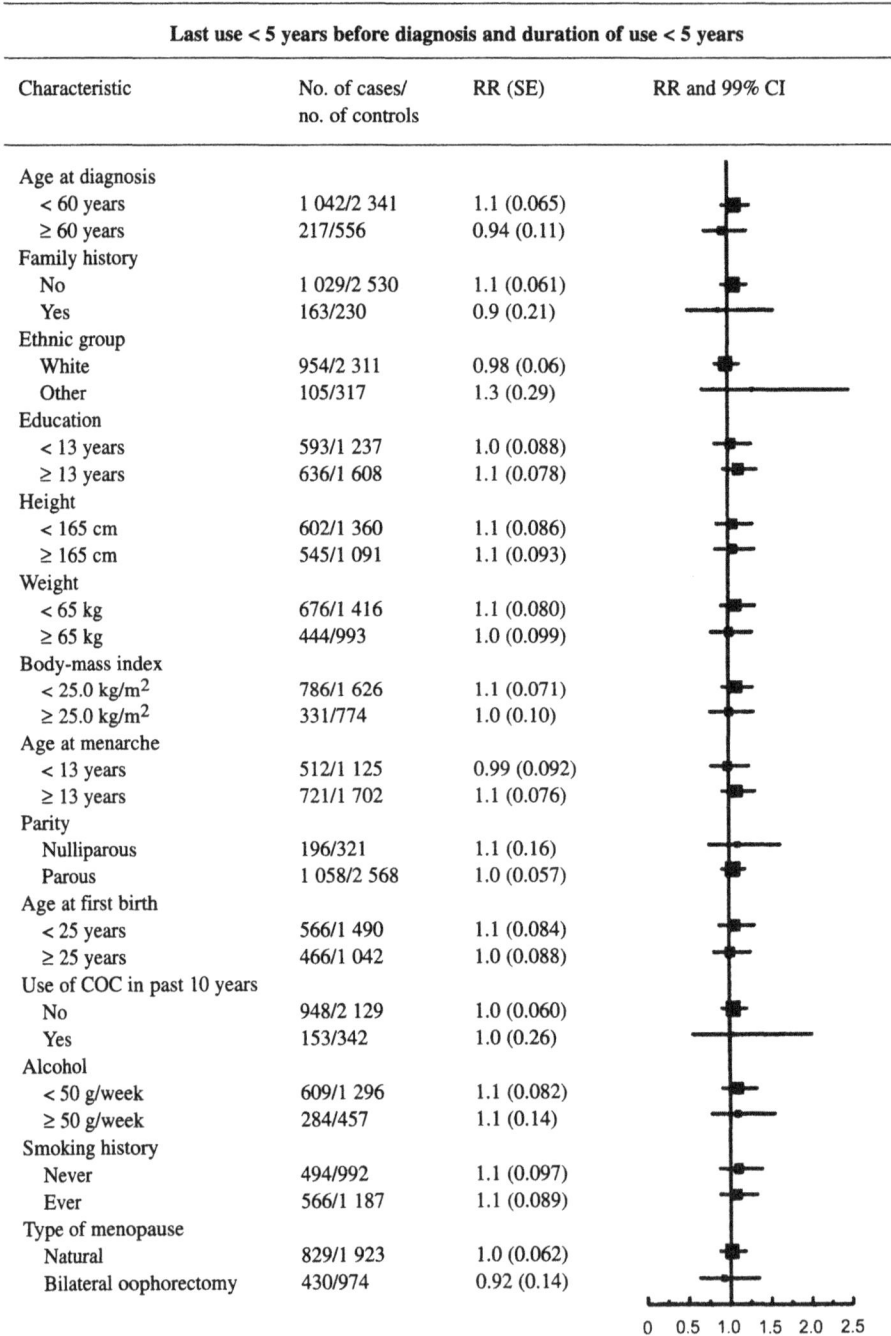

	Last use < 5 years before diagnosis and duration of use < 5 years		
Characteristic	No. of cases/ no. of controls	RR (SE)	RR and 99% CI
Age at diagnosis			
< 60 years	1 042/2 341	1.1 (0.065)	
≥ 60 years	217/556	0.94 (0.11)	
Family history			
No	1 029/2 530	1.1 (0.061)	
Yes	163/230	0.9 (0.21)	
Ethnic group			
White	954/2 311	0.98 (0.06)	
Other	105/317	1.3 (0.29)	
Education			
< 13 years	593/1 237	1.0 (0.088)	
≥ 13 years	636/1 608	1.1 (0.078)	
Height			
< 165 cm	602/1 360	1.1 (0.086)	
≥ 165 cm	545/1 091	1.1 (0.093)	
Weight			
< 65 kg	676/1 416	1.1 (0.080)	
≥ 65 kg	444/993	1.0 (0.099)	
Body-mass index			
< 25.0 kg/m^2	786/1 626	1.1 (0.071)	
≥ 25.0 kg/m^2	331/774	1.0 (0.10)	
Age at menarche			
< 13 years	512/1 125	0.99 (0.092)	
≥ 13 years	721/1 702	1.1 (0.076)	
Parity			
Nulliparous	196/321	1.1 (0.16)	
Parous	1 058/2 568	1.0 (0.057)	
Age at first birth			
< 25 years	566/1 490	1.1 (0.084)	
≥ 25 years	466/1 042	1.0 (0.088)	
Use of COC in past 10 years			
No	948/2 129	1.0 (0.060)	
Yes	153/342	1.0 (0.26)	
Alcohol			
< 50 g/week	609/1 296	1.1 (0.082)	
≥ 50 g/week	284/457	1.1 (0.14)	
Smoking history			
Never	494/992	1.1 (0.097)	
Ever	566/1 187	1.1 (0.089)	
Type of menopause			
Natural	829/1 923	1.0 (0.062)	
Bilateral oophorectomy	430/974	0.92 (0.14)	

0   0.5   1.0   1.5   2.0   2.5

Figure 3 (contd)

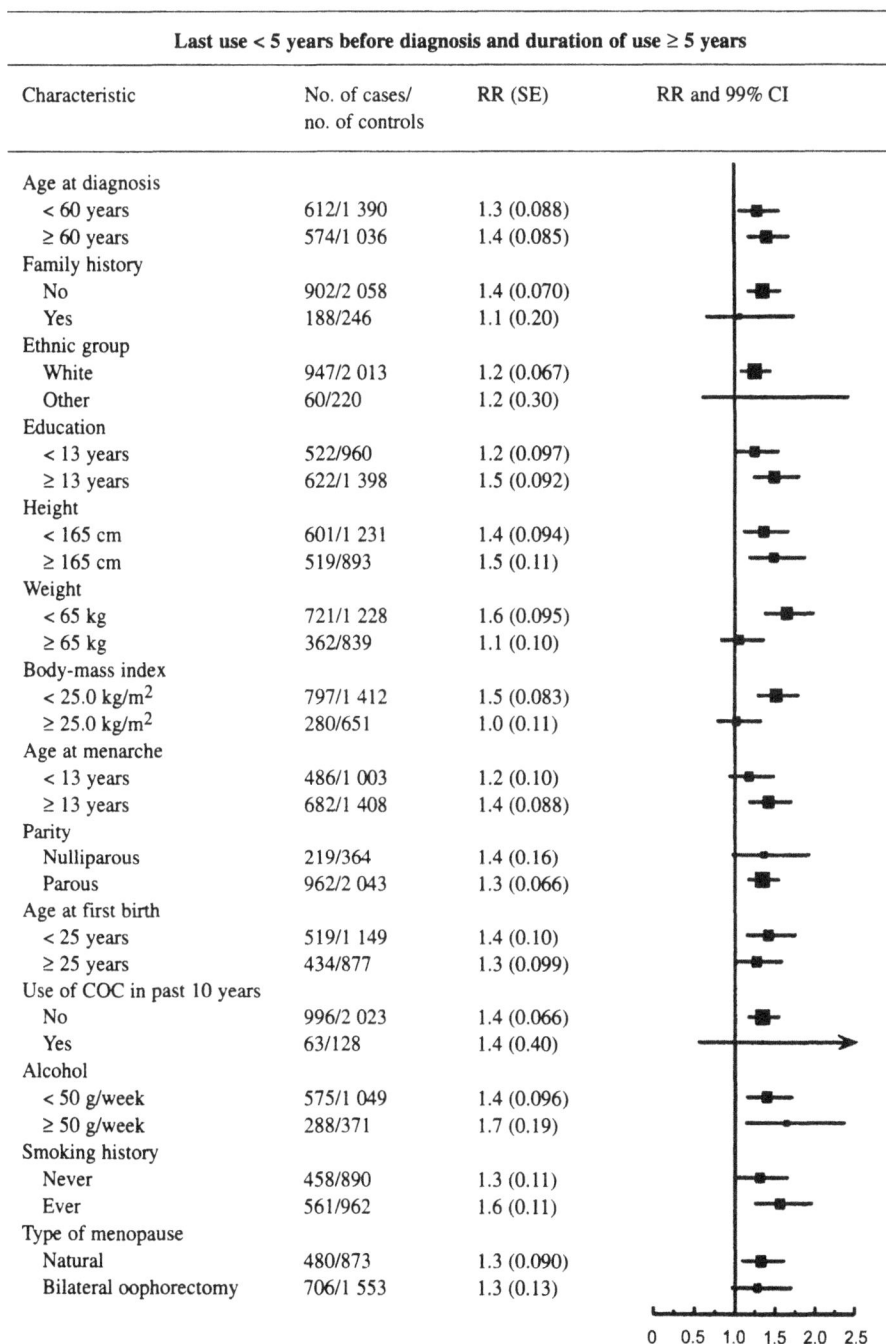

Last use < 5 years before diagnosis and duration of use ≥ 5 years			
Characteristic	No. of cases/ no. of controls	RR (SE)	RR and 99% CI
Age at diagnosis			
< 60 years	612/1 390	1.3 (0.088)	
≥ 60 years	574/1 036	1.4 (0.085)	
Family history			
No	902/2 058	1.4 (0.070)	
Yes	188/246	1.1 (0.20)	
Ethnic group			
White	947/2 013	1.2 (0.067)	
Other	60/220	1.2 (0.30)	
Education			
< 13 years	522/960	1.2 (0.097)	
≥ 13 years	622/1 398	1.5 (0.092)	
Height			
< 165 cm	601/1 231	1.4 (0.094)	
≥ 165 cm	519/893	1.5 (0.11)	
Weight			
< 65 kg	721/1 228	1.6 (0.095)	
≥ 65 kg	362/839	1.1 (0.10)	
Body-mass index			
< 25.0 kg/m^2	797/1 412	1.5 (0.083)	
≥ 25.0 kg/m^2	280/651	1.0 (0.11)	
Age at menarche			
< 13 years	486/1 003	1.2 (0.10)	
≥ 13 years	682/1 408	1.4 (0.088)	
Parity			
Nulliparous	219/364	1.4 (0.16)	
Parous	962/2 043	1.3 (0.066)	
Age at first birth			
< 25 years	519/1 149	1.4 (0.10)	
≥ 25 years	434/877	1.3 (0.099)	
Use of COC in past 10 years			
No	996/2 023	1.4 (0.066)	
Yes	63/128	1.4 (0.40)	
Alcohol			
< 50 g/week	575/1 049	1.4 (0.096)	
≥ 50 g/week	288/371	1.7 (0.19)	
Smoking history			
Never	458/890	1.3 (0.11)	
Ever	561/962	1.6 (0.11)	
Type of menopause			
Natural	480/873	1.3 (0.090)	
Bilateral oophorectomy	706/1 553	1.3 (0.13)	

0   0.5   1.0   1.5   2.0   2.5

Figure 3 (contd)

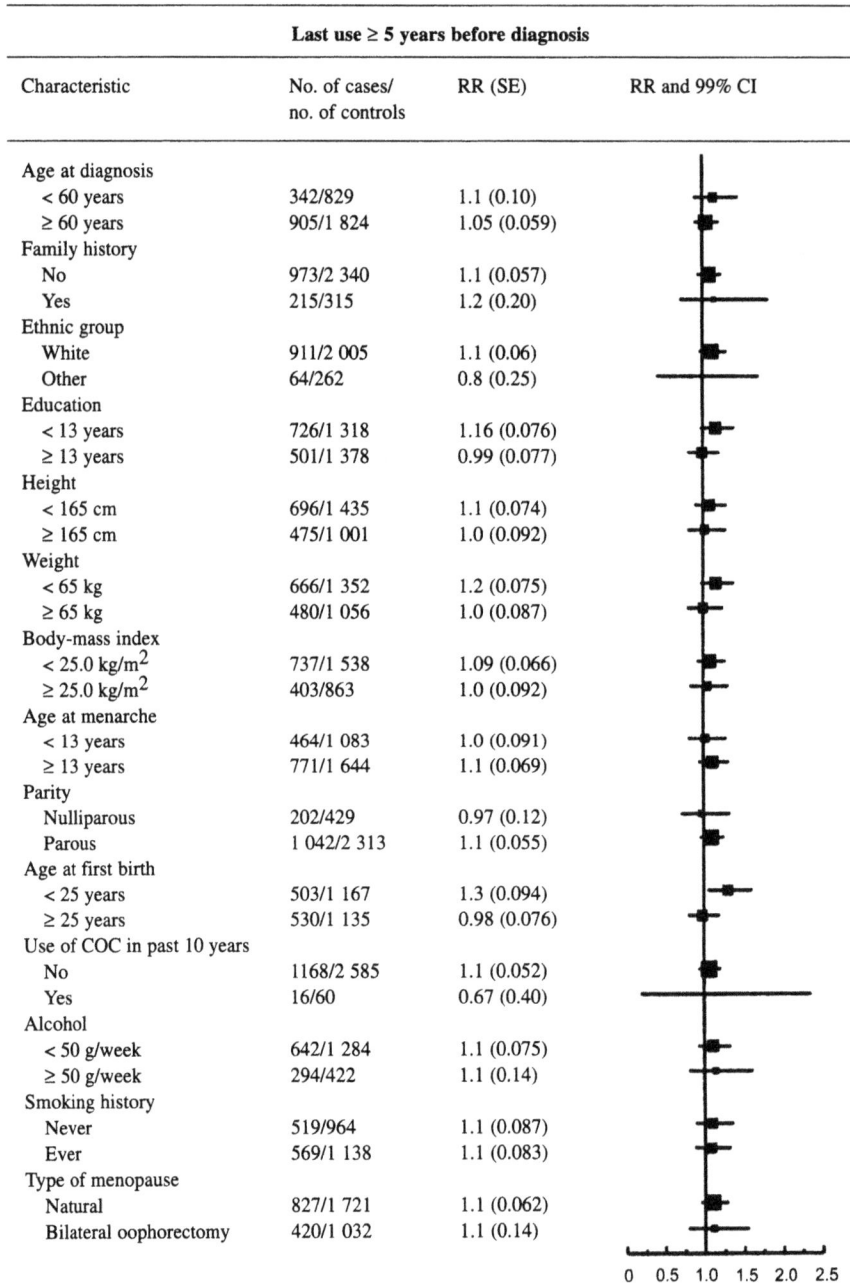

Characteristic	No. of cases/ no. of controls	RR (SE)	RR and 99% CI
Last use ≥ 5 years before diagnosis			
Age at diagnosis			
< 60 years	342/829	1.1 (0.10)	
≥ 60 years	905/1 824	1.05 (0.059)	
Family history			
No	973/2 340	1.1 (0.057)	
Yes	215/315	1.2 (0.20)	
Ethnic group			
White	911/2 005	1.1 (0.06)	
Other	64/262	0.8 (0.25)	
Education			
< 13 years	726/1 318	1.16 (0.076)	
≥ 13 years	501/1 378	0.99 (0.077)	
Height			
< 165 cm	696/1 435	1.1 (0.074)	
≥ 165 cm	475/1 001	1.0 (0.092)	
Weight			
< 65 kg	666/1 352	1.2 (0.075)	
≥ 65 kg	480/1 056	1.0 (0.087)	
Body-mass index			
< 25.0 kg/m^2	737/1 538	1.09 (0.066)	
≥ 25.0 kg/m^2	403/863	1.0 (0.092)	
Age at menarche			
< 13 years	464/1 083	1.0 (0.091)	
≥ 13 years	771/1 644	1.1 (0.069)	
Parity			
Nulliparous	202/429	0.97 (0.12)	
Parous	1 042/2 313	1.1 (0.055)	
Age at first birth			
< 25 years	503/1 167	1.3 (0.094)	
≥ 25 years	530/1 135	0.98 (0.076)	
Use of COC in past 10 years			
No	1168/2 585	1.1 (0.052)	
Yes	16/60	0.67 (0.40)	
Alcohol			
< 50 g/week	642/1 284	1.1 (0.075)	
≥ 50 g/week	294/422	1.1 (0.14)	
Smoking history			
Never	519/964	1.1 (0.087)	
Ever	569/1 138	1.1 (0.083)	
Type of menopause			
Natural	827/1 721	1.1 (0.062)	
Bilateral oophorectomy	420/1 032	1.1 (0.14)	

0   0.5   1.0   1.5   2.0   2.5

Adapted from Collaborative Group on Hormonal Factors in Breast Cancer (1997)

RR, relative risk; CI, confidence interval; SE, standard error

Family history, mother or sister with breast cancer; COC, combined oral contraceptives

[a] Relative to no use, stratified by study, age at diagnosis, time since menopause, body-mass index, parity and age when her first child was born.

Table 4. Summary of cohort studies on post-menopausal oestrogen therapy and breast cancer

Reference	Study base	Design: cohort, follow-up, data	Risk relationships: relative risk (RR) and 95% confidence intervals (95% CI)	Comments
Hoover et al. (1976)	Records of private practice, Kentucky, USA, 1969–72	Retrospective cohort, 1 891 women; follow-up through individual contacts and medical records for 12 years; 22 717 person–years; comparison with external incidence rates	**Incidence:** 49 cases observed Conjugated oestrogens: Any use: **RR**, 1.3 (95% CI, 1.0–1.7) Time since inclusion: increasing trend, ≥ 15 years, **RR**, 2.0 (95% CI, 1.1–3.4) Increasing risk with increasing dose and number of prescriptions Similar risk relationships for age at start and ovarian status	Confounding difficult to assess Proxy variables of dose–response relationship
Buring et al. (1987)	Nurses in 11 US states, 1976–80, 30–55 years	Cohort, 33 335 women; follow-up questionnaires sent after 4 years	**Incidence:** 221 new cases Any use: **RR**, 1.1 (95% CI, 0.8–1.4) Current: **RR**, 1.0 (95% CI, 0.7–1.4) Past: **RR**, 1.3 (95% CI, 0.9–1.8) Duration: < 1 year: **RR**, 1.0 (95% CI, 0.6–1.7) 1–< 3 years: **RR**, 1.0 (95% CI, 0.7–1.6) 3–5 years: **RR**, 1.0 (95% CI, 0.6–1.6) > 5 years: **RR**, 1.3 (95% CI, 0.9–2.1)	Only exposure at baseline Short follow-up
Hunt et al. (1987)	Menopause clinics in UK, 1978–82, counsel for menopausal symptoms	Cohort of 4 544 women who used hormones ≥ 1 year; 17 830 person–years; follow-up through contact letters and medical records; exposure data from baseline interview	**Incidence:** 50 cases. **Mortality:** 12 deaths Various kinds of hormones Any use - incidence: **RR**, 1.6 (95% CI, 1.2–2.1) - mortality: **SMR**, 0.6 (95% CI, 0.3–1.0) Time since first intake: trend for incidence ≥ 10 years: **RR**, 3.1 (95% CI, 1.5–5.6)	Possible selection bias in study of mortality Heterogeneous exposure regimens

Table 4 (contd)

Reference	Study base	Design: cohort, follow-up, data	Risk relationships: relative risk (RR) and 95% confidence intervals (95% CI)	Comments
Bergkvist et al. (1989)	Six counties in Sweden 1977–83, women prescribed hormones	Population-based cohort; 23 244 ≥ 35 years; 133 375 person–years; follow-up through record linkage with national cancer registry; exposure data from prescriptions; questionnaire data in a random sample; cohort, case–cohort and case–control analyses	**Incidence**: 253 cases Hormone regimens prevalent in Sweden: Any use: **RR**, 1.1 (95% CI, 1.0–1.3) Duration of intake: - all compounds; ≥ 9 years: **RR**, 1.7 (95% CI, 1.1–2.7) - oestradiol: trend, ≥ 9 years: **RR**, 1.8 (95% CI, 0.7–4.6) - conjugated oestrogens: no trend, ≥ 6 years: **RR**, 1.3 (95% CI, 0.6–2.9) Regimens, duration ≥ 9 years - oestrogens alone: **RR**, 1.8 (95% CI, 1.0–3.1)	Adjustment for confounders led to higher risk estimates Low power to examine conjugated oestrogens
Mills et al. (1989)	Seventh-day Adventists, California, USA, 1976–82, Caucasians	Cohort of 20 341 women; internal comparisons; 115 619 person-years; individual follow-up through registry linkage; baseline questionnaire in 1976	**Incidence**: 6 years follow-up, 215 cases Conjugated oestrogens: Any use: **RR**, 1.7 (95% CI, 1.2–2.4) - current: **RR**, 2.5 (95% CI, 1.6–4.0) - former: **RR**, 1.4 (95% CI, 1.0–2.2) Duration: - significant trend, after 6–10 years: **RR**, 2.8 (95% CI, 1.7–4.6) Effect modification: - previous COC intake: **RR**, 1.4 (95% CI, 0.7–2.9)	Data on exposure duration incomplete (only baseline)

Table 4 (contd)

Reference	Study base	Design: cohort, follow-up, data	Risk relationships: relative risk (RR) and 95% confidence intervals (95% CI)	Comments
Colditz et al. (1992)	Nurses' Health Cohort, USA, 1976–88, 30–55 years at entry	Cohort, 118 300 nurses at post-menopausal ages; 480 665 person-years; individual follow-up through questionnaires, 95% complete for incidence and 98% for deaths; internal comparisons; baseline questionnaire 1976; up-date questionnaires every 2 years	**Incidence:** 12 years' follow-up, 1015 cases Conjugated oestrogens, combinations with progestogens: - any use: RR, 0.9 (95% CI, 0.8–1.1) - current use: RR, 1.3 (95% CI, 1.1–1.6) - previous use: RR, 0.9 (95% CI, 0.8–1.0) Duration, current intake 5–< 10 years: RR, 1.6 (95% CI, 1.3–2.1) Effect modification: - none with other risk factors - previous COC-intake: RR, 1.5	Mainly relationship with current intake, possibly also duration effect: current use: 2–< 5 years: RR, 1.3 (95% CI, 1.0–1.7) 5–10 years: RR, 1.6 (95% CI, 1.25–2.06) > 10 years: RR, 1.5 (95% CI, 1.1–2.0)
Yuen et al. (1993)	Uppsala health care region, Sweden, 1977–80; women prescribed hormonal therapy	See Bergkvist et al. above. Follow-up through record-linkages with causes of death registry; comparison with external, corrected mortality rates; exposure data from prescriptions	**Mortality**, 12 years' follow-up, 73 deaths Various hormone regimens Any use: SMR, 0.8 (95% CI, 0.6–1.0) Prescribed compounds: - oestradiol and/or conjugated oestrogens: SMR, 0.8 (95% CI, 0.2–1.1) - other oestrogens: SMR, 0.9 (95% CI, 0.5-1.3)	Exposure data only from prescriptions Correction for possible bias due to healthy drug use (population rates corrected for prevalent cases)
Schairer et al. (1994)	Populations in 27 cities in the USA, breast cancer screening programme, 1980–89	Cohort of 49 017 participants; 313 902 person–years; follow-up through interviews and questionnaires; information on exposure and risk factors through questionnaires	**Incidence**, both in-situ and invasive tumours, 1 185 cases Conjugated oestrogens, combinations with progestogens Any use: - oestrogens only: RR, 1.0 (95% CI, 0.9–1.2) In-situ tumours: - oestrogens only: RR, 1.4 (95% CI, 1.0–2.0) Duration: 10–14 years, oestrogens only/ in-situ tumours: RR, 2.1 (95% CI, 1.2–3.7)	Detection bias minimized Risk relationship limited to in-situ tumours Low power to assess long-term duration of oestrogen plus progestogen regimens

Table 4 (contd)

Reference	Study base	Design: cohort, follow-up, data	Risk relationships: relative risk (RR) and 95% confidence intervals (95% CI)	Comments
Risch & Howe (1994)	Inhabitants of Saskatchewan, Canada, 43–49 years, start in 1976	Registry-based cohort, 32 790 women followed-up through linkage to cancer registry; 448 716 person–years; exposure data from prescription roster	**Incidence:** 742 cases Conjugated oestrogens, added progestogens Oestrogens only: increasing RR 7% per year (RR, 1.07; 95% CI, 1.02–1.13)	Limited power to look at long-term treatment
Colditz et al. (1995)	Nurses' Health Cohort (see above)	Cohort of 121 700 nurses; 725 550 person-years; baseline questionnaire in 1976, biannual questionnaires, updates on exposure and outcome (follow-up)	**Incidence:** 16 years' follow-up, 1 935 cases Conjugated oestrogens and added progestogens Current intake: - oestrogens alone: **RR**, 1.3 (95% CI, 1.1–1.5) - 5–9 years' oestrogens: **RR**, 1.5 (95% CI, 1.2–1.7) - oestrogen plus progestogen: **RR**, 1.4 (95% CI, 1.2–1.7) By age at diagnosis/≥ 5 years' current hormones: - 50–54 years: **RR**, 1.5 (95% CI, 0.91–2.3) - 55–59 years: **RR**, 1.5 (95% CI, 1.2–2.0) - 60–64 years: **RR**, 1.7 (95% CI, 1.3–2.2) **Mortality:** 359 deaths: Current use, ≥ 5 years: **RR**, 1.4 (95% CI, 1.0–2.1)	No relationship with past use Detection bias unlikely as explanation First study to show an increased risk of death with post-menopausal oestrogen therapy
Schuurman et al. (1995)	The Netherlands, random selection from 204 municipal population registries, age 55–69 years	62 573 women responding to mailed questionnaire; record linkage follow-up; case-cohort approach (subcohort, 1 812 women)	**Incidence:** 3.3 years' follow-up, 471 cases 'Replacement hormones': Any use: **RR**, 1.0 (95% CI, 0.7–1.4) Duration: no trend Any use of COC and post-menopausal oestrogen therapy: **RR**, 1.0 (95% CI, 0.51–1.9)	Low power in duration categories No data on compounds or regimens Short latency

Table 4 (contd)

Reference	Study base	Design: cohort, follow-up, data	Risk relationships: relative risk (RR) and 95% confidence intervals (95% CI)	Comments
Folsom *et al.* (1995)	Iowa 'Women's Health Study', USA, 55–69 years, 1986–92	41 070 post-menopausal women; 129 149 person-years; record linkage for incident cases	**Incidence**, 6 years' follow-up: 468 cases 'Replacement hormones': Former use: **RR**, 0.96 (95% CI, 0.81–1.1) Current use: **RR**, 1.2 (95% CI, 0.99–1.6) ≤ 5 years: **RR**, 1.4 (95% CI, 1.0–2.1) > 5 years: **RR**, 1.2 (95% CI, 0.92–1.6)	General cancer mortality: **RR**, 1.1 (95% CI, 0.81–1.5) Insufficient power for cause-specific mortality No data on duration of compounds or regimens
Willis *et al.* (1996)	Women volunteers in 50 states in the USA, 1982–91	422 373 post-menopausal women; follow-up through record linkage for cause-specific deaths; data in baseline questionnaires; fatal breast cancers	**Mortality**, 9 years' follow-up: 1469 breast cancer deaths Oestrogens: Any use: **RR**, 0.84 (95% CI, 0.75–0.94) Recent use: **RR**, 0.90 (95% CI, 0.75–1.1) Duration: ≥ 11 years: **RR**, 0.93 (95% CI, 0.75–1.2) (no trend)	Exposure data only at baseline No specific data on exposure Mortality only
Persson *et al.* (1996)	See Yuen *et al.* above	22 597 women with registered hormone prescriptions; record linkage follow-up of incidence and mortality; risk factors from questionnaire survey	**Incidence**, 13 years' follow-up, 634 cases Prescriptions for various regimens Any post-menopausal oestrogen therapy: **RR**, 1.0 (95% CI, 0.9–1.1) Oestradiol or conjugated oestrogens: **RR**, 0.9 (95% CI, 0.8–1.1) **Mortality**: 102 deaths Any post-menopausal oestrogen therapy: **RR**, 0.5 (95% CI, 0.4–0.6)	No direct adjustment for covariates 'Healthy drug user' bias in mortality analyses

Table 4 (contd)

Reference	Study base	Design: cohort, follow-up, data	Risk relationships: relative risk (RR) and 95% confidence intervals (95% CI)	Comments
Persson *et al.* (1997b)	Participants in mammography screening, Uppsala, Sweden, 1990–95, 46–74 years	Cohort of 30 982 women participating in two screening rounds; follow-up through screening and in diagnostic registry of pathology department; questionnaires at visits; nested case–control approach	Five-year follow-up: 435 cases (87% invasive), 1 740 controls. Any post-menopausal oestrogen therapy: odds ratio, 1.1 (95% CI, 0.8–1.4). Duration ≥ 11 years: odds ratio, 2.1 (95% CI, 1.1–4.0). Oestradiol or conjugated oestrogen ≥ 11 years: odds ratio, 1.3 (95% CI, 0.5–3.7)	Duration of intake significantly associated. Low power in regimen subgroups

SMR, standardized mortality ratio; COC, combined oral contraceptives

Table 5. Summary of case–control studies of post-menopausal oestrogen therapy and breast cancer

Reference	Study base	Design: number of cases and controls, data	Risk relationships: relative risk (RR) and 95% confidence intervals (95% CI)	Comments
Ross et al. (1980)	Los Angeles, USA, retirement community, 1971–77, Caucasians, age 50–74	Population-based; 131 cases, 262 controls; data from interviews, pharmacy and medical records	Conjugated oestrogens: Any use: RR, 1.1 (95% CI, 0.8–1.9) Cumulative dose > 1 500 mg: RR, 1.9 (95% CI, 1.0–3.3) Ovaries retained: RR, 2.5 (95% CI, 1.2–5.6)	Dose and duration could not be separated
Hoover et al. (1981)	Portland, USA, members of insurance programme (prepaid health plan), 1969–75	Population-based; 345 cases, 611 controls; data from medical records, e.g. number of prescriptions	Conjugated oestrogens: Any use: RR, 1.4 (95% CI, 1.0–2.0) ovaries retained: RR, 1.3 ovaries removed: RR, 1.5 No. of prescriptions: trend, highest RR, 1.8 Dose: trend, highest RR, 1.8 Duration: trend, highest RR, 1.7 Effect modification: higher risk if family history	Only medical record data Adjustment only for type of menopause
Brinton et al. (1981)	Multicentre screening programme, 29 centres in the USA, age 35–74 years	Population-based; 881 cases, 863 controls; interviews	Conjugated oestrogens: Any use: RR, 1.2 (95% CI, 1.0–1.5) Oophorectomy: Any use: RR, 1.5 (95% CI, 0.9–2.8) ≥ 10 years: RR, 1.7 (NS)	Higher risks with higher-dose compounds Possible interaction with nulliparity, family history and benign breast disease
Hulka et al. (1982)	North Carolina, USA, city hospitals, 1977–78, post-menopausal women	Population- and hospital-based; 199 cases, 451 and 852 controls; data from interviews	Oestrogens: Any use: RR, 1.2 (NS) - natural menopause: RR, 1.8 (95% CI, 1.2–2.7) - surgical menopause: RR, 1.3 (NS) No relationship to duration or timing of exposure	Two control groups Speculations on higher risk with injectable oestrogens

Table 5 (contd)

Reference	Study base	Design: number of cases and controls, data	Risk relationships: relative risk (RR) and 95% confidence intervals (95% CI)	Comments
Hiatt et al. (1984)	Kaiser Foundation Health Plan, oophorecto-mized women, 1971–79	Population-based; 119 cases, 119 controls (matched); medical records	Oestrogens: Any use: RR, 0.7 (95% CI, 0.3–1.6) ≥ 5 notations: RR, 2.1 (95 % CI, 1.2–3.6) (significant trend)	No effect modification No trend with years of use
Kaufman et al. (1984)	Large cities, USA and Canada, 1976–81, < 70 years	Hospital-based; 1 610 cases, 1 606 controls; data from interviews	Conjugated oestrogens: Any use: RR, 1.0 (95% CI, 0.8–1.2) Duration: ≥ 10 years: RR, 1.3 (0.6–2.8) (no trend) Subgroup analysis: no risk relationships	Discussion on selection bias due to hospital controls
La Vecchia et al. (1986)	Northern Italy, 1983–85, age 26–74	Hospital-based; 1 108 cases, 1 281 controls; data from interviews	Non-contraceptive oestrogens: Any use: RR, 1.8 (95% CI, 1.3–2.7) Duration - ≤ 2 years: RR, 1.7 (95% CI, 1.1–2.6) - > 2 years : RR, 2.0 (95% CI, 1.0–4.1) Recency, latency: no relationship	Low prevalence of exposure in population
Brinton et al. (1986)	Nationwide screening programme, USA, 1977–80, Caucasians, post-menopausal; extension of study reported by Brinton et al. (1981), see above	Population-based; 1 960 cases, 2 258 controls (random); interviews	Conjugated oestrogens: Any use: RR, 1.0 (95% CI, 0.9–1.2) Duration: significant trend of increase; ≥ 20 years: RR, 1.5 (95% CI, 0.9–2.3) By menopause types: similar relationships Effect modification: benign breast disease, RR, 3.0 (95% CI, 1.6–5.5) for hormone use of ≥ 10 years Tumour stage: highest risk for in-situ and small tumours	Large study Diagnostic bias unlikely

Table 5 (contd)

Reference	Study base	Design: number of cases and controls, data	Risk relationships: relative risk (RR) and 95% confidence intervals (95% CI)	Comments
Nomura et al. (1986)	Patients in Hawaiian hospitals, 1975–80, age 45–74	Hospital and neighbourhood controls; 183/183 Japanese; 161/161 Caucasians	Oestrogen use: Caucasians/Japanese analysed separately: Any use: - Caucasians: RR, 0.9 (95% CI, 0.5–1.3) - Japanese, RR, 1.1 (95% CI, 0.7–1.6) Duration: no trend	Low response rates among cases Low power in subgroup analyses
Wingo et al. (1987)	Large cities, USA, 1980–82, age 25–54	Population-based; 1 369 cases, 1 645 controls; random-digit dialling; interviews	Conjugated oestrogens: Any use: RR, 1.0 (95% CI, 0.9–1.2) - natural menopause: RR, 0.8 (95% CI, 0.6–1.1) - 'surgical menopause': RR, 1.3 (95% CI, 0.9–1.9) Duration, latency, recency: no pattern	Limited to early post-menopausal women Low power for long-term treatment
Rohan & McMichael (1988)	Adelaide, Australia, 1982–84, post-menopausal women, < 74 years	281 cases, 288 controls; interviews	Exogenous oestrogens: Any use: RR, 1.0 (95% CI, 0.6–1.7) Duration, latency, recency: no pattern	Small numbers in duration categories
Ewertz (1988)	Denmark, nationwide, 1983–84, > 70 years	Population-based; 1 486 cases, 1 336 controls (random); self-administered, mailed questionnaire	Oestradiol and oestradiol-progestogen combinations: Any use: RR 1.0–1.3 (NS) depending on menopause status Duration: trend with increasing years of intake: RR, 0.9–2.3 after 3–13 years (p > 0.002)	Chiefly exposure to oestradiol compounds

Table 5 (contd)

Reference	Study base	Design: number of cases and controls, data	Risk relationships: relative risk (RR) and 95% confidence intervals (95% CI)	Comments
Kaufman et al. (1991)	Large cities, east coast, USA, 1980–86, post-menopausal women, 40–69 years	Hospital-based; 1 686 cases, 2 077 controls; interviews	Mostly conjugated oestrogens: Any use: RR, 1.2 (95% CI, 1.0–1.6) Duration: > 15 years RR, 0.9 (95% CI, 0.4–2.1) - conjugated oestrogens, current intake: RR, 1.2 (95% CI, 0.8–1.8) Dose: no pattern	Low power for long-term treatment
Palmer et al. (1991)	Toronto, Canada, one cancer hospital, 1982–86, < 70 years	Population-based: 607 cases, 1 214 controls; interviews	Conjugated oestrogens: Any use: RR, 0.9 (95% CI, 0.6–1.2) Duration ≥ 15 years: RR, 1.5 (95% CI, 0.6–3.8) (no significant trend) Current use and ≥ 5 years use: RR, 0.9 (95% CI, 0.4–1.9)	Low power in long duration categories Response rate of controls, 65%
Yang et al. (1992)	British Columbia, Canada, 1988–89, post-menopausal women < 75 years	Population-based: 699 cases, 685 controls; mailed questionnaire	Mainly conjugated oestrogens: Any use: RR, 1.0 (95% CI, 0.8–1.3) Current intake: RR, 1.4 (95% CI, 1.0–2.0) Duration ≥ 10 years: RR, 1.6 (95% CI, 1.1–2.5) Effect modification: highest risk after oophorectomy: RR, 1.9 (95% CI, 0.8–5.3)	Low response rate
Harris et al. (1992a)	New York city area, USA, 1987–89	Hospital-based; 604 cases, 520 controls; interviews in hospitals	'Use of oestrogens': lean, post-menopausal women: odds ratio, 2.0 (95% CI, 1.1–3.5) (body mass index, < 22) - < 5 years: odds ratio, 2.0 (95% CI, 1.0–3.8) - ≥ 5 years: odds ratio, 2.2 (95% CI, 0.8–5.6)	Risk increase with high body mass index and weight gain Few subjects with long duration of hormone therapy

Table 5 (contd)

Reference	Study base	Design: number of cases and controls, data	Risk relationships: relative risk (RR) and 95% confidence intervals (95% CI)	Comments
Weinstein et al. (1993)	Long Island, New York, USA, 1984–86	Population-based; 1 436 cases, 1 419 controls; telephone interviews	'Use of oestrogens': Any use: RR = 1.1 (0.86–1.4) No trend with duration. Current use: RR = 1.3 (0.76–2.3) Former use: no trend	Interaction with body mass index
La Vecchia et al. (1995)	Six areas in northern Italy, 1991–94, ≤ 74 years	Hospital-based; 2 569 cases, 2 588 controls; structured questionnaire at interview	'Conjugated and other oestrogens': Trend with duration: odds ratios, 1.0, 1.3 and 1.5 for < 1 year, 1–4 and > 5 years of intake (NS) Recency < 10 years: odds ratio, 2.0 (95% CI, 1.3–2.9)	Low power in long-duration categories
Stanford et al. (1995)	13 counties, Washington State, USA, 1998–90, cancer survey system, Caucasian, 50–64 years	Population-based; 537 cases, 492 controls (random-digit dialling); personal interviews	Any use: Oestrogen alone: RR, 0.9 (95% CI, 0.6–1.1) Oestrogen with progestogen: RR, 0.9 (95% CI, 0.7–1.3) Duration, recency: no association	Response rate 81% for cases and 73% for controls Low power for long-term use
Newcomb et al. (1995)	Four states in northern and eastern USA, tumour registries, 1988–91, age 65–74	Population-based; 3 130 cases, 3 698 controls; personal interviews	'Non-contraceptive hormones, oestrogens and progestogen combinations': Any use: RR, 1.1 (95% CI, 0.9–1.2) Duration: > 15 years: RR, 1.1 (95% CI, 0.9–1.4)	Response rates 81% for cases and 84% for controls Reasonable power for long-duration categories No effects in subgroups

Table 5 (contd)

Reference	Study base	Design: number of cases and controls, data	Risk relationships: relative risk (RR) and 95% confidence intervals (95% CI)	Comments
Levi *et al.* (1996)	Vaud, Switzerland, 1990–95, < 75 years	Hospital-based; 230 cases, 507 controls; interviews in hospitals	'Hormonal therapy': Any use: odds ratio, 1.2 (95% CI, 0.8–1.8) Recency < 10 years: odds ratio, 1.7 (95% CI, 1.1–2.9) Duration ≥ 10 years: odds ratio, 1.0 (95% CI, 0.4–2.4)	No information on participation rates Power limitations
Tavani *et al.* (1997)	Greater Milan area 1983–91, six areas in northern Italy, 1991–94, age 15–74	Two hospital-based studies; 5 984 cases, 5 504 controls; interviews	'Hormonal therapy': Any use: odds ratio, 1.2 (95% CI, 1.0–1.4) Duration > 5 years: odds ratio, 1.3 (95% CI, 0.8–2.0) Significant trend with duration Any use, age at diagnosis: trend of increasing risk with increasing age	Pooled data Low prevalence of any use of hormones Low power for long-duration categories
Lipworth *et al.* (1995)	Residents of greater Athens area, Greece, 4 major hospitals, 1989–91, all ages	Hospital-based; 820 cases, 795 orthopaedic patients; 753 healthy visitors; data from interviews in hospital	'Menopausal oestrogens': Any use: RR, 1.5 (95% CI, 1.2–2.3) Duration: - ≤ 11 months: RR, 1.8 (95% CI, 1.0–3.0) - 12–35 months: RR, 1.3 (95% CI, 0.6–2.5) - ≥ 36 months: RR, 1.4 (95% CI, 0.6–3.3) (no trend)	No information on details of exposure, oestrogen–progestogen use rare Low prevalence of hormone use

NS, not significant

The pooled analysis of individual data showed a relationship of increasing risk with increasing duration only for women with current use or use ended within the previous four years. There was no significant variation in results across the individual studies (Collaborative Group on Hormonal Factors in Breast Cancer, 1997).

(c) Recency of intake

Several of the studies suggest that recency of exposure is the most important determinant of risk (Mills *et al.*, 1989; Colditz *et al.*, 1992, 1995; Folsom *et al.*, 1995; La Vecchia *et al.*, 1995; Levi *et al.*, 1996). The investigators in the Nurses' Health Study in particular reported that their finding of a 50% increase in risk is best explained in this way (Colditz *et al.*, 1995); however, numerous other studies found no relationship between excess risk and current or recent intake (Hulka *et al.* 1982; Kaufman *et al.*, 1984; Wingo *et al.*, 1987; Ewertz, 1988; Rohan & McMichael, 1988; Kaufman *et al.*, 1991; Palmer *et al.*, 1991; Stanford *et al.*, 1995). Several of the studies did not include an analysis by recency of intake. The main results of the pooled analysis of individual data was an excess risk related to current use or use terminated within five years

(d) Latency of intake

Most studies showed no independent association with the number of years since first use (Hulka *et al.*, 1982; Hiatt *et al.*, 1984; Kaufman *et al.*, 1984; Nomura *et al.*, 1986; Wingo *et al.*, 1987; Rohan & McMichael, 1988; Palmer *et al.*, 1991; La Vecchia *et al.*, 1995; Stanford *et al.*, 1995; Brinton, 1997).

(e) Compound, dose and route of administration

Studies in the United States reflect use almost exclusively of conjugated oestrogens, while studies in Europe give results of exposure mainly to the other oestrogens, such as oestradiol valerate, oestradiol and, to a minor extent, the synthetic oestrogen ethinyl-oestradiol. In the European studies (Hunt *et al.*, 1987; Ewertz, 1988; Bergkvist *et al.*, 1989; La Vecchia *et al.*, 1995), the infrequent use of conjugated oestrogens provided insufficient power for comparative analyses. Oestradiol compounds and conjugated oestrogens seem to have similar oestrogenic effects on the target organs, e.g. with regard to endometrial cancer (Persson *et al.*, 1989; Beresford *et al.*, 1997) and breast cancer in studies in Europe and the United States (Bergkvist *et al.*, 1989; Colditz *et al.*, 1995). Neither the pooled analysis of individual data nor studies in the United States (Hulka *et al.*, 1982; Hiatt *et al.*, 1984; Kaufman *et al.*, 1984; Brinton *et al.*, 1986; Wingo *et al.*, 1987; Stanford *et al.*, 1995) showed a difference in risk with dose of conjugated oestrogens (i.e. 0.625 versus 1.25 mg).

Data on risk by type of administration are scarce. No pattern of risk has been related to cyclic versus continuous intake of oestrogens (Hulka *et al.*, 1982; Brinton *et al.*, 1986). Vaginal application of oestrogen was not related to the risk for breast cancer (Colditz *et al.*, 1992), whereas parenteral administration was linked to an increased risk in one study (Hulka *et al.*, 1982).

(f)   *Susceptibility factors*

In epidemiological research, interest has focused on whether certain sub-groups of women are more likely to develop breast cancer after post-menopausal hormonal therapy. Such analyses are often hampered by lack of power. In the pooled analysis of individual data, the only significant effect modifier was body mass index: the adverse effect of hormone treatment was greater for women with a body mass index < 25 kg/m². Other types of factor addressed in individual studies are described below.

(i)   *Type of menopause*

Since oophorectomy and time of natural menopause are powerful determinants of breast cancer, menopausal status has been examined as a modifier of the risk associated with hormonal therapy. The association in oophorectomized women has been found to be strong in some studies (Hoover *et al.*, 1981; Wingo *et al.*, 1987; Yang *et al.*, 1992; Stanford *et al.*, 1995), whereas in other studies, higher risks have been noted for women who had a natural menopause and have intact ovaries (Ross *et al.*, 1980; Hulka *et al.*, 1982; Ewertz, 1988); some studies found no difference in effect with ovarian status (Kaufman *et al.*, 1991; Palmer *et al.*, 1991; Newcomb *et al.*, 1995).

(ii)   *Age at diagnosis*

In the Nurses' Health Study, the increased risk with current intake became progressively more pronounced with increasing age at diagnosis (Colditz *et al.*, 1995). An effect of age at diagnosis has also been suggested in some case–control studies (Brinton *et al.*, 1981; Wingo *et al.*, 1987; Kaufman *et al.*, 1991; Palmer *et al.*, 1991; La Vecchia *et al.*, 1992a). One difficulty in interpreting the data is that the effect of age could be mixed with duration of intake.

(iii)   *Body build*

The relative contribution of treatment to post-menopausal oestrogen concentrations is likely to be greater in lean than obese women, since endogenous oestrogen production is enhanced by the amount of fat tissue (Siiteri, 1987). The findings of some epidemiological studies corroborate this hypothesis by showing stronger or unique associations in lean women (Kaufman *et al.*, 1991; Palmer *et al.*, 1991; Colditz *et al.*, 1992; Harris *et al.*, 1992a; Newcomb *et al.*, 1995; Collaborative Group on Hormonal Factors in Breast Cancer, 1997); conversely, in other studies, the effect was more marked in obese women (Mills *et al.*, 1989; La Vecchia *et al.*, 1992a).

(iv)   *Previous use of combined oral contraceptives*

Current and recent use of combined oral contraceptives has been linked to an increased risk for breast cancer (see the monograph on 'Oral contraceptives, combined'). Few studies have yet been able to address whether the risk associated with hormonal therapy is modified by previous use of combined oral contraceptives, especially for women who have taken high-dose pills. There is no evidence of such an interaction;

however, few data are available (Mills *et al.*, 1989; Colditz *et al.*, 1992; Schuurman *et al.*, 1995; Stanford *et al.*, 1995; Collaborative Group on Hormonal Factors in Breast Cancer, 1997). Since cohorts of women who were commonly exposed to combined oral contraceptives are increasingly being treated with hormonal therapy, the possibility of a combined effect becomes an important issue.

(v) *Hereditary breast cancer*

Inherited breast cancer has been studied through the proxy variable of family history, i.e. according to closeness of relationship and age at onset. Further, the share of cancers caused by dominant inheritance is lower for post-menopausal women than for women with breast cancer before the menopause. These circumstances may explain why the findings on the joint effect of family history and hormone use are inconsistent: about as many studies show an increased risk (Hoover *et al.*, 1981; Hulka *et al.*, 1982; Nomura *et al.*, 1986; Wingo *et al.*, 1987; Kaufman *et al.*, 1991; Newcomb *et al.*, 1995) as show an absence of an effect modification (Kaufman *et al.*, 1984; Brinton *et al.*, 1986; Rohan & McMichael, 1988; Mills *et al.*, 1989; Palmer *et al.*, 1991; Yang *et al.*, 1992; Stanford *et al.*, 1995).

(vi) *Benign breast disease*

Women with a history of so-called benign breast disease may have a higher risk of developing breast cancer after post-menopausal hormonal therapy (Ross *et al.*, 1980; Brinton *et al.*, 1986; Nomura *et al.*, 1986; Mills *et al.*, 1989), but numerous other studies do not support the association (Hoover *et al.*, 1981; Hulka *et al.*, 1982; Kaufman *et al.*, 1984; Wingo *et al.*, 1987; Rohan & McMichael, 1988; Kaufman *et al.*, 1991; Palmer *et al.*, 1991; Yang *et al.*, 1992; La Vecchia *et al.*, 1995; Newcomb *et al.*, 1995; Stanford *et al.*, 1995). Many uncertainties hamper the interpretation of the data, e.g. whether a risk-increasing effect applies to specific types of benign lesions (hyperplasia or atypia) or whether it is use of post-menopausal hormonal therapy before or after diagnosis that is important.

(vii) *Alcohol, reproductive factors*

A few studies have shown an increased risk in association with heavy alcohol consumption (Colditz *et al.*, 1992; Gapstur *et al.*, 1992). Studies of the combined effects of hormonal therapy and age at menarche, age at first birth, parity and age at menopause have generally yielded null results (Kaufman *et al.*, 1984; Nomura *et al.*, 1986; Palmer *et al.*, 1991; Yang *et al.*, 1992; Stanford *et al.*, 1995), whereas a few others found stronger associations among users who were older at the time of the birth of their first child (Colditz *et al.*, 1992), with multiparity (La Vecchia *et al.*, 1992a) and with late menopause (Wingo *et al.*, 1987; Ewertz, 1988; Mills *et al.*, 1989).

(g) *Tumour characteristics*

More intense surveillance of users of hormonal therapy may lead to earlier detection and bias with regard to latency. There is evidence of an increased risk for breast cancer after hormone treatment in two studies performed in a population of women participating in a breast cancer screening programme in the United States, in which the impact of detection bias should be low. Thus, in a case–control study (Brinton et al., 1986), the positive duration-dependent relationship was significant and strongest for in-situ or small (≤ 1 cm) tumours. In a subsequent follow-up study (Schairer et al., 1994), a doubling of the relative risk with oestrogen use for more than 10 years was limited to in-situ tumours. Further, in a Swedish record-linkage study, the odds ratio of having a small tumour (≤ 2 cm) and spread to axillary lymph nodes was lower for women prescribed oestrogens (in combination with progestogens), even when adjustment was made for mode of detection (mammography screening or examinations because of symptoms) (Magnusson et al., 1996).

In the pooled analysis of individual data, the adverse effect of hormone use was stronger for women with cancers localized to the breast than for those with cancers that had spread beyond the breast (Collaborative Group on Hormonal Factors in Breast Cancer, 1997).

(h)   Survival and mortality

Mortality rates due to breast cancer were analysed during a 12-year follow-up, after correction for the comparative external mortality rates for prevalent breast disease (Yuen et al., 1993). The standardized mortality ratio estimates were still slightly below baseline (0.8). A reduction in the rate of mortality from breast cancer among women using hormone treatment as compared with those who were not has been found in other cohort studies (Petitti et al., 1987; Hunt et al., 1990; Henderson et al., 1991; Willis et al., 1996). In the Nurses' Health Study, the relative risks for death from breast cancer were 0.76 (95% CI, 0.56–1.02) for current use and 0.83 (95% CI, 0.63–1.1) for past use, but rose to 1.4 (95% CI, 0.82–2.5) for current use for 10 or more years (Grodstein et al., 1997). These data should be interpreted cautiously.

In summary, the preponderance of evidence suggests an increase in risk for breast cancer with increasing duration of use of post-menopausal oestrogen therapy for current and recent users.

2.2   Endometrial cancer

2.2.1   Descriptive studies

In the United States, use of oestrogens at menopause increased during the 1960s. With increasing evidence of an association between post-menopausal oestrogen therapy and endometrial cancer, the United States Food and Drug Administration issued a warning to physicians in 1976. A decline in post-menopausal oestrogen therapy use ensued and was later followed by an increase in the use of post-menopausal oestrogen–progestogen therapy (Austin & Roe, 1982; Standeven et al., 1986; Gruber & Luciani, 1986; Ross et al., 1988). The incidence of uterine corpus cancer (as a proxy for endometrial cancer) began to rise in the 1960s, reached a peak in the mid-1970s and then declined until the 1990s (Persky et al., 1990). The increased incidence was found primarily among post-menopausal women and followed and then paralleled the increase in the use of post-menopausal oestrogen therapy.

2.2.2 Cohort studies

The impact of post-menopausal oestrogen therapy on the occurrence of endometrial cancer has been investigated in eight cohort studies (Table 6). Six of the studies (Hammond *et al.*, 1979; Gambrell *et al.*, 1980; Vakil *et al.*, 1983; Lafferty & Helmuth, 1985; Hunt *et al.*, 1987; Ettinger *et al.*, 1988) showed an elevated risk associated with any use of post-menopausal oestrogen therapy, without specifying the risk by duration or dose, while two others (Paganini-Hill *et al.*, 1989; Persson *et al.*, 1989) also provided risk estimates related to the duration of use. Women who had ever used post-menopausal oestrogen therapy were more likely to develop endometrial cancer than non-users in all these studies (relative risk, 1.3–10). In three cohort studies (Hammond *et al.*, 1979; Hunt *et al.*, 1987; Persson *et al,*. 1989), the increased risk was significant; in two reports (Paganini-Hill *et al.*, 1989; Persson *et al.*, 1989) described in detail below, the risk estimates for duration of use were given.

In the study of Paganini-Hill *et al.* (1989), the risk for endometrial cancer increased from 5.2 [95% CI not provided] for ≤ 2 years of use to 20 for ≥ 15 years of use (95% CI, 7.2–54; p for trend, < 0.0001). A sustained increase in risk was noted after the cessation of therapy. Women who had stopped post-menopausal oestrogen therapy 15 or more years previously still had a nearly sixfold increase in risk (5.8; 95% CI, 2.0–17) relative to women who had never used them. In an analysis of oestrogen dose in this study, the risk for women using higher doses (≥ 1.25 mg; relative risk, 11.0 [95% CI not provided]) did not differ from that of women using lower doses (≤ 0.625 mg; relative risk, 15.0 [95% CI not provided]).

In the case–cohort study of Persson *et al.* (1989), the risk increased with increasing duration of use, from 1.1 (95% CI, 0.5–2.5) among users for six months or fewer to 1.8 (95% CI, 1.1–3.2) among women who had used post-menopausal oestrogen therapy for 73 months or more. Use of either conjugated oestrogen or oestradiol was associated with an increase in risk, with a relative risk of 1.7 (95% CI, 1.1–2.7) for conjugated oestrogen and 2.1 (95% CI, 1.4–3.0) for oestradiol.

2.2.3 Case–control studies

Over 30 studies have been conducted to investigate the association between post-menopausal oestrogen therapy and endometrial cancer (Table 7); all except one (Salmi, 1980) reported an elevated risk for women with any use of post-menopausal oestrogen therapy relative to those who had never used it (relative risks, 1.3–12.0), and in 22 studies the excess was statistically significant. Both qualitative reviews (Herrinton & Weiss, 1993) and a meta-analysis of the published results (Grady *et al.*, 1995) have found an overall excess, with increasing risk with increasing duration of use.

The risk for endometrial cancer has been evaluated in relation to the duration of use, the time since last use (recency), oestrogenic potency (dose), type (conjugated, synthetic) and regimen (continuous versus cyclic with breaks) of therapy.

Over 20 studies that provide information on the duration of post-menopausal oestrogen therapy showed that duration is one of the strongest determinants of risk; the risk continues to increase with continuing duration of use (Ziel & Finkle, 1975; Mack *et al.*,

Table 6. Cohort studies on use of unopposed post-menopausal oestrogen therapy and risk for endometrial cancer

Reference, country	Age at beginning of follow-up (years)	Study group of source population	Comparison group	Approximate duration of follow-up (years)	No. of observed cases	No. of expected cases or person–years	Relative risk or SIR	95% CI
Hammond et al. (1979), USA	NR	301 women attending hospital clinic, use of OT ≥ 5 years	Rates from Third National Cancer Survey	NR	11	1.18	9.3	4.7–17
Gambrell et al. (1980), USA	NR	Women attending medical centre, any use of OT	Women attending medical centre, no use of OT	≤ 11	NR	NR	[1.6]	NR
Vakil et al. (1983), Canada	32–62	1 483 women attending gynaecology clinics	Rates from Ontario	≤ 17	8	6.2	1.3	NR, NS
Lafferty & Helmuth (1985), USA	45–60	61 women attending a private clinic, use of OT ≥ 3 years	63 women attending a private clinic, no OT use	3–16	NR	NR	[2.7]	NR
Hunt et al. (1987), UK	NR	4 544 women attending 21 menopause clinics	Rates from Birmingham Cancer Registry	5	12	4.2	2.8	1.5–5.0
Ettinger et al. (1988)	≥ 53	181 members of health maintenance organization with ≥ 5 years of OT	220 members with ≤ 1 year use of OT	≤ 24	5 years of use: 18; ≤ 1 year of use: 3	2 705 person–years 4 197 person–years	[9.3]	NR
Paganini-Hill et al. (1989), USA	44–100	5 160 women in a retirement community	Internal comparison	5	Never use: 45 Any use: 5	11 281 person–years 12 472 person–years	10	NR

Table 6 (contd)

Reference, country	Age at beginning of follow-up (years)	Study group of source population	Comparison group	Approximate duration of follow-up (years)	No. of observed cases	No. of expected cases or person–years	Relative risk or SIR	95% CI
Persson et al. (1989), Sweden	≥ 35	23 244 women with ≥ 1 prescription for any OT use	Rates from the Uppsala health care region	6	48	34.3	1.5	1.1–1.9

SIR, standardized incidence ratio; CI, confidence interval; NR, not reported; OT, oestrogen therapy; NS, not significant

Table 7. Case–control studies on any use of oestrogen alone and the risk for endometrial cancer

Reference, country	Age (years)	No. of cases/ no. of controls	Proportion (%) of cases/controls exposed	Odds ratio (95% CI)	Longest duration of OT use (years)	Odds ratio (95% CI) for longest duration of OT use
Smith et al. (1975), USA	≥48	317/317	48/17	4.5 [3.1–6.6]	NR	NR
Ziel & Finkle (1975), USA	57	94/188	57/15	7.6 [4.7–11]	≥7	14 (NR)
Mack et al. (1976), USA	≥52	63/252	NR/43	5.6 (2.8–11)	≥8	8.8 (NR)
Gray et al. (1977), USA	57	205/205	16/6	3.1 (1.5–6.8)	≥10	12 (1.5–240)
McDonald et al. (1977), USA	≥25	145/580	27/28	0.9 (0.6–1.4)	≥3	7.9 (2.9–21)
Horwitz & Feinstein (1978), USA	62	119/119	29/3	12 (4.0–48)	NR	NR
Hoogerland et al. (1978), USA	NR	587/587	18/9	2.2 (1.6–3.2)	≥10	6.7 (NR)
Antunes et al. (1979), USA	NR	451/888	17/4	5.5 (2.3–13)	≥5	15 (4.9–45)
Weiss et al. (1979), USA	50–74	322/289	69/25	[6.3] (NR)	≥20	8.3 (2.8–25)
Hulka et al. (1980), USA	61	256/861	33/35[a]	1.4 (0.9–2.1)	≥9.5	5.5 (1.9–16)[a]
Jelovsek et al. (1980), USA	58	431/431	12/6	2.4 (1.4–3.9)	≥10	2.6 (1.1–5.9)
Salmi (1980), Finland	35–60	282/282	6/15	0.4[b] (0.2–0.7)	NR	NR
Spengler et al. (1981), Canada	40–74	88/177	45/22	2.9 (1.7–5.1)	≥5	8.6 (3.2–23)
Stavraky et al. (1981), Canada	40–80	206/199[c]	47/29	4.8 (2.7–8.4)	≥10	14 (5.0–42)
Kelsey et al. (1982), USA	45–74	167/903	36/19	1.6 (1.3–2.0)[c]	≥10	2.7 (NR)
Henderson et al. (1983), USA	≤45	127/127	12/7	[1.8] (NR)	≥2	3.1 (NR)
La Vecchia et al. (1984), Italy	33–74	283/566	25/17	2.3 (1.6–3.2)	≥5	'Trend'
Ewertz et al. (1984), Denmark	NR	115/115	18/13	4.9 (2.0–12)	≥1	1.7 (0.4–6.9)
Shapiro et al. (1985), USA/Canada	50–69	425/792	31/15	3.5 (2.6–4.7)	NR	NR
Petterson et al. (1986), Sweden	34–90	254/254	16/12	1.3 (0.8–2.1)	≥4	4.3 (1.3–14)
Buring et al. (1986), USA	40–80	188/428	39/20	2.4 (1.7–3.6)	≥10	7.6 (NR)
Ewertz (1988), Denmark	44–89	149/154	56/21	4.7 (2.9–7.7)	NR	NR
Koumantaki et al. (1989), Greece	40–79	83/164	10/6	2.0 (0.8–5.1)	NR	NR
Rubin et al. (1990), USA	20–54	196/986	24/14	1.9 (1.3–2.8)	≥6	3.5 (1.7–7.4)
Voigt et al. (1991), USA	40–64	158/182	19/7	3.1 (1.6–5.8)	>3	5.7 (2.5–13)
Jick (1993), USA	50–64	172/172	75/49	6.5 (3.1–13)	≥5	22 (6.5–74)
Levi et al. (1993a), Switzerland	32–74	158/468	38/20	2.7 (1.7–4.1)	≥5	5.1 (2.7–9.8)

Table 7 (contd)

Reference, country	Age (years)	No. of cases/ no. of controls	Proportion (%) of cases/controls exposed	Odds ratio (95% CI)	Longest duration of OT use (years)	Odds ratio (95% CI) for longest duration of OT use
Brinton et al. (1993), USA	20–74	300/207	24/14	3.0 (1.7–5.1)	≥ 5	6.0 (2.7–13)
Finkle et al. (1995), USA	29–85	NR	54/44	5.0 (2.9–9.8)	NR	NR
Green et al. (1996), USA	45–74	661/865	49/21	[2.0] [1.7–2.5]	> 12	16 (10–26)
Beresford et al. (1997), USA	45–74	832/1 114	15/13	2.7 (1.9–4.0)	NR	NR
Goodman et al. (1997b), USA	18–84	332/511	50/32	2.6 (1.8–3.8)	≥ 3	3.6 (2.2–6.0)
Pike et al. (1997), USA	50–74	833/791	51/33	2.2[d] (1.9–2.5)	NR	NR
Cushing et al. (1998), USA	45–64	484/780	30/12	5.4 (2.3–13)	> 8	8.4[e] (4.0–18)

CI, confidence interval; OT, oestrogen therapy; NR, not reported
[a] Only for 321 community controls
[b] Risk for oestriol use; risk for conjugated oestrogen use, 5.0 [CI not reported]
[c] Controls without gynaecological disorders
[d] Risk per five years of use
[e] > 1.25 mg/day

1976; Gray *et al.*, 1977; McDonald *et al.*, 1977; Hoogerland *et al.*, 1978; Antunes *et al.*, 1979; Hulka *et al.*, 1980; Jelovsek *et al.*, 1980; Shapiro *et al.*, 1980; Spengler *et al.*, 1981; Stavraky *et al.*, 1981; Kelsey *et al*, 1982; La Vecchia *et al.*, 1984; Shapiro *et al.*, 1985; Buring *et al.*, 1986; Rubin *et al.*, 1990; Brinton *et al.*, 1993; Pike *et al.*, 1997). Use for less than six months was found not to increase the risk in four studies (McDonald *et al.*, 1977; Hoogerland *et al.*, 1978; Hulka *et al.*, 1980; Spengler *et al.*, 1981), while two studies that included the risk of use for six months to one year (McDonald *et al.*, 1977; Hoogerland *et al.*, 1978) found increased risks in this category of duration also. In the meta-analysis of the published results (Grady *et al.*, 1995), the overall relative risk was 2.3 (95% CI, 2.1–2.5) for oestrogen users when compared with non-users. The summary relative risk for less than one year of use was 1.4 (95% CI, 1.0–1.8), whereas that for use for more than 10 years was 9.5 (95% CI, 7.4–12).

In some studies, but not all (Brinton *et al.*, 1993; Finkle *et al.*, 1995), that addressed the risk associated with recency of post-menopausal oestrogen therapy, the risk for endometrial cancer remained higher than in non-users even 10 years after cessation (Shapiro *et al.*, 1985; Levi *et al.*, 1993a; Finkle *et al.*, 1995; Green *et al.*, 1996). Women with the longest durations of post-menopausal oestrogen therapy had especially high excess risks after discontinuation of use (Rubin *et al.*, 1990; Green *et al.*, 1996). In the meta-analysis of the published results (Grady *et al.*, 1995), the summary relative risk was largest for the group of women who had ceased use within one year or less (relative risk, 4.1; 95% CI, 2.9–5.7) but remained elevated (2.3; 95% CI, 1.8–3.1) five years or more after cessation.

An elevated risk for endometrial cancer is associated with all commonly prescribed doses of conjugated oestrogens (Gray *et al.*, 1977; Antunes *et al.*, 1979; Weiss *et al.*, 1979; Hulka *et al.*, 1980; Stavraky *et al.*, 1981; Jick *et al.*, 1993; Cushing *et al.*, 1998). Four studies that addressed the effect of a low dose (0.3 mg/day) on the risk for endometrial cancer (Gray *et al.*, 1977; Weiss *et al.*, 1979; Jick *et al.*, 1993; Cushing *et al.*, 1998) yielded consistent results: the risk of women using low doses did not differ from that of women using high doses (0.625 mg). In the meta-analysis of the published studies (Grady *et al.*, 1995), the summary relative risks were 3.9 (95% CI, 1.6–9.5) for any use of low doses (0.3 mg), 3.4 (95% CI, 2.0–5.6) for intermediate doses (0.625 mg) and 5.8 (95% CI, 4.5–7.5) for high doses (≥ 1.25 mg), but these values did not differ significantly.

Use of oestrogens other than conjugated ones (e.g. oestradiol) was commoner in Europe than in the United States (Persson *et al.*, 1989). Other oestrogens have been shown to be related to an increased risk for endometrial cancer in most (Mack *et al.*, 1976; Weiss *et al.*, 1979; Antunes *et al.*, 1979; Buring *et al.*, 1986) but not all (Shapiro *et al.*, 1980) studies of the type of post-menopausal oestrogen therapy. In the meta-analysis of the published results (Grady *et al.*, 1995), users of conjugated oestrogens had greater risk for endometrial cancer (relative risk, 2.5; 95% CI, 2.1–2.9) than users of other oestrogens (1.3; 95% CI, 1.1–1.6).

Most cases of endometrial cancer related to post-menopausal oestrogen therapy have been of the well-differentiated histological type and at an early clinical stage (McDonald *et al.*, 1977; Antunes *et al*,. 1979; Buring *et al.*, 1986; Rubin *et al.*, 1990). Myometrial invasion has been reported in only a few cases (Mack *et al.*, 1976; McDonald *et al.*, 1977; Antunes *et al.*, 1979; Weiss *et al.*, 1979; Jelovsek *et al.*, 1980; Buring *et al.*, 1986). In the meta-analysis of the published results (Grady *et al.*, 1995), the summary relative risk for early-stage (0–1) cancer was higher (4.2; 95% CI, 3.1–5.7) than that for later stages (2–4) (1.4; 95% CI, 0.8–2.4). Similarly, the summary risk estimate for non-invasive cancer was higher (6.2; 95% CI, 4.5–8.4) than that for invasive cancer (3.8; 95% CI, 2.9–5.1) (Grady *et al.*, 1995). Post-menopausal oestrogen therapy was related to the risk for death from endometrial cancer in four studies (Lafferty & Helmuth, 1985; Petitti *et al.*, 1987; Ettinger *et al.*, 1988; Paganini-Hill *et al.*, 1989) and in the meta-analysis (Grady *et al.*, 1995). Each of these studies reported at least a doubling of the risk for death from endometrial cancer among women who had ever used post-menopausal oestrogen therapy as compared with those who had never done so.

An increased risk for endometrial cancer has been associated with both continuous and cyclic oestrogen use (Mack *et al.*, 1976; McDonald *et al.*, 1977; Antunes *et al.*, 1979; Weiss *et al.*, 1979; Hulka *et al.*, 1980; Buring *et al.*, 1986) as well as with intermittent regimens (McDonald *et al.*, 1977; Antunes *et al.*, 1979). There were no differences in the summary relative risk estimates for the continuous regimen (2.9; 95% CI, 2.2–3.8) and intermittent and cyclic regimens (3.0; 95% CI, 2.4–3.8) in the meta-analysis (Grady *et al.*, 1995).

Weight and smoking have been reported to modify the relationship between post-menopausal oestrogen therapy and the risk for endometrial cancer. Some studies (Kelsey *et al.*, 1982; Ewertz *et al.*, 1984; La Vecchia *et al.*, 1984; Ewertz *et al.*, 1988; Levi *et al.*, 1993a) indicate that the effects of obesity and oestrogen use are not multiplicative; leaner women have a higher risk for endometrial cancer than women with higher body mass indices (La Vecchia *et al.*, 1982a). Smoking modified the relationship between post-menopausal oestrogen therapy and endometrial cancer in three case–control studies (Franks *et al.*, 1987; Koumantaki *et al.*, 1989; Levi *et al.*, 1993a). Franks *et al.* (1987) presented risks for endometrial cancer stratified by smoking: post-menopausal non-smoking women using oestrogen therapy had a higher relative risk (3.8; 95% CI, 1.7–8.2) than smokers using such therapy (1.0; 95% CI, 0.4–2.6). Levi *et al.* (1993a) and Koumantaki *et al.* (1989) reported similar risk estimates. [Although the effect of smoking is biologically plausible, it cannot be regarded as protective against endometrial cancer.]

2.3 Cervical cancer

2.3.1 *Methodological considerations*

The methodological issues that arise in studies of oral contraceptives and cervical cancer also apply to studies of post-menopausal oestrogen therapy and this disease (see section 2.3 of the monograph on 'Oral contraceptives, combined'). Briefly, exogenous oestrogens may affect various stages in the development of cervical cancer, and epidemiological studies of intraepithelial lesions and invasive lesions should therefore be considered separately. There are also two main histological types of invasive disease, squamous-cell carcinoma and adenocarcinoma, and ideally these also should be considered separately. In assessing associations between exogenous oestrogens and cervical cancer, the potentially confounding effects of sexual factors and infection by oncogenic strains of the human papillomavirus should be considered. Finally, the influence of Papanicolaou (Pap) smear screening should be considered, as women on post-menopausal hormonal therapy may be more likely to have Pap smears than women not on this therapy.

In the study of Persson *et al.* (1997a) in Sweden, women taking post-menopausal hormonal therapy tended to be of lower parity, older at the birth of their first child and have a higher prevalence of hysterectomy or oophorectomy than women who did not receive such therapy. In addition, a higher level of education was associated with long-term exposure to post-menopausal hormonal therapy, as were heavy physical exercise and diets rich in fibre. Women who had used oral contraceptives were more likely to use oestrogens both with and without progestogen than women who had not used oral contraceptives. These observations serve to demonstrate the importance of considering potentially confounding variables when assessing observed relationships between post-menopausal hormonal therapy and the risks for various neoplasms.

2.3.2   Cohort studies

The risk for cervical carcinoma in relation to post-menopausal hormonal therapy has been considered in two cohort studies. Adami *et al.* (1989) reported results for a cohort of 23 244 Swedish women who had been given prescriptions for such therapy. The cohort was assembled between 1977 and 1980 and followed through to the end of 1984. The observed numbers of women with various cancers were compared with expected numbers based on the incidence rates in the population from which the cohort members were accrued. Women who had ever used post-menopausal oestrogen therapy had a relative risk for cervical cancer of 0.8 (95% CI, 0.5–1.2) in comparison with women who had never used oestrogens (27 observed and 34.05 expected cases). The risk in relation to duration of use was not calculated. The risk was lower for women who had used conjugated oestrogens or oestradiol (0.6; 95% CI, 0.3–1.0) than for women who had used other compounds, mainly oestriol (1.3; 95% CI, 0.7–2.3), although oestriol is a less potent oestrogen than conjugated oestrogens or oestradiol. Women who were under 60 years of age at entry into the cohort had a relative risk of 0.6 (95% CI, 0.4–1.0) when compared with older women, whose relative risk was 1.2 (95% CI, 0.6–2.3). This difference was observed for use of either conjugated oestrogens or oestradiol and for use of oestriol. The risk was also somewhat lower for women who were followed for more than five years than for women who were followed for a shorter period: the relative risk of women followed from 0–4 years was 0.9 (95% CI, 0.6–1.3) and that for women followed for five or more years was 0.6 (95% CI, 0.2–1.3). The investigators were unable to control for sexual variables, prior Pap smear screening or human papillomavirus infection. An updated report of the same study (Schairer *et al.*, 1997) gave a relative risk for dying of cervical cancer in relation to use of post-menopausal hormonal therapy of 1.2 (95% CI, 0.8–1.7), based on 23 deaths after follow-up through the end of 1986.

In a study in Britain (Hunt *et al.*, 1990), 4544 women who had received continuous post-menopausal hormone treatment for at least one year were recruited from 21 pre-menopause clinics around the country between 1974 and 1982, and were followed through 1988. During this period, two women died of cervical cancer, whereas the expected number was 6.8 on the basis of mortality rates for England and Wales. This gave a rate ratio of 0.3 (95% CI, 0.0–1.1).

2.3.3 *Case–control studies*

The results of only one case–control study of post-menopausal oestrogen therapy and cervical cancer have been published (Parazzini *et al.*, 1997). In this hospital-based study conducted in northern Italy, 645 women with invasive cervical cancer were compared with 749 women admitted to the same hospitals with acute conditions. After adjustment for age, calendar year of interview, number of sexual partners, parity, oral contraceptive use, lifetime number of cervical smears, social class, smoking and menopausal status, the relative risk for women who had ever used post-menopausal oestrogen therapy was estimated to be 0.5 (95% CI, 0.3–0.8). The risk of women who had used post-meno-pausal oestrogen therapy for fewer than 12 months was 0.6 (95% CI, 0.4–1.1) and that for women who had used it for 12 or more months was 0.5 (95% CI, 0.2–1.0) (*p* value for trend, < 0.01). Consistent with the results of Adami *et al.* (1989) described above, the risk of women who had last used post-menopausal oestrogen therapy more than 10 years previously was 0.4 (95% CI, 0.2–0.7), whereas that for women who had last used these products within the past 10 years was 0.9 (95% CI, 0.5–1.7); the risk was lower for women who had first used these products before the age of 50 (0.4; 95% CI, 0.2–0.7) than for women who had first used them at a greater age (0.8; 95% CI, 0.4–1.5).

2.4 Ovarian cancer

2.4.1 *Descriptive studies*

Over the last few decades, no major or systematic trend in incidence or mortality rates has been observed for ovarian cancer in elderly women (Adami *et al.*, 1990; La Vecchia *et al.*, 1992b; Koper *et al.*, 1996; La Vecchia *et al.*, 1998). Consequently, des-criptive data on the incidence of and mortality from ovarian cancer do not indicate an effect of post-menopausal oestrogen therapy.

2.4.2 *Cohort studies*

The main findings of cohort studies on post-menopausal oestrogen therapy and ovarian cancer risk are given in Table 8.

In a 13-year follow-up for mortality, between recruitment in 1968–72 and 1983, in a study in the United States on contraception use in 16 638 women aged 18–59, six deaths from ovarian cancer were observed among women who had ever used post-menopausal oestrogen therapy (relative risk, 0.9; 95% CI, 0.3–2.8) (Petitti *et al.*, 1987).

The relationship between post-menopausal oestrogen therapy and ovarian cancer was also analysed in the data from the American Cancer Society's cancer prevention study (II)

Table 8. Selected cohort studies on post-menopausal oestrogen therapy and ovarian cancer, 1980–97

Reference, country	Outcome	No. of cases	Relative risk for any use (95% CI)	Comments
Petitti *et al.* (1987), USA	Mortality	6	0.9 (0.3–2.8)	13-year mortality follow-up of the study on contraception
Rodriguez *et al.* (1995), USA	Mortality	436	1.2 (0.9–1.4)	Significant: direct relationship with duration ($p = 0.03$). RR, 1.4 (95% CI, 0.9–2.1) for 6–10 years and RR, 1.7 (95% CI, 1.1–2.8) for ≥ 11 years of use
Adami *et al.* (1989), Sweden	Incidence	64	1.0 (0.7–1.2)	Cohort of 23 246 women prescribed post-menopausal oestrogen therapy, followed for an average of 6.7 years
Schairer *et al.* (1997), Sweden	Mortality	52	1.0 (0.8–1.3)	Same cohort as Adami *et al.* (1989); follow-up for mortality, 8.6 years

CI, confidence interval; RR, relative risk

for 240 073 peri- and post-menopausal women enrolled in 1982; 436 deaths from ovarian cancer were registered over seven years of follow-up (Rodriguez *et al.*, 1995). The relative risk was 1.2 (95% CI, 0.9–1.4) for any use of oestrogen and rose to 1.4 (95% CI, 0.9–2.1) for 6–10 years of use and to 1.7 (95% CI, 1.1–2.8) for ≥ 11 years of use. This elevated risk was not explained by allowance for other known or likely risk factors for ovarian cancer.

In a Swedish record-linkage prospective study of 23 246 women who were prescribed menopausal oestrogens, recruited between 1977 and 1980 and followed-up for an average of 6.7 years (Adami *et al.*, 1989), 64 cases of ovarian cancer were observed versus 66.64 expected (relative risk, 1.0; 95% CI, 0.7–1.2). After 8.6 years of follow-up (Schairer *et al.*, 1997), 52 deaths from ovarian cancer were observed versus 52.7 expected (relative risk, 1.0; 95% CI, 0.8–1.3).

2.4.3   Case–control studies

At least 12 case–control studies published after 1979 and a pooled analysis of individual data from 12 studies of ovarian cancer have provided data on post-menopausal oestrogen therapy (Table 9). Of these, seven studies, including an investigation of 205 cases in the United States (Weiss *et al.*, 1982), a multicentre case–control study of 377 cases in various areas of Canada, Israel and the United States (Kaufman *et al.*, 1989), a population-based case–control investigation of 367 cases and 564 controls in Ontario,

Table 9. Selected case–control studies on post-menopausal oestrogen therapy and ovarian cancer, 1980–97

Reference, country	Type of study	No. of cases	Age (years)	Relative risk for any use (95% CI)	Comments
Hildreth et al. (1981), USA	Hospital-based	62	45–74	0.9 (0.5–1.6)	
Weiss et al. (1982), USA	Population-based	205	36–75	1.3 (0.9–1.5)	Stronger association for endometrioid ovarian cancer (3.1; 95% CI, 1.0–9.8)
Franceschi et al. (1982), Italy	Hospital-based	161	19–69	[1.0]	No effect
Tzonou et al. (1984), Greece	Hospital-based	150	All	1.6 (post-menopausal)	Not significant
Harlow et al. (1988), USA	Population-based	116	20–79	0.9	Ovarian neoplasms of borderline malignancy
Kaufman et al. (1989), Canada, Israel, USA	Hospital-based	377	18–69	1.1 (0.8–1.6)	Unopposed oestrogens only. No association with combined treatment (RR, 0.7; 95% CI, 0.2–1.8) or with specific histotypes
Booth et al. (1989), UK	Hospital-based	225	< 65	1.5 (0.9–2.6)	No association with specific histotypes
Polychronopoulou et al. (1993), Greece	Hospital-based	189	< 75	1.4 (0.4–4.9)	Based on 6 exposed cases and 4 controls only
Parazzini et al. (1994), Italy	Hospital-based	953	23–74	1.6 (1.2–2.4)	Adjusted for major covariates, including combined oral contraceptive use
Purdie et al. (1995), Australia	Population-based	824	18–79	1.0 (0.8–1.3)	Adjusted for major covariates, including oral contraceptive use
Risch et al. (1996), Ontario, Canada	Population-based	367	35–79	1.3 (0.9–2.0)	Multivariate RR, 2.0 (95% CI, 1.0–4.0) for serous and 2.8 (95% CI, 1.2–6.9) for endometrioid for ≥ 5 years of use. No association with mucinous tumours

Table 9 (contd)

Reference, country	Type of study	No. of cases	Age (years)	Relative risk for any use (95% CI)	Comments
Hempling et al. (1997), USA	Hospital-based	491	NR	0.9 (0.6–1.2)	Other cancers as controls
Re-analysis of original data					
Whittemore et al. (1992), USA	Pooled analysis of 12 US hospital- and population-based case-control studies	2 197	All	0.9 (0.7–1.3) (hospital-based) 1.1 (0.9–1.4) (population-based)	Invasive cancers. No trend in risk with duration. RR per year of use, 1.0 for both hospital- and population-based studies
Harris et al. (1992b), USA	Pooled analysis of same 12 studies as Whittemore et al. (1992) but for tumours of low malignant potential	327	All	1.1 (0.7–1.9)	Ovarian neoplasms of borderline malignancy. No difference between hospital-based and population-based studies. No trend in risk with duration

CI, confidence interval; RR, relative risk; NR, not reported

Canada (Risch, 1996), and four European studies, from the United Kingdom (Booth *et al.*, 1989), Greece (Tzonou *et al.*, 1984; Polychronopoulou *et al.*, 1993) and Italy (Parazzini *et al.*, 1994), reported relative risks between 1.2 and 1.6. Other case–control studies, including the pooled analysis of individual data from the United States studies (Whittemore *et al.*, 1992), however, showed no consistent association.

Hildreth *et al.* (1981) provided data on 62 cases of ovarian cancer and 1068 controls in seven hospitals in Connecticut, United States, between 1977 and 1979. The response rate was 71% for both cases and controls. The relative risk for any use of post-menopausal oestrogen therapy was 0.9 (95% CI, 0.5–1.6).

Weiss *et al.* (1982) considered 205 cases of epithelial ovarian cancer diagnosed between 1975 and 1979 and 611 population controls in Washington State and Utah, United States. The overall relative risk for any use of post-menopausal oestrogen therapy was 1.3 (95% CI, 0.9–1.8), and there was no consistent time–risk relationship; however, the relative risk was 3.1 (95% CI, 1.0–9.8) for the 17 endometrioid tumours. Allowance was made for age, state of residence and hysterectomy.

Franceschi *et al.* (1982) reported data on 161 cases and 561 population controls interviewed in 1979–80 in greater Milan, northern Italy. Any use of non-contraceptive oestrogens was reported by 17% of cases and 17% of controls, corresponding to an age-adjusted relative risk of [1.0]. The duration of use was also similar in cases and controls.

In a hospital-based case–control investigation of 150 case and 250 control women interviewed in 1980–81 in Athens, Greece (Tzonou *et al.*, 1984), the relative risk for any use of post-menopausal oestrogen therapy was 1.6 (not significant). No information was available on duration of use or other time factors.

Harlow *et al.* (1988) considered 116 cases of ovarian cancer of borderline malignancy and 158 hospital controls in western Washington, United States, diagnosed between 1980 and 1985. The response rate was 68% for cases and 74% for controls. The relative risk for any use of post-menopausal oestrogen therapy was 0.9, in the absence of a consistent duration–risk relationship.

Kaufman *et al.* (1989) conducted a multicentre case–control study in Canada, Israel and the United States on 377 cases of epithelial ovarian cancer and 2030 hospital controls interviewed between 1976 and 1985. The multivariate relative risk for any use of post-menopausal oestrogen therapy was 1.1 (95% CI, 0.8–1.6), after allowance for socio-demographic factors, age at menarche, parity, menopausal status, age at menopause and oral contraceptive use, but it rose to 1.6 (95% CI, 0.8–3.2) for ≥ 10 years of use. The trend in risk with duration was not significant. No appreciable heterogeneity was observed across different histological types.

A study of 235 cases and 451 hospital controls conducted between 1978 and 1983 in London and Oxford, England (Booth *et al.*, 1989), gave a multivariate relative risk for any use of post-menopausal oestrogen therapy of 1.5 (95% CI, 0.9–2.6) after adjustment for age and social class. No data were available on duration of use.

A study of 189 cases and 200 controls conducted in 1989–91 in greater Athens, Greece (Polychronopoulou *et al.*, 1993) gave a relative risk for any use of post-menopausal oestrogen therapy of 1.4 (95% CI, 0.4–4.9). No information was given on duration or other time–risk relationships. The response rate of cases was almost 90%. Allowance was made for age, education, weight, age at menarche, parity and age at the birth of the first child.

A study of 953 cases diagnosed between 1983 and 1992 in northern Italy and 2503 hospital controls (Parazzini *et al.*, 1994) found a multivariate relative risk (after allowance for socio-demographic factors, parity, age at menarche, type of menopause, age at meno-pause and oral contraceptive use) of 1.6 (95% CI, 1.2–2.4) for any use of post-menopausal oestrogen therapy. The relative risk for ≥ 2 years of use was 1.7 (95% CI, 0.9–3.4).

Purdie *et al.* (1995) provided data on 824 cases diagnosed between 1990 and 1993 and 860 population controls in three Australian states. The response rate was 90% for cases and 73% for controls. The multivariate relative risk (adjusted for socio-demographic factors, family history of cancers, talc use, smoking and reproductive and hormonal factors) for any use of post-menopausal oestrogen therapy was 1.0 (95% CI, 0.8–1.3). No information was given on duration of use or any other time–risk relationship.

Risch (1996) reported data on post-menopausal oestrogen therapy for 367 patients with invasive epithelial ovarian cancer and 564 population controls in Ontario, Canada, interviewed during 1989–92. The response rate was 71% for cases and 65% for controls. The relative risk for any use of post-menopausal oestrogen therapy was 1.3 (95% CI, 0.9–2.0) for non-mucinous neoplasms and 0.7 (95% CI, 0.2–2.1) for mucinous ones. The association was apparently strongest (1.9; 95% CI, 1.0–3.5) for endometrioid neoplasms, with a significant duration–risk relationship. Allowance was made in the analysis for age, parity, lactation, combined oral contraceptive use, tubal ligation, hysterectomy and family history of breast cancer.

In a study based on data collected between 1982 and 1995 at the Roswell Park Cancer Institute, United States (Hempling *et al.*, 1997), 491 patients with epithelial ova-rian cancer were compared with 741 women admitted for non-hormone-related mali-gnancies. The overall relative risk for any use of post-menopausal oestrogen therapy was 0.9 (95% CI, 0.6–1.2); there was no significant trend with duration of use. The relative risk was 0.6 (95% CI , 0.3–1.4) for ≥ 10 years of use. Further, there was no appreciable heterogeneity across histological types. Allowance was made for age, parity, combined oral contraceptive use, smoking, family history of ovarian cancer, age at menarche, menopausal status and socio-demographic factors.

A pooled analysis of individual data from 12 studies of 2197 white cases of invasive epithelial ovarian cancer and 8893 white controls in the United States (Whittemore *et al.*, 1992) gave a pooled multivariate relative risk for invasive ovarian cancer associated with any use of post-menopausal oestrogen therapy for more than three months of 0.9 (95% CI, 0.7–1.3) for hospital-based studies and 1.1 (95% CI, 0.9–1.4) for population-based studies; there was no consistent duration–risk relationship. The relative risk for use for > 15 years was 0.5 (95% CI, 0.2–1.3) for hospital-based and 1.5 (95% CI, 0.8–3.1) for population-based studies. The overall trend per year of use was 1.0 for both types of study; neither risk estimate was significant. Allowance was made in the analysis for age, study, parity and combined oral contraceptive use.

In a similar pooled analysis of individual data on 327 cases of epithelial ovarian tumours of borderline malignancy, the relative risk for any use of post-menopausal oestrogen therapy was 1.1 (95% CI, 0.7–1.9) (Harris *et al.*, 1992b).

Earlier studies (La Vecchia *et al.*, 1982b; Weiss *et al.*, 1982) had suggested that endometrioid neoplasms are related to post-menopausal oestrogen therapy, but this suggestion was not confirmed in several subsequent studies (Kaufman *et al.*, 1989; Whittemore *et al.*, 1992). It was thus unclear whether post-menopausal oestrogen therapy is consistently related to any specific histotype of ovarian cancer; however, a recent Canadian study (Risch, 1996) gave relative risks of 1.4 for serous, 1.9 for endometrioid and 0.7 for mucinous tumours, and significant trends in risk with duration of use for serous and endometrioid tumours. The issue of a potential histotype-specific relationship is therefore still open to discussion, although it remains possible that ovarian cancer cases in women who had used post-menopausal oestrogen therapy are more often classified as endometrioid. The available data therefore suggest that there is little or no association between use of post-menopausal oestrogen therapy and invasive epithelial ovarian neoplasms or those of borderline malignancy. No adequate data were available on post-menopausal oestrogen therapy and non-epithelial (germ-cell or sex-cord-stromal) ovarian neoplasms.

2.5   Liver cancer
2.5.1   *Cohort studies*

Goodman *et al.* (1995) reported the results of a study of risk factors for liver cancer in Hiroshima and Nagasaki, Japan. Information was collected by questionnaire from 36 133 men and women between 1978 and 1981, who were followed through population-based cancer registries until 1989. There were 242 cases of hepatocellular carcinoma in the two cities, of which 86 were in women; information on use of female hormone preparations was available for 76 of these cases. Details of the type of female hormones used were not collected, but oral contraceptive use is very rare in Japan and it is likely that the hormones were largely given as post-menopausal hormonal therapy. Sixty-nine of the case women had never used hormones, and seven had used these preparations. The risk for any use relative to no use of hormones, adjusted for city, age at the time of the atomic bombing, attained age and radiation dose to the liver, was 1.3 (95% CI, 0.6–2.8). There was no information on infection with hepatitis viruses, but infection with hepatitis B virus is common in western Japan.

Persson *et al.* (1996) studied the cancer risk after post-menopausal hormonal therapy in a population-based cohort of 22 579 women aged 35 or more and living in the Uppsala health care region, Sweden. Women who had ever received a prescription for post-menopausal hormonal therapy between 1977 and 1980 were identified and followed-up until 1991. Information on hormone use was obtained from pharmacy records. The expected numbers of cases were calculated from national incidence rates. There was no information on smoking or alcohol consumption. The standardized incidence ratio for all cancers was

1.0 (95% CI, 0.9–1.0). There were 43 cancers of the hepatobiliary tract, comprising 14 hepatocellular carcinomas, five cholangiocarcinomas, 23 gall-bladder cancers and one unclassified; the expected number was 73.2, giving a standardized incidence ratio of 0.6 (95% CI, 0.4–0.8) for any type of post-menopausal hormonal therapy. The ratios for hepatocellular carcinoma were 0.8 (95% CI, 0.4–1.6) for treatment with oestradiol or conjugated oestrogens and 0.5 (95% CI, 0.2–1.4) for treatment with oestriol and other oestrogens. The relative risks for cholangiocarcinoma were 0.7 (95% CI, 0.1–2.0) for treatment with oestradiol or conjugated oestrogens and 0.3 (95% CI, 0.0–1.7) for treatment with oestriol and other oestrogens. There was no information on infection with hepatitis viruses.

2.5.2   *Case–control studies*

Yu *et al.* (1991) used a population-based cancer registry to identify histologically confirmed hepatocellular carcinomas diagnosed in women aged 18–74 between 1984 and 1990 who were black or white residents of Los Angeles County, United States. Two neighbourhood controls were sought for each case and matched on sex, year of birth and race. Eighty-four of 412 (20.4%) eligible patients were interviewed (70.6% died before attempted contact), of which 10 were excluded from the analysis because the diagnosis of hepatocellular carcinoma was not confirmed. The response rate among the initially selected controls was 71%. Adjustment for smoking and alcohol did not alter the results. Ten of the 25 case women (40.0%) had used Premarin® or other oestrogens, in comparison with 19 of the 58 female controls (32.8%). The relative risks, adjusted for duration of use of oral contraceptives, were 1.1 (95% CI, 0.3–3.6) for any use and 0.8 (95% CI, 0.2–4.5) for use for up to 12 months, 1.0 (95% CI, 0.2–5.1) for 13–60 months and 1.0 (95% CI, 0.2–6.0) for 61 months or more. Seven case women had one or more markers of hepatitis B and C viral infections; when these cases were excluded, use of Premarin® was still not related to hepatocellular carcinoma after adjustment for duration of use of oral contraceptives.

Tavani *et al.* (1996) studied the relationship between the risk for biliary cancer and factors related to female hormones in Milan, northern Italy, between 1984 and 1993. The cases were in 31 women aged 27–76 with histologically confirmed cancers of the biliary tract (of whom 17 had gall-bladder cancers); the controls were 377 women, age frequency-matched with cases, who were in hospital for acute, non-neoplastic, non-digestive conditions. Post-menopausal oestrogen therapy was used by 4 of 31 cases and 21 of 377 controls, yielding a relative risk, adjusted for age and history of cholelithiasis, of 2.2 (95% CI, 0.7–7.2).

2.6   Colorectal cancer

2.6.1   *Descriptive studies*

The incidence of colon cancer is similar for men and women, while a male predominance is found for rectal cancer. The female:male ratio of colon cancer incidence is relatively higher at pre-menopausal ages, suggesting an influence of some biological correlate of sex. Over the last two decades, mortality rates from these cancers in many developed countries have declined in women but not in men (La Vecchia *et al.*, 1998).

2.6.2 Cohort studies

(a) Colorectal adenomas

Grodstein *et al.* (1998) reported that 838 of 59 002 post-menopausal women had developed colorectal adenomas. There was no association between hormonal therapy and the incidence of adenomas overall, but current users had a lower risk for large (≥ 1 cm) adenomas than women who had never used hormones (relative risk, 0.74; 95% CI, 0.55–0.99).

(b) Colorectal cancer

Cohort studies on post-menopausal oestrogen therapy and cancers of the colon and rectum are summarized in Table 10.

Wu *et al.* (1987) followed a cohort of 7345 women in a large retirement community in California, United States, representing 62% of those to whom a questionnaire had been mailed; 4060 women reported ever having used post-menopausal oestrogen therapy of any type. After a four-year follow-up, 68 incident cases of colorectal cancer were identified. No association with risk for colorectal cancer was found (age-adjusted relative risk, 0.98; 95% CI, 0.5–1.8, for < 8 years of use and 1.0, 95% CI, 0.6–1.8 for ≥ 8 years' use).

A cohort of 22 597 Swedish women (mean age, 55 years) who received a prescription for post-menopausal oestrogen therapy were followed-up for cancer incidence and deaths through national cancer registries for an average of 6.7 years (Adami *et al.*, 1989) and, subsequently, for 13 years from 1977 through 1991 (Persson *et al.*, 1996). Overall, 153 incident cases and 62 deaths due to cancer of the colon and 80 incident cases of rectal cancer were observed. Information on exposure to post-menopausal oestrogen therapy was available only from accumulated pharmacy records; women were categorized into three exclusive compound groups according to the formulation prescribed: any oestradiol compounds or conjugated oestrogens, 11% of whom also received a progestogen; other oestrogens, chiefly a weak oestriol compound; and a fixed oestrogen–progestogen combination. For those for whom oestradiol compounds or conjugated oestrogens had ever been prescribed, the relative risk was 0.9 (95% CI, 0.7–1.1) for incident colorectal cancer and 0.9 (95% CI, 0.7–1.2) for incident rectal cancer (Persson *et al.*, 1996); a significant decrease in risk for mortality from colon cancer was observed (0.6; 95% CI, 0.4–0.9). The corresponding relative risks for women who had received only other oestrogens were 1.0 (95% CI, 0.8–1.3) for new cases of colon cancer, 0.8 (95% CI, 0.5–1.2) for new cases of rectal cancer and 0.8 (95% CI, 0.5–1.2) for death from colon cancer. The relative risk for exposure to any type of oestrogen was 0.9 for the incidence of either colon or rectal cancer and 0.7 (95% CI, 0.5–0.9) for mortality from colon cancer.

In an initial report from the Nurses' Health Study (Chute *et al.*, 1991), there was no significant association between hormonal therapy and colon or rectal cancer after an

Table 10. Cohort studies of use of post-menopausal oestrogen therapy and colorectal cancer

Reference, country	Size of cohort	Follow-up (years)	No. of cases of colorectal cancer	Type of use	Relative risk (RR; 95% confidence interval) (any versus no use)					Duration of use	Recency of use	Adjustment, comments
					Colon–rectum	Colon	Right colon	Left colon	Rectum			
Wu et al. (1987), California, USA	7 345	4	68	–	1.00 (NS)	–	–	–	–	No effect (RR ≥ 8 years' use, 1.0; 0.6–1.8)	NR	Age
Adami et al. (1989); Persson et al. (1996), Sweden	23 244	13	233, 62 deaths	OT / Oestriol / Any type	0.9 (0.7–1.1) / 1.0 (0.8–1.3) / 0.9 (0.7–1.2)	–	–	–	0.9 (0.7–1.2) / 0.8 (0.5–1.2) / 0.9 (0.7–1.1)	No effect	NR	Age; RR for colon mortality, 0.6 (0.4–0.9)
Chute et al. (1991); Grodstein et al. (1998), USA	59 002	14	262	Current users / Past users		0.64 (0.48–0.85) / 0.65 (0.50–0.83) / 0.86 (0.67–1.1)	0.56 (0.35–0.91)	0.79 (0.50–1.2)	0.67 (0.40–1.1)	No effect (RR ≥ 5 years' use, 0.72; 0.53–0.96)	No risk reduction after 5 years' duration (RR, 0.92; 0.70–1.2)	Age, body mass index, COC use, family history of cancer, diet, alcohol, smoking and age at menopause
Bostick et al. (1994); Folsom et al. (1995), Iowa, USA	41 837	6	293	Current users / Past users		0.73 (0.47–1.1) / 0.80 (0.61–1.1)	–	–	–	Inverse trend (RR, 0.31 for ≤ 5 years' use)	No effect	Age, body mass index, weight:height ratio, alcohol, exercise and medical history

Table 10 (contd)

Reference, country	Size of cohort	Follow-up (years)	No. of cases of colorectal cancer	Type of use	Relative risk (RR; 95% confidence interval) (any versus no use)					Duration of use	Recency of use	Adjustment, comments
					Colon–rectum	Colon	Right colon	Left colon	Rectum			
Calle *et al.* (1995), USA	422 373	7	897 deaths	—	—	0.71 (0.61–0.83)	—	—	—	Significant trend (RR for > 11 years' use, 0.54; 0.39–0.76)	Stronger effect among current users (RR, 0.55; 0.40–0.76)	Age, body mass index, parity, menopause, COC, diet, exercise, race and smoking
Risch & Howe (1995), Canada	33 003	14	230	—	1.0 (0.74–1.5)	1.3 (0.86–1.9)	—	—	0.64 (0.33–1.2)	RR, 0.65 (0.21–2.6) for ≥ 5 years)	Not shown	Age Linkage study
Troisi *et al.* (1997), USA	33 779	7.7	313	Un-opposed OT	—	1.1 (0.7–1.5)	1.6 (1.0–2.7)	0.8 (0.5–1.5)	1.2 (0.7–2.3)	No effect	RR for recent use, 0.78 (0.55–1.1)	Age (but unaltered by education, body mass index, parity and COC use)
				Any OT	0.99 (0.79–1.2)	1.1 (0.81–1.6)	1.7 (1.0–2.7)	0.98 (0.58–1.7)	1.1 (0.59–1.9)			

NS, not significant; OT, oestrogen therapy; NR, not reported; COC, combined oral contraceptives

eight-year follow-up. After 14 years, however, Grodstein *et al.* (1998) reported that 262 of 59 002 post-menopausal women had developed colorectal cancer. In this analysis, current use was associated with a decreased risk, the relative risk adjusted for several potential confounding variables being 0.65 (95% CI, 0.50–0.83). The results were not changed (relative risk, 0.64; 95% CI, 0.49–0.82) after exclusion of women who had undergone a screening sigmoidoscopy, suggesting that the lower risk was not due to more intensive screening of women who had used hormones. This association disappeared five years after hormone use was discontinued (relative risk, 0.92; 95% CI, 0.70–1.2).

In a prospective cohort study of 35 215 women aged 55–69 years with a driver's licence and without a history of cancer in Iowa, United States, from 1986 through 1990 (Bostick *et al.*, 1994), 212 new cases of colon cancer were documented. The relative risk for colon cancer associated with post-menopausal oestrogen therapy use, adjusted for age, parity, height, energy and vitamin intake, was 0.93 (95% CI, 0.68–1.3) for former users and 0.82 (95% CI, 0.50–1.3) for current users. The study cohort was updated by Folsom *et al.* (1995), who followed-up 41 837 women aged 55–69 years for two additional years. The relative risk for colon cancer (293 observed cases), adjusted for age, body mass index, waist-to-hip ratio, exercise, alcohol and medical history, was 0.80 (95% CI, 0.61–1.1) in former users and 0.73 (95% CI, 0.47–1.1) in current users. The lowest relative risk was seen for short-term (≤ 5 years) current post-menopausal oestrogen therapy use (relative risk, 0.3; 95% CI, 0.10–0.98).

A cohort of 676 526 female participants (median age, 56) in the Cancer Prevention Study II was recruited in 1982 from all over the United States (Calle *et al.*, 1995). By the end of 1989, 43 862 (6.5%) of the women had died. A total of 897 deaths from colon cancer occurred among 422 373 post-menopausal women who had not had cancer at entry to the study. The relative risk associated with any use of post-menopausal oestrogen therapy, adjusted for age, race, body mass index, parity, menopause, combined oral contraceptive use, dietary habits, exercise, smoking and aspirin use, was 0.71 (95% CI, 0.61–0.83). The risk reduction was strongest for women who were current users at the time of entry to the cohort (0.55; 95% CI, 0.40–0.76), and there was a significant trend of decreasing risk with increasing years of use (at entry) among all users (relative risk for users of > 11 years, 0.54; 95% CI, 0.39–0.76). No data on incidence were available.

A record linkage cohort study was carried out in Saskatchewan, Canada, between the Prescription Drug Plan Database (1976–87) and the Provincial Cancer Registry Database (1960–90) on all 33 003 resident women aged 43–49 (Risch & Howe, 1995). Of 32 973 women who did not have colorectal cancer at the beginning of the study, 230 developed this cancer. For users of post-menopausal oestrogen therapy, the age-adjusted relative risk was 1.3 (95% CI, 0.86–1.9) for colon cancer, 0.64 (95% CI, 0.33–1.2) for rectal cancer and 1.0 (95% CI, 0.74–1.5) for both together.

A cohort of 64 182 women was selected for follow-up within the Breast Cancer Detection Demonstration project between 1973 and 1980 in 27 cities of the United States (Troisi *et al.*, 1997). Telephone interviews were conducted between 1979 and 1986 with 61 434 women. The analyses were restricted to 33 779 post-menopausal women (41–80 years of age; mean age, 59) who completed the follow-up questionnaire between 1987 and 1989. After an average follow-up of 7.7 years, 313 cases of colorectal cancer were identified (84 from death certificates). Any use of post-menopausal oestrogen therapy was not related to the risk for colorectal cancer (age-adjusted relative risk, 0.99; 95% CI, 0.79–1.2). The relative risk for recent use of five or more years' duration was 0.75 (95% CI, 0.50–1.1). The risks were similar for colon cancer and rectal cancer. Eighty-four per cent of the person–years of post-menopausal oestrogen therapy use were accounted for by oestrogen use alone: the relative risks for any use of oestrogen alone were similar to those for any use of post-menopausal oestrogen therapy (relative risk, 1.1; 95% CI, 0.7–1.5 for colon; and 1.2; 95% CI, 0.7–2.3 for rectum).

2.6.3 Case–control studies

(a) Colorectal polyps

Potter et al. (1996) undertook a case–control study in Minnesota, United States, between 1991 and 1994 of cases in 219 women, aged 30–74, with colonoscopy-proven, pathology-confirmed, adenomatous polyps of the colon and rectum. Two control groups were selected: 438 women without polyps at colonoscopy and 247 community controls matched on age and postal code; the response rates of all three groups were around 65%. The multivariate relative risks for use of post-menopausal oestrogen therapy for fewer than five years, compared with no use, among post-menopausal women were 0.52 (0.32–0.85) in comparison with colonoscopy-negative controls and 0.74 (0.44–1.3) in comparison with community controls. For five or more years of use, the corresponding figures were 0.39 (0.23–0.67) and 0.61 (0.34–1.1).

Jacobson et al. (1995) studied patients with colorectal adenomatous polyps between 1986 and 1988 in New York, United States. The cases (128) were in cancer-free women aged 35–84 years in whom an adenoma was detected at the index colonoscopy. The 283 controls were cancer-free women with a normal index colonoscopy at the same institution as the cases. The adjusted relative risk associated with post-menopausal oestrogen therapy was 0.7 (95% CI, 0.3–1.2).

Chen et al. (1998) studied 187 women with colorectal polyps and 188 controls, aged 50–75 years, who were members of a prepaid health plan and underwent sigmoidoscopy in 1991–93. For women who used post-menopausal oestrogen therapy in the year before sigmoidoscopy relative to women who did not (37 cases and 38 controls), the relative risk adjusted for age, sigmoidoscopy date, physical activity, bone mass index, smoking and ethnicity was 0.57 (95% CI, 0.35–0.94). The risk for > 5 years of use (16 cases and 30 controls) was 0.49 (95% CI, 0.25–0.97).

(b) Colorectal cancer

Case–control studies of use of post-menopausal oestrogen therapy and the risks for cancers of the colon and rectum are summarized in Table 11.

A case–control study was conducted in 1976–77 in Washington State, United States, on 143 white women with colorectal cancer, aged 45–74 years, and 707 white women of

Table 11. Case–control studies of use of post-menopausal oestrogen therapy and colorectal cancer

Reference, country	No. of cases/ no. of controls	Type of controls	Type of use	Relative risk (RR; 95% confidence interval) (any versus no use)					Duration of use	Recency of use	Adjustment, coments
				Colon-rectum	Colon	Right colon	Left colon	Rectum			
Weiss et al. (1981), Washington, USA	143/707	Population	≤ 5 years ≥ 6 years	1.1 (0.7–1.9) 1.0 (0.6–1.6)	–	–	–	–	No trend	NR	Age
Potter & McMichael (1983), Adelaide, Australia	155/311	Population		–	0.8 (0.4–1.5)	–	–	1.5 (0.8–3.0)			Reproductive variables (diet had no effect); use of hormones other than COC
Davis et al. (1989), Canada	720/349	Cancer patients	Current users Past users	1.5 (0.8–2.7) 1.1 (0.7–1.9)	–	–	–	–	NR	NR	Age and parity No distinction possible between OT and COC use
Furner et al. (1989), Chicago, USA	90/208	Spouses		0.5 (0.27–0.90)	–	0.8 (0.27–2.6)	0.6 (0.27–1.3)	0.2 (0.03–0.77)	No trend	NR	Age, parity, hysterectomy
Fernandez et al. (1998), including data from Negri et al. (1989); Fernandez et al. (1996), Italy	1 536/3 110	Hospital		0.58 (0.44–0.76)	0.59 (0.43–0.82)	0.35 (0.15–0.80)	0.67 (0.44–1.0)	0.48 (0.31–0.75)	Significant (RR for ≥ 2 years' use, 0.46; 0.26–0.81)	RR for ≥ 10 years since last use, 0.52 (0.27–0.99)	Age, education, family history of cancer, body mass index, parity, menopause, COC and energy intake

Table 11 (contd)

Reference, country	No. of cases/ no. of controls	Type of controls	Type of use	Relative risk (RR; 95% confidence interval) (any versus no use)					Duration of use	Recency of use	Adjustment, comments
				Colon-rectum	Colon	Right colon	Left colon	Rectum			
Peters et al. (1990), Los Angeles, USA	327/327	Neighbours	< 5 years	–	1.3 (0.88–2.0)	1.4 (0.80–2.6)	1.2 (0.69–2.3)	–	No effect	NR	Family history of cancer, parity, menopause, exercise, fat, alcohol and calcium intake
			5–14 years		1.1 (0.64–1.8)	1.1 (0.47–2.6)	1.1 (0.55–2.2)				
			≥ 15 years		1.1 (0.58–1.9)	1.2 (0.51–2.8)	0.75 (0.30–1.8)				
Wu-Williams et al. (1991), North America	189/494 (North America)	Neighbours			2.1 p = 0.14	–	–	0.5 p = 0.23	NR; mostly short duration of use	NR	Use of 'other hormones' Unadjusted but unaltered by exercise, saturated fat intake and years in the USA Artificial menopause was a risk factor in China
	206/618 (China)				2.9 p = 0.01	–	–	1.3 p = 0.56			
Gerhardsson de Verdier & London (1992), Sweden	299/276	Population		–	0.6 (0.4–1.0)	0.4 (0.2–0.8)	1.0 (0.5–1.9)	0.7 (0.4–1.3)	No trend	NR	Age Hormone use included both OT and COC, but mostly OT
Jacobs et al. (1994), Seattle, USA	148/138	Population		–	0.60 (0.35–1.0)	0.46 (0.23–0.91)	0.74 (0.39–1.4)	–	Significant trend (RR ≥ 5 years' use, 0.47; 0.24–0.91)	RR of current users, 0.53 (0.29–0.96)	Age, vitamin intake and hysterectomy Greater protection for multiparous women

Table 11 (contd)

Reference, country	No. of cases/ no. of controls	Type of controls	Type of use	Relative risk (RR; 95% confidence interval) (any versus no use)					Duration of use	Recency of use	Adjustment, coments
				Colon-rectum	Colon	Right colon	Left colon	Rectum			
Newcomb & Storer (1995), Wisconsin, USA	694/1 622	Population	Unopposed oestrogen (recent use)	–	0.54 (0.34–0.88)	–	–	0.90 (0.46–1.76)	Significant trend (p = 0.002)	Lower RR for < 10 years since last use, 0.54 (0.36–0.80) for colon	Age, alcohol, body mass index, family history of cancer and sigmoidoscopy
			Any OT		0.73 (0.56–0.94)	0.43 (0.22–0.84) (recent use)	0.64 (0.39–1.0) (recent use)	1.2 (0.83–1.6)			
Kampman et al. (1997), USA	815/1 019	Members of medical care organization		–	0.82 (0.67–0.99)	NR	NR	–	No trend (RR ≥ 10 years' use, 0.86)	RR for recent use, 0.71 (0.56–0.89)	Age, family history of cancer, aspirin, energy intake, COC and exercise
Yood et al. (1998), Detroit, USA	60/143	Members of health maintenance organization	Current use	0.34 (0.11–0.99)	–	0.55 (0.14–2.2)	0.32 (0.30–1.7)	–	NR	NR	Age, race, reproductive variables, dietary habits and colonoscopy
			Past use	0.40 (0.12–1.4)							

NR, not reported; COC, combined oral contraceptives; OT, oestrogen therapy

the same ages drawn from a population survey in the area (Weiss *et al.*, 1981). Use of post-menopausal oestrogen therapy of any type was not related to cancer risk (age-adjusted relative risk, 1.1; 95% CI, 0.7–1.9 for ≤ 5 years' use; and 1.0; 95% CI, 0.6–1.6 for ≥ 6 years' use).

Potter and McMichael (1983) conducted a case–control study in Adelaide, Australia, between 1979 and 1980 on 155 cases of colorectal cancer (out of 212 eligible cases) and 311 control women selected from the local electoral roll. The relative risk, adjusted for reproductive variables, for use of oestrogen therapy of any type, apart from oral contraceptives, was 0.8 (95% CI, 0.4–1.5) for colon cancer and 1.5 (95% CI, 0.8–3.0) for rectal cancer.

A case–control study conducted in Alberta, Canada, between 1969 and 1973 included data on 528 cases of colon cancer, 192 of rectal cancer (i.e. 69% of identified colorectal cancers in the study area) and 349 control women aged 35 and more (Davis *et al.*, 1989). The controls were women with cancers at sites not associated with endocrine factors (chiefly cancers of the mouth and stomach). The estimated relative risk for use of exogenous hormones (including post-menopausal oestrogen therapy and combined oral contraceptives) among women over 50, as a surrogate for post-menopausal oestrogen therapy, adjusted for age and parity, was 1.5 (95% CI, 0.8–2.7) for current use and 1.1 (95% CI, 0.7–1.9) for past use.

Ninety women with colorectal cancer and 208 controls who were the wives of colorectal cancer patients were interviewed between 1980 and 1983 in Chicago, United States, representing 63% of the subjects initially contacted (Furner *et al.*, 1989). The relative risk associated with post-menopausal oestrogen therapy [not otherwise specified] adjusted for age, parity and hysterectomy was 0.5 (95% CI, 0.27–0.90). The inverse association was stronger for cancer of the rectum (relative risk, 0.2; 95% CI, 0.03–0.77; two cases) than for cancers of the right colon (0.8; 0.27–2.63; six cases) or left colon (0.6; 0.03–0.77; 12 cases). No trend in risk emerged with duration of post-menopausal oestrogen therapy.

A hospital-based case–control study conducted in Milan, Italy, between 1985 and 1992 (Negri *et al.*, 1989; Fernandez *et al.*, 1996) included 709 women with colon cancer (median age, 61 years) and 992 women in hospital for acute, non-digestive, non-hormone-related disorders. The relative risk for women who had ever used post-menopausal oestrogen therapy, adjusted for age, social class, family history of cancer, menarche and parity was 0.40 (95% CI, 0.25–0.66). The risk decreased with increasing duration of use (0.46 for ≤ 2 years; 0.25 for > 2 years of use). No consistent trend was observed with time since first or last use. Another case–control study conducted with a similar protocol in six Italian areas between 1992 and 1996 (Talamini *et al.*, 1998) included 537 women with colon cancer, 291 women with rectal cancer and 2081 control women in hospital for acute conditions unrelated to hormonal or gynaecological diseases. The relative risk for any use of post-menopausal oestrogen therapy, adjusted for age, centre, education, exercise and energy intake, was 0.6 (95% CI, 0.3–1.0) for rectal cancer and 1.0 (95% CI, 0.69–1.5) for colon cancer; however, only about 10% of post-menopausal women had had post-menopausal oestrogen therapy. A pooled analysis of the two Italian studies described by Fernandez *et al.* (1996) and Talamini *et al.* (1998) included 994 women with cancer of the colon and 542 with cancer of the rectum, in addition to 3110 hospital controls (Fernandez *et al.*, 1998). The relative risks for any use, adjusted for age, education, family history of cancer, body mass index, parity, menopause, combined oral contraceptive use and energy intake, were 0.59 (95% CI, 0.43–0.82) for colon cancer and 0.48 (95% CI, 0.31–0.75) for rectal cancer. The inverse association was stronger for cancer of the right colon (0.35; 0.15–0.80) than for that of the left colon (0.67; 0.44–1.03). Significant trends in risk by duration of use emerged for all subsites. The decrease in the relative risk associated with post-menopausal oestrogen therapy was greater 10 or more years after cessation of use (relative risk, 0.50 for colon and 0.54 for rectum) than earlier.

Peters *et al.* (1990) conducted a population-based case–control study in Los Angeles, United States, between 1983 and 1986. A total of 327 white women with colon cancer (out of 472 eligible cases) and 327 individually matched neighbourhood controls were interviewed. The relative risks, adjusted for age, family history of cancer, parity, meno-pause, exercise, fat, calcium and alcohol intake, for < 5, 5–14 and ≥ 15 years' duration of use, were 1.3 (95% CI, 0.88–2.0), 1.1 (95% CI, 0.64–1.8) and 1.0 (95% CI, 0.58–1.9), respectively. The risk estimates were similar for cancers of the right and left colon.

A population-based case–control study was conducted among Chinese women in western North America and China between 1981 and 1986 with a common protocol (Wu-Williams *et al.*, 1991). It included 395 women with colorectal cancer, 189 from North America and 206 from China, and 1112 age-matched controls, 494 and 618, respectively. The unadjusted relative risk for rectal cancer associated with the use of hormones other than combined oral contraceptives was 0.5 in North America and 1.3 in China (neither significant). The relative risk for colon cancer was 2.1 ($p = 0.14$) in North America and 2.9 ($p = 0.01$) in China. About 90% of the post-menopausal oestrogen therapy users had used hormones for one year or less.

A population-based case–control study was performed in Stockholm, Sweden, in 1986–88, which included 299 cases and 276 controls (i.e. about 80% of eligible subjects) (Gerhardsson de Verdier & London, 1992). The questionnaire used did not allow distinc-tion between post-menopausal oestrogen therapy and combined oral contraceptives. The age-adjusted relative risk for hormone use was 0.6 (95% CI, 0.4–1.0) for colon cancer, 0.7 (95% CI, 0.4–1.3) for rectal cancer, 0.4 (95% CI, 0.4–1.0) for cancer of the right colon and 1.0 (95% CI, 0.5–1.9) for cancer of the left colon.

Jacobs *et al.* (1994) conducted a case–control study among women aged 30–62 years in Seattle, United States, between 1985 and 1989. It included 193 new cases of colon cancer (out of 295 eligible cases) and 194 controls (out of 227 eligible controls) selected by random-digit dialling. Among post-menopausal women aged ≥ 45 years (i.e. 148 cases and 138 controls), the relative risk associated with use of post-menopausal oestrogen therapy, adjusted for age, vitamin intake and hysterectomy, was 0.60 (95% CI, 0.35–1.0) for colon cancer, with estimates of 0.47 (95% CI, 0.24–0.91) for ≥ 5 years' use and 0.53 (95% CI, 0.29–0.96) for current use.

A case–control study was conducted between 1990 and 1991 in Wisconsin, United States (Newcomb & Storer, 1995). After exclusion of pre-menopausal women, 694 women with colorectal cancer (480 colon and 214 rectum) and 1622 control women (randomly selected from lists of licensed drivers and Medicare beneficiaries) were included. The relative risk for any use of post-menopausal oestrogen therapy, adjusted for age, alcohol, body mass index, family history of cancer and history of sigmoidoscopy, was 0.73 (95% CI, 0.56–0.94) for colon cancer and 1.2 (95% CI, 0.83–1.6) for rectal cancer. Among recent users, the relative risk for colon cancer was 0.54 for both use of post-menopausal oestrogen therapy of any type and use of oestrogens only. The inverse association was stronger for recent use ($p < 0.001$).

Kampman et al. (1997) conducted a case–control study between 1992 and 1995 in the United States among women aged 30–79 who were members of a medical care programme, covering 894 cases of colon cancer (out of 1521 eligible cases) and 1120 control women (63% of those who were contacted). The relative risk for colon cancer (adjusted for age, family history of cancer, aspirin and energy intake) of post-menopausal women (i.e. 815 cases and 1019 controls) for use of oestrogen therapy for longer than three months was 0.82 (95% CI, 0.67–0.99). The inverse assocation was confined to recent users (i.e. < 1 year before diagnosis) (relative risk, 0.71; 95% CI, 0.56–0.89). No trend with duration of post-menopausal oestrogen therapy was observed (relative risk for ≥ 10 years of use, 0.86). The reduced relative risk associated with post-menopausal oestrogen therapy use did not appear to be explained by confounding factors such as dietary habits, body mass index or physical activity. Although the number of routine sigmoidoscopies did not differ significantly between women who had ever and never had post-menopausal oestrogen therapy, those who had used it had undergone more sigmoidoscopies because of symptoms.

A case–control study was conducted among members of a large health maintenance organization in Detroit, United States. The preliminary results (Yood et al., 1998) on 60 women with colorectal cancer and 143 population controls showed an adjusted relative risk associated with post-menopausal oestrogen therapy of 0.34 (95% CI, 0.11–0.99) for current users and 0.40 (95% CI, 0.12–1.40) for past users.

2.7 Cutaneous malignant melanoma

2.7.1 Descriptive studies

The incidence of melanoma has increased at a rate of 3–7% per year in most Caucasian populations in the last decades (Armstrong & Kricker, 1994). Changes in recreational patterns of exposure to the sun and, to some extent, increasing detection account for the observed rises. The incidence rates are similar in men and women, although a female excess is found in some countries, e.g. the United Kingdom and the Nordic countries.

Cohort and case–control studies of cutaneous and ocular malignant melanoma and post-menopausal oestrogen therapy are summarized in Table 12.

Table 12. Studies on use of post-menopausal oestrogen therapy (OT) or combined hormonal therapy (HT) and cutaneous malignant melanoma

Reference, country	No. of cases/ no. of controls	Type of controls	Type of use	RR (95% CI) for any versus no use	Duration of use	Recency of use	Adjustment, comments
Cohort							
Persson et al. (1996), Sweden	22 597 (60 cases)		Any OT HT	0.9 (0.7–1.1) 0.6 (0.3–1.1)	NR	NR	Age 13 years' follow-up. Standardized mortality ratio, 0.5 (95% CI, 0.2–1.0) No association with non-melanomatous skin cancer
Case–control							
Holly et al. (1983) Seattle, USA	87/863	Population	1–3 years 4–7 years ≥ 8 years	1.1 0.85 1.0	No effect	NR	Age RR very similar for 61 cases of SSM
Lew et al. (1983), Massachusetts, USA	111/107	Friends of cases	–	–	–	–	No difference in OT use
Beral et al. (1984), Sydney, Australia	287/574	Hospital and population		1.4 (0.78–2.6)	NR	NR	Age
Holman et al. (1984), Western Australia	276/276	Population		1.5 (0.87–2.7)	No trend	NR	Age and residence RR very similar for SSM (1.9; 0.88–4.2)
Gallagher et al. (1985), Canada	361/361	Members of health plans	< 1 year 1–4 years ≥ 5 years	1.0 1.0 0.9	No trend	No effect	Age, education, phenotype and freckling RR similar for SSM
Green & Bain (1985), Queensland, Australia	91/91	Population		–	–	–	Age 11 cases and 11 controls reported use of hormonal therapy other than COC

Table 12 (contd)

Reference, country	No. of cases/ no. of controls	Type of controls	Type of use	RR (95% CI) for any versus no use	Duration of use	Recency of use	Adjustment, comments
Østerlind et al. (1988), Denmark	151/297	Population	Oestrogen, unopposed	1.3 (0.8–2.1)	No trend (RR for > 7 years' use, 1.2; 0.7–2.2)	NR	Age, naevi and sunbathing No difference in risk between histological subtypes
			Oestrogen, opposed	1.5 (0.8–2.8)			
Holly et al. (1994), San Francisco, USA	452/935	Population	Conjugated oestrogens, after oophorectomy	2.4 (1.1–5.2)	No trend	NR	Age and education but unaltered by phenotype and sun Similar risks for SSM
			Any OT, after natural menopause	0.88 (0.50–1.6)			
			Hysterectomy with no or one ovary removed	2.0 (0.8–5.0)			
			Any OT after bilateral oophorectomy	2.2 (1.0–4.7)			
Westerdahl et al. (1996), Sweden	403/707	Population	HT, any	1.0 (0.5–1.8)	No trend	No effect of age at first or last use	Phenotype, naevi and sunburns Risks were similar at different anatomical sites
Ocular melanoma							
Hartge et al. (1989), Philadelphia, USA	214/209	Detached retina		2.0 (1.2–3.0)	No effect (RR for ≥ 6 years' use, 2.2; 0.9–5.8)	NR	Age and oophorectomy Similar risks for users of conjugated oestrogens and users of other formulations

RR, relative risk; CI, confidence interval; NR, not reported; SSM, superficial spreading melanoma; COC, combined oral contraceptives

2.7.2   Cohort studies

One cohort investigation (see section 2.6.2) provided information on post-menopausal oestrogen therapy and the risk for cutaneous malignant melanoma (Persson *et al.*, 1996), expressed as incidence and mortality rates, among 22 597 Swedish women. After 13 years of follow-up, 60 new cases and eight deaths from cutaneous malignant melanoma were recorded. The age-adjusted standardized incidence ratios for any use of post-menopausal oestrogen therapy were 0.9 (95% CI, 0.7–1.1) for a diagnosis of cutaneous malignant melanoma and 0.5 (95% CI, 0.2–1.0) for death from this condition.

2.7.3   Case–control studies

Holly *et al.* (1983) conducted a case–control study in Seattle, United States, between 1976 and 1979 of 87 women aged 37–74 years (out of 124 eligible) with histologically confirmed cutaneous malignant melanoma, 61 of whom had superficial spreading melanomas. The controls were 863 age-matched women (response rate, 93%), who represented a random sample of the population from which the cases were derived. The age-adjusted relative risks for any use of post-menopausal oestrogen therapy among women ≥ 45 were close to unity: 1.1, 0.85 and 1.0 for 1–3, 4–7 and ≥ 8 years of use, respectively, for all histological types combined. Very similar risks were found when the analysis was restricted to women with superficial spreading melanomas (1.1, 1.1 and 0.98, respectively).

Lew *et al.* (1983) studied 111 women with cutaneous malignant melanoma in Massachusetts, United States, during 1978–79 and 107 controls chosen among friends of the cases. No difference in the frequency of post-menopausal oestrogen therapy use was reported between cases and controls, but detailed data were not shown.

Beral *et al.* (1984) investigated 287 women aged 15–54 years in Sydney, Australia, between 1978 and 1980, who had received a diagnosis of cutaneous malignant melanoma (new and prevalent cases) between 1974 and 1980, and 574 age-matched controls, who were hospital patients for the new cases and from the population for prevalent cases. Post-menopausal oestrogen therapy use was slightly more frequent among cases (6.6%) than controls (4.7%; unadjusted relative risk, 1.4; 95% CI, 0.78–2.6).

In another case–control study carried out in Western Australia between 1980 and 1981 (Holman *et al.*, 1984), the cases were those of 276 women under the age of 80 (mean age, 45) with histologically proven pre-invasive or invasive cutaneous malignant melanoma (out of 373 eligible women). The controls were 276 age-matched women extracted from the electoral roll (out of 458 sampled women). Fourteen percent of subjects had ever taken hormone tablets or injections containing an oestrogen but no progestogen; of these, 59% had taken them for menopausal symptoms. The relative risk associated with any post-menopausal oestrogen therapy, adjusted for age and area of residence, were 1.5 (95% CI, 0.87–2.7) for all cutaneous malignant melanoma and 1.9 (95% CI, 0.88–4.2) for superficial spreading melanoma. No trend in risk with duration of use was seen.

Gallagher *et al.* (1985) conducted a case–control study in western Canada between 1979 and 1981 that included 361 women aged 20–79 years (out of 412 eligible cases) with cutaneous malignant melanoma, of whom 269 had superficial spreading melanoma, and

361 age-matched control women selected from medical plan listings (59% response rate). No association was found with any post-menopausal oestrogen therapy; the relative risks, adjusted for age, education, skin colour, hair colour and freckling, were 1.0 for < 1 or 1–4 years of use and 0.9 for ≥ 5 years of use. The risks for superficial spreading melanoma were identical.

Green and Bain (1985) studied the effect of female hormones on the incidence of cutaneous malignant melanoma in Queensland, Australia, between 1979 and 1980 in 91 women aged 15–81 years (92% of eligible women) with a first cutaneous malignant melanoma; lentigo maligna melanomas were not included. The control women consisted of a random sample of 91 women drawn from the electoral rolls, who were matched with cases by age and residence. The frequency of use of hormones other than oral contraceptives was low, and it was the same in cases and controls.

A case–control study on cutaneous malignant melanoma was carried out in Denmark between 1982 and 1985 (Østerlind et al., 1988). The case series consisted of 280 women aged 20–79 with newly diagnosed cutaneous malignant melanoma, of whom 207 had superficial spreading melanoma (out of 304 eligible women); lentigo maligna melanomas were not included. The controls consisted of 536 women selected from the National Population Register (out of 677 originally identified). Among post-menopausal women (i.e. 151 cases and 297 controls), the relative risk for cutaneous malignant melanoma among users of unopposed post-menopausal oestrogen therapy (adjusted for age, naevi and sunbathing) was 1.3 (95% CI, 0.8–2.1). For users of post-menopausal oestrogen therapy of any type, the relative risk was 1.1 (95% CI, 0.7–1.7). No trend in risk with increasing duration of use was found (relative risk for ≥ 7 years of use, 1.2; 95% CI, 0.7–2.2). There was no difference in risk for subtypes of melanoma, including superficial spreading melanoma.

Holly et al. (1994) carried out a case–control study of cutaneous malignant melanoma between 1981 and 1987 in San Francisco, United States, among 452 white women aged 25–59, 355 of whom had superficial spreading melanoma; 79% of those eligible were interviewed. Random-digit dialling was used to identify 935 control women of the same age (77% of those contacted). The relative risks associated with post-menopausal oestrogen therapy in pre-menopausal or naturally menopaused women were close to 1.0: for women with a natural menopause, the relative risk was 0.88 (95% CI, 0.50–1.6). The relative risk of women who had undergone a hysterectomy without removal of both ovaries was 2.0 (95% CI, 0.85–4.5), and that for women who had had bilateral oophorectomy was 2.2 (95% CI, 1.0–4.7). No difference was found according to the dose of conjugated oestrogens.

Westerdahl et al. (1996) carried out a case–control study on exposure to hormones in southern Sweden between 1988 and 1990. The cases were those of 403 women with a first histopathological diagnosis of cutaneous malignant melanoma, and the 707 age-matched control women were randomly selected from the National Population Registry. Post-menopausal oestrogen therapy had been used by 13% of the cases and 14% of the controls, giving a relative risk, adjusted for phenotype, naevi and sunburns, of 1.0 (95% CI, 0.5–1.8). No associations were found between cutaneous malignant melanoma and duration of post-menopausal oestrogen therapy, age at first use or age at latest use. Consistent results were found for cutaneous malignant melanoma at different anatomical sites.

2.8   Intraocular malignant melanoma

A case–control study carried out between 1979 and 1980 in Philadelphia, United States, of ocular melanoma included 239 women (mean age, 58) with intraocular malignant melanoma (out of 444 eligible cases) and 223 control matched by age and race (Hartge *et al.*, 1989). The controls were patients with detached retinas. The relative risk for post-menopausal women who reported using oestrogen therapy, adjusted for age and history of oophorectomy, was 2.0 (95% CI, 1.2–3.0) and that for ≥ 6 years of use was 2.2 (95% CI, 0.9–5.8) (Table 12).

2.9   Thyroid cancer

2.9.1   *Descriptive studies*

Cancer of the thyroid is a rare, very heterogeneous disease. The rate of mortality from this cancer has been falling slowly, whereas the incidence has been increasing in most developed countries over the last three decades (Franceschi & La Vecchia, 1994). The incidence rates are two- to threefold higher for women than for men, and the difference is greatest for well-differentiated papillary carcinomas for women aged 25–44 (Franceschi & Dal Maso, 1998). A positive correlation between parity and the incidence of thyroid cancer was reported from individual data on all (1.1 million) Norwegian women born 1935–69 (Kravdal *et al.*, 1991).

2.9.2   *Case–control studies*

These studies are summarized in Table 13.

The case–control study of McTiernan *et al.* (1984) was carried out in Seattle, United States, between 1980 and 1981. The cases were those of 183 women aged 18–80 with papillary, follicular and mixed thyroid carcinomas, diagnosed between 1974 and 1979, who represented 65% of those identified through the cancer surveillance system of western Washington, United States. The controls were women aged 18–80 identified through random-digit dialling; of 478 eligible controls, 394 were interviewed. The majority of the patients and controls (87%) were white. Among women over 30 years of age (153 cases and 281 controls), the age-adjusted relative risk for any use of post-menopausal oestrogen therapy (34% of cases and 27% controls) was 1.4 (95% CI, 0.89–2.3) for thyroid cancer overall and 1.9 (95% CI, 1.1–3.4) for tumours of the papillary type. The relative risk for ≥ 3 years' duration of use was 1.2 for all thyroid cancers and 1.6 for papillary thyroid cancer. The association was slightly stronger when only women whose tumours were found by a physician (rather than by the woman herself) were included.

A case–control study carried out in Connecticut, United States, between 1978 and 1980 by Ron *et al.* (1987) included 159 women aged 20–76 with thyroid cancer, i.e. 80% of those identified through the Connecticut Tumor Registry. Tumour slides were reviewed centrally. The controls were 285 women frequency-matched to the cases on age. Random-digit

Table 13. Case–control studies on use of oestrogen therapy and thyroid cancer

Reference, country	No. of cases/ no. of controls	Type of controls	RR (95% CI) for any versus no use	Duration of use	Adjustment, comments
McTiernan et al. (1984), Seattle, USA	153/281	Population	All 1.4 (0.89–2.3) Papillary 1.9 (1.1–3.4)	No trend (RR for ≥ 3 years' use, 1.2)	Age Risk slightly higher for cases found by physicians
Ron et al. (1987), Connecticut, USA	71/123	Population, ≥ 35 years	0.5 (NS)	NR	Age, parity, radiotherapy and benign thyroid disease
Franceschi et al. (1990), Italy	71/94	Hospital	0.3 (0.1–1.1)	NR	Age and residence
Kolonel et al. (1990), Hawaii, USA	140/328	Population	0.9 (0.5–1.7)	NR	Age and ethnic group
Levi et al. (1993b), Switzerland	91/306	Hospital	1.8 (0.6–5.2)	NR	Age and history of benign thyroid disease
Hallquist et al. (1994), northern Sweden	123/140		1.1 (0.3–3.7)	NR	Age
Galanti et al. (1996), Norway and Sweden	74/134	Population, post-menopausal	0.98 (0.39–2.5)	No effect (RR for > 2 years' duration, 1.2; 0.25–5.3)	Age and parity

RR, relative risk; CI, confidence interval; NS, not significant; NR, not reported

dialling was used to select controls under 65 years of age, while controls over 65 years were chosen from the Medicare roster. Post-menopausal oestrogen therapy had ever been used by 8/71 cases and 23/123 controls over the age of 35. The relative risk, adjusted for age, parity and history of radiotherapy and benign thyroid diseases was 0.5 (not significant).

Franceschi *et al.* (1990) conducted a case–control study in the provinces of Pordenone, Padua and Milan, northern Italy, between 1986 and 1992, which included 165 women under 75 years old with newly diagnosed, histologically confirmed thyroid cancer. The control women, frequency-matched by age to the cases, were 214 in-patients identified in the same network of hospitals with diagnoses of acute, non-neoplastic, non-hormonal diseases. The response rates exceeded 95% among both cases and controls. All of the study subjects were interviewed during their hospital stay. Among post-menopausal women, any use of oestrogen therapy was reported by five of 71 cases and 17 of 94 controls (relative risk adjusted for age and area of residence, 0.3; 95% CI, 0.1–1.1).

A case–control study of thyroid cancer was conducted between 1980 and 1987 in Hawaii, United States (Kolonel *et al.*, 1990), and consisted of 140 women from five ethnic groups, 18 years or older, with thyroid cancer identified through the Hawaii Tumour Registry. The histological type of the tumours was reviewed centrally. The controls were 328 women, age-matched to cases, selected from among people participating in a con-current health surveillance programme. Questionnaires were administered at home, with response rates of 79% for cases and 74% for controls. The relative risk for women who had ever used post-menopausal oestrogen therapy (15% of control women), adjusted for age and ethnic group, was 0.9 (95% CI, 0.5–1.7).

Levi *et al.* (1993b) studied risk factors for thyroid cancer in the Canton of Vaud, Switzerland, between 1988 and 1990. The cases were those of 91 women, aged 12–72, with histologically confirmed thyroid cancer. The controls were 306 women admitted to the same hospital as the cases for acute conditions. Post-menopausal oestrogen therapy had ever been used by seven of 91 cases and 31 of 306 controls. The relative risk, adjusted for age and history of benign thyroid diseases, was 1.8 (95% CI, 0.6–5.2).

Hallquist *et al.* (1994) conducted a case–control study on thyroid cancer in northern Sweden between 1980 and 1989. The cases were those of 123 women, aged 20–70, with histopathologically confirmed thyroid cancer, identified through the Swedish Cancer Registry. The controls were 240 women randomly drawn from the National Population Registry of the same counties as the cases. All of the study subjects returned a mailed questionnaire. Use of post-menopausal oestrogen therapy was uncommon (five cases and nine controls) and unrelated to the risk for thyroid cancer; the age-adjusted relative risk was 1.1 (95% CI, 0.3–3.7).

Galanti *et al.* (1996) carried out a case–control study on thyroid cancer in northern Norway and central Sweden between 1985 and 1993. The cases were those of 191 women aged 17–72 years with histologically confirmed papillary, follicular or mixed carcinoma of the thyroid gland. The controls were 341 age-matched women selected from the national population registries. Information was based on a mailed questionnaire, with a response rate of over 90%. Among post-menopausal women, use of any type of oestrogen therapy was reported by 13 of 74 cases and 24 of 134 controls; the relative risk, adjusted for age and parity, was 0.98 (95% CI, 0.39–2.5). The relative risk for use for more than two years was 1.2 (95% CI, 0.25–5.3).

2.10 Other cancers

La Vecchia *et al.* (1994) assessed the role of female hormones in gastric cancer in Milan, Italy, between 1985 and 1993. The cases were those of 229 post-menopausal women with newly diagnosed, histologically confirmed gastric cancer. The controls were 614 post-menopausal women in hospital for acute, non-neoplastic, non-digestive tract conditions. The relative risk for users of post-menopausal oestrogen therapy, adjusted for age, education, family history of cancer and dietary habits, was 0.54 (95% CI, 0.3–1.1).

Chow *et al.* (1995) studied 165 cases of renal-cell cancer in women aged 20–79 and 227 age- and frequency-matched population controls in Minnesota, United States, between 1988 and 1990. Among post-menopausal women (134 cases and 173 controls), the relative risk for any use of post-menopausal oestrogen therapy, adjusted for age, smoking and body mass index, was 1.8 (95% CI, 1.1–3.0). There was no trend with duration of use.

Lindblad *et al.* (1995) evaluated the effect of exogenous hormones on the incidence of renal-cell cancer in Australia, Denmark, Germany, Sweden and the United States during 1989–91. The cases were those of 608 women aged 20–79 with histologically confirmed renal-cell cancer identified mainly through local cancer registries. The controls were 766 women sampled from local residential lists and frequency-matched by age to the cancer cases. The relative risk of post-menopausal oestrogen therapy users, adjusted for age, smoking and body mass index, was 1.0 (95% CI, 0.8–1.4). For > 7 years of use, the relative risk was 1.2 (95% CI, 0.7–2.0). The risk did not vary with the age at starting post-menopausal oestrogen therapy.

In the record-linkage study of a cohort of 22 597 Swedish women to whom post-menopausal oestrogen therapy had ever been prescribed (Persson *et al.*, 1996), a 13-year follow-up showed the following standardized incidence ratios for cancer: vulva/vagina, 1.2 (95% CI, 0.7–1.8); pancreas, 1.1 (95% CI, 0.9–1.4); brain, 0.8 (95% CI, 0.6–1.0); lung, 1.0 (95% CI, 0.8–1.2); urinary bladder, 0.9 (95% CI, 0.7–1.1); other skin cancers, 0.9 (95% CI, 0.7–1.3); endocrine glands other than thyroid, 1.0 (95% CI, 0.8–1.3) and connective tissue, 1.6 (95% CI, 1.0–2.4).

3. Studies of Cancer in Experimental Animals

3.1 Studies reviewed previously

The conclusions with regard to carcinogenicity in experimental animals for oestrogens used in post-menopausal oestrogen therapy in the previous monograph (IARC, 1979) are summarized below.

Conjugated oestrogens (Premarin®) were tested in only one experiment in rats by oral administration. The data were insufficient to evaluate the carcinogenicity of this compound.

Oestradiol and its esters were tested in mice, rats, hamsters, guinea-pigs and monkeys by subcutaneous injection or implantation and in mice by oral administration. Subcutaneous administration of oestradiol resulted in increased incidences of mammary, pituitary, uterine, cervical, vaginal and lymphoid tumours and interstitial-cell tumours of the testis in mice. In rats, there was an increased incidence of mammary and/or pituitary tumours. In hamsters, a high incidence of malignant kidney tumours occurred in intact and castrated males and in ovariectomized females, but not in intact females. In guinea-pigs, diffuse fibromyomatous uterine and abdominal lesions were observed. Oral administration of oestradiol to mice led to an increased incidence of mammary tumours. Subcutaneous injections to neonatal mice resulted in precancerous and cancerous cervical and vaginal lesions in later life and an increased incidence of mammary tumours.

Oestriol was tested by subcutaneous implantation in castrated mice and in rats and hamsters. It increased the incidence and accelerated the appearance of mammary tumours in both male and female mice and produced kidney tumours in hamsters.

Oestrone was tested in mice by oral administration; in mice, rats and hamsters by subcutaneous injection and implantation and in mice by skin painting. Its administration resulted in an increased incidence of mammary tumours in mice; in pituitary, adrenal and mammary tumours, as well as bladder tumours in association with stones, in rats and in renal tumours in both castrated and intact male hamsters.

Oestrone benzoate increased the incidence of mammary tumours in mice following its subcutaneous injection.

3.2   New studies of oestrogens used in post-menopausal oestrogen therapy

3.2.1   *Conjugated oestrogens*

(a)   *Subcutaneous implantation*

Hamster: Groups of eight or nine adult, castrated, male Syrian golden hamsters, 50–55 days of age, were administered equilin or d-equilenin by subcutaneous implantation of a pure pellet (20 ± 1.4 mg) in the shoulder region; to maintain constant levels, the pellets were reimplantated at three-month intervals. The mean daily absorption of equilin and d-equilenin was 147 ± 22 µg and 145 ± 15 µg, respectively. After nine months of treatment, renal adenocarcinomas were detected microscopically in frozen serial sections (at least 25–30 sections from each kidney) stained histochemically for esterase. Equilin produced renal carcinoma in 6/8 hamsters (number of tumours per animal, 5.5 ± 0.9), whereas no detectable tumours were found in nine hamsters after d-equilenin treatment (Li *et al.*, 1983). [The Working Group noted the small number of animals, that only a single dose was used and that only the kidney was examined microscopically.]

Groups of six to eight adult, castrated, male Syrian golden hamsters (weighing 85–95 g) were implanted with pellets containing deconjugated hormones designed to provide absorption of 111 ± 11 µg oestrogen per day. Additional pellets were implanted every 2.5 months. The duration of treatment was nine months. Renal tumours were detected in frozen sections stained for nonspecific esterase activity (Li *et al.*, 1995). The incidence in untreated controls was not reported; historically, it was 0 under these experimental conditions (Liehr *et al.*, 1986a). All animals developed microscopic renal carcinomas. The numbers of tumours in the two kidneys combined were 15 ± 3 in animals given oestrone, 18 ± 1 in those given equilin plus d-equilenin and 16 ± 2 in those given Premarin®.

(b) Administration with known carcinogens

Rat: In a study reported in more detail in the monograph on 'Post-menopausal oestrogen–progestogen therapy', one group of seven ovariectomized rats treated with 7,12-dimethylbenz[*a*]anthracene (DMBA) received Premarin® at a concentration of 18.75 mg/kg diet (ppm) for 285 days. Mammary tumours occurred in 0/7 ovariectomized controls given DMBA, 6/7 intact controls given DMBA and 5/7 ovariectomized rats given both DMBA and Premarin® (Sakamoto *et al.*, 1997).

3.2.2 Oestradiol

(a) Oral administration

Mouse: Groups of 200–227 female C3H/HeJ mice, six weeks of age, with a high titre of antibodies to the mouse mammary tumour virus (MTV+) factor were fed diets containing 0, 100, 1000 or 5000 μg/kg diet (ppb) oestradiol for 104 weeks. Interim kills were carried out at 26, 52 and 78 weeks, and all surviving animals were killed at 104 weeks. At that time, the incidence of cervical adenosis was increased in 8/20 mice at 1000 ppb and 3/6 at 5000 ppb, and the incidence of uterine adenocarcinomas was increased in the latter group (5/207 compared with 0/227 controls). Mammary hyperplastic alveolar nodules were increased by this dose, from 0/57 in controls to 5/78 at weeks 40–65, 3/29 in controls to 5/19 at weeks 66–91 and 6/50 in controls to 6/17 at weeks 92–105; the time to development of mammary adenocarcinomas was also shortened, the tumour incidences being 4/91 in controls and 5/93 at the high dose at weeks 0–39, 15/57 in controls and 34/78 at the high dose at weeks 40–65, 13/29 in controls and 11/19 at the high dose at weeks 66–91 and 19/50 in controls and 8/17 at the high dose at weeks 92–105 (Highman *et al.*, 1980).

(b) Subcutaneous and/or intramuscular administration

Rat: Groups of 2–16 female Fischer 344 rats, seven weeks of age, were each injected subcutaneously with 5 mg oestradiol dipropionate once every two weeks for 13 weeks. Treated animals were killed at two-week intervals during the study. Ten untreated female rats were used as controls, five rats being killed at week 7 and at week 13. No pituitary tumour was observed in control animals, but pituitary adenomas were observed in 1/2 treated animals killed at week 5 and 11/12 killed at week 7, and carcinomas were observed in 1/12 rats killed at week 7, 6/6 at week 9, 4/4 at week 11 and 16/16 at week 13 (Satoh *et al.*, 1997).

(c)   Subcutaneous implantation

Rat: A group of 21 intact ACI rats, 61–63 days of age, received subcutaneous implants of Silastic tubing containing 27.5 mg crystalline oestradiol. A group of three untreated females served as controls. Treatment with oestradiol resulted in rapid development of palpable mammary tumours, which were first observed 99 days after treatment; 100% of the treated group developed tumours within 197 days. The mean time to appearance of the first palpable tumour was 145 ± 26 days. All of the mammary tumours were classified as carcinomas, and invasive features were observed. The average concentration of circulating oestradiol in the serum of treated animals at the time of killing was 185 pg/mL. Mammary tumours were not observed in intact controls or in 11 ovariectomized female rats treated at 45 days of age with oestradiol for 140 days. Intact and ovariectomized rats had similar incidences of oestradiol-induced pituitary tumours (Shull *et al.*, 1997).

Hamster: Male Syrian golden hamsters were orchiectomized at seven weeks of age; then, four weeks later, they received implants every three months of pellets containing 20 mg oestradiol. After 5.3 months, renal-cell dysplasia and infiltrating and non-infiltrating renal carcinoma were observed in 5/5 oestradiol-treated animals. No tumour was observed in untreated control hamsters (Goldfarb & Pugh, 1990).

Li *et al.* (1983) reported renal carcinomas in 6/6 castrated male hamsters treated similarly with pellets of 20 mg oestradiol for 8.3 months.

(d)   Administration with known carcinogens

Mouse: Groups of virgin female Swiss mice, 12–13 weeks of age, receive no treatment (10 mice), beeswax-impregnated cotton threads inserted into the cervix (10 mice), 0.1 mL olive oil weekly by injection (4 mice), an intracervical insertion of beeswax-impregnated threads containing approximately 600 µg 3-methylcholanthrene (MCA) and weekly injections of 0, 0.01, 0.1, 5 or 50 µg oestradiol for 16 weeks (18–25 mice), insertion of beeswax-impregnated threads and weekly injections of 0.01, 0.1, 5 and 50 µg oestradiol throughout the period of observation (6–9 mice) or weekly injections of 0.01, 0.1, 5 and 50 µg oestradiol alone (5–8 mice). Placement of thread containing MCA resulted in the emergence of precancerous and cancerous lesions in the cervical epithelium. Weekly administration of oestradiol resulted in incidences of cervical squamous-cell carcinomas of 16/24, 16/26, 10/18 and 8/19 at the four doses, respectively, as compared with 16/21 mice given only MCA by the same regimen. The decrease in the incidence of carcinomas was significant ($p < 0.05$) with the high dose of oestradiol. The occurrence of hyperplastic and dysplastic changes was not correlated with treatment (Das *et al.*, 1988). [The Working Group noted that the effect could have been due to interference with the metabolism of MCA.]

Groups of 30 or 31 female ICR mice, 10 weeks of age, were given 10 mg/kg bw *N*-methyl-*N*-nitrosourea (MNU) by intravaginal instillation once a week for three weeks and then fed a diet containing 0 or 5 ppm oestradiol for 20 weeks, starting one week after the last exposure to MNU; a third group of 31 mice was given oestradiol in the diet, and a fourth group of 15 mice received basal diet. At the termination of the experiment at week 23, the incidence of endometrial adenocarcinomas in the groups receiving both MNU and oestradiol (15/31) was significantly higher ($p = 0.001$) than that in the group given MNU alone (2/29) and significantly higher ($p = 0.001$) than that given oestradiol alone (7/31). The incidence of endometrial preneoplastic lesions in the group receiving oestradiol alone was 48%. No endometrial lesions or carcinomas were observed in the 15 controls on basal diet. Small numbers of squamous-cell carcinomas and preneoplastic lesions (dysplasia and hyperplasia) were also seen in the uterine cervix of mice given MNU alone or MNU plus oestradiol (Niwa *et al.*, 1991). [The Working Group noted that no statistical comparison was presented between the untreated controls and the group receiving oestradiol alone.]

Groups of 30 female ICR mice, 10 weeks of age, were given 10 mg/kg bw MNU into the left uterine corpus and normal saline into the right. One week later, the animals received a diet containing 0 or 5 ppm oestradiol for 30 weeks. At that time, the incidence of endometrial adenocarcinomas in the group given MNU plus oestradiol (8/24) was higher than that in mice given MNU alone (3/26), but the difference was not statistically significant. The incidence of preneoplastic endometrial lesions (atypical and adenomatous hyperplasia) was somewhat increased in the group given MNU plus oestradiol in comparison with those given MNU alone (Niwa *et al.*, 1993).

Groups of 24–73 female ICR mice, 10 weeks of age, were fed a diet containing 0 or 5 ppm oestradiol from the beginning of the experiment up to 16 weeks and an intravaginal instillation of 10 mg/kg bw MNU once a week for three weeks from week 4 (73 mice), oestradiol only (41 mice), MNU only (41 mice) or were untreated (24 mice). Mice from each group were killed and necropsied at weeks 8, 12, 16, 23 and 30. Oestradiol induced cystic glandular hyperplasia and adenomatous and atypical hyperplasia of the endometrium, and MNU induced adenomatous and atypical hyperplasia. Oestradiol did not induce endometrial carcinoma. Data presented in bar graphs indicate that the incidence of endometrial adenocarcinoma was approximately 10% in the mice given MNU alone and approximately 30% in those given MNU plus oestradiol [no statistics specified] (Niwa *et al.*, 1996).

Three groups of 25–29 CD-1 mice, 10 weeks of age and in persistent oestrous, were given either a single intrauterine administration of polyethylene glycol, 12.5 mg/kg bw *N*-ethyl-*N*-nitrosourea (ENU) dissolved in polyethylene glycol or ENU in the same manner plus subcutaneously implanted oestradiol pellets one week before ENU administration, the pellets being renewed after eight weeks of the experiment. At termination of the experiment at week 15 after ENU treatment, all surviving mice were killed for assessment of proliferative uterine lesions. All groups had endometrial hyperplasia, the severity being greatest in mice given oestradiol plus ENU. The incidence of adenocarcinomas in this group (20/29) was significantly greater ($p < 0.01$) than that in mice given the vehicle (0/25) or in mice given ENU alone (0/29) (Takahashi *et al.*, 1996).

Rat: Groups of 19 female Sprague-Dawley rats were ovariectomized at 60 days of age and given a single dose of 0 or 0.25 mg MNU by vaginal instillation, followed one week later by subcutaneous implantation of long-term release Silastic pellets containing

5 mg/mL oestradiol in sesame oil. After 16 months, an increase in the incidence of benign vaginal stromal polyps (4/19) was found in the MNU plus oestradiol group. No vaginal polyps were seen in groups given either MNU alone (0/19) or oestradiol alone (0/17). A number of non-neoplastic changes also seen in the vagina and uterus were due to oestradiol treatment either with or without MNU (Sheehan *et al.*, 1982).

Groups of 29–30 female Sprague-Dawley rats, 50 days of age, received an intravenous injection of 50 mg/kg bw MNU and, 10 days later, subcutaneous injections of 20 µg oestradiol, 4 mg progesterone, 20 µg oestradiol plus 4 mg progesterone or sesame oil on five days a week for 40 days. A further group were ovariectomized at 60 days of age and received no further treatment. Administration of oestradiol delayed the appearance of mammary carcinomas, reduced the incidence (13/30 compared with 27/30 with MNU alone) and decreased the number of tumours per rat (0.6 versus 3.5). Concomitant administration of oestradiol and progesterone after initiation with MNU was as effective as ovariectomy in inhibiting mammary carcinogenesis after initiation with MNU: 4/29 and 4/29, respectively, compared with 27/30 with MNU alone (Grubbs *et al.*, 1983).

Groups of 10 male Fischer 344 rats, weighing 130–150 g, were given 0 or 0.05 mg/kg bw oestradiol after partial hepatectomy. After a 13-day recovery phase, all animals received 0.02% 2-acetylaminofluorene in the diet for two weeks, with a further growth stimulus in the form of 2 mL/kg bw carbon tetrachloride given by intragastric instillation on day 7 of the feeding period. There was no significant difference in the incidence of γ-glutamyl-transpeptidase-positive foci [putative preneoplasic lesions] in oestradiol and control groups (Schuppler *et al.*, 1983).

Groups of 12 or 14 male Wistar Furth rats were castrated at 40 days of age and received subcutaneous implants of pellets containing 5 mg oestradiol, which were replaced every two months throughout the 12-month experiment. Twelve rats at 50–55 days of age were further given 5 mg/kg bw *N*-butyl-*N*-nitrosourea. None of the 14 castrated rats given oestradiol alone developed hepatic tumours. Treatment with the nitrosourea plus oestradiol did not elicit any hepatic tumours; however, oestradiol alone or in combination with the nitrosourea resulted in high incidences of pituitary adenomas (9/14 and 8/11, respectively). No control data were reported (Sumi *et al.*, 1984).

Groups of 12 or 13 female Sprague-Dawley rats, seven weeks of age, were subjected to partial hepatectomy; 24 h later, they received 5 mg/kg bw *N*-nitrosodiethylamine (NDEA) and then 0 or 0.6 ppm oestradiol in the diet for nine months. In NDEA-initiated rats, oestradiol did not increase the number of γ-glutamyltranspeptidase-positive lesions per liver or the incidence of hepatic nodules or hepatocellular carcinoma (Yager *et al.*, 1984).

A group of 30 female Sprague-Dawley rats, 50–55 days of age, received implants of 3 mg oestradiol-containing silicone wafers; 48 h later, all animals were given 20 mg DMBA by oral gavage. The animals were palpated for mammary tumours after one month and twice weekly thereafter. Oestradiol treatment was continued for 160 days in 15 animals, and the implants from 15 rats were removed after 14 days. After 160 days, 90% of the surviving animals treated continuously with oestradiol had developed palpable mammary tumours; this incidence was similar to that in rats from which the implant had been removed at 14 days (Wotiz *et al.*, 1984).

Groups of 24–31 female Sprague-Dawley rats, 40 days of age, were given 0 or 20 µg oestradiol and/or 4 mg progesterone by subcutaneous injection on five days a week for five weeks. A dose of 50 mg/kg bw MNU was administered at 96 and 103 days of age, three and four weeks, respectively, after the last hormone injection. The incidence of mammary adenocarcinomas was 48% in the MNU plus oestradiol group, 42% in the MNU plus progesterone group, 13% in the MNU plus oestradiol plus progesterone group ($p < 0.05$) and 61% in the group given MNU alone (Grubbs *et al.*, 1985).

Groups of six female Sprague-Dawley rats, weighing 200–250 g, received 5 mg/kg bw oestradiol 1 or 24 h before an intraperitoneal injection of 0 or 50 mg/kg bw NDEA and were killed after eight weeks. The numbers of γ-glutamyltranspeptidase-positive foci per cm³ of liver increased from 364 ± 57 in animals given only NDEA to 1149 ± 186 in those receiving oestradiol 24 h before NDEA ($p < 0.01$); the number was increased to 3779 ± 280 ($p < 0.001$) when the hormone was injected 1 h before the carcinogen, i.e. about 25% of the number of foci scored in control rats receiving NDEA 24 h after partial hepatectomy (Taton *et al.*, 1990).

Female Wistar MS rats were ovariectomized at 23 days of age and, at 60 days of age, were divided into groups of 20–25 rats. The animals were given subcutaneous injections of 50 µg oestradiol benzoate in 0.2 mL olive oil, 5 mg progesterone in 0.2 mL olive oil or 50 µg oestradiol benzoate plus 5 mg progesterone daily for 14 days. At this time, rats were irradiated with 260 cGy γ-rays, followed 30 days later by subcutaneous implantation of pellets containing diethylstilboestrol (estimated release rate, 0.38 µg per day). The rats were observed for the appearance of palpable mammary tumours for up to one year. The tumour incidences were 6/23 in the controls, 12/21 in rats given oestradiol benzoate alone ($p < 0.05$), 8/25 in rats given progesterone alone and 9/23 in those given oestradiol plus progesterone. These increases were accompanied by significant increases in DNA synthesis in the mammary gland, as determined on the final day of oestrogen or progestogen at the time of radiation treatment (Inano *et al.*, 1995).

(e)   Carcinogenicity of metabolites

Hamster: In two studies, castrated male Syrian golden hamsters were given the 2-hydroxy- and 4-hydroxy metabolites of oestradiol. In the first study, the oestrogen-containing pellets (25 mg) were implanted at 0 and three months and left for six months. In the second study, the oestrogen-containing pellets were implanted every three months and left for 9–10 months. Oestradiol produced renal-cell carcinomas in 4/5 and 6/6 hamsters, respectively; 2-hydroxyoestradiol in 0/5 and 0/6 hamsters, respectively; and 4-hydroxy-oestradiol in 4/5 and 5/5 hamsters, respectively (Liehr *et al.*, 1986a; Li & Li, 1987).

3.2.3   Oestriol

Mouse: Groups of 30 female ICR mice, 10 weeks of age, received 10 mg/kg bw MNU solution into the left uterine corpus and saline into the right. One week later, animals received a diet containing 0 or 25 mg/kg diet (ppm) oestriol for 30 weeks. At that time, all surviving mice were necropsied and underwent histological examination. Endometrial adenocarcinomas developed in both groups: the incidence was 7/25 in mice given MNU plus oestriol and 3/26 in controls, but the difference was not statistically significant (Niwa *et al.*, 1993).

Rat: Two groups of 30 female Sprague-Dawley rats, 55 days old, received subcutaneous implants of Silastic wafers containing 0 or 5 mg oestriol; 48 h later, all rats were given 20 mg DMBA by oral gavage. The animals were examined one month after DMBA treatment and thereafter once weekly. Seven weeks after the onset of the first mammary tumour (day 42 after DMBA treatment), palpable mammary tumours were found in all of the 28 surviving animals given DMBA alone and in 6/26 given DMBA plus oestriol; 180 days after the onset of the first mammary tumour, 13/26 given DMBA plus oestriol had palpable mammary tumours (Wotiz *et al.*, 1984).

Thirty female Sprague-Dawley rats, 50–55 days old, received subcutaneous implants of Silastic wafers containing 5 mg oestriol; 48 h later, all animals received 20 mg DMBA by oral gavage. The implants were removed from 15 animals after 14 days. At the termination of the experiment at 180 days, the incidence of mammary tumours was 60% after two weeks of oestriol treatment and 20% with continuous oestriol treatment (Wotiz *et al.*, 1984).

Groups of 19 female Sprague-Dawley rats, 35–50 days of age, received 20 mg DMBA in 1.5 mL sesame oil by oral gavage; two weeks later, one group received subcutaneous implants of crystalline pellets containing 638 µg oestriol each month for 10 months. The incidences of mammary carcinomas at one year were 12/19 in the group receiving DMBA plus oestriol and 18/19 in those given DMBA alone ($p < 0.05$, χ^2 test) (Lemon, 1987).

Groups of 8–26 virgin female Sprague-Dawley rats, 40–50 days of age, were irradiated from a cobalt-60 gamma source delivering 3.5 Gy to the dorsal area of the rats. Crystalline sodium chloride pellets containing oestriol (638 ± 175 µg per month) were implanted subcutaneously into the anterior dorsal area each month for life. Control rats were irradiated without oestriol treatment. Oestriol treatment was begun one to three days before irradiation or 5, 13 or 15 days after irradiation. The rats were weighed and examined every 10–14 days during their natural life span after irradiation. Biopsies were performed on persistent and growing tumours within two to four weeks of discovery, and biopsy tissues were examined histopathologically. Tumour-free rats were observed until death, at which time they underwent necropsy. Of 142 irradiated controls, 93 developed mammary carcinomas; two-thirds of the tumours appeared more than 300 days after irradiation. When oestriol administration was begun one to three days before or five days after irradiation, no significant reduction in mammary carcinoma incidence (29/54 controls versus 50/113 oestriol-treated) was observed. When oestriol administration was further delayed, a significant reduction in mammary carcinogenesis was observed: 7/12 controls versus 6/14 given oestriol 15 days after irradiation ($p < 0.07$) and 14/20 controls versus 6/18 rats given oestriol 13 days after irradiation ($p < 0.02$). This inhibition was stated to be associated with the rapid differentiation of the mammary gland (Lemon *et al.*, 1989).

3.2.4   *Oestrone*

(*a*)   *Subcutaneous implantation*

Hamster: Implantation of 20-mg pellets of oestrone resulted in microscopic renal carcinomas in 8/10 male castrated Syrian hamsters after 8.5 months of treatment (Li *et al.*,
1983).

(*b*)   *Administration with known carcinogens*

Mouse: Groups of 30 female ICR mice, 10 weeks of age, were given 10 mg/kg bw
MNU into the left uterine corpus and normal saline into the right. One week later, the mice
received a diet containing 0 or 25 mg/kg diet (ppm) oestrone for 29 weeks. At that time,
the incidence of adenocarcinoma in the group given MNU plus oestrone (9/23) was significantly higher ($p < 0.05$) than that in mice given MNU alone (3/26). In addition, the incidences of preneoplastic endometrial lesions (atypical and adenomatous glandular hyperplasia) in mice receiving oestrone with or without MNU were higher than that in controls
(Niwa *et al.*, 1993).

Toad: Groups of 100 female toads (*Bufo regularis*), weighing approximately 50 g,
received either subcutaneous injections of 1 mL amphibian saline containing 3 mg *N*-nitro-
sodimethylamine (NDMA) into the dorsal lymph sac once a week, subcutaneous injections
of 0.1 mg oestrone dissolved in 1 mL corn oil once a week or 3 mg NDMA followed by
direct injection of 0.1 mg oestrone in 1 mL corn oil once a week. The duration of the
experiment was 14 weeks. The incidence of hepatocellular carcinomas was 17/99 in toads
given NDMA alone, the first tumour appearing at week 8. In toads treated with oestrone
alone, the incidence was 4/97, the first tumour appearing at week 12 after the first injection.
The incidence of liver tumours was 23/94 in toads treated with NDMA plus oestrone, the
first tumour appearing at week 6 after initiation (Sakr *et al.*, 1989).

(*c*)   *Carcinogenicity of metabolites*

Rat: Groups of 20 female Crl:CD(SD)BR rats, 30 days of age, were given 100 μL
dimethyl sulfoxide (DMSO) containing 30 μmol/rat oestrone-3,4-quinone [purity not
specified], DMSO alone or 1.2 μmol/rat *trans*-3,4-dihydroxy-*anti*-1,2-epoxy-1,2,3,4-
tetrahydrobenzo[*c*]phenanthrene (purity, > 99%), which were used as vehicle and positive controls, respectively. One-sixth of the total dose was injected under each of six
nipples on the left side of each rat, whereas DMSO only was injected under the nipples
on the right side. The thoracic mammary glands of the rats were treated at 30 days of age,
and those located in the inguinal area were treated on the following day. Rats were fed a
high-fat AIN76A diet (23.5% corn oil) throughout the course of the experiment. The
experiment was terminated 44 weeks after treatment. The positive control induced mammary tumours in 20/20 rats, but there was no difference in tumour incidence or multiplicity among rats receiving DMSO (3/20) and those treated with oestrone-3,4-quinone
(4/20) (El-Bayoumy *et al.*, 1996).

Hamster: Li and Li (1987) investigated the carcinogenicity of the 2-hydroxy and 4-
hydroxy metabolites of oestrone in castrated male Syrian golden hamsters given implants

of oestrogen-containing pellets every three months for 9–10 months. Renal tumours were found in 8/10 hamsters given oestrone, 0/6 given 2-hydroxyoestrone and 2/6 given 4-hydroxyoestrone.

4. Other Data Relevant to an Evaluation of Carcinogenicity and its Mechanisms

4.1 Absorption, distribution, metabolism and excretion

The disposition of oestradiol, oestrone and oestriol is considered together, because there is interconversion between oestradiol and oestrone *in vivo* in both humans and other mammals, and the latter is converted to oestriol (Figure 4).

Various preparations of oestradiol, such as crystalline oestradiol, micronized oestradiol and esterified oestradiol (e.g. oestradiol valerate, oestradiol 3-benzoate, oestradiol dipropionate), are used for post-menopausal hormonal therapy. The absorption of these oestradiol preparations differs, while the route of exposure remains the same. For example, crystalline oestradiol applied dermally in a cream diffuses more readily through the skin to the systemic circulation than esterified oestradiol, because oestradiol is more lipophilic than its ester derivative. Similarly, micronized oestradiol is absorbed more rapidly than crystalline oestradiol because of its small particle size. The absorption of these oestradiol preparations also depends on the dose administered and the route of administration.

The pharmacokinetics of conjugated equine oestrogens is complicated because so many different kinds of oestrogens are present, including oestrone sulfate (15%), equilin sulfate (25%), dihydroequilin sulfate (15%) and several other oestrogen sulfates. All of these oestrogens undergo metabolic conversions in the gastrointestinal tract and liver. Equilin sulfate and oestrone sulfate are the major components (approximately 40%) of the equine oestrogen preparation Premarin®, which is the most widely prescribed oestrogen used in therapy for post-menopausal women in the United States.

4.1.1 Humans

The absorption of oestradiol in humans has been studied extensively; however, the results are difficult to compare as different preparations of oestradiol and different routes of administration have been used.

Daily oral administration of oestradiol tablets results in large pulses of oestradiol and oestrone and exposes women to high concentrations of these compounds. Oral administration of the first oestradiol tablet, 2 mg micronized oestradiol, to 32 healthy post-menopausal women resulted in a maximal plasma oestradiol concentration of 1084 pg/mL 49 min after administration, which decreased rapidly during the subsequent 3 h. Progressive accumulation of oestradiol occurred until a steady state was reached. After the fifth tablet, the average concentration of oestradiol was about 418 pg/mL, which was 12 times greater than that found when a transdermal patch was used. The oestrone concentration reached a peak of 334 pg/mL 4.3 h after the first administration and reached a steady state

Figure 4. Pathways for the metabolism and redox cycling of oestradiol, oestriol and oestrone

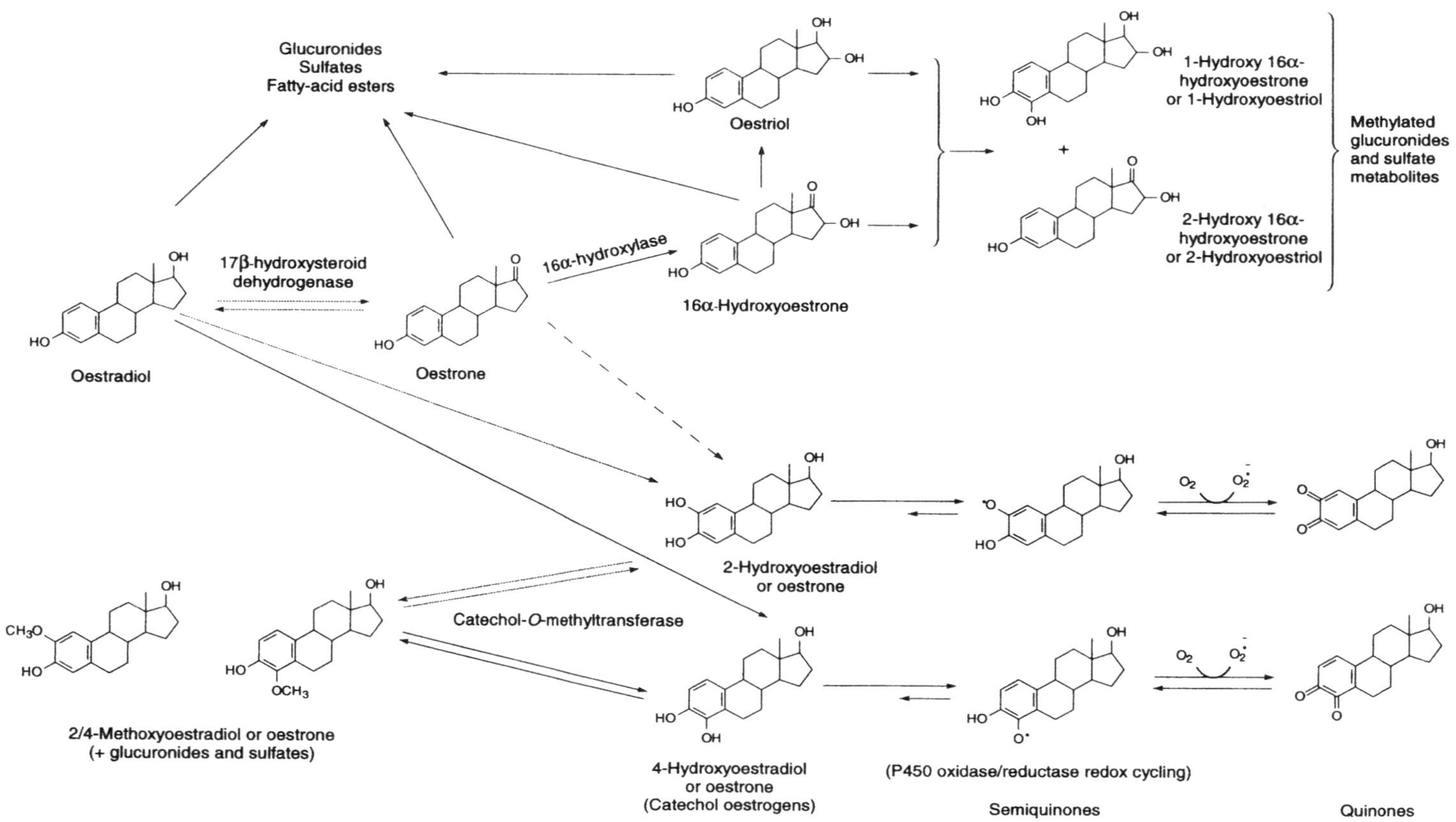

Modified from Yager & Liehn (1996)

after the 14th daily administration. This average concentration of oestrone was 9.4 times greater than that found when a transdermal patch was used (Setnikar *et al.*, 1996).

After a single oral dose of 2.0 mg/day oestradiol valerate to post-menopausal women, the maximal plasma concentrations were 0.96 nmol/L oestrone, 0.19 nmol/L oestradiol, 44.4 nmol/L oestrone sulfate, 0.6 nmol/L oestradiol sulfate and 0.19 nmol/L oestriol sulfate. The times to reach the maximal concentration were 5.2 h for oestrone, 3.2 h for oestradiol, 4.1 h for oestrone sulfate, 5.0 h for oestradiol sulfate and 8.8 h for oestriol sulfate (Aedo *et al.*, 1990).

A comparison of the pharmacokinetic parameters of oral and sublingual adminis-tration of micronized oestradiol to post-menopausal women revealed that the time to the maximal concentration of oestradiol was significantly different by the two routes of administration, being 1 h or less for sublingual administration and 6.5–7.6 h for oral administration. The maximal plasma concentration, terminal half-life, area under the curve for the integral of the serum concentration over time (area under the curve) and oral clearance were also different with the two routes of administration. For example, after sublingual administration of 1 mg micronized oestradiol, the maximal plasma oestradiol concentration was 451 pg/mL, the terminal half-life was 18 h, the area under the curve was 2109 pg/mL per h and the oral clearance was 7.6 L/h per kg bw; after oral adminis-tration, these values were 34 pg/mL, 20.1 h, 823 pg/mL per h and 27.2 L/h per kg bw, respectively. The concentrations of oestrone were not dependent on route of adminis-tration. Sublingual administration resulted in a significantly lower ratio of oestrone to oestradiol than oral administration during the 24-h period (Price *et al.*, 1997).

Because oestrogen penetrates normal skin easily (Jewelewicz, 1997), various prepa-rations based on this property have been evaluated, including subcutaneous implants, vaginal creams and rings, percutaneous gels and transdermal therapeutic systems. Trans-dermal oestradiol provides physiological levels of oestradiol at a constant rate; the trans-dermal route avoids loss of drug by the hepatic first-pass effect and minimally affects hepatic protein metabolism. As a result, the oestradiol:oestrone ratios more closely resemble those of pre-menopausal women. Maximal serum concentrations of oestradiol are reached within 2–8 h of application of a transdermal system. When 50 µg/day trans-dermal therapy is used on a long-term basis, the mean steady-state serum concentrations can be 20–50 pg/mL. In a study of 100 µg/day transdermal therapy, the mean oestradiol concentration was 46–152 pg/mL. Within 24 h of removal of the transdermal delivery system, the plasma concentrations of oestradiol and oestrone and the urinary excretion of oestradiol and oestrone conjugates generally returned to pre-treatment levels (Balfour & Heel, 1990).

The pharmacokinetic profiles of oestradiol and oestrone have been reported in 16 healthy post-menopausal women after twice weekly applications for three weeks of an oestradiol transdermal patch, which contains 4 mg oestradiol and delivers 50 µg oestradiol daily. During the first application, oestradiol reached effective concentrations of 30 pg/mL or more 12 h after application; during the following five applications, the concentration remained constant at an average of 35 pg/mL. After removal of the patch, the concentration returned to basal level within 12 h. The oestrone concentration reached a maximum of 48 pg/mL 41 h after the first application and then remained constant (Setnikar *et al.*, 1996).

Seven days' use of patches containing 0.1 or 0.05 mg/day oestradiol resulted in peak average blood concentrations of 100 and 50 pg/mL, respectively. Values approximating 90% of the maximal level were achieved within 12 h after patch application and were maintained for up to 48 h. The mean steady-state blood concentrations over seven days were approximately 70 and 35 pg/mL, respectively. After removal of the patch, the concentrations fell to near baseline within 12 h (Gordon, 1995).

Subcutaneous administration of oestradiol pellets containing 25–200 μg pure crystalline oestradiol resulted in good bioavailability, as seen from the oestradiol:oestrone ratios, because minimal metabolism occurs in subcutaneous tissues (Jewelewicz, 1997). Pellets of 25 mg and 50 mg oestradiol produced serum concentrations of oestradiol of approximately 50–70 pg/mL and 100–120 pg/mL, respectively, for up to several months (Stumpf, 1990). Although the serum oestradiol concentrations were reported to be stable with this route of administration, 12 women of similar age and body weight in one small open study showed striking variations in hormone concentrations over 12 months of follow-up (Jewelewicz, 1997).

In a study of 24 women with vaginal atrophy treated daily with vaginal tablets containing 10 or 25 μg oestradiol, the oestradiol plasma concentrations reached 45 and 60 pmol/L after two weeks, respectively. The plasma oestrone concentration was unchanged by treatment (Johnston, 1996).

Oestradiol-containing polydimethylsiloxane rings inserted into the vagina release oestradiol continuously, and the substance is readily absorbed by the vaginal mucosa. Relatively constant serum concentrations of approximately 150 pg/mL oestradiol and oestrone were achieved for 21 days from a ring containing 400 mg oestradiol (Kuhl, 1990). The bioavailability of oestradiol from vaginal rings has been reported to be 13 ± 7% (range, 7–27%) in post-menopausal women (Gabrielsson *et al.*, 1995).

After intramuscular injection of oestradiol esters in oily solution, the compound is released slowly from the primary depot at the injection site and/or from secondary depots in fat tissue (Kuhl, 1990).

Oral intake of 8 mg oestriol resulted in a maximum plasma concentration of 75 pg/mL unconjugated oestriol after 2 h, and the concentrations increased to up to 130 pg/mL after continued daily ingestion of 8 mg oestriol for 30 days, although the serum concentration of conjugated oestriol remained unaltered (Schiff *et al.*, 1978). Orally administered oestriol was almost completely conjugated in the intestine to glucuronides (80–90%) and sulfates (10–20%); only 1–2% of the parent steroid reached the circulation (Kuhl, 1990).

Oestriol undergoes much less metabolism after vaginal application than after oral ingestion, and 20% of the dose appears as unconjugated steroid in the blood. At a dose of 0.5 mg, peak levels of 100–150 pg/mL were observed within 2 h. The maximal concentrations of oestriol after vaginal application of 0.5 mg were similar to those obtained after oral intake of 8–12 mg oestriol (Kuhl, 1990). There was no significant difference in the plasma oestriol concentrations after vaginal administration of 1 mg and oral administration of 10 mg oestriol (Heimer, 1987). Daily administration of 1 g of a cream containing 500 µg oestriol to 11 post-menopausal women for eight weeks caused a mean rise in plasma oestriol from unmeasurable (< 35 pmol/L) to 87 pmol/L (Haspels *et al.*, 1981). Treatment with a low dose of oestriol by the vaginal route may therefore induce systemic effects comparable to those achieved with high oral doses.

After a single oral dose of 2.5 mg/day piperazine oestrone sulfate to post-menopausal women, the maximal plasma concentrations were 1.3 nmol/L oestrone, 0.25 nmol/L oestradiol, 54 nmol/L oestrone sulfate, 0.9 nmol/L oestradiol sulfate and 0.23 nmol/L oestriol sulfate. The time to reach the maximal plasma concentration was 6.4 h for oestrone, 9.8 h for oestradiol, 4.4 h for oestrone sulfate, 6.5 h for oestradiol sulfate and 4.9 h for oestriol sulfate (Aedo *et al.*, 1990).

Most of the available data on distribution are based on studies of intravenous administration. After intravenous administration of oestradiol to post-menopausal women, a high clearance (1.8 ± 0.6 L/min) and a low distribution volume (51 ± 28 L) were found. Oestrogens circulate in the blood bound to albumin (about 60%), sex hormone-binding globulin (about 38%), α_1-glycoproteins and transcortin. Oestradiol binds weakly to albumin (low affinity/high capacity; plasma concentration, 40 g/L), about one-third is tightly bound to sex hormone-binding globulin (high affinity/low capacity) and a small fraction (< 3%) is 'free'. After intravenous administration, the distribution volume of oestradiol at steady state was only about 70 L, representing 1.5–2 times the total body water in fertile women. Its low level of distribution is consistent with its high level of binding to plasma proteins. The production of sex hormone-binding globulin is stimulated by increasing oestrogen concentration. Because of the high concentration of albumin (about five orders of magnitude higher than sex hormone-binding globulin) and its rapid dissociation, albumin may serve a more important regulating role (Gabrielsson *et al.*, 1996).

After daily transdermal treatment of post-menopausal women with 0.1 mg oestradiol for three consecutive cycles, there was no significant difference in the distribution of oestradiol and oestrone between free and protein-bound oestrogen fractions in peripheral plasma (Jasonni *et al.*, 1988).

Oestrone is not tightly bound to plasma proteins and therefore has a higher clearance rate than oestradiol. Oestrone sulfate is quantitatively the most important plasma oestrogen metabolite and is bound with high affinity to albumin, 90% circulating in bound form. Oestrone sulfate is considered to have a large, slowly metabolized reservoir, with 90% of its mass bound to albumin; accordingly, it has a low metabolic clearance rate (about 150 L/24 h) and low renal clearance (Anderson, 1993).

Few studies have addressed the accumulation and storage of oestradiol, oestrone and oestriol after exogenous administration. All three are distributed to various target and non-target organs through the systemic circulation but are also produced locally and accumulate in target tissues particularly rich in fat. Knowledge about the metabolism of oestradiol, oestrone and oestriol in humans has not advanced much since the last evaluation (IARC, 1979), except for hydroxylation of oestradiol.

The metabolic disposition of oestrogens includes oxidative metabolism (largely hydroxylation) and conjugative metabolism by glucuronidation, sulfonation and/or *O*-methylation (reviewed by Zhu & Conney, 1998). Oestradiol is converted to oestrone by a 17β-hydroxysteroid dehydrogenase; the oestrone produced is further metabolized to 16α-hydroxyoestrone and then to oestriol (Johnston, 1996). Hydroxylation of oestradiol at the 2 position is a major metabolic pathway in the liver (Kerlan *et al.*, 1992). There are large inter-individual differences in oestradiol 2-hydroxylation in human liver samples, which may be reflected by differences in oestrogenic action. 4-Hydroxylation of oestradiol to a catechol is a minor pathway (usually < 15% of 2-hydroxylation) in the liver. Recent studies have shown that 4-hydroxylation of oestradiol is the dominant pathway of catechol oestrogen formation in human breast and uterus (Figure 4; Liehr *et al.*, 1995; Liehr & Ricco, 1996). In humans, 4-hydroxylation of oestradiol is catalysed by the cytochrome P450 enzyme CYP1B1 (Hayes *et al.*, 1996). Oestradiol and oestrone hydroxylated can undergo metabolic redox cycling *in vitro* to generate free radicals such as superoxide and the chemically reactive oestrogen semiquinone/quinone intermediates (Liehr & Roy, 1990). In the presence of fatty acid acyl-coenzyme A, oestradiol can be converted at the C-17 position to very lipophilic oestrogen fatty acid esters by enzymes present in liver and in oestrogen target organs such as breast and placenta (Adams *et al.*, 1986).

Oestrone sulfate is the oestrogen found at the highest concentration in plasma and seems to constitute a storage form for circulating oestrogens. Oestrone sulfate can be hydrolysed to oestrone by arylsulfatases, which are widely distributed in human tissues (Rozenbaum, 1996).

There is a reversible equilibrium between oestradiol, oestrone and oestrone sulfate, which are interconverted by oestradiol dehydrogenase, sulfotransferase and aryl sulfatase. The two pathways of phase I oestrone inactivation are ring A metabolism, which produces catechol–oestrogens and is favoured in underweight women and hyperthyroid patients, and ring D metabolism, which leads to oestriol production and is increased in obese women and hypothyroid patients. Phase II metabolism involves the formation of several oestrogen conjugates; the sulfates circulate in high concentrations in the blood, and the glucuronides are excreted with the bile and in urine. After oral administration of micronized oestradiol, the serum oestrone:oestradiol ratio, which is 1:2 in fertile women and 2:1 in post-menopausal women, increased to 4:1. Prolonged percutaneous or transdermal treatment with oestradiol in conjunction with subcutaneous implantation of oestradiol pellets has been reported to lead to continuously elevated oestrogen levels and an oestrone:oestradiol ratio of 1:1 to 1:2 (Kuhl, 1990).

Conjugated equine oestrogens are hydrolysed to their active form in the gastrointestinal tract and also undergo considerable hepatic metabolism before entering the bloodstream in an active form (Ansbacher, 1993). Most sulfate esters are hydrolysed to free or unconjugated oestrogen by enzymes in the lower gut; the free oestrogen is absorbed by intestinal tissue, where it can be reconjugated with sulfate. Therefore, the oestrogen sulfate found in the bloodstream is not the same sulfate that was administered. The rate of dissolution is important because it influences where the active ingredients of the product are released in the gastrointestinal tract, a factor which may affect the amounts of the oestrogen that are activated and the patterns of active and inactive metabolites. Equilin and equilenin are interconverted to 17β-dihydroequilin and 17β-dihydroequilenin and correspond to the interrelation between oestrone and oestradiol. As in the case of natural oestrogen in women, there is an equilibrium between equilin, equilenin and their metabolites and the respective sulfates (Kuhl, 1990).

The sulfate esters of equilin, oestrone and oestradiol do not bind sex hormone-binding globulin; however, equilin sulfate and oestrone sulfate interact with serum albumin with high affinity ($0.9–1.1 \times 10^5$/mol per L). Up to 74% of total equilin sulfate and 85–90% of oestrone sulfate were bound to serum albumin (Bhavnani, 1998). The peak concentration of equilin sulfate is found after 4 h. Equilin is rapidly absorbed and converted to 17β-dihydroequilin. The volume of distribution at steady state was 6 ± 0.5 L for 17β-dihydroequilin sulfate, 23 ± 1.3 L for 17β-dihydroequilin and 12.4 ± 1.6 L for equilin sulfate (O'Connell, 1995).

Six healthy post-menopausal women were seen each month during a six-month trial of cyclic therapy with conjugated equine oestrogens (Premarin®), ingested at 1.25 mg per day for 21 days followed by seven days without therapy. The average serum concentrations in samples taken within 2 h of the last ingestion of drug in a given cycle were 1850 pg/mL unconjugated equilin, 162 pg/mL oestrone and 106 pg/mL oestradiol. Three months after completion of therapy, the oestrone and oestradiol concentrations had returned to pre-treatment levels, but equilin was still detected in serum at a concentration of 144 pg/mL in all three of the women who were investigated (Whittaker *et al.*, 1980).

After administration of ^{3}H-equilin sulfate and ^{3}H-17β-dihydroequilin sulfate to post-menopausal women, less than 50% of the administered dose was excreted in the urine. The majority (63–74%) of the radiolabelled metabolites excreted were in the form of glucuronides, whereas 16–17% were found as sulfates and 1–2% in the unconjugated fractions (Bhavnani, 1998). About 40–50% of the radiolabel from injected oestradiol is excreted in the bile (Sandberg & Slaunwhite, 1957).

These studies show that the bioavailability of oestrone, oestradiol and oestriol depends on the formulation, route of exposure and dose of oestradiol administered. Generalizations cannot be made about the disposition of oestrogen because of differences in the regimens, products and route of exposure and other factors such as age and inter- and intra-individual variations. It can be concluded, however, that transdermal administration by patch, percutaneous administration or transvaginal administration allow more circulating oestrogen for a longer time than oral administration. Comparative trials of various oestrogen products are urgently needed, keeping in consideration the route of exposure and the composition of the different products, to allow quantitative evaluation of the disposition of oestrogens.

4.1.2 *Experimental systems*

Few studies have been carried out in experimental systems on the disposition of oestrone, oestradiol and oestriol products since the previous evaluation (IARC, 1979), and limited experimental studies are available on the absorption, distribution and excretion of oestradiol. Oestrone, oestradiol and oestriol undergo various phase I and phase II metabolic reactions in humans and animals (reviewed by Zhu & Conney, 1998). During phase I metabolism, oestrone, oestradiol and oestriol serve as substrates for aromatic hydroxylation, and these reactions are catalysed by cytochrome P450 enzymes. Oestrone and oestradiol are converted to 2- and 4-hydroxyoestrone and 2- and 4-hydroxyoestradiol, respectively, the ratio of hydroxylated products depending on the target tissues and animal species. Oestradiol and its metabolites serve as substrates for sulfation, methylation and glutathione conjugation. The metabolism depends on the species, strain and sex of the experimental animals and on the experimental conditions.

In the early 1970s and 1980s, it was postulated that oestradiol is converted to reactive intermediates during its metabolism, and direct evidence of reactive metabolites of oestradiol has now been obtained (Liehr et al., 1986b; Roy et al., 1991). Catechol oestrogens undergo microsomal cytochrome P450-mediated redox cycling reactions (Liehr et al., 1986b; Liehr & Roy, 1990; Roy et al., 1991), resulting in the formation of reactive metabolites. Both catechols of oestradiol are converted to their respective quinones in the presence of metabolic activation systems. Nuclei can also catalyse redox cycling of oestrogens (Roy & Thomas, 1994). In vitro, oestradiol in the presence of a metabolic activation system can be converted to DNA-binding oestrogen quinone metabolite(s) (Liehr et al., 1993), but DNA binding has not been detected in vivo.

Oestrone, oestradiol and oestriol are excreted in the bile as glucuronides and undergo enterohepatic recirculation. Their glucuronides are hydrolysed in the intestine, and unconjugated oestradiol or oestrone is reabsorbed from the intestine by enterohepatic cycling (Zhu & Conney, 1998).

Topical application of radiolabelled oestradiol to shaved skin of the dorsal neck of rats at a dose of 30.1, 120.4 or 301 pmol/cm² and autoradiography revealed the presence of oestradiol in epidermis, sebaceous glands, dermal papillae of hair and fibroblasts 2 h after application. A high concentration and retention of oestradiol in sebaceous glands was observed for more than 24 h, suggesting that sebaceous glands serve as a second storage site for oestradiol (Bidmon et al., 1990). An effect of dose and the area of topical application of oestradiol has also been observed in a hairless strain of rats. After a single dose of 50 nmol applied topically, the bioavailability, determined by urinary and faecal excretion of radiolabel after four days, was not affected by the area of the application surface. When the applied doses were increased from 50 to 1000 and 10 000 nmol, the percentage of percutaneous absorption decreased with reduction in the area of application (Chanez et al., 1989). Nasal administration of oestradiol to rats resulted in significantly higher blood levels than after intraduodenal administration, the bioavailability being 50% after a dose of 5 µg, 71% after 10 µg and 84% after 20 µg/rat compared with 2–5% via the intraduodenal route for the same doses (Bawarshi-Nassar et al., 1989). In rats and rabbits, nasal administration of oestradiol with dimethyl-β-cyclodextrin as a solubilizer and absorption enhancer resulted in significantly more absorption of the oestrogen than when it was given in suspension. Nasal administration of oestradiol–dimethyl-β-cyclodextrin resulted in an absolute bioavailability of 94.6% in rabbits and 67.2% in rats in relation to an intravenous injection (Hermens *et al.*, 1990).

In a study in rats given oestradiol–bisphosphonate conjugates with different esterase-sensitive linkers between the two molecular moieties, the conjugate with the low-cleavage resistance doubled the serum half-life of oestradiol (3.78 h), and the high-cleavage resistance conjugate resulted in a serum half-life approximately four times higher (8.36 h) than that of free oestradiol (Bauss *et al.*, 1996).

After administration of oestriol to rats, glucuronides and sulfates of 16-keto-oestradiol and of 2- and 3-methyl esters of 2-hydroxyoestriol and 2-hydroxy-16-ketooestradiol were excreted in the bile (Bolt, 1979).

Oestradiol represented only 6% of the total oestrogen detected in the hepatic portal vein after oestradiol was placed in the stomach of a prepubertal pig; thus, most of the oestradiol was converted or conjugated before entering the hepatic portal vein. The blood concentrations of oestradiol glucuronide, oestrone glucuronide and oestrone sulfate but not of oestradiol or oestrone in the jugular vein rose and remained elevated for several hours, indicating that oestradiol and oestrone are completely converted and/or removed by the liver (Ruoff & Dziuk, 1994a).

In a comparison of the serum and tissue concentrations of oestradiol in fertile female and in castrated male Syrian golden hamsters, oestradiol pellets (20 mg) were implanted into the shoulder region of groups of four to six hamsters every 45 days to maintain the hormone concentration, and the animals were killed after 15 days and at 30-day intervals. The average serum oestradiol concentration in the cycling female hamsters was 79 pg/mL on days 1–2 and 311 pg/mL on days 3–4, attaining a maximum of 358 pg/mL on day 4 of the cycle. The concentrations on days 3–4 of the cycle were threefold higher than those on day 1 in uterine tissue, twofold higher in renal tissue and 2.6-fold higher in hepatic tissue. As was to be expected, the serum oestradiol concentrations of untreated castrated male hamsters did not vary appreciably over the six months of the study, and the average was about 32 pg/mL. Under conditions that produced essentially 100% renal tumour incidence, the serum oestradiol concentration rose rapidly to an average of 71-fold the untreated level. A steady-state serum concentration of 2400–2700 pg/mL was maintained during 45–180 days of continuous oestrogen treatment. The renal concentration of oestradiol in hamsters given this hormone rose by an average of only 5.4-fold between days 15 and 180 of treatment, and the serum concentrations were 5.7- to 8.0-fold higher than those in cycling female hamsters on days 3 and 4, with, however, no apparent effect on weight or mortality rate (Li *et al.* 1994).

A 10-mg dose of crystalline oestradiol placed in the rectum of prepubertal gilts resulted in increased concentrations of oestradiol, oestrone, oestradiol glucuronide, oestrone glucuronide and oestrone sulfate in the hepatic portal vein within 30 min, and the concentrations remained elevated for several hours (Ruoff & Dziuk, 1994b). After oestradiol was placed in the stomach of the prepubertal gilts, the concentrations of oestradiol, oestrone, oestradiol glucuronide, oestrone glucuronide and oestrone sulfate in the hepatic portal vein rose within 5 min and remained elevated for several hours (Ruoff &

Dziuk, 1994a). Most of the conjugated metabolites in liver and kidney of cattle are glucuronides (85–95%) (Kaltenbach *et al.*, 1976).

In pregnant rhesus monkeys, oestradiol was eliminated from the maternal circulation principally by conversion to glucuronide conjugates (Hill *et al.*, 1980; Slikker *et al.*, 1982). After pulse injection of ^{3}H-oestrone sulfate to adult female rhesus monkeys, the initial volume of distribution was 4.6 ± 0.9 L, and the metabolic clearance rate was 42 ± 2.9 L/day. Infusion of ^{3}H-oestrone sulfate or ^{14}C-oestrone resulted in a metabolic clearance rate of 67.5 ± 8.3 L/day. The conversion ratio of oestradiol to oestrone sulfate was 0.054 ± 0.016; the interconversion value was $43.6 \pm 3.4\%$ for oestrone sulfate to oestrone and $33.5 \pm 6.6\%$ for oestrone to oestrone sulfate. Thus, oestrone sulfate is cleared slowly and is converted to both oestrone and oestradiol (Longcope *et al.*, 1994).

The disposition of equilin sulfate was determined in female dogs receiving 2.5 mg/kg bw ^{3}H-equilin sulfate orally. The drug was rapidly absorbed (time to reach maximal concentration in plasma, 1 h) and had a moderate half-life (16.3 ± 9.6 h) in plasma. An average of $26.7 \pm 4.4\%$ of the administered radiolabel was excreted in urine. When ^{3}H-equilin sulfate was administered as part of a conjugated equine oestrogen preparation, a lower peak concentration, a lower area under the curve, a longer terminal half-life and a lower elimination percentage in urine were observed, indicating that the absorption of equilin sulfate was altered by other components in the preparation. Both plasma and urine contained equilin, equilenin, 17β-dihydroequilenin, 17β-dihydroequilin, 17α-dihydroequilenin and 17α-dihydroequilin. 17β-Dihydroequilin and equilin were the two major chromatographic peaks in plasma, whereas 17β-dihydroequilenin and 17β-dihydroequilin were the major metabolites in urine. The reduction of the 17-keto group and aromatization of ring-B are the major metabolic pathways of equilin in dogs (Chandrasekaran *et al.*, 1995).

Uptake of oestrone sulfate has been reported by isolated rat hepatocytes. Accumulation in the cell remained linear with time up to 1 min and then began to decrease. The K_m was 16 ± 6 μmol/L, and the V_m was 0.85 ± 0.56 nmol/min per 10^6 cells. The uptake of oestrone sulfate involves a Na^+- and energy-dependent transport protein and a Na^+-independent anionic transport or multiple organic anion transport (Hassen *et al.*, 1996).

4-Hydroxylation of equilenin was reported in hamster liver microsomes (Sarabia *et al.*, 1997). *In vitro*, 4-hydroxyequilenin can participate in redox cycling, and its quinone metabolite (4-hydroxyequilenin-*ortho*-quinone) is more reactive than 4-hydroxyoestrone-*ortho*-quinone (Shen *et al.*, 1997).

4.2   Receptor-mediated effects

4.2.1   *Humans*

In hyperplastic endometrial samples from four women who had been exposed to oestrogen [not further specified], the expression of keratinocyte growth factor mRNA was suppressed to the concentrations found in endometrial samples from unexposed women during the late proliferative phase of the menstrual cycle, whereas the expression of keratinocyte growth factor receptor mRNA was increased by approximately 35% over the enhanced levels found in the same control women (Siegfried *et al.*, 1995).

In endometrial biopsy samples from post-menopausal women who had received 1.25 mg Premarin® daily for at least three months, the in-vitro DNA labelling index (incorporation of tritiated thymidine) in glandular epithelial cells and the nuclear oestradiol receptor content were increased and were similar to those found in proliferative-phase endometrium from eight unexposed women. The number of tritiated thymidine-labelled cells per microscopic high-power field was increased threefold by the treatment (four women) in comparison with the pre-menopausal control values (eight women) (Siddle *et al.*, 1982).

Groups of post-menopausal women continuously received either oral doses of 2 mg per day oestradiol valerate, 1.5 mg per day oestropipate, 0.625 or 1.25 mg per day conjugated equine oestrogens (Premarin®), 50-mg oestradiol implants or 5 g of a skin cream containing 3 mg oestradiol; most women received a progestogen during the last 7–10 days of each month. Endometrial biopsy samples were obtained, and the receptor content was measured. The content of soluble progesterone receptor was not affected in 13 women taking Premarin® when compared with the level in proliferative-phase endometrium from 12 unexposed women. The nuclear oestradiol receptor content was slightly elevated (by 30%) in the endometrial samples from the 15 women who had received the high dose of Premarin® (1.25 mg/day) as compared with the level in proliferative-phase endometrium from 16 unexposed women. The percentage of endometrial glandular cells that had incorporated tritiated thymidine *in vitro*, examined only in cells from five women given 1.25 mg per day Premarin®, appeared to be minimally elevated (by approximately 10%) over the labelling index observed in proliferative-phase endometrium of 12 women; the endometrial oestrogen receptor content was increased by approximately 25% in these samples. All of the studies indicated a slight increase in cell proliferation in Premarin®-exposed women (Whitehead *et al.*, 1981).

The effect of oral treatment for 90 days with 0.2 mg/day of a constituent of conjugated equine oestrogens, 17α-dihydroequilin sulfate, or 1.25 mg per day oestrone sulfate or a combination of these two steroids was examined in groups of seven women in whom menopause had been surgically induced. The serum concentration of sex hormone-binding globulin, measured as an indicator of oestrogenic activity, was increased after the oestrone sulfate treatment, by 20% after 30 days and by 60% after 90 days. Exposure to 17α-dihydroequilin, however, caused a 21 and 12% reduction of this parameter after these time intervals, whereas the combined treatment synergistically increased the concentrations of sex hormone-binding globulin by approximately 100% after 30 or 90 days (Wilcox *et al.*, 1996). Ingestion by post-menopausal women of conjugated equine oestrogens at doses of 0.9–1.25 mg/day significantly increased the cortisol-binding capacity of transcortin, whereas lower doses of conjugated equine oestrogens (0.3 and 0.6 mg/day) did not (Schwartz *et al.*, 1983).

Post-menopausal women received oral doses of conjugated equine oestrogens (0.625 mg per day Premarin®) for 24 days each month or transdermal doses of oestradiol via adhesive patches delivering 0.05 mg/day every fourth day for the first 24 days of each month. Some women also received a progestogen (dydrogesterone) during the last 12 days of each month. The serum concentrations of insulin-like growth factor-I were decreased as compared with the pre-treatment levels in the Premarin®-treated group only. The growth hormone and sex hormone-binding globulin concentrations were increased in this group but not in the women receiving transdermal oestrogen (Campagnoli *et al.*, 1993).

4.2.2   *Experimental systems*
(a)   *Conjugated oestrogens*

The equine oestrogens equilin and equilenin bound to the oestrogen receptor with low affinity (less than oestrone) when examined by displacement of radiolabelled 17β-dihydroequilin in rat and human uterine tissue (Bhavnani & Woolever, 1991).

Oestrone sulfate at concentrations of 10^{-7} mol/L and higher stimulated the growth of MCF-7 human breast cancer cells determined after six days; however, when the mitotic index was used as the indicator of cell proliferation, stimulation was already maximal at a concentration of 10^{-10} mol/L, reaching the same level as that achieved with oestradiol at 10^{-12}–10^{-11} mol/L. This effect of oestrone sulfate was inhibited by simultaneous exposure of the cells to the pure anti-oestrogen ICI164,384. Induction of progesterone receptor or production of the pS2 protein, both indicators of cellular oestrogenic effects, occurred only at a concentration of 10^{-6} mol/L and was weaker than that after oestradiol treatment. Three days of treatment of MCF-7 cells with 10^{-7} or 10^{-9} mol/L oestrone sulfate resulted in concentrations in the medium of 4.4×10^{-9} mol/L oestrone and 1.0×10^{-9} mol/L oestradiol (average of two experiments at the high dose) in comparison with 3.3×10^{-11} mol/L oestrone and 4.4×10^{-12} mol/L oestradiol (at the low dose). Importantly, treatment of MCF-7 cells with 10^{-7} mol/L oestrone sulfate resulted in considerable accumulation in isolated nuclei of free oestrone (560 pg/mg DNA) and oestradiol (180 pg/mg DNA) but very litte oestrone sulfate (13 pg/mg DNA) (Santner *et al.*, 1993).

Twenty-two adult female cynomolgus monkeys that had undergone surgical meno-pause were given Premarin® in a diet in which 40% of the calories were from fat; 26 animals received control diet. The daily dose of Premarin® was approximately 7.2 μg per animal for the first eight months of the experiment and 166 μg per animal for the sub-sequent duration of the 30-month study; the latter dose was stated by the authors to be equivalent to a human dose of 0.625 mg per day. The oestrogen treatment increased the concentration of circulating oestradiol from 5 to 167 pg/mL, increased the thickness of the mammary tissue by 50% and significantly enlarged the estimated surface area of lobular tissue. The mean percentage of epithelial breast cells that stained for Ki-67 MIB-1 antibody (a marker of cell proliferation) was increased from 2.5 to 5.4% in alveoli, from 0.6 to 2.1% in terminal ducts and from 1.2 to 3.0% in major mammary ducts. The mean percentage of epithelial breast cells that stained for progesterone receptors (with antibody techniques) was increased four- to sixfold in these mammary glands, but the percentage of cells that stained for oestrogen receptor was not significantly affected. Oestrogen treatment induced mammary gland hyperplasia in 9/22 of the monkeys as compared with none of the control group (Cline *et al.*, 1996).

Hydrolysed Premarin® stimulated cell proliferation in primary cultures of renal proximal tubular cells isolated from castrated male Syrian golden hamsters at concentrations of 10^{-9} and 10^{-8} mol/L, with no effect at either higher or lower concentrations. Treatment of these hamsters with pellets that released 111 ± 11 µg hydrolysed Premarin® per animal per day resulted in a 100% tumour incidence in the kidney within approximately nine months (Li *et al.*, 1995).

Equilin bound to sex hormone-binding globulin, displacing 5α-dihydrotestosterone with an affinity that was 50% that of oestradiol and 5.6% that of testosterone (Pan *et al.*, 1985).

(b)   Oestradiol

Oestradiol is the natural ligand for the oestrogen receptor. It drives the oestrogen responses of the uterus and mammary gland, which are typical oestrogen-sensitive organs, and in many other tissues. Classical responses to oestradiol mediated by the oestrogen receptor include uterine growth in immature or ovariectomized rodents and transcriptional activation of the progesterone receptor (see, e.g., Musgrove & Sutherland, 1997; Rutanen, 1997). The response of these tissues to oestradiol and the effects observed in cells and with oestrogen-responsive reporter gene constructs, are usually taken as a standard against which the oestrogenicity of other compounds is measured (see, e.g., Jeng *et al.*, 1992; Katzenellenbogen *et al.*, 1993; Parker, 1995; Kuiper *et al.*, 1996). Similarly, displacement of radiolabelled oestradiol is the standard by which binding affinity to the oestrogen receptor is determined. The nature of these oestrogen responses depends mainly on the stage of development of the tissues and the age of the organism. Two high-affinity–low-capacity forms of the receptor have been identified: the oestrogen receptors α and β (Koike *et al.*, 1987; Parker, 1995; Kuiper *et al.*, 1996). Both types are widely distributed and have been isolated from several mammalian tissues (Greene *et al.*, 1986; Krust *et al.*, 1986). The role of the oestrogen receptor-β is still largely unclear, and almost all of the reports in the literature about oestrogen binding, oestrogen receptor–ligand interactions and transcriptional regulation by the oestrogen receptor–ligand complex pertain to the oestrogen receptor-α. The oestrogen responses that have been observed in many tissues and cells are probably, however, a result of the compound involvement of the oestrogen receptors α and β, although the relative contribution of each is still unknown. Anti-oestrogens, such as tamoxifen, which also has weak agonist activity, and pure anti-oestrogens, such as ICI164,384 and ICI182,780, compete with oestradiol for oestrogen receptor binding and are typically used to demonstrate that oestrogenic responses are mediated by this receptor (Jeng *et al.*, 1992; McDonnell *et al.*, 1995). In the context of this monograph, the responses to exogenous oestradiol in various tissues of pre- and post-menopausal women and the effects of oestradiol in appropriate animal or in-vitro models are the most relevant and are summarized here.

Oestradiol strongly induced growth of both MCF-7 and T47D human breast cancer cell lines and other human breast cancer cell lines that contain oestrogen receptors, but it did not stimulate growth of oestrogen receptor-negative breast cancer cell lines (Jeng *et al.*, 1992; Catherino & Jordan, 1995; Schoonen *et al.*, 1995a,b). In MCF-7 cells, the growth-stimulating effect of oestradiol was already observed at a concentration of 10^{-12} mol/L; it increased to a maximum at a concentration of about 10^{-10} mol/L and decreased at concentrations higher than 10^{-9} mol/L (Jeng *et al.*, 1992). These growth-stimulating effects were abolished not only by anti-oestrogens such as tamoxifen and ICI182,780 but also by anti-progestogens such as RU486 (Catherino & Jordan, 1995; Schoonen *et al.*, 1995a,b). The effects were demonstrated in experiments performed with breast cancer cell lines grown in phenol red-free medium which contained steroid-free (dextran-coated charcoal-stripped) serum (Jeng *et al.*, 1992; Schoonen *et al.*, 1995a,b).

At concentrations that stimulate growth of human breast cancer cells, oestradiol induced expression of oestrogen-responsive genes, such as the *pS2* gene, at the transcriptional level (Brown *et al.*, 1984; Kalkhoven *et al.*, 1994) and *trans*-activated oestradiol-responsive reporter constructs containing oestrogen response elements in oestrogen receptor-positive cells (Jeng *et al.*, 1992; Kalkhoven *et al.*, 1994; Catherino & Jordan, 1995). These effects were inhibited by anti-oestrogens. Most of the effects of oestradiol are believed to be mediated by triggering of the secretion of growth factors by autocrine and paracrine action (Lippman & Dickson, 1989). Transforming growth factor (TGF)-α and epidermal growth factor are the most extensively studied mediators of the cell growth-stimulating effects of oestradiol in breast and uterine tissues (see for reviews Boyd, 1996; McLachlan & Newbold, 1996; Snedeker & Diaugustine, 1996). Both up-regulation of these growth-enhancing factors and down-regulation of growth-inhibiting factors may be involved in the action of oestradiol. For example, oestradiol was shown to affect the production of the growth inhibitor TGF-β by human breast cancer cells (Knabbe *et al.*, 1987; Arrick *et al.*, 1990). It markedly down-regulated the mRNA expression of growth-inhibiting TGF-β2 and -β3 in MCF-7 cells at a concentration of oestradiol that stimulated the growth of these cells (10^{-8} mol/L), but it did not affect the mRNA expression of TGF-β1 (Arrick *et al.*, 1990; Jeng & Jordan, 1991). Other cytokines that are not under oestrogen regulation may also influence the growth of breast cancer cells, but oestradiol may affect the responsiveness of the cells to these factors. For example, a six-day exposure of oestrogen receptor-positive ZR-75-1 human breast cancer cells to 10^{-9} mol/L oestradiol reduced by 20–40% the expression of binding sites for interferon, which has anti-proliferative activity for these cells (Martin *et al.*, 1991).

Oestradiol at 10^{-10}–10^{-9} mol/L increased the reductive activity of 17β-hydroxy-steroid oxidoreductase [17-hydroxysteroid dehydrogenase] in an oestrogen- and progestogen-sensitive MCF-7 cell line in phenol red-free medium (Coldham & James, 1990). This activity may be involved in the mechanism of breast cancer cell growth stimulation through the induction of oestradiol formation.

Oestradiol at concentrations of 5×10^{-12}–10^{-7} mol/L stimulated alkaline phosphatase activity in Ishikawa human endometrial cancer cells, which is an oestrogen-specific response inhibited by 4-hydroxytamoxifen (Markiewicz *et al.*, 1992; Markiewicz & Gurpide, 1994; Botella *et al.*, 1995). This assay has been used as a marker for oestrogenic activity in endometrial cells.

Oestradiol at a concentration of 10^{-8} mol/L increased anchorage-independent growth of an SV40-immortalized human endometrial stromal cell line by almost 80% (Xu et al., 1995).

Oestradiol given subcutaneously to ovariectomized rats at a dose of 200 μg/kg bw per day for four days slightly decreased the gene expression of mitogen-activated protein kinase (MAPK) and increased MAPK tyrosine phosphorylation and membrane-associated MAPK enzymatic activity in uterine smooth-muscle tissue (Ruzycky, 1996). In the same model, oestradiol increased the membrane-associated protein expression of seven protein kinase C isozymes by 1.5–2.25-fold, whereas no such change occurred in cardiac muscle. These studies indicate that MAPK and protein kinase C play a role in two of the signal transduction pathways that regulate cell proliferation and are affected by oestradiol (Ruzycky & Kulick, 1996).

Groups of 10 female rats received 20 g DMBA by gavage over two weeks to induce mammary tumours. Ovariectomy suppressed MAPK expression in these tumours, and daily subcutaneous injections of oestradiol (10 μg/rat) induced activation of this enzyme in tumours in ovariectomized rats (Koibuchi et al., 1997).

In ovariectomized BALB/c mice, a single subcutaneous dose of 20 μg oestradiol 3-benzoate induced an approximately threefold induction of mRNA expression of the RXRα and RARγ retinoic acid receptor subtypes in cervical tissue within 0.5 and 4 h, respectively (Celli et al., 1996).

Treatment of cultures of normal human endometrial stromal cells with 10^{-8} mol/L oestradiol with or without 10^{-7} mol/L medroxyprogesterone acetate increased mRNA expression of vascular endothelial growth factor by 4.7- and 3.1-fold, respectively, over control values (Shifren et al., 1996); however, in ovariectomized nude mice carrying a human endometrial carcinoma xenograft, implantation of oestradiol pellets that maintained serum levels of this steroid at 200–300 pg/mL did not alter the expression of vascular endothelial growth factor in the tumour tissue (Kim et al., 1996). Oestradiol did not alter the secretion of vascular endothelial growth factor by T47D human breast cancer cells (Hyder et al., 1998) and had no effect on angiogenesis induction by basic fibroblast growth factor or TGF-α in rabbit cornea in vitro (Yamamoto et al., 1994).

Oestradiol decreased by approximately 50–60% the growth of decidual endothelial cells derived from human endometrium at concentrations of 0.5 and 2.5 ng/mL, increased the growth of these cells by approximately 30% at 5 ng/mL and had no effect at concentrations of 10 ng/mL and higher (Peek et al., 1995).

Oestradiol at concentrations above 10^{-10} mol/L stimulated the migration of human endometrial cancer cells (Ishikawa, HEC-1 or HHUA cells) through an artificial basement membrane and suppressed the mRNA expression of the cell adhesion-related molecules E-cadherin and α- and β-catenin in Ishikawa cells (Fujimoto et al., 1996a,b). At concentrations of 10^{-10} mol/L and higher, oestradiol up-regulated the mRNA expression of fibroblast growth factors-1 and -2 but not of fibroblast growth factor-4 in Ishikawa human endometrial cancer cells, with a maximal effect at 10^{-8} mol/L (Fujimoto et al., 1997). In contrast, no effect of oestradiol was found on endometrial adenocarcinoma SNG-M cells in migration and invasion assays, which involve cell growth along a fibronectin gradient, or on their growth or locomotion as determined in a monolayer wounding model *in vitro*. The secretion of matrix metalloproteinases and stromelysin by these cells was not affected (Ueda *et al.*, 1996).

Oestradiol has been shown to induce liver cell growth, increasing both liver weight and hepatic DNA content in female Wistar rats when given by subcutaneous injection (1–200 μg/kg bw per day) or in the diet (30–300 μg/kg bw per day) for seven days. The relationship between dose and response for these two parameters was approximately linear over the range of subcutaneous doses (Ochs *et al.*, 1986; Schulte-Hermann *et al.*, 1988). Oral administration of oestradiol was less effective than subcutaneous injection (Ochs *et al.*, 1986).

Oestradiol at 3×10^{-5} mol/L for 48 h induced a two- to threefold increase in tritiated thymidine incorporation into DNA of cultured primary female rat hepatocytes. Although oestradiol by itself thus appeared to have only weak mitogenic effects on primary rat hepatocytes, it strongly enhanced the induction of hepatic DNA synthesis by epidermal growth factor or TGF-α (Ni & Yager, 1994a,b). Epidermal growth factor-induced growth of male rat hepatocytes, however, was inhibited by concomitant oestradiol treatment at concentrations of 2.5×10^{-6}–10^{-5} mol/L (Francavilla *et al.*, 1989), suggesting marked sex differences in the mitogenic effects of epidermal growth factor and oestrogens on rat liver. Differences in culture medium composition may also have contributed to these discrepancies (Yager & Liehr, 1996).

Within 6–12 h after oestradiol was given at a dose of 5 mg/kg bw to castrated Syrian golden hamsters by intraperitoneal injection, renal ornithine decarboxylase activities were increased threefold above the control level. Similarly, in hamsters that received subcutaneous implants of pellets of 20 mg oestradiol to maintain chronically high oestrogen levels, the renal activity of ornithine decarboxylase was 1.5–1.9 times the corresponding activity in control animals after 60–80 days of treatment. With a series of oestrogen analogues, there was a direct correlation between the increase in renal ornithine decarboxylase activity *in vivo* and binding to renal oestradiol receptor sites *in vitro*. The concentrations of the polyamines putrescine, spermidine and spermine in hamster kidney all declined during the 180-day experimental period (Nawata *et al.*, 1981).

(c) Oestriol

Oestriol bound with low affinity to oestrogen receptors in calf, rat and human uterine tissue and in Ishikawa human endometrial cancer cells (Katzenellenbogen, 1984; Lubahn *et al.*, 1985; Botella *et al.*, 1995), with a relative binding affinity about 5–12% that of oestradiol (Batra *et al.*, 1984; Katzenellenbogen, 1984; Botella *et al.*, 1995).

Incorporation of tritiated thymidine by primary cultures of hepatocytes from female Fischer 344 or Lewis rats was minimally (1.5-fold) stimulated by addition of oestriol to the medium for 48 h at a concentration of 3×10^{-5} mol/L. Simultaneous addition of 15 ng/mL TGF-α stimulated DNA synthesis in these cells by approximately 100-fold in a synergistic fashion, while TGF-α alone at this concentration stimulated DNA synthesis by 54-fold (Ni & Yager, 1994a,b).

(d) Oestrone

Oestrone bound with low affinity to the oestrogen receptor in calf, rat and human uterine tissue (Lubahn *et al.*, 1985; Bhavnani & Woolever, 1991) and in Ishikawa human endometrial cancer cells (Botella *et al.*, 1995). Its relative binding affinity to the receptor in human endometrial cytosol is 2–10% that of oestradiol (Lubahn *et al.*, 1985; Bhavnani & Woolever, 1991; Botella *et al.*, 1995).

Oestrone stimulated the incorporation of tritiated thymidine into the DNA of MCF-7 human breast cancer cells at concentrations of 10^{-11} mol/L and higher, reaching a plateau of stimulation at 10^{-9} mol/L; this was approximately 20% lower than the maximal stimulation achieved by oestradiol at a concentration of 10^{-10} mol/L (Kitawaki *et al.*, 1992). Oestrone treatment of MCF-7 human breast cancer cells stimulated their growth, as seen from the increase in cell number, over a six-day period at concentrations of 10^{-10} mol/L and higher, reaching a maximum at between 10^{-9} and 10^{-8} mol/L. When the mitotic index was used as an indicator of cell proliferation, however, stimulation was already maximal at an oestrone concentration of 10^{-13} mol/L and was similar to that achieved by oestradiol at 10^{-11} mol/L. This effect of oestrone was inhibited by simultaneous exposure of the cells to the pure anti-oestrogen ICI164,384. Three days of treatment of MCF-7 cells with 10^{-8} mol/L oestrone resulted in a concentration of 3.3×10^{-9} mol/L oestradiol in the culture medium (Santner *et al.*, 1993).

Oestrone given to female Sprague Dawley rats after ovariectomy at a subcutaneous dose of 1 µg/rat twice daily stimulated the growth of DMBA-induced mammary tumours by 225% after 65 days of treatment; this effect was abolished by simultaneous administration of an anti-oestrogen, EM-800, at 2.5 mg/kg bw per day or medroxyprogesterone acetate at 1 mg/rat subcutaneously twice daily (Luo *et al.*, 1997).

Incorporation of tritiated thymidine by cultured primary hepatocytes from female Fischer 344 or Lewis rats was stimulated threefold by addition of oestrone to the medium for 48 h at a concentration of 3×10^{-5} mol/L. Simultaneous addition of 15 ng/mL TGF-α stimulated DNA synthesis by approximately 100-fold in a synergistic fashion, while TGF-α alone at this concentration stimulated DNA synthesis by 54-fold (Ni & Yager, 1994b).

Oestrone at concentrations of 10^{-10}–10^{-8} mol/L stimulated cell proliferation in primary cultures of renal proximal tubular cells isolated from castrated male Syrian hamsters, being maximally effective at 10^{-9} mol/L and not effective at higher or lower concentrations. Treatment of these hamsters with pellets that released 111 ± 11 µg oestrone per animal per day resulted in a 100% tumour incidence in the kidney in approximately nine months (Li *et al.* (1995).

Oestrone bound to sex hormone-binding globulin, displacing 5α-dihydrotestosterone with an affinity that was 25% that of oestradiol and 1.8% that of testosterone (Pan *et al.*, 1985).

4.3   Genetic and related effects

Receptor mechanisms are fundamental to the responses to oestrogens (King, 1991), although non-receptor mechanisms may also be important (Duval *et al.*, 1983; Yager & Liehr, 1996).

4.3.1   *Humans*

No data were available on the genetic effects of unopposed oestrogens in humans.

4.3.2   *Experimental systems*

The genetic and related effects of oestrogens are summarized in Table 14.

In one study, oestradiol decreased the formation of single- and double-strand breaks in ΦX-174 RFI DNA induced by hydrogen peroxide alone or with Cu^{2+} (Tang & Subbiah, 1996). Gene mutations were not induced in *Salmonella typhimurium* by oestradiol. DNA strand breaks were not induced by oestradiol in rat hepatocytes or hamster ovary cells in the absence or presence of a metabolic activation system. Oestradiol weakly induced DNA breakage in mouse brain cells. It did not induce DNA repair in a mouse mammary cell line and did not give rise to unscheduled DNA synthesis in hamster embryo cells. It did not induce gene mutations at either the *hprt* or Na^+/K^+ ATPase loci, or sister chromatid exchange or chromosomal aberrations in hamster embryo cells, whereas the formation of micronuclei was increased in these cells in a single study. In several studies, aneuploidy was induced in hamster embryo cells, male hamster cells and human foreskin fibroblasts. In rodent cells, oestradiol was shown to cause cell transformation in five studies with different experimental designs, but it gave negative results in two studies. In hamster cells, it gave rise to the formation of DNA adducts, but it did not cause oxidative DNA damage. In human lymphocytes, oestradiol caused micronucleus formation but no chromosomal aberrations or sister chromatid exchange; it weakly induced aneuploidy.

Studies conducted with oestrogens *in vivo* allow the examination of sex- and organ-specific effects. Induction of covalent modifications in DNA was demonstrated by ^{32}P-postlabelling in the kidneys and liver of hamsters and rats after a subcutaneous implant of oestradiol. In a single study, apparent covalent binding to DNA was not induced in the kidneys or liver of rats or hamsters treated by oral administration with oestradiol; the authors of the study reported that the radiolabel detected in some DNA samples could have been due to protein contamination.

DNA strand breakage was induced in the kidneys but not the livers of hamsters after subcutaneous implantation of oestradiol at low doses and in both liver and kidney after a much higher dose; an even higher dose of oestradiol administered to male hamsters intraperitoneally had no effect on either kidneys or liver.

Oestradiol induced sister chromatid exchange in mouse uterine cells but not in kidney cells *in vivo*, but it did not cause aneuploidy in either cell type. It gave rise to chromosomal aberrations and aneuploidy in renal cells of hamsters exposed *in vivo*.

In a single study, K-, H- or N-*ras* and *p53* gene mutations were not found in endometrial lesions of mice fed a diet containing MNU and oestradiol (Murase *et al.*, 1995).

Table 14. Genetic and related effects of oestradiol and oestrone and their derivatives and of oestriol

Test system	Result[a] Without exogenous metabolic system	With exogenous metabolic system	Dose[b] (LED or HID)	Reference
Oestradiol				
Salmonella typhimurium TA100, TA1535, TA1537, TA1538, TA98, reverse mutation	–	–	2500 µg/plate	Lang & Redman (1979)
Salmonella typhimurium TA1535, TA1537, reverse mutation	–	–	500 µg/plate	Ingerowski et al. (1981)
Salmonella typhimurium TA100, TA1535, TA1537, TA1538, TA98, reverse mutation	–	–	500 µg/plate[c]	Lang & Reimann (1993)
DNA strand breaks, cross-links or related damage, mouse brain DNA in vitro	(+)	NT	27.2	Yamafuji et al. (1971)
DNA strand breaks, cross-links or related damage, Chinese hamster V79 cells in vitro	–	–	816	Swenberg (1981)
DNA single-strand breaks, rat hepatocytes in vitro	–	NT	82	Sina et al. (1983)
DNA repair exclusive of unscheduled DNA synthesis, female C57BL mouse mammary epithelial cells in vitro	–	NT	0.2	Telang et al. (1992)
Unscheduled DNA synthesis, Syrian hamster embryo cells in vitro	–	NT	10	Tsutsui et al. (1987)
Gene mutation, Chinese hamster lung V79 cells, hprt locus in vitro	–	–	27.2	Drevon et al. (1981)
Gene mutation, Chinese hamster lung V79 cells, ouabain in vitro	–	–	27.2	Drevon et al. (1981)
Gene mutation, Syrian hamster embryo cells, hprt and Na+/K+ ATPase loci in vitro	–	NT	10	Tsutsui et al. (1987)
Sister chromatid exchange, mouse cervical fibroblasts and kidney cells in vitro	–	NT	2.7	Hillbertz-Nilsson & Forsberg (1985)
Sister chromatid exchange, Syrian hamster embryo cells in vitro	–	NT	10	Tsutsui et al. (1987)
Micronucleus formation, Syrian hamster embryo cells in vitro	+[c]	NT	2.72	Schnitzler et al. (1994)
Micronucleus formation, ovine seminal vesicle cells in vitro	+[c]	NT	2.72	Schnitzler et al. (1994)
Chromosomal aberrations, Syrian hamster embryo cells in vitro	–	NT	10	Tsutsui et al. (1987)
Chromosomal aberrations, Syrian hamster embryo cells in vitro	–	NT	8.17	Tsutsui et al. (1997)

Table 14 (contd)

Test system	Result[a]		Dose[b] (LED or HID)	Reference
	Without exogenous metabolic system	With exogenous metabolic system		
Aneuploidy, male Chinese hamster DON cells *in vitro*	+	NT	13.6	Wheeler *et al.* (1986)
Aneuploidy, Syrian hamster embryo cells *in vitro*	+	NT	10	Tsutsui *et al.* (1987, 1990)
Aneuploidy, Syrian hamster embryo cells *in vitro*	+	NT	0.82	Tsutsui *et al.* (1997)
Cell transformation, BALB/c 3T3 embryo-derived mouse fibroblasts	+	NT	5.5	Liehr *et al.* (1987a)
Cell transformation, C3H 10T1/2 mouse cells	+	NT	0.27	Kennedy & Weichselbaum (1981)
Cell transformation, Syrian hamster embryo cells	+	NT	3	Tsutsui *et al.* (1987)
Cell transformation, Syrian hamster embryo cells	NT	+	3	Hayashi *et al.* (1996)
Cell transformation, Syrian hamster embryo cells	+	NT	2.72	Tsutsui *et al.* (1997)
Cell transformation, female C57BL mouse mammary epithelial cells	−	NT	0.2	Telang *et al.* (1992)
Cell transformation, primary baby rat kidney + HPV16 + *ras*	−	NT	0.27	Pater *et al.* (1990)
Sister chromatid exchange, human lymphocytes *in vitro*	−	NT	13.6	Hill & Wolff (1983)
Sister chromatid exchange, human lymphocytes *in vitro*	−	−	27.2	Banduhn & Obe (1985)
Micronucleus formation, human lymphocytes *in vitro*	+	NT	1.3	Banduhn & Obe (1985)
Chromosomal aberrations, human lymphocytes *in vitro*	−	NT	100	Stenchever *et al.* (1969)
Chromosomal aberrations, human lymphocytes *in vitro*	−	−	27.2	Banduhn & Obe (1985)
Aneuploidy, human lymphocytes *in vitro*	(+)	NT	13.6	Banduhn & Obe (1985)
Aneuploidy, human foreskin JHU-1 fibroblasts *in vitro*	+	NT	20	Tsutsui *et al.* (1990)
DNA strand breaks, cross-links or related damage, male Syrian hamster kidney and liver *in vivo*	(+)	NT	22.5 mg imp × 1, 2 wk	Han & Liehr (1994)
DNA strand breaks, cross-links or related damage, male Syrian hamster kidney *in vivo*	+		250 µg/d imp × 1, 7 d	Han & Liehr (1994)
DNA strand breaks, cross-links or related damage, male Syrian hamster liver *in vivo*	−		250 µg/d imp × 1, 7 d	Han & Liehr (1994)

Table 14 (contd)

Test system	Result[a] Without exogenous metabolic system	Result[a] With exogenous metabolic system	Dose[b] (LED or HID)	Reference
DNA strand breaks, cross-links or related damage, male Syrian hamster kidney and liver in vivo	−		150 ip × 1	Han & Liehr (1994)
Sister chromatid exchange, female NMRI mouse uterine cervix and uterine horn epithelial cells in vivo	+		5 µg sc × 1	Forsberg (1991)
Sister chromatid exchange, female NMRI kidney cells in vivo	−		5 µg sc × 1	Forsberg (1991)
Chromosomal aberrations, male Syrian hamster renal cortical cells in vivo	+		125 µg/d imp × 1, 5 mo	Banerjee et al. (1994)
Aneuploidy, female NMRI mouse uterine cervix and uterine horn epithelial cells in vivo	−		5 µg sc × 1	Forsberg (1991)
Aneuploidy, female NMRI mouse kidney cells in vivo	−		5 µg sc × 1	Forsberg (1991)
Aneuploidy, male Syrian hamster renal tubular cells in vivo	+		20 mg imp × 1, 3.5 mo	Li et al. (1993)
Increase in nuclear DNA content (aneuploidy), female BALB/c mouse cervicovaginal epithelium in vivo	+		25 µg sc × 5	Hajek et al. (1993)
Binding (covalent) to DNA, male Syrian hamster liver, 8-hydroxy-2'-deoxyguanosine formation in vitro	NT	−	54.5	Han & Liehr (1995)
Binding (covalent) to DNA, Syrian hamster embryo cells in vitro	NT	(+)	1	Hayashi et al. (1996)
Binding (covalent) to DNA, female Sprague-Dawley rat liver in vivo	−		0.3 po × 1	Caviezel et al. (1984)
Binding (covalent) to DNA, male and female Syrian hamster kidney and liver in vivo	−		0.3 po × 1	Caviezel et al. (1984)
Binding (covalent) to DNA, male Syrian hamster kidney cortex in vivo	+		31 mg imp × 1, 2.5 mo	Liehr et al. (1986c)

Table 14 (contd)

Test system	Result[a]		Dose[b] (LED or HID)	Reference
	Without exogenous metabolic system	With exogenous metabolic system		
Binding (covalent) to DNA, male Syrian hamster kidney *in vivo*	+		22.5 mg imp × 1, 7 mo	Lu *et al.* (1988)
Oestradiol + testosterone				
Binding (covalent) to DNA, male NBL/Cr rat dorsolateral prostate *in vivo*	+		NR	Han *et al.* (1995)
Binding (covalent) to DNA, male NBL/Cr rat ventral and anterior prostate *in vivo*	−		NR	Han *et al.* (1995)
17α-Oestradiol				
Chromosomal aberrations, male Syrian hamster renal cortical cells *in vivo*	−		105 μg/d imp × 1, 5 mo	Banerjee *et al.* (1994)
4-Hydroxyoestradiol				
Cell transformation, Syrian hamster embryo cells	NT	+	0.3	Hayashi *et al.* (1996)
DNA strand breaks, cross-links or related damage, male Syrian hamster kidney cells *in vivo*	+		250 μg/d imp × 1, 7 d	Han & Liehr (1994)
Binding (covalent) to DNA, male Syrian hamster liver, 8-hydroxy-2′-deoxyguanosine formation *in vitro*	NT	+	57.9	Han & Liehr (1995)
Binding (covalent) to DNA, Syrian hamster embryo cells *in vitro*	NT	+	1	Hayashi *et al.* (1996)
Binding (covalent) to calf thymus DNA *in vitro*	NT	+[d]	66.7	Cavalieri *et al.* (1997)
Binding (covalent) to DNA, female Sprague-Dawley rat mammary cells *in vivo*	+		250 μg i-mam × 1	Cavalieri *et al.* (1997)

Table 14 (contd)

Test system	Result[a] Without exogenous metabolic system	Result[a] With exogenous metabolic system	Dose[b] (LED or HID)	Reference
2-Hydroxyoestradiol				
Cell transformation, Syrian hamster embryo cells	NT	+	1	Hayashi et al. (1996)
DNA strand breaks, cross-links or related damage, male Syrian hamster kidney cells in vivo	-		250 µg/d imp × 1, 7 d	Han & Liehr (1994)
Binding (covalent) to DNA, male Syrian hamster liver, 8-hydroxy-2′-deoxyguanosine formation in vitro	NT	-	57.9	Han & Liehr (1995)
Binding (covalent) to DNA, Syrian hamster embryo cells in vitro	NT	+	1	Hayashi et al. (1996)
Oestradiol-3,4-quinone				
Binding (covalent) to calf thymus DNA in vitro	+	NT	200	Cavalieri et al. (1997)
Binding (covalent) to DNA, female Sprague-Dawley rat mammary cells in vivo	+		250 µg i-mam × 1	Cavalieri et al. (1997)
Oestrone				
Gene mutation, Chinese hamster lung V79 cells, hprt locus in vitro	-	-	27	Drevon et al. (1981)
Gene mutation, Chinese hamster lung V79 cells, ouabain in vitro	-	-	27	Drevon et al. (1981)
Binding (covalent) to DNA, male Syrian hamster liver, 8-hydroxy-2′-deoxyguanosine formation in vitro	NT	-	54.1	Han & Liehr (1995)
Binding (covalent) to DNA, female Sprague-Dawley rat liver in vivo	-		0.3 po × 1	Caviezel et al. (1984)
Binding (covalent) to DNA, male Syrian hamster kidney and liver in vivo	-		0.3 po × 1	Caviezel et al. (1984)
Oestrone-3,4 quinone				
DNA strand breaks, cross-links or related damage, human MCF-7 cells in vitro	+	NT	7.1	Nutter et al. (1994)
Binding (covalent) to calf thymus DNA in vitro	(+)	NT	200	Cavalieri et al. (1997)

Table 14 (contd)

Test system	Result[a] Without exogenous metabolic system	Result[a] With exogenous metabolic system	Dose[b] (LED or HID)	Reference
16α-Hydroxyoestrone				
DNA repair exclusive of unscheduled DNA synthesis, female C57BL mouse mammary epithelial cells in vitro	+	NT	0.2	Telang et al. (1992)
Cell transformation, female C57BL mouse mammary epithelial cells	+	NT	0.2	Telang et al. (1992)
2-Hydroxyoestrone				
Binding (covalent) to DNA, male Syrian hamster liver, 8-hydroxy-2'-deoxyguanosine formation in vitro	NT	–	57.5	Han & Liehr (1995)
4-Hydroxyoestrone				
Binding (covalent) to calf thymus DNA in vitro	NT	+[d]	66.7	Cavalieri et al. (1997)
Binding (covalent) to DNA, male Syrian hamster liver, 8-hydroxy-2'-deoxyguanosine formation in vitro	NT	+	57.5	Han & Liehr (1995)
Oestriol				
DNA repair exclusive of unscheduled DNA synthesis, female C57BL mouse mammary epithelial cells in vitro	–	NT	0.2	Telang et al. (1992)
Aneuploidy, male Chinese hamster DON cells in vitro	+	NT	21.6	Wheeler et al. (1986)
Cell transformation, female C57BL mouse mammary epithelial cells	–	NT	0.2	Telang et al. (1992)
Sister chromatid exchange, human lymphocytes in vitro	(+)	NT	14	Hill & Wolff (1983)

[a] +, positive; (+), weak positive; –, negative; NT, not tested

[b] LED, lowest effective dose; HID, highest ineffective dose; in-vitro tests, μg/mL; in-vivo tests, mg/kg bw per day; wk, week; d, day; mo, months; imp, subcutaneous implant; ip, intraperitoneal injection; sc, subcutaneous injection; po, oral; i-mam, intramammary; NR, not reported

[c] 41–68% of the induced micronuclei contained CREST-reactive kinetochores

[d] Horeradish peroxidase-activated or lactoperoxidase-activated or S9 activated system

A combination of oestradiol and testosterone administered to male rats resulted in DNA binding in the dorsolateral prostate but not in the ventral or anterior prostate.

In a single study, the frequency of chromosomal aberrations was not increased in renal proximal convoluted tubules of male hamsters treated with 17α-oestradiol.

DNA strand breakage was demonstrated in kidney cells of male hamsters treated subcutaneously with 4-hydroxyoestradiol. In hamster cells *in vitro*, 4-hydroxyoestradiol caused cell transformation and formation of DNA adducts in the presence of exogenous metabolic activation. Induction of oxidative damage in male hamster liver DNA and binding to calf thymus DNA were seen after in-vitro treatment with 4-hydroxyoestradiol, and similar results were observed *in vivo* in mammary cells of rats treated with this compound.

DNA strand breakage was not demonstrated in kidney cells from male hamsters treated subcutaneously with 2-hydroxyoestradiol, and this compound did not bind to liver DNA of hamsters *in vitro* in one study. In hamster cells, 2-hydroxyoestradiol caused cell transformation and formation of DNA adducts in the presence of exogenous metabolic activation.

Oestradiol-3,4-quinone bound to DNA both *in vitro* and *in vivo* in rat mammary cells.

Oestrone did not cause gene mutation at various loci in hamster ovary cells. It did not induce oxidative damage in hamster liver DNA, nor did it bind to kidney or liver DNA of male hamsters or to liver DNA of rats treated *in vivo*.

In vitro, oestrone-3,4-quinone induced DNA strand breaks in human MCF-7 cells and bound weakly to calf thymus DNA.

In a mammary cell line derived from mice, DNA repair and cell transformation were induced by treatment with 16α-hydroxyoestrone.

No induction of oxidative DNA damage was seen in the presence of an exogenous metabolic activation system in male hamster liver cells treated *in vitro* with 2-hydroxyoestrone, but 4-hydroxyoestrone was active in this assay. Furthermore, the latter compound bound to calf thymus DNA under these conditions.

Neither DNA repair nor cell transformation was induced in mouse mammary epithelial cells treated with oestriol, whereas aneuploidy was induced in male hamster DON cells. Oestriol weakly induced sister chromatid exchange in human lymphocytes *in vitro*.

In one study, equilin and equilenin decreased the formation of single- and double-strand DNA breaks induced by hydrogen peroxide alone or with Cu^{2+} (Tang & Subbiah, 1996).

5.   Summary of Data Reported and Evaluation

5.1   Exposure

The numbers of women who have used post-menopausal oestrogen therapy vary between countries and within regions of individual countries. The prevalence of use has been greater in the United States than in most other countries; use of oestrogen therapy after the menopause is rare in developing countries but is increasing. Conjugated equine oestrogens are the most widely prescribed preparation for oestrogen therapy for women in the United States, but oestradiol and its esters have greater use in most of Europe. Oral administration is the most popular route, but percutaneous methods are becoming commoner; use of injections, the first form of post-menopausal oestrogen therapy, has been declining.

5.2   Human carcinogenicity

Breast cancer

Information on the relationship between post-menopausal oestrogen therapy and risk for breast cancer is available from many epidemiological studies. A pooled analysis of the original data from 51 of those studies and a review of data from 15 cohort and 23 case–control studies showed that in the majority of the studies there is a small increase in risk with longer duration of use (five years or more) in current and recent users. Although there is far less information about women who used post-menopausal oestrogen therapy and then ceased use, the increase in risk appears to cease several years after use has stopped. The increase in risk is predominantly for small localized carcinomas of the breast. There are insufficient data to determine whether the risk varies with type of compound or dose.

Endometrial cancer

Three cohort and more than 30 case–control studies consistently showed an association between use of post-menopausal oestrogen therapy and an increased risk for endometrial cancer. The risk increases with increasing duration of use. It decreases with time since last use but remains higher than that of untreated women for at least 10 years.

Cervical cancer

Only one cohort and two case–control studies were available on the relationship between use of post-menopausal oestrogen therapy and the risk for invasive cervical cancer; in none of them were the possible confounding effects of oncogenic human papillomaviruses considered. On balance, the limited evidence available suggests that post-menopausal oestrogen therapy is not associated with an increased risk for invasive cervical carcinoma. The results provide some suggestion that post-menopausal oestrogen therapy is associated with a reduced risk for cervical cancer, but the finding could be due to more active screening for pre-invasive disease among women who have received post-menopausal oestrogen therapy.

Ovarian cancer

The four cohort and 12 case–control studies that addressed the risk for ovarian cancer (largely epithelial) among women undergoing post-menopausal oestrogen therapy gave mixed results. One cohort study and one large case–control study showed a significant excess risk for ovarian cancer in women who used this therapy, but a pooled analysis of the individual data from case–control studies showed no excess risk. There is therefore no clear association between post-menopausal oestrogen therapy and the risk for ovarian cancer.

Cancers of the liver and gall-bladder

The two cohort and two case–control studies that addressed the association between use of post-menopausal oestrogen therapy and the risk for cancers of the liver or biliary tract showed no alteration in risk.

Colorectal cancer

Seven cohort and 12 case–control studies have provided information on use of post-menopausal oestrogen therapy and the risk for colorectal cancer. The risk was not increased and appeared to be reduced in one-half of the studies. The reduced risk tended to be observed among recent users and did not appear to be related to duration of use.

Cutaneous malignant melanoma

One cohort and nine case–control studies addressed the risk for cutaneous malignant melanoma in relation to use of post-menopausal oestrogen therapy. Most suggested no alteration in risk.

Thyroid cancer

Seven case–control studies that provided information on thyroid cancer and use of post-menopausal oestrogen therapy suggested no effect on risk.

5.3   Carcinogenicity in experimental animals

Conjugated oestrogens

Hydrolysed conjugated equine oestrogens, equilin and d-equilenin were tested in male hamsters by subcutaneous implantation. The hydrolysed oestrogens and equilin induced microscopic renal carcinomas, whereas d-equilenin was inactive.

Oestradiol

Oestradiol and its esters were tested in mice by oral administration, in mice, rats, hamsters, guinea-pigs and monkeys by subcutaneous injection or implantation and in mice by neonatal exposure.

Oral administration of oestradiol to mice bearing murine mammary tumour virus increased the incidences of uterine (endometrial and cervical) adenocarcinomas and mammary tumours. Its subcutaneous administration to mice resulted in increased incidences of mammary, pituitary, uterine, cervical, vaginal and lymphoid tumours and interstitial-cell tumours of the testis.

Invasive pituitary tumours were induced in rats treated with oestradiol dipropionate. In hamsters, a high incidence of malignant kidney tumours occurred in intact and castrated males and in ovariectomized females treated with oestradiol, but not in intact females. In guinea-pigs, diffuse fibromyomatous uterine and abdominal lesions were observed. Subcutaneous injections to neonatal mice resulted in precancerous and cancerous cervical and vaginal lesions in later life and an increased incidence of mammary tumours. The 4-hydroxy metabolite of oestradiol induced renal-cell carcinomas in castrated male hamsters.

Oestradiol was tested in two-stage carcinogenesis models in mice with the known carcinogens N-methyl-N-nitrosourea, N-ethyl-N-nitrosourea or 3-methylcholanthrene and in two-stage carcinogenesis models in rats with N-methyl-N-nitrosourea, 2-acetylamino-fluorene, N-nitrosodiethylamine, 7,12-dimethylbenz[a]anthracene or N-butyl-N-nitroso-urea. In mice, oestradiol enhanced the incidences of endometrial adenomatous hyper-plasia, atypical hyperplasia and adenocarcinomas induced by N-methyl-N-nitrosourea and N-ethyl-N-nitrosourea. A continuously high serum concentration of oestradiol and a low concentration of progesterone appeared to be important for the development of endo-metrial adenocarcinomas in mice. Oestradiol suppressed the development of uterine cervical carcinomas induced by 3-methylcholanthrene. In rats, large doses of oestradiol alone or oestradiol with progesterone suppressed the development of mammary carci-nomas induced by N-methyl-N-nitrosourea. Combined treatment of ovariectomized rats with oestradiol and N-methyl-N-nitrosourea induced vaginal polyps. In a two-stage model of liver carcinogenesis in rats, oestradiol showed no initiating activity. It did not show pro-moting effects in the livers of rats initiated with N-nitrosodiethylamine. In one study pre-treatment with oestradiol increased the number of liver foci positive for γ-glutamyl trans-ferase induced by N-nitrosodiethylamine. Oestradiol did not affect mammary tumour development in intact or ovariectomized female rats treated with 7,12-dimethylbenz[a]-anthracene. Oestradiol benzoate enhanced the incidence of mammary tumours in rats treated with γ-rays.

Oestriol

Oestriol was tested for carcinogenicity by subcutaneous implantation in one study in castrated mice and in one study in hamsters. In mice, oestriol increased the incidence and accelerated the appearance of mammary tumours in both male and female mice. In hamsters, oestriol produced kidney tumours.

In female mice, oestriol slightly increased the incidence of N-methyl-N-nitrosourea-induced endometrial adenocarcinomas. In several studies in female rats, oestriol inhibited the induction of mammary tumours by 7,12-dimethylbenz[a]anthracene when adminis-tered before the carcinogen; continuous treatment with oestriol resulted in a decreased inci-dence of mammary tumours. In one study in female rats, oestriol inhibited the induction of mammary carcinomas when administered 13–15 days after irradiation with γ-rays.

Oestrone

Oestrone was tested for carcinogenicity by oral administration in two studies in castrated male mice. The incidence of mammary tumours was increased. In one study in which oestrone was administered by skin application to mice, the incidence of mammary tumours was increased in males and that of pituitary tumours in animals of each sex. In studies in which oestrone was tested by subcutaneous and/or intramuscular adminis-tration, mammary tumours were induced in male mice, and the average age at the time of appearance of mammary tumours in female mice was reduced. In castrated male and female rats, subcutaneous injection of oestrone resulted in mammary tumours.

In three studies of subcutaneous or intramuscular administration, oestrone benzoate induced mammary tumours in male mice. In one study in rats, subcutaneous injection of oestrone benzoate induced mammary and pituitary tumours in animals of each sex. In several studies involving subcutaneous implantation of oestrone, the incidences of mammary and lymphoid tumours were increased in mice, and those of mammary and pituitary tumours were increased in rats. In one study in rats, implantation of low-dose oestrone pellets induced adrenal cortical tumours, but high-dose pellets reduced the incidence. In intact and castrated male hamsters, implantation of oestrone resulted in malignant kidney tumours. The oestrone metabolite, 4-hydroxyoestrone, induced kidney tumours at a low incidence in castrated male hamsters.

Oestrone-3,4-quinone, a metabolite of oestrone, was tested for carcinogenicity by direct injection into the mammary glands of rats fed a high-fat diet. There were no significant differences in mammary tumour incidence or multiplicity in comparison with controls that did not receive the metabolite.

The incidence of endometrial adenocarcinomas induced by N-methyl-N-nitrosourea in the uterine corpus of mice was significantly increased in those receiving an oestrone-containing diet; furthermore, the incidences of preneoplastic endometrial lesions in the N-methyl-N-nitrosourea-treated and untreated uterine corpora were significantly increased in mice receiving the oestrone-containing diet. In one study in female toads, subcutaneous administration of oestrone enhanced the incidence of hepatocellular carcinomas induced by subcutaneous injection of N-nitrosodimethylamine.

5.4   Other relevant data

Oestrogens administered orally are absorbed rapidly and achieve maximum serum levels quickly. Although the major route of metabolism for oestrogens inactivates them and facilitates their excretion, a minor metabolic pathway activates a small proportion of oestrogen to catechol intermediates, with significant potential for damaging DNA, and may also yield reactive oxygen species that damage DNA. Some oestrogens, including conjugated oestrogens, have been reported to have genotoxic activity in experimental systems. At higher concentrations, which may or may not involve receptor mediation, oestrogens have been reported to induce changes in DNA and chromosomes. Oestradiol binds to oestrogen receptors with higher affinity than oestriol or oestrone. Oestrogens can increase the number of proliferating cells in the human endometrium *in vivo*. It has been reported that oestrogens increase cell proliferation in normal breast cells in monkeys and in cultured human breast cancer cells. At higher concentrations, oestrogens stimulated cell proliferation in rat liver *in vivo* and in cultured rat hepatocytes *in vitro*. No information was available on whether the effect of oestrogens on the mammary gland is modified by body weight or by the recency or duration of exposure to oestrogens in experimental systems. Similarly, no information was available on the possible relationship between exposure to oestrogens and the degree of malignancy of breast tumours.

5.5 Evaluation

There is *sufficient evidence* in humans for the carcinogenicity of post-menopausal oestrogen therapy.

There is *sufficient evidence* in experimental animals for the carcinogenicity of oestradiol and oestrone.

There is *limited evidence* in experimental animals for the carcinogenicity of conjugated equine oestrogens, equilin and oestriol.

There is *inadequate evidence* in experimental animals for the carcinogenicity of d-equilenin.

Overall evaluation

Post-menopausal oestrogen therapy is *carcinogenic to humans (Group 1).*

6. References

Adami, H.-O., Persson, I., Hoover, R., Schairer, C. & Bergkvist, L. (1989) Risk of cancer in women receiving hormone replacement therapy. *Int. J. Cancer*, **44**, 833–839

Adami, H.-O., Bergström, R., Persson, I. & Sparén, P. (1990) The incidence of ovarian cancer in Sweden, 1960–1984. *Am. J. Epidemiol.*, **132**, 446–452

Adams, J.B., Hall, R.T. & Nott, S. (1986) Esterification–deesterification of estradiol by human mammary cancer cells in culture. *J. Steroid Biochem.*, **24**, 1159–1162

Aedo, A.-R., Landgren, B.-M. & Diczfalusy, E. (1990) Pharmacokinetics and biotransformation of orally administered oestrone sulphate and oestradiol valerate in post-menopausal women. *Maturitas*, **12**, 333–343

Alexander, F.E., Roberts, M.M. & Huggins, A. (1987) Risk factors for breast cancer with applications to selection for the prevalence screen. *J. Epidemiol. Community Health*, **41**, 101–106

American College of Physicians (1992) Guidelines for counseling postmenopausal women about preventive hormone therapy. *Ann. intern. Med.*, **117**, 1038–1041

Anderson, F. (1993) Kinetics and pharmacology of estrogens in pre- and postmenopausal women. *Int. J. Fertil.*, **38** (Suppl. 1), 53–64

Anon. (1996) Hormone replacement therapy. *Drugs Ther. Bull.*, **34**, 81–84

Ansbacher, R. (1993) Bioequivalence of conjugated estrogen products. *Clin. Pharmacokinet.*, **24**, 271–274

Antunes, C.M.F., Stolley, P.D., Rosenshein, N.B., Davies, J.L., Tonascia, J.A., Brown, C., Burnett, L., Rutledge, A., Pokempner, M. & Garcia, R. (1979) Endometrial cancer and estrogen use. Report of a large case–control study. *New Engl. J. Med.*, **300**, 9–13

Armstrong, B.K. & Kricker, A. (1994) Cutaneous melanoma. *Cancer Surv.*, **19**, 219–240

Arrick, B.A., Korc, M. & Derynck, R. (1990) Differential regulation of expression of three transforming growth factor β species in human breast cancer cell lines by estradiol. *Cancer Res.*, **50**, 299–303

Austin, D.F. & Roe, K.M. (1982) The decreasing incidence of endometrial cancer: Public health implications. *Am. J. public Health*, **72**, 65–68

Balfour, J.A. & Heel, R.C. (1990) Transdermal estradiol: A review of its pharmacodynamic and pharmacokinetic properties, and therapeutic efficacy in the treatment of menopausal complaints. *Drugs*, **40**, 561–582

Banduhn, N. & Obe, G. (1985) Mutagenicity of methyl 2-benzimidazolecarbamate, diethylstilbestrol and estradiol: Structural chromosomal aberrations, sister-chromatid exchanges, C-mitoses, polyploidies and micronuclei. *Mutat. Res.*, **156**, 199–218

Banerjee, S.K., Banerjee, S., Li, S.A. & Li, J.J. (1994) Induction of chromosome aberrations in Syrian hamster renal cortical cells by various estrogens. *Mutat. Res.*, **311**, 191–197

Banks, E., Crossley, B., English, R. & Richardson, A. (1996) Women doctors' use of hormone replacement therapy: High prevalence of use is not confined to doctors (Letter to the Editor). *Br. med. J.*, **312**, 638

Barrett-Connor, E.L., Brown, W.V., Turner, J., Austin, M. & Criqui, M.H. (1979) Heart disease risk factors and hormone use in postmenopausal women. *J. Am. med. Assoc*, **241**, 2167–2169

Barrett-Connor, E.L., Wingard, D.L. & Criqui, M.H. (1989) Postmenopausal estrogen use and heart disease risk factors in the 1980s. *J. Am. med. Assoc.*, **261**, 2095–2100

Batra, S., Bjork, P. & Sjogren, C. (1984) Binding of estradiol-17 beta and estriol in cytosolic and nuclear fractions from urogenital tissues. *J. Steroid Biochem.*, **21**, 163–168

Bauss, F., Esswein, A., Reiff, K., Sponer, G. & Müller-Beckmann, B. (1996) Effect of 17β-estra-diol–bisphosphonate conjugates, potential bone-seeking estrogen pro-drugs, on 17β-estradiol serum kinetics and bone mass in rats. *Calcified Tissue int.*, **59**, 168–173

Bawarshi-Nassar, R.N., Hussain, A.A. & Crooks, P.A. (1989) Nasal absorption and metabolism of progesterone and 17 beta-estradiol in the rat. *Drug Metab. Disposition*, **17**, 248–254

Beral, V., Evans, S., Shaw, H. & Milton, G. (1984) Oral contraceptive use and malignant melanoma in Australia. *Br. J. Cancer*, **50**, 681–685

Beresford, S.A.A., Weiss, N.S., Voigt, L.F. & McKnight, B. (1997) Risk of endometrial cancer in relation to use of oestrogen combined with cyclic progestagen therapy in postmenopausal women. *Lancet*, **349**, 458–461

Bergkvist, L., Adami, H.-O., Persson, I., Hoover, R. & Schairer, C. (1989) The risk of breast cancer after estrogen and estrogen–progestin replacement. *New Engl. J. Med.*, **321**, 293–297

Bhavnani, B.R. (1998) Pharmacokinetics and pharmacodynamics of conjugated equine estrogens: Chemistry and metabolism. *Proc. Soc. exp. Med. Biol.*, **217**, 6–16

Bhavnani, B.R. & Woolever, C.A. (1991) Interaction of ring B unsaturated estrogens with estrogen receptors of human endometrium and rat uterus. *Steroids*, **56**, 201–210

Bidmon, H.J., Pitts, J.D., Solomon, H.F., Bondi, J.V. & Stumpf, W.E. (1990) Estradiol distribution and penetration in the rat skin after topical application, studied by high resolution autoradiography. *Histochemistry*, **95**, 43–54

Bishop, P.M.F. (1938) A clinical experiment in oestrin therapy. *Br. med. J.*, **i**, 939–941

Bolt, H.M. (1979) Metabolism of estrogens—natural and synthetic. *Pharmacol. Ther.*, **4**, 155–181

Booth, M., Beral, V. & Smith, P. (1989) Risk factors for ovarian cancer: A case–control study. *Br. J. Cancer*, **60**, 592–598

Bostick, R.M., Potter, J.D., Kushi, L.H., Sellers, T.A., Steinmetz, K.A., McKenzie, D.R., Gapstur, S.M. & Folsom, A.R. (1994) Sugar, meat, and fat intake, and non-dietary risk factors for colon cancer incidence in Iowa women (United States). *Cancer Causes Control*, **5**, 38–52

Botella, J., Duranti, E., Viader, V., Duc, I., Delansorne, R. & Paris, J. (1995) Lack of estrogenic potential of progesterone- or 19-nor-progesterone-derived progestins as opposed to testosterone or 19-nortestosterone derivatives on endometrial Ishikawa cells. *J. Steroid Biochem. mol. Biol.*, **55**, 77–84

Boyd, J. (1996) Estrogen as a carcinogen: The genetics and molecular biology of human endometrial carcinoma. In: Huff, J., Boyd, J. & Barrett, J.C., eds, *Cellular and Molecular Mechanisms of Hormonal Carcinogenesis: Environmental Influences*, New York, Wiley-Liss, pp. 151–173

Brett, K.M. & Madans, J.H. (1997) Use of postmenopausal hormone replacement therapy: Estimates from a nationally representative cohort study. *Am. J. Epidemiol.*, **145**, 536–545

Brinton, L.A. (1997) Hormone replacement therapy and risk for breast cancer. *Endocrinol. Metab. Clin. N. Am.*, **26**, 361–378

Brinton, L.A., Hoover, R.N., Szklo, M. & Fraumeni, J.F., Jr (1981) Menopausal estrogen use and risk of breast cancer. *Cancer*, **47**, 2517–2522

Brinton, L.A., Hoover, R. & Fraumeni, J.F., Jr (1986) Menopausal oestrogens and breast cancer risk: An expanded case–control study. *Br. J. Cancer*, **54**, 825–832

Brinton, L.A., Hoover, R.N. & the Endometrial Cancer Collaborative Group (1993) Estrogen replacement therapy and endometrial cancer risk: Unresolved issues. *Obstet. Gynecol.*, **81**, 265–271

Brinton, L.A., Dalling, J.R., Liff, J.M., Schoenberg, J.B., Malone, K.E., Stanford, J.L., Coates, R.J., Gammon, M.D., Hanson, L. & Hoover, R.N. (1995) Oral contraceptives and breast cancer risk among younger women. *J. natl Cancer Inst.*, **87**, 827–835

British Medical Association (1997) *British National Formulary*, No. 34, London, Royal Pharmaceutical Society of Great Britain, pp. 345–349

Brown, A.M.C., Jeltsch, J.-M., Roberts, M. & Chambon, P. (1984) Activation of *pS2* gene transcription is a primary response to estrogen in the human breast cancer cell line MCF-7. *Proc. natl Acad. Sci. USA*, **81**, 6344–6348

Buring, J.E., Bain, C.J. & Ehrmann, R.L. (1986) Conjugated estrogen use and risk of endometrial cancer. *Am. J. Epidemiol.*, **124**, 434–441

Buring, J.E., Hennekens, C.H., Lipnick, R.J., Willett, W., Stampfer, M.J., Rosner, B., Peto, R. & Speizer, F.E. (1987) A prospective cohort study of postmenopausal hormone use and risk of breast cancer in US women. *Am. J. Epidemiol.*, **125**, 939–947

Bush, T.L. & Barrett-Connor, E. (1985) Noncontraceptive estrogen use and cardiovascular disease. *Epidemiol. Rev.*, **7**, 80–104

Calle, E.E., Miracle-McMahill, H.L., Thun, M.J. & Heath, C.W., Jr (1995) Estrogen replacement therapy and risk of fatal colon cancer in a prospective cohort of postmenopausal women. *J. natl Cancer Inst.*, **87**, 517–523

Campagnoli, C., Biglia, N., Altare, F., Lanza, M.G., Lesca, L., Cantamessa, C., Peris, C., Fiorucci, G.C. & Sismondi, P. (1993) Differential effects of oral conjugated estrogens and transdermal estradiol on insulin-like growth factor 1, growth hormone and sex hormone binding globulin serum levels. *Gynecol. Endocrinol.*, **7**, 251–258

Campbell, A.D. & Collip, J.B. (1930) Notes on the clinical use of certain placental extracts. *Can. med. Assoc. J.*, **23**, 633–641

Catherino, W.H. & Jordan, V.C. (1995) Nomegestrol acetate, a clinically useful 19-norprogesterone derivative which lacks estrogenic activity. *J. Steroid Biochem. mol. Biol.*, **55**, 239–246

Cauley, J.A., Cummings, S.R., Black, D.M., Mascioli, S.R. & Seeley, D.G. (1990) Prevalence and determinants of estrogen replacement therapy in elderly women. *Am. J. Obstet. Gynecol.*, **163**, 1438–1444

Cavalieri, E.L., Stack, D.E., Devanesan, P.D., Todorovic, R., Dwivedy, I., Higginbotham, S., Johansson, S.L., Patil, K.D., Gross, M.L., Gooden, J.K., Ramanathan, R., Cerny, R.L. & Rogan, E.G. (1997) Molecular origin of cancer: Catechol estrogen-3,4-quinones as endogenous tumour initiators. *Proc. natl Acad. Sci. USA*, **94**, 10937–10942

Caviezel, M., Lutz, W.K. & Minini, C. (1984) Interaction of estrone and estradiol with DNA and protein of liver and kidney in rat and hamster *in vivo* and *in vitro*. *Arch. Toxicol.*, **55**, 97–103

Celli, G., Darwiche, N. & De Luca, L.M. (1996) Estrogen induces retinoid receptor expression in mouse cervical epithelia. *Exp. Cell Res.*, **226**, 273–282

Chandrasekaran, A., Osman, M., Scatina, J.A. & Sisenwine, S.F. (1995) Metabolism of equilin sulfate in the dog. *J. Steroid Biochem. mol. Biol.*, **55**, 271–278

Chanez, J.F., de Lignières, B., Marty, J.P. & Wepierre, J. (1989) Influence of the size of the area of treatment on percutaneous absorption of estradiol in the rat. *Skin Pharmacol.*, **2**, 15–21

Chen, M.J., Longnecker, M.P., Morgenstern, H., Lee, E.R., Frankl, H.D. & Haile, R.W. (1998) Recent use of hormone replacement therapy and the prevalence of colorectal adenomas. *Cancer Epidemiol. Biomarkers Prev.*, **7**, 227–230

Chow, W.-H., McLaughlin, J.K., Mandel, J.S., Blot, W.J., Niwa, S. & Fraumeni, J.F., Jr (1995) Reproductive factors and the risk of renal cell cancer among women. *Int. J. Cancer*, **60**, 321–324

Chute, C.G., Willett, W.C., Colditz, G.A., Stampfer, M.J., Rosner, B. & Speizer, F.E. (1991) A prospective study of reproductive history and exogenous estrogens on the risk of colorectal cancer in women. *Epidemiology*, **2**, 201–207

Cline, J.M., Soderqvist, G., von Schoultz, E., Skoog, L. & von Schoultz, B. (1996) Effects of hormone replacement therapy on the mammary gland of surgically postmenopausal cynomolgus macaques. *Am. J. Obstet. Glynecol.*, **174**, 93–100

Coldham, N.G. & James, V.H.T. (1990) A possible mechanism for increased breast cell proliferation by progestins through increased reductive 17β-hydroxysteroid dehydrogenase activity. *Int. J. Cancer*, **45**, 174–178

Colditz, G.A. (1996) Postmenopausal estrogens and breast cancer. *J. Soc. gynecol. Invest.*, **3**, 50–56

Colditz, G.A., Stampfer, M.J., Willett, W.C., Hunter, D.J., Manson, J.E., Hennekens, C.H., Rosner, B.A. & Speizer, F.E. (1992) Type of postmenopausal hormone use and risk of breast cancer: 12-year follow-up from the Nurses' Health Study. *Cancer Causes Control*, **3**, 433–439

Colditz, G.A., Hankinson, S.E., Hunter, D.J., Willett, W.C., Manson, J.E., Stampfer, M.J., Hennekens, C.H., Rosner, B.A. & Speizer, F.E. (1995) The use of estrogens and progestins and the risk of breast cancer in postmenopausal women. *New Engl. J. Med.*, **332**, 1589–1593

Collaborative Group on Hormonal Factors in Breast Cancer (1997) Breast cancer and hormone replacement therapy: Collaborative reanalysis of data from 51 epidemiological studies of 52 705 women with breast cancer and 108 411 women without breast cancer. *Lancet*, **350**, 1047–1059

Cushing, K.L., Weiss, N.S., Voigt, L.F., McKnight, B. & Beresford, S.A.A. (1998) Risk of endometrial cancer in relation to use of low-dose, unopposed estrogens. *Obstet. Gynecol.*, **91**, 35–39

Das, P., Rao, A.R. & Srivastava, P.N. (1988) Modulatory influences of exogenous estrogen on MCA-induced carcinogenesis in the uterine cervix of mouse. *Cancer Lett.*, **43**, 73–77

Davis, F.G., Furner, S.E., Persky, V. & Koch, M. (1989) The influence of parity and exogenous female hormones on the risk of colorectal cancer. *Int. J. Cancer*, **43**, 587–590

Derby, C.A., Hume, A.L., Barbour, M.M., McPhillips, J.B., Lasater, T.M. & Carleton, R.A. (1993) Correlates of postmenopausal estrogen use and trends through the 1980s in two southeastern New England communities. *Am. J. Epidemiol.*, **137**, 1125–1135

Devesa, S.S., Silverman, D.T., Young, J.L., Jr, Pollack, E.S., Brown, C.C., Horm, J.W., Percy, C.L., Myers, M.H., McKay, F.W. & Fraumeni, J.F., Jr (1987) Cancer incidence and mortality trends among whites in the United States, 1947–84. *J. natl Cancer Inst.*, **79**, 701–770

Drevon, C., Piccoli, C. & Montesano, R. (1981) Mutagenicity assays of estrogenic hormones in mammalian cells. *Mutat. Res.*, **89**, 83–90

Duval, D., Durant, S. & Homo-Delarche, F. (1983) Non-genomic effects of steroids: Interactions of steroid molecules with membrane structures and functions. *Biochim. biophys. Acta*, **737**, 409–442

Egeland, G.M., Matthews, K.A., Kuller, L.H. & Kelsey, S.F. (1988) Characteristics of non-contraceptive hormone users. *Prev. Med.*, **17**, 403–411

El-Bayoumy, K., Ji, B.-Y., Upadhyaya, P., Chac, Y.-H., Kurtzke, C., Riverson, A., Reddy, B.S., Amin, S. & Hecht, S.S. (1996) Lack of tumorigenicity of cholesterol epoxides and estrone-3,4-quinone in the rat mammary gland. *Cancer Res.*, **56**, 1970–1973

Ettinger, B., Golditch, I.M. & Friedman, G. (1988) Gynecologic consequences of long-term, unopposed estrogen replacement therapy. *Maturitas*, **10**, 271–282

Ewertz, M. (1988) Influence of non-contraceptive exogenous and endogenous sex hormones on breast cancer risk in Denmark. *Int. J. Cancer*, **42**, 832–838

Ewertz, M., Machado, S.G., Boice, J.D. & Jensen, O.M. (1984) Endometrial cancer following treatment for breast cancer: A case–control study in Denmark. *Br. J. Cancer*, **50**, 687–692

Ewertz, M., Schou, G. & Boice, J.D. (1988) The joint effect of risk factors on endometrial cancer. *Eur. J. Cancer clin. Oncol.*, **24**, 189–194

Fernandez, E., La Vecchia, C., D'Avanzo, B., Franceschi, S., Negri E. & Parazzini, F. (1996) Oral contraceptives, hormone replacement therapy and the risk of colorectal cancer. *Br. J. Cancer*, **73**, 1431–1435

Fernandez, E., La Vecchia, C., Braga, C., Talamini, R., Negri, E., Parazzini, F. & Franceschi, S. (1998) Hormone replacement therapy and risk of colon and rectal cancer. *Cancer Epidemiol. Biomarkers Prev.*, **7**, 329–333

Finkle, W.D., Greenland, S., Miettinen, O.S. & Ziel, H.K. (1995) Endometrial cancer risk after discontinuing use of unopposed conjugated estrogens (California, United States). *Cancer Causes Control*, **6**, 99–102

Finnegan, L.P., Rossouw, J. & Harlan, W.R. (1995) A peppy response to PEPI results. *Nature Med.*, **1**, 205–206

Folsom, A.R., Mink, P.J., Sellers, T.A., Hong, C.P., Zheng, W. & Potter, J.D. (1995) Hormonal replacement therapy and morbidity and mortality in a prospective study of postmenopausal women. *Am. J. public Health*, **85**, 1128–1132

Forsberg, J.G. (1991) Estrogen effects on chromosome number and sister chromatid exchanges in uterine epithelial cells and kidney cells from neonatal mice. *Teratog. Carcinog. Mutag.*, **11**, 135–146

Francavilla, A., Polimeno, L. DiLeo, A., Barone, M., Ove, P., Coetzee, M., Eagon, P., Makowka, L., Ambrosino, G., Mazzaferro, V. & Starzl, T.E. (1989) The effect of estrogen and tamoxifen on hepatocyte proliferation *in vivo* and *in vitro*. *Hepatology*, **9**, 614–620

Franceschi, S. & Dal Maso, L. (1999) Hormonal imbalance and thyroid cancers in humans. In: Capen, C.C., Dybing, E., Rice, J.M. & Wilbourn, J.D., eds, *Species Differences in Thyroid, Kidney and Urinary Bladder Carcinogenesis* (IARC Scientific Publications No. 147), Lyon, IARC, pp. 33–44

Franceschi, S. & La Vecchia, C. (1994) Thyroid cancer. *Cancer Surv.*, **19**, 393–422

Franceschi, S., La Vecchia, C., Helmrich, S.P., Mangioni, C. & Tognoni, G. (1982) Risk factors for epithelial ovarian cancer in Italy. *Am. J. Epidemiol.*, **115**, 714–719

Franceschi, S., Fassina, A., Talamini, R., Mazzolini, A., Vianello, S., Bidoli, E., Cizza, G. & La Vecchia C. (1990) The influence of reproductive and hormonal factors on thyroid cancer in women. *Rev. Epidémiol. Santé publique*, **38**, 27–34

Franks, A.L., Kendrick, J.S., Tyler, C.W. & the Cancer and Steroid Hormone Study Group (1987) Postmenopausal smoking, estrogen replacement therapy, and the risk of endometrial cancer. *Am. J. Obstet. Gynecol.*, **156**, 20–23

Fujimoto, J., Hori, M., Ichigo, S., Morishita, S. & Tamaya, T. (1996a) Estrogen activates migration potential of endometrial cancer cells through basement membrane. *Tumor Biol.*, **17**, 48–57

Fujimoto, J., Ichigo, S., Hori, M., Morishita, S. & Tamaya, T. (1996b) Progestins and danazol effect on cell-to-cell adhesion, and E-cadherin and α- and β-catenin mRNA expressions. *J. Steroid Biochem. mol. Biol.*, **57**, 275–282

Fujimoto, J., Hori, M., Ichigo, S. & Tamaya, T. (1997) Antiestrogenic compounds inhibit estrogen-induced expression of fibroblast growth factor family (FGF-1, 2, and 4) mRNA in well-differentiated endometrial cancer cells. *Eur. J. gynaecol. Oncol.*, **18**, 497–501

Furner, S.E., Davis, F.G., Nelson, R.L. & Haenszel, W. (1989) A case–control study of large bowel cancer and hormone exposure in women. *Cancer Res.*, **49**, 4936–4940

Gabrielsson, J., Wallenbeck, I., Larsson, G., Birgerson, L. & Heimer, G. (1995) New kinetic data on estradiol in light of the vaginal ring concept. *Maturitas*, **22** (Suppl.) S35–S39

Gabrielsson, J., Wallenbeck, I. & Birgerson, L. (1996) Pharmacokinetic data on estradiol in light of the Estring® concept. Estradiol and estring pharmacokinetics. *Acta obstet. gynecol. scand.*, **163** (Suppl.), 26–31

Galanti, M.R., Hansson, L., Lund, E., Bergström, R., Grimelius, L., Stalsberg, H., Carlsen, E., Baron, J.A., Persson, I. & Ekbom, A. (1996) Reproductive history and cigarette smoking as risk factors for thyroid cancer in women: A population-based case–control study. *Cancer Epidemiol. Biomarkers Prev.*, **5**, 425–431

Gallagher, R.P., Elwood, J.M., Hill, G.B., Coldman, A.J., Threlfall, W.J. & Spinelli, J.J. (1985) Reproductive factors, oral contraceptives and risk of malignant melanoma: Western Canada melanoma study. *Br. J. Cancer*, **52**, 901–907

Gambrell, R.D., Jr, Massey, F.M., Castaneda, T.A., Ugenas, A.J., Ricci, C.A. & Wright, J.M. (1980) Use of the progestogen challenge test to reduce the risk of endometrial cancer. *Obstet. Gynecol.*, **55**, 732–738

Gapstur, S.M., Potter, J.D., Sellers, T.A. & Folsom, A.R. (1992) Increased risk of breast cancer with alcohol consumption in postmenopausal women. *Am. J. Epidemiol.*, **136**, 1221–1231

Gerhardsson de Verdier, M. & London, S. (1992) Reproductive factors, exogenous female hormones, and colorectal cancer by subsite. *Cancer Causes Control*, **3**, 355–360

Godfree, V. (1994) Which oestrogen? Does the oestrogen you prescribe as hormone replacement therapy (HRT) make a difference to the patient? *Change*, **4**, 1–2

Goldfarb, S. & Pugh, T.D. (1990) Morphology and anatomic localization of renal microneoplasms and proximal tubule dysplasias induced by four different estrogens in the hamster. *Cancer Res.*, **50**, 113–119

Goodman, M.T., Moriwaki, H., Vaeth, M., Akiba, S., Hayabuchi, H. & Mabuchi, K. (1995) Prospective cohort study of risk factors for primary liver cancer in Hiroshima and Nagasaki, Japan. *Epidemiology*, **6**, 36–41

Goodman, M.T., Cologne, J., Moriwaki, H., Vaeth, M. & Mabuchi, K. (1997a) Risk factors for primary breast cancer in Japan: 8-year follow-up of atomic-bomb survivors. *Prevent. Med.*, **26**, 144–153

Goodman, M.T., Wilkens, L.R., Hankin, J.H., Lyu, L.-C., Wu, A.H. & Kolonel, L.N. (1997b) Association of soy and fiber consumption with the risk of endometrial cancer. *Am. J. Epidemiol.*, **146**, 294–306

Gordon, S.F. (1995) Clinical experience with a seven-day estradiol transdermal system for estrogen replacement therapy. *Am. J. Obstet. Gynecol.*, **173**, 998–1004

Grady, D., Gebretsadik, T., Kerlikowske, K., Ernster, V. & Petitti, D. (1995) Hormone replacement therapy and endometrial cancer risk: A meta-analysis. *Obstet. Gynecol.*, **85**, 304–313

Gray, L.A., Christopherson, W.M. & Hoover, R.N. (1977) Estrogens and endometrial carcinoma. *Obstet. Gynecol.*, **49**, 385–389

Green, A. & Bain, C. (1985) Hormonal factors and melanoma in women. *Med. J. Austr.*, **142**, 446–448

Green, P.K., Weiss, N.S., McKnight, B., Voigt, L.F. & Beresford, S.A.A. (1996) Risk of endometrial cancer following cessation of menopausal hormone use (Washington, United States). *Cancer Causes Control*, **7**, 575–580

Greene, G.L., Gilna, P., Waterfield, M., Baker, A., Hort, Y. & Shine, J. (1986) Sequence and expression of human estrogen receptor complementary DNA. *Science*, **231**, 1150–1154

Griffiths, F. & Jones, K. (1995) The use of hormone replacement therapy: Results of a community survey. *Fam. Pract.*, **12**, 163–165

Grodstein, F., Stampfer, M.J,. Colditz, G.A., Willett, W.C., Manson, J.E., Joffe, M., Rosner, B., Fuchs, C., Hankinson, S.E., Hunter, D.J., Hennekens, C.H. & Speizer, F.E. (1997) Postmenopausal hormone therapy and mortality. *New Engl. J. Med.*, **336**, 1769–1775

Grodstein, F., Martinez, E., Platz, E.A., Giovannucci, E., Colditz, G.A., Kautzky, M., Fuchs, C. & Stampfer, M.J. (1998) Postmenopausal hormone use and risk for colorectal cancer and adenoma. *Ann. intern. Med.*, **128**, 705–712

Grubbs, C.J., Peckham, J.C. & McDonough, K.D. (1983) Effect of ovarian hormones on the induction of 1-methyl-1-nitrosourea-induced mammary cancer. *Carcinogenesis*, **4**, 495–497

Grubbs, C.J., Farnell, D.R., Hill, D.L. & McDonough K.C. (1985) Chemoprevention of *N*-nitroso-*N*-methylurea-induced mammary cancers by pretreatment with 17β-estradiol and progesterone. *J. natl Cancer Inst.*, **74**, 927–931

Gruber, J.S. & Luciani, C.T. (1986) Physicians changing postmenopausal sex hormone prescribing regimens. *Prog. clin. biol. Res.*, **216**, 325–335

Hajek, R.A., Van, N.T., Johnston, D.A. & Jones, L.A. (1993) In vivo induction of increased DNA ploidy of mouse cervicovaginal epithelium by neonatal estrogen treatment. *Biol. Reprod.*, **49**, 908–917

Hallquist, A., Hardell, L., Degerman, A. & Boquist, L. (1994) Thyroid cancer: Reproductive factors, previous diseases, drug intake, family history and diet. A case–control study. *Eur. J. Cancer Prev.*, **3**, 481–488

Hammar, M., Brynhildsen, J., Dabrosin, L., Frisk, J., Lindgren, R., Nedstrand, E. & Wyon, Y. (1996) Hormone replacement therapy and previous use of oral contraceptives among Swedish women. *Maturitas*, **25**, 193–199

Hammond, C.B., Jelovsek, F.R., Lee, K.L., Creasman, W.T. & Parker, R.T. (1979) Effects of long-term estrogen replacement therapy. II. Neoplasia. *Am. J. Obstet. Gynecol.*, **133**, 537–547

Han, X. & Liehr, J.G. (1994) DNA single-strand breaks in kidneys of Syrian hamsters treated with steroidal estrogens: Hormone-induced free radical damage preceding renal malignancy. *Carcinogenesis*, **15**, 997–1000

Han, X. & Liehr, J.G. (1995) Microsome-mediated 8-hydroxylation of guanine bases of DNA by steroid estrogens: Correlation of DNA damage by free radicals with metabolic activation to quinones. *Carcinogenesis*, **16**, 2571–2574

Han, X., Liehr, J.G. & Bosland, M.C. (1995) Induction of a DNA adduct detectable by ^{32}P-post-labelling in the dorsolateral prostate of NBL/Cr rats treated with estradiol-17β and testosterone. *Carcinogenesis*, **16**, 951–954

Handa, V.L., Landerman, R., Hanlon, J.T., Harris, T. & Cohen, H.J. (1996) Do older women use estrogen replacement? Data from the Duke Established Populations for Epidemiologic Studies of the Elderly (EPESE). *J. Am. geriatr. Soc.*, **44**, 1–6

Harlow, B.L., Weiss, N.S., Roth, G.J., Chu, J. & Daling, J.R. (1988) Case–control study of border-line ovarian tumors: Reproductive history and exposure to exogenous female hormones. *Cancer Res.*, **48**, 5849–5852

Harris, R.B., Laws, A., Reddy, V.M., King, A. & Haskell, W.L. (1990) Are women using post-menopausal estrogens? A community survey. *Am. J. public Health*, **80**, 1266–1268

Harris, R.E., Namboodin, K.K. & Wynder, E.L. (1992a) Breast cancer risk: Effects of estrogen replacement therapy and body mass. *J. natl Cancer Inst.*, **84**, 1575–1582

Harris, R., Whittemore, A.S., Itnyre, J. & the Collaborative Ovarian Cancer Group (1992b) Characteristics relating to ovarian cancer risk: Collaborative analysis of 12 US case–control studies. III. Epithelial tumors of low malignant potential in white women. *Am. J. Epidemiol.*, **136**, 1204–1211

Hartge, P., Tucker, M.A., Shields, J.A., Augsburger, J., Hoover, R.N. & Fraumeni, J.F., Jr (1989) Case–control study of female hormones and eye melanoma. *Cancer Res.*, **49**, 4622–4625

Haspels, A.A., Luisi, M. & Kicovic, P.M. (1981) Endocrinological and clinical investigations in post-menopausal women following administration of vaginal cream containing oestriol. *Maturitas*, **3**, 321–327

Hassen, A.M., Lam, D., Chiba, M., Tan, E., Geng, W. & Pang, K.S. (1996) Uptake of sulfate conjugates by isolated rat hepatocytes. *Drug Metab. Disposition*, **24**, 792–798

Hayashi, N., Hasegawa, K., Komine, A., Tanaka, Y., McLachlan, J.A., Barrett, J.C. & Tsutsui, T. (1996) Estrogen-induced cell transformation and DNA adduct formation in cultured Syrian hamster embryo cells. *Mol. Carcinogen.*, **16**, 149–156

Hayes, C.L., Spink, D.C., Spink, B.C., Cao, J.Q., Walker, N.J. & Sutter, T.R. (1996) 17β-Estradiol hydroxylation catalyzed by human cytochrome P450 1B1. *Proc. natl Acad. Sci. USA*, **93**, 9776–9781

Heimer, G.M. (1987) Estriol in the postmenopause. *Acta obstet. gynecol. scand.*, **139** (Suppl.), 1–23

Hemminki, E., Kennedy, D.L., Baum, C. & McKinlay, S.M. (1988) Prescribing of noncontraceptive estrogens and progestins in the United States, 1974–86. *Am. J. public Health*, **78**, 1479–1481

Hempling, R.E., Wong, C., Piver, M.S., Natarajan, N. & Mettlin, C.J. (1997) Hormone replacement therapy as a risk factor for epithelial ovarian cancer: Results of a case–control study. *Obstet. Gynecol.*, **89**, 1012–1216

Henderson, B.E., Paganini-Hill, A. & Ross, R.K. (1991) Decreased mortality in users of estrogen replacement therapy. *Arch. intern. Med.*, **151**, 75–78

Hermens, W.A., Deurloo, M.J., Romeyn, S.G., Verhoef, J.C. & Merkus, F.W. (1990) Nasal absorption enhancement of 17 beta-estradiol by dimethyl-beta-cyclodextrin in rabbits and rats. *Pharmacol. Res.*, **7**, 500–503

Herrinton, L.J. & Weiss, N.S. (1993) Postmenopausal unopposed estrogens. Characteristics of use in relation to the risk of endometrial carcinoma. *Ann. Epidemiol.*, **3**, 308–318

Hiatt, R.A., Bawol, R., Friedman, G.D. & Hoover, R. (1984) Exogenous estrogen and breast cancer after bilateral oophorectomy. *Cancer*, **54**, 139–144

Highman, B., Greenman, D.L., Norvell, M.J., Farmer, J. & Shellenberger, T.E. (1980) Neoplastic and preneoplastic lesions induced in female C3H mice by diets containing diethylstilbestrol or 17 beta-estradiol. *J. environ. Pathol. Toxicol.*, **4**, 81–95

Hildreth, N.G., Kelsey, J.L., LiVolsi, V.A., Fischer, D.B., Holford, T.R., Mostow, E.D., Schwartz, P.E. & White, C. (1981) An epidemiologic study of epithelial carcinoma of the ovary. *Am. J. Epidemiol.*, **114**, 398–405

Hill, A. & Wolff, S. (1983) Sister chromatid exchanges and cell division delays induced by diethylstilbestrol, estradiol, and estriol in human lymphocytes. *Cancer Res.*, **43**, 4114–4118

Hill, D.E., Slikker, W., Helton, E.D., Lipe, G.W., Newport, G.D., Sziszak, T.J. & Bailey, J.R. (1980) Transplacental pharmacokinetics and metabolism of diethylstilbestrol and 17β-estradiol in the pregnant rhesus monkey. *J. clin. Endocrinol. Metab.*, **50**, 811–818

Hillbertz-Nilsson, K. & Forsberg, J.-G. (1985) Estrogen effects on sister chromatid exchanges in mouse uterine cervical and kidney cells. *J. natl Cancer Inst.*, **75**, 575–580

Hislop, T.G., Coldman, A.J., Elwood, J.M., Brauer, G. & Kan, L. (1986) Childhood and recent eating patterns and risk of breast cancer. *Cancer Detect. Prevent.*, **9**, 47–58

Holford, T.R., Roush, G.C. & McKay, L.A. (1991) Trends in female breast cancer in Connecticut and the United States. *J. clin. Epidemiol.*, **44**, 29–39

Holly, E.A., Weiss, N.S. & Liff, J.M. (1983) Cutaneous melanoma in relation to exogenous hormones and reproductive factors. *J. natl Cancer Inst.*, **70**, 827–831

Holly, E.A., Cress, R.D. & Ahn, D.K. (1994) Cutaneous melanoma in women: Ovulatory life, menopause, and use of exogenous estrogens. *Cancer Epidemiol. Biomarkers Prev.*, **3**, 661–668

Holman, C.D.J., Armstrong, B.K. & Heenan, P.J. (1984) Cutaneous malignant melanoma in women: Exogenous sex hormones and reproductive factors. *Br. J. Cancer*, **50**, 673–680

Hoogerland, D.L., Buchler, D.A., Crowley, J.J. & Carr, W.F. (1978) Estrogen use—risk of endometrial carcinoma. *Gynecol. Oncol.*, **6**, 451–458

Hoover, R., Gray, L.A., Sr, Cole, P. & MacMahon, B. (1976) Menopausal estrogens and breast cancer. *New Engl. J. Med.*, **295**, 401–405

Hoover, R., Glass, A., Finkle, W.D., Azevedo, D. & Milne, K. (1981) Conjugated estrogens and breast cancer risk in women. *J. natl Cancer Inst.*, **67**, 815–820

Hulka, B.S., Fowler, W.C., Jr, Kaufman, D.G., Grimson, R.C., Greenberg, B.G., Hogue, C.J., Berger, G.S. & Pulliam, C.C. (1980) Estrogen and endometrial cancer: Cases and two control groups from North Carolina. *Am. J. Obstet. Gynecol.*, **137**, 92–101

Hulka, B.S., Chambless, L.E., Deubner, D.C. & Wilkinson, W.E. (1982) Breast cancer and estrogen replacement therapy. *Am. J. Obstet. Gynecol.*, **143**, 638–644

Hunt, K., Vessey, M., McPherson, K. & Coleman, M. (1987) Long-term surveillance of mortality and cancer incidence in women receiving hormone replacement therapy. *Br. J. Obstet. Gynaecol.*, **94**, 620–635

Hunt, K., Vessey, M. & McPherson, K. (1990) Mortality in a cohort of long-term users of hormone replacement therapy: An updated analysis. *Br. J. Obstet. Gynaecol.*, **97**, 1080–1086

Hyder, S.M., Murthy, L. & Stancel, G.M. (1998) Progestin regulation of vascular endothelial growth factor in human breast cancer cells. *Cancer Res.*, **58**, 392–395

IARC (1979) *IARC Monographs on the Evaluation of the Carcinogenic Risk of Chemicals to Humans*, Vol. 21, *Sex Hormones (II)*, Lyon, pp. 279–326, 327–341, 343–362, 491–515

Inano, H., Yamanouchi, H., Suzuki, K., Onoda, M. & Wakabayashi, K. (1995) Estradiol-17β as an intiation modifier for radiation-induced mammary tumorigenesis of rats ovariectomized before puberty. *Carcinogenesis*, **16**, 1871–1877

Ingerowski, G.H., Scheutwinkel-Reich, M. & Stan, H.-J. (1981) Mutagenicity studies on veterinary anabolic drugs with the *Salmonella*/microsome test. *Mutat. Res.*, **91**, 93–98

Jacobs, E.J., White, E. & Weiss, N.S. (1994) Exogenous hormones, reproductive history, and colon cancer (Seattle, Washington, USA). *Cancer Causes Control*, **5**, 359–366

Jacobson, J.S., Neugut, A.I., Garbowski, G.D., Ahsan, H., Waye, J.D., Treat, M.R. & Forde, K.A. (1995) Reproductive risk factors for colorectal adenomatous polyps (New York City, NY, United States). *Cancer Causes Control*, **6**, 513–518

Jasonni, V.M., Bulleti, C., Naldi, S., Ciotti, P., Di Cosmo, D., Lazaretto, R. & Flamigni, C. (1988) Biological and endocrine aspects of transdermal 17β-oestradiol administration in postmenopausal women. *Maturitus*, **10**, 263–270

Jelovsek, F.R., Hammond, C.B., Woodard, B.H., Draffin, R., Lev, K.L., Craesman, W.T. & Parker, R.T. (1980) Risk of exogenous estrogen therapy and endometrial cancer. *Am. J. Obstet. Gynecol.*, **137**, 85–91

Jeng, M.-H. & Jordan V.C. (1991) Growth stimulation and differential regulation of transforming growth factor-β1 (TGF β1), TGF β2, and TGF β3 messenger RNA levels by norethindrone in MCF-7 human breast cancer cells. *Mol. Endocrinol.*, **8**, 1120–1128

Jeng, M.-H., Parker, C.J. & Jordan, V.C. (1992) Estrogenic potential of progestins in oral contraceptives to stimulate human breast cancer cell proliferation. *Cancer Res.*, **52**, 6539–6546

Jewelewicz, R. (1997) New developments in topical estrogen therapy. *Fertil. Steril.*, **67**, 1–12

Jick, S.S., Walker, A.M. & Jick, H. (1993) Estrogens, progesterone, and endometrial cancer. *Epidemiology*, **4**, 20–24

Johannes, C.B., Crawford, S.L., Posner, J.G. & McKinlay, S.M. (1994) Longitudinal patterns and correlates of hormone replacement therapy use in middle-aged women. *Am. J. Epidemiol.*, **140**, 439–452

Johnston, A. (1996) Estrogens—Pharmacokinetics and pharmacodynamics with special reference to vaginal administration and the new estradiol formulation—Estring®. *Acta obstet. gynecol. scand.*, **75**, 16–25

Jolleys, J.V. & Olesen, F. (1996) A comparative study of prescribing of hormone replacement therapy in USA and Europe. *Maturitas*, **23**, 47–53

Kalkhoven, E., Kwakkenbos-Isbrücker, L., de Laat, S.W., van der Saag, P.T. & Van der Burg, B. (1994) Synthetic progestins induce proliferation of breast tumor cell lines via the progesterone or estrogen receptor. *Mol. cell. Endocrinol.*, **102**, 45–52

Kaltenbach, C.C., Dunn, T.G., Koritnik, D.R., Tucker, W.F., Batson, D.B., Staigmiller, R.B. & Niswender, G.D. (1976) Isolation and identification of metabolites of ^{14}C-labeled estradiol in cattle. *J. Toxicol. environ. Health*, **1**, 607–616

Kampman, E., Potter, J.D., Slattery, M.L., Caan, B.J. & Edward, S. (1997) Hormone replacement therapy, reproductive history, and colon cancer: A multicenter, case–control study in the United States. *Cancer Causes Control*, **8**, 146–158

Katzenellenbogen, B.S. (1984) Biology and receptor interactions of estriol and estriol derivatives *in vitro* and *in vivo*. *J. Steroid Biochem.*, **20**, 1033–1037

Katzenellenbogen, B.S., Bhardwaj, B., Fang, H., Ince, B.A., Pakdel, F., Reese, J.C., Schodin, D. & Wrenn, C.K. (1993) Hormone binding and transcription activation by estrogen receptors: Analyses using mammalian and yeast systems. *J. Steroid Biochem. mol. Biol.*, **47**, 39–48

Kaufman, D.W., Miller, D.R., Rosenberg, L., Helmrich, S.P., Stolley, P., Schottenfeld, D. & Shapiro, S. (1984) Noncontraceptive estrogen use and the risk of breast cancer. *J. Am. med. Assoc.*, **252**, 63–67

Kaufman, D.W., Kelly, J.P., Welch, W.R., Rosenberg, L., Stolley, P.D., Warshauer, M.E., Lewis, J., Woodruff, J. & Shapiro, S. (1989) Noncontraceptive estrogen use and epithelial ovarian cancer. *Am. J. Epidemiol.*, **130**, 1142–1151

Kaufman, D.W., Palmer, J.R., de Mouzon, J., Rosenberg, L., Stolley, P.D., Warshauer, M.E., Zauber, A.G. & Shapiro, S. (1991) Estrogen replacement therapy and the risk of breast cancer: Results from the case–control surveillance study. *Am. J. Epidemiol.*, **134**, 1375–1385

Kay, C.R. & Hannaford, P.C. (1988) Breast cancer and the pill—A further report from the Royal College of General Practitioners' Oral Contraception Study. *Br. J. Cancer*, **58**, 675–680

Keating, N.L., Cleary, P.D., Rossi, A.S. & Ayanian, J.Z. (1997) Use of hormone replacement therapy in a national sample of postmenopausal women (Abstract). *J. gen. intern. Med.*, **12** (Suppl.), 127

Kelsey, J.L., Livolsi, V.A., Holford, T.R., Fisher, D.B., Mostow, E.D., Schwartz, P.E., O'Connor, T. & White, C. (1982) A case–control study of cancer of the endometrium. *Am. J. Epidemiol.*, **116**, 333–342

Kelsey, J.L., Gammon, M.D. & John, E.M. (1993) Reproductive factors and breast cancer. *Epidemiol. Rev.*, **15**, 36–47

Kennedy, A.R. & Wiechselbaum, R.R. (1981) Effects of 17β-estradiol on radiation transformation *in vitro*; inhibition of effects by protease inhibitors. *Carcinogenesis*, **2**, 67–69

Kennedy, D.L., Baum, C. & Forbes, M.B. (1985) Noncontraceptive estrogens and progestins: Use patterns over time. *Obstet. Gynecol.*, **65**, 441–446

Kerlan, V., Dreano, Y., Bercovici, J.P., Beaune, P.H., Floch, H.H. & Berthou, F. (1992) Nature of cytochrome P450 involved in 2-/4-hydroxylations of estradiol in human liver microsomes. *Biochem. Pharmacol.*, **44**, 1745–1756

Kim, Y.B., Berek, J.S., Martinez-Maza, O. & Satyaswaroop, P.G. (1996) Vascular endothelial growth factor expression is not regulated by estradiol or medroxyprogesterone acetate in endometrial carcinoma. *Gynecol. Oncol.*, **61**, 97–100

King, R.J.B. (1991) Biology of female sex hormone action in relation to contraceptive agents and neoplasia. *Contraception*, **43**, 527–542

Kitawaki, J., Fukuoka, M., Yamamoto, T., Honjo, H. & Okada, H. (1992) Contribution of aromatase to the deoxyribonucleic acid synthesis of MCF-7 human breast cancer cells and its suppression by aromatase inhibitors. *J. Steroid Biochem. mol. Biol.*, **42**, 267–277

Knabbe, C., Lippman, M.E., Wakefield, L.M., Flanders, K.C., Kasid, A., Derynck, R. & Dickson, R.B. (1987) Evidence that transforming growth factor-β is a hormonally regulated negative growth factor in human breast cancer cells. *Cell*, **48**, 417–428

Koibuchi, Y., Iino, Y., Uchida, T., Nagasawa, M. & Morishita, Y. (1997) Effects of estrogen and tamoxifen on the MAP kinase cascade in experimental rat breast cancer. *Int. J. Oncol.*, **11**, 583–589

Koike, S., Sakai, M. & Muramatsu, M. (1987) Molecular cloning and characterization of rat estrogen receptor cDNA. *Nucleic Acids Res.*, **15**, 2499–2513

Kolonel, L.N., Hankin, J.H., Wilkens, L.R., Fukunaga, F.H. & Hinds, M.W. (1990) An epidemiologic study of thyroid cancer in Hawaii. *Cancer Cases Control*, **1**, 223–234

Koper, N.P., Kiemeney, L.A.L.M., Massuger, L.F.A.G., Thomas, C.M.G., Schijf, C.P.T. & Verbeek, A.L.M. (1996) Ovarian cancer incidence (1989–1991) and mortality (1954–1993) in The Netherlands. *Obstet. Gynecol.*, **88**, 387–393

Kopera, H. & van Keep, P.A. (1991) Development and present state of hormone replacement therapy. *Int. J. clin. Pharmacol.*, **29**, 412–417

Køster, A. (1990) Hormone replacement therapy: Use patterns in 51-year-old Danish women. *Maturitas*, **12**, 345–356

Koumantaki, Y., Tzonou, A., Koumantakis, E., Kaklamani, E., Aravantinos, D. & Trichopoulos, D. (1989) A case–control study of cancer of endometrium in Athens. *Int. J. Cancer*, **43**, 795–799

Kravdal, Ø., Glattre, E. & Haldorsen, T. (1991) Positive correlation between parity and incidence of thyroid cancer: New evidence based on complete Norwegian birth cohorts. *Int. J. Cancer*, **49**, 831–836

Krust, A., Green, S., Argos, P., Kumar, V., Walter, P., Bornert, J.-M. & Chambon, P. (1986) The chicken oestrogen receptor sequence: Homology with v-*erbA* and the human oestrogen and glucocorticoid receptors. *EMBO J.*, **5**, 891–897

Kuh, D.L., Wadsworth, M. & Hardy, R. (1997) Women's health in midlife: The influence of the menopause, social factors and health in earlier life. *Br. J. Obstet. Gynaecol.*, **104**, 923–933

Kuhl, H. (1990) Pharmacokinetics of oestrogens and progestogens. *Maturitas*, **12**, 171–197

Kuiper, G.G.J.M., Enmark, E., Pelto-Huikko, M., Nilsson, S. & Gustafsson, J.-Å. (1996) Cloning of a novel estrogen receptor expressed in rat prostate and ovary. *Proc. natl Acad. Sci. USA*, **93**, 5925–5930

Lafferty, F.W. & Helmuth, D.O. (1985) Post-menopausal estrogen replacement: The prevention of osteoporosis and systemic effects. *Maturitas*, **7**, 147–159

Lancaster, T., Surman, G., Lawrence, M., Mant, D., Vessey, M., Thorogood, M., Yudkin, P. & Daly, E. (1995) Hormone replacement therapy: Characteristics of users and non-users in a British general practice cohort identified through computerised prescribing records. *J. Epidemiol. Community Health*, **49**, 389–394

Lang, R. & Redmann, U. (1979) Non-mutagenicity of some sex hormones in the Ames *Salmonella*/microsome mutagenicity test. *Mutat. Res.*, **67**, 361–365

Lang, R. & Reimann, R. (1993) Studies for a genotoxic potential of some endogenous and exogenous steroids. I. Communication: Examination for the induction of gene mutations using the Ames *Salmonella*/microsome test and the HGPRT test in V79 cells. *Environ. mol. Mutag.*, **21**, 272–304

La Vecchia, C., Franceschi, S., Gallus, G., Decarli, A., Colombo, E., Mangioni, C. & Tognoni, G. (1982a) Oestrogens and obesity as risk factors for endometrial cancer in Italy. *Int. J. Epidemiol.*, **11**, 120–126

La Vecchia, C., Liberati, A. & Franceschi, S. (1982b) Noncontraceptive estrogen use and the occurrence of ovarian cancer (Letter to the Editor). *J. natl Cancer Inst.*, **69**, 1207

La Vecchia, C., Franceschi, S., Decarli, A., Gallus, G. & Tognoni, G. (1984) Risk factors for endometrial cancer at different ages. *J. natl Cancer Inst.*, **73**, 667–671

La Vecchia, C., Decarli, A., Parazzini, F., Gentile, A., Liberati, C. & Franceschi, S. (1986) Noncontraceptive oestrogens and the risk of breast cancer in women. *Int. J. Cancer*, **38**, 853–858

La Vecchia, C., Negri, E., Franceschi, S. & Parazzini, F. (1992a) Non-contraceptive oestrogens and breast cancer. *Int. J. Cancer*, **50**, 161–162

La Vecchia, C., Lucchini, F., Negri, E., Boyle, P., Maisonneuve, P. & Levi, F. (1992b) Trends of cancer mortality in Europe, 1955–1989: III. Breast and genital sites. *Eur. J. Cancer*, **28A**, 927–998

La Vecchia, C., D'Avanzo, B., Franceschi, S., Negri, E., Parazzini, F., Decarli, A. (1994) Menstrual and reproductive factors and gastric-cancer risk in women. *Int. J. Cancer*, **59**, 761–764

La Vecchia, C., Negri, E., Franceschi, S., Favero, A., Nanni, O., Filiberti, R., Conti, E., Montella, M., Veronesi, A., Ferranoni, M. & Decarli, A. (1995) Hormone replacement treatment and breast cancer risk: A cooperative Italian study. *Br. J. Cancer*, **72**, 244–248

La Vecchia, C., Negri, E., Levi, F., Decarli, A. & Boyle, P. (1998) Cancer mortality in Europe: Effects of age, cohort of birth and period of death. *Eur. J. Cancer*, **34**, 118–141

Lee, N.C., Rosero-Bixby, L., Oberle, M.W., Grimaldo, C., Whatley, A.S. & Rovira, E.Z. (1987) A case–control study of breast cancer and hormonal contraception in Costa Rica. *J. natl Cancer Inst.*, **79**, 1247–1254

Lemon, H.M. (1987) Antimammary carcinogenic activity of 17-alpha-ethinyl estriol. *Cancer*, **60**, 2873–2881

Lemon, H.M., Kumar, P.F., Peterson, C., Rodriguez-Sierra, J.F. & Abbo, K.M. (1989) Inhibition of radiogenic mammary carcinoma in rats by estriol or tamoxifen. *Cancer*, **63**, 1685–1692

Levi, F., La Vecchia, C., Gulie, C., Franceschi, S. & Negri, E. (1993a) Oestrogen replacement treatment and the risk of endometrial cancer: An assessment of the role of covariates. *Eur. J. Cancer*, **29A**, 1445–1449

Levi, F., Franceschi, S., Gulie, C., Negri, E. & La Vecchia, C. (1993b) Female thyroid cancer: The role of reproductive and hormonal factors in Switzerland. *Oncology*, **50**, 309–315

Levi, F., Lucchini, F., Pasche, C. & La Vecchia, C. (1996) Oral contraceptives, menopausal hormone replacement treatment and breast cancer risk. *Eur. J. Cancer Prev.*, **5**, 259–266

Lew, R.A., Sober, A.J., Cook, N., Marvell, R. & Fitzpatrick, T.B. (1983) Sun exposure habits in patients with cutaneous melanoma: A case–control study. *J. Dermatol. surg. Oncol.*, **9**, 981–986

Li, J.J. & Li, S.A. (1987) Estrogen carcinogenesis in Syrian hamster tissues: Role of metabolism. *Fed. Proc.*, **46**, 1858–1863

Li, J.J., Li, S.A., Klicka, J.K., Parsons, J.A. & Lam, L.K. (1983) Relative carcinogenic activity of various synthetic and natural estrogens in the Syrian hamster kidney. *Cancer Res.*, **43**, 5200–5204

Li, J.J., Gonzalez, A., Banerjee, S., Banerjee, S.K. & Li, S.A. (1993) Estrogen carcinogenesis in the hamster kidney: Role of cytotoxicity and cell proliferation. *Environ. Health Perspectives*, **101** (Suppl. 5), 259–264

Li, S.A., Xue, Y., Xie, Q., Li, C.I. & Li, J.J. (1994) Serum and tissue levels of estradiol during estrogen-induced renal tumorigenesis in the Syrian hamster. *J. Steroid Biochem. mol. Biol.*, **48**, 283–286

Li, J.J., Li, S.A., Oberley, T.D. & Parsons, J.A. (1995) Carcinogenic activities of various steroidal and nonsteroidal estrogens in the hamster kidney: Relation to hormonal activity and cell proliferation. *Cancer Res.*, **55**, 4347–4351

Liehr, J.G. & Ricco, M.J. (1996) 4-Hydroxylation of estrogens as marker of human mammary tumors. *Proc. natl Acad. Sci. USA*, **93**, 3294–3296

Liehr, J.G. & Roy, D. (1990) Free radical generation by redox cycling of estrogen. *Free Rad. Biol. Med.*, **8**, 415–423

Liehr, J.G., Fang, W.-F., Sirbasku, D.A. & Ari-Ulubelen, A. (1986a) Carcinogenicity of catechol estrogens in Syrian hamsters. *J. Steroid Biochem.*, **24**, 353–356

Liehr, J.G., Ulubelen, A.A. & Strobel, H.W. (1986b) Cytochrome P450-mediated redox cycling of estrogens. *J. biol. Chem.*, **261**, 16865–16870

Liehr, J.G., Avitts, T.A., Randerath, E. & Randerath, K. (1986c) Estrogen-induced endogenous DNA adduction: Possible mechanism of hormonal cancer. *Proc. natl Acad. Sci. USA*, **83**, 5302–5305

Liehr, J.G., Purdy, R.H., Baran, J.S., Nutting, E.F., Colton, F., Randerath, E. & Randerath, K. (1987a) Correlation of aromatic hydroxylation of 11β-substituted estrogens with morphological transformation *in vitro* but not with in vivo tumour induction by these hormones. *Cancer Res.*, **47**, 2583–2588

Liehr, J.G., Hall, E.R., Avitts, T.A., Randerath, E. & Randerath, K. (1987b) Localisation of estrogen-induced DNA adducts and cytochrome P-450 activity at the site of renal carcinogenesis in the hamster kidney. *Cancer Res.*, **47**, 2156–2159

Liehr, J.G., Han, X. & Bhat, H.K. (1993) ^{32}P-Postlabelling in studies of hormonal carcinogenesis. In: Phillips, D.H., Castegnaro, M. & Bartsch, H., eds, *Postlabelling Methods for Detection of DNA Adducts* (IARC Scientific Publications No. 124), Lyon, IARC, pp. 149–155

Liehr, J.G., Ricci, M.J., Jefcoate, C.R., Hannigan, E.V., Hokanson, J.A. & Zhu, B.T. (1995) 4-Hydroxylation of estradiol by human uterine myometrium and myoma microsomes: Implication for the mechanism of uterine tumorigenesis. *Proc. natl Acad. Sci. USA*, **92**, 9220–9224

Lindblad, P., Mellemgaard, A., Schlehofer, B., Adami, H.-O., McCredie, M., McLaughlin, J.K. & Mandel, J.S. (1995) International renal-cell cancer study. V. Reproductive factors, gynecologic operations and exogenous hormones. *Int. J. Cancer*, **61**, 192–198

Lindgren, R., Berg, G., Hammarm, M. & Zuccon, E. (1993) Hormonal replacement therapy and sexuality in a population of Swedish postmenopausal women. *Acta obstet. gynecol. scand.*, **72**, 292–297

Lippman, M.E. & Dickson, R.B. (1989) Mechanisms of normal and malignant breast epithelial growth regulation. *J. Steroid Biochem.*, **34**, 107–121

Lipworth, L., Katsouyanni, K., Stuver, S., Samoli, E., Hankinson, S. & Trichopoulos, D. (1995) Oral contraceptives, menopausal oestrogens and the risk of breast cancer: A case–control study in Greece. *Int. J. Cancer*, **62**, 548–551

Longcope, C., Flood, C. & Tast, J. (1994) The metabolism of estrone sulfate in the female rhesus monkey. *Steroids*, **59**, 270–273

Lu, L.J.W., Liehr, J.G., Sirbasku, D.A., Randerath, E. & Randerath, K. (1988) Hypomethylation of DNA in estrogen-induced and -dependent hamster kidney tumours. *Carcinogenesis*, **9**, 925–929

Lubahn, D.B., McCarty, K.S., Jr & McCarty, K.S., Sr (1985) Electrophoretic characterization of purified bovine, porcine, murine, rat, and human uterine estrogen receptors. *J. biol. Chem.*, **260**, 2515–2526

Luo, S., Stojanovic, M., Labrie, C. & Labrie, F. (1997) Inhibitory effect of the novel anti-estrogen EM-800 and medroxyprogesterone acetate on estrone-stimulated growth of dimethylbenz[a]-anthracene-induced mammary carcinoma in rats. *Int. J. Cancer*, **73**, 580–586

Mack, T.M., Pike, M.C., Henderson, B.E., Pfeffer, R.I., Gerkins, V.R., Arthur, M. & Brown, S.E. (1976) Estrogens and endometrial cancer in a retirement community. *New Engl. J. Med.*, **294**, 1262–1267

MacLennan, A.H., MacLennan, A. & Wilson, D. (1993) The prevalence of oestrogen replacement therapy in South Australia. *Maturitas*, **16**, 175–183

Maddison, J. (1973) Hormone replacement therapy for menopausal symptoms (Letter to the Editor). *Lancet*, **i**, 1507

Magnusson, C., Holmberg, L., Norden, T., Lindgren, A. & Persson, I. (1996) Prognostic charac-teristics in breast cancers after hormone replacement therapy. *Breast Cancer Res. Treat.*, **38**, 325–334

Markiewicz, L. & Gurpide, E. (1994) Estrogenic and progestagenic activities coexisting in steroi-dal drugs: Quantitative evaluation by *in vitro* bioassays with human cells. *J. Steroid Biochem. mol. Biol.*, **48**, 89–94

Markiewicz, L., Hochberg, R.B. & Gurpide, E. (1992) Intrinsic estrogenicity of some progesta-genic drugs. *J. Steroid Biochem. mol. Biol.*, **41**, 53–58

Martin, J.H.J., McKibben, B.M., Lynch, M. & van den Berg, H.W. (1991) Modulation by oestro-gen and progestins/antiprogestins of alpha interferon receptor expression in human breast cancer cells. *Eur. J. Cancer*, **27**, 143–146

Marubini, E., Decarli, A., Costa, A., Marroleni, C., Andreoli, C., Barbieri, A., Capitelli, E., Carlucci, M., Cavallo, F., Monferroni, N., Pastorino, U. & Salvini, S. (1988) The relationship of dietary intake and serum levels of retinol and beta-carotene with breast cancer: Results of a case–control study. *Cancer*, **61**, 173–180

McDonald, T.W., Annegers, J.F., O'Fallon, W.M., Dockerty, M.B., Malkasian, G.D., Jr & Kurland, L.T. (1977) Exogenous estrogen and endometrial carcinoma: Case–control and incidence study. *Am. J. Obstet. Gynecol.*, **127**, 572–580

McDonnell, D.P., Clemm, D.L., Hermann, T., Goldman, M.E. & Pike, J.W. (1995) Analysis of estrogen receptor function *in vitro* reveals three distinct classes of antiestrogens. *Mol. Endocrinol.*, **9**, 659–669

McLachlan, J.A. & Newbold, R.R. (1996) Cellular and molecular mechanisms of cancers of the uterus in animals. In: Huff, J., Boyd, J. & Barrett, J.C., eds, *Cellular and Molecular Mechanisms of Hormonal Carcinogenesis: Environmental Influences*, New York, Wiley-Liss, pp. 175–182

McPherson, K., Vessey, M.P., Neil, A., Doll, R., Jones, L. & Roberts, M. (1987) Early oral contraceptive use and breast cancer: Results of another case–control study. *Br. J. Cancer*, **56**, 653–660

McTiernan, A.M., Weiss, N.S. & Daling, J.R. (1984) Incidence of thyroid cancer in women in relation to reproductive and hormonal factors. *Am. J. Epidemiol.*, **120**, 423–435

Miller, A.B., Baines, C.J., To, T. & Wall, C. (1992) Canadian National Breast Screening Study. I. Breast cancer detection and death rates among women aged 40–49 years. *Can. med. Assoc. J.*, **147**, 1459–1476

Mills, P.K., Beeson, W.L., Phillips, R.L. & Fraser, G.E. (1989) Prospective study of exogenous hormone use and breast cancer in Seventh-day Adventists. *Cancer*, **64**, 591–597

Morabia, A., Szklo, M., Stewart, W., Schuman, L. & Thomas, D.B. (1993) Consistent lack of association between breast cancer and oral contraceptives using either hospital or neighbourhood controls. *Prev. Med.*, **22**, 178–186

Murase, T., Niwa, K., Morishita, S., Itoh, N., Mori, H., Tanaka, T. & Tamaya, T. (1995) Rare occurrence of *p53* and *ras* gene mutations in preneoplastic and neoplastic mouse endometrial lesions induced by *N*-methyl-*N*-nitrosourea and 17β-estradiol. *Cancer Lett.*, **92**, 223–227

Musgrove, E.A. & Sutherland, R.L. (1997) Steroidal control of cell proliferation in the breast and breast cancer. In: Wren, B.G., ed., *Progress in the Management of the Menopause*, New York, Parthenon Publishing Group, pp. 194–202

Nabulsi, A.A., Folsom, A.R., White, A., Patsch, W., Heiss, G., Wu, K.K. & Szklo, M. (1993) Association of hormone-replacement therapy with various cardiovascular risk factors in post-menopausal women. The Atherosclerosis Risk in Communities study investigators. *New Engl. J. Med.*, **328**, 1069–1075

Nagata, C., Matsushita, Y. & Shimizu, H. (1996) Prevalence of hormone replacement therapy and user's characteristics: A community survey in Japan. *Maturitas*, **25**, 201–207

National Corporation of Pharmacies (1997) *Sales Statistics of Defined Daily Doses/1000 Women, 1947–1997*, Stockholm, Apoteket AB

Nawata, H., Yamamoto, R.S. & Poirer, L.A. (1981) Elevated levels of ornithine decarboxylase and polyamines in the kidneys of estradiol-treated male hamsters. *Carcinogenesis*, **11**, 1207–1211

Negri, E., La Vecchia, C., Parazzini, F., Savoldelli, R., Gentile, A., D'Avanzo, B., Gramenzi, A. & Franceschi, S. (1989) Reproductive and menstrual factors and risk of colorectal cancer. *Cancer Res.*, **49**, 7158–7161

Newcomb, P.A. & Storer, B.E. (1995) Postmenopausal hormone use and risk of large-bowel cancer. *J. natl Cancer Inst.*, **87**, 1067–1071

Newcomb, P.A., Longnecker, M.P., Storer, B.E., Mittendorf, R., Baron, J., Clapp, R.W., Trentham-Dietz, A. & Willett, W.C. (1995) Long-term hormone replacement therapy and risk of breast cancer in postmenopausal women. *Am. J. Epidemiol.*, **142**, 788–795

Ngelangel, C.A., Lacaya, L.B., Cordero, C. & Laudico, A.V. (1994) Risk factors for breast cancer among Filipino women. *Phil. J. intern. Med.*, **32**, 231–236

Ni, N. & Yager, J.D. (1994a) Comitogenic effects of estrogens on DNA synthesis induced by various growth factors in cultured female rat hepatocytes. *Hepatology*, **19**, 183–192

Ni, N. & Yager, J.D. (1994b) The comitogenic effects of various estrogens for TGF-α-induced DNA synthesis in cultured female rat hepatocytes. *Cancer Lett.*, **84**, 133–140

Niwa, K., Tanaka, T., Mori, H., Yokoyama, Y., Furui, T., Mori, H. & Tamaya, T. (1991) Rapid induction of endometrial carcinoma in ICR mice treated with N-methyl-N-nitrosourea and 17β-estradiol. *Jpn. J. Cancer Res.*, **82**, 1391–1396

Niwa, K., Murase, T., Furui, T., Morishita, S., Mori, H., Tanaka, T., Mori, H. & Tamaya, T. (1993) Enhancing effects of estrogens on endometrial carcinogenesis initiated by *N*-methyl-*N*-nitrosourea in ICR mice. *Jpn. J. Cancer Res.*, **84**, 951–955

Niwa, K., Morishita, S., Murase, T., Mudigdo, A., Tanaka, T., Mori, H. & Tamaya, T. (1996) Chronological observation of mouse endometrial carcinogenesis induced by *N*-methyl-*N*-nitrosourea and 17beta-estradiol. *Cancer Lett.*, **104**, 115–119

Nomura, A.M., Kolonel, L.N., Hirohata, T. & Lee, J. (1986) The association of replacement estrogens with breast cancer. *Int. J. Cancer*, **37**, 49–53

Nutter, L.M., Wu, Y.Y., Ngo, E.O., Sierra, E.E., Gutierrez, P.L. & Abul-Hajj, Y.J. (1994) An *o*-quinone form of estrogen produces free radicals in human breast cancer cells: Correlation with DNA damage. *Chem. Res. Toxicol.*, **7**, 23–28

Ochs, H., Dusterberg, B., Gunzel, P. & Schulte-Hermann, R. (1986) Effect of tumor promoting contraceptive steroids on growth and drug metabolizing enzymes in rat liver. *Cancer Res.*, **46**, 1224–1232

O'Connell, M.B. (1995) Pharmacokinetic and pharmacologic variation between different estrogen products. *J. clin. Pharmacol.*, **35**, 18S–24S

Oddens, B.J. & Boulet, M.J. (1997) Hormone replacement therapy among Danish women aged 45–65 years: Prevalence, determinants and compliance. *Obstet. Gynecol.*, **90**, 269–277

Østerlind, A., Tucker, M.A., Stone, B.J. & Jensen, O.M. (1988) The Danish case–control study of cutaneous malignant melanoma. III. Hormonal and reproductive factors in women. *Int. J. Cancer*, **42**, 821–824

Paganini-Hill, A., Ross, R.K. & Henderson, B.E. (1989) Endometrial cancer and patterns of use of oestrogen replacement therapy: A cohort study. *Br. J. Cancer*, **59**, 445–447

Palmer, J.R., Rosenberg, L., Clarke, E.A., Miller, D.R. & Shapiro, S. (1991) Breast cancer risk after estrogen replacement therapy: Results from the Toronto breast cancer study. *Am. J. Epidemiol.*, **134**, 1386–1395

Pan, C.C., Woolever, C.A. & Bhavnani, B.R. (1985) Transport of equine estrogens: Binding of conjugated and unconjugated equine estrogens with human serum proteins. *J. clin. Endocrinol. Metab.*, **61**, 499–507

Parazzini, F., La Vecchia, C., Negri, E. & Villa, A. (1994) Estrogen replacement therapy and ovarian cancer risk. *Int. J. Cancer*, **57**, 135–136

Parazzini, F., La Vecchia, C., Negri, E., Franceschi, S., Moroni, S., Chatenoud, L. & Bolis, G. (1997) Case–control study of oestrogen replacement therapy and risk of cervical cancer. *Br. med. J.*, **315**, 85–88

Parker, M.G. (1995) Structure and function of estrogen receptors. *Vitam. Horm.*, **51**, 267–287

Pater, A., Bayatpour, M. & Pater, M.M. (1990) Oncogenic transformation by human papilloma virus type 16 deoxyribonucleic acid in the presence of progesterone or progestins from oral contraceptives. *Am. J. Obstet. Gynecol.*, **162**, 1099–1103

Paul, C., Skegg, D.C.G. & Spears, G.F.S. (1990) Oral contraceptives and risk of breast cancer. *Int. J. Cancer*, **46**, 366–373

Pedersen, S.H. & Jeune, B. (1988) Prevalence of hormone replacement therapy in a sample of middle-aged women. *Maturitas*, **9**, 339–345

Peek, M.J, Markham, R. & Fraser, I.S. (1995) The effects of natural and synthetic sex steroids on human decidual endothelial cell proliferation. *Hum. Reprod.*, **10**, 2238–2243

Persky, V., Davis, F., Barrett, R., Ruby, E., Sailer, C. & Levy, P. (1990) Recent time trends in uterine cancer. *Am. J. public Health*, **80**, 935–939

Persson, I., Adami, H.-O, Lindberg, B.S., Johansson, E.D.B. & Manell, P. (1983) Practice and patterns of estrogen treatment in climacteric women in a Swedish population. *Acta obstet. gynecol. scand.*, **62**, 289–296

Persson, I., Adami, H.-O., Bergkvist, L., Lindgren, A., Pettersson, B., Hoover, R. & Schairer, C. (1989) Risk of endometrial cancer after treatment with oestrogens alone or in conjunction with progestogens: Results of a prospective study. *Br. med. J.*, **298**, 147–151

Persson, I., Bergström, R., Sparén, P., Thörn, M. & Adami, H.-O. (1993) Trends in breast cancer incidence in Sweden 1958–1988 by time period and birth cohort. *Br. J. Cancer*, **68**, 1247–1253

Persson, I., Yuen, J., Bergkvist, L. & Schairer, C. (1996) Cancer incidence and mortality in women receiving estrogen and estrogen–progestin replacement therapy—Long-term follow-up of a Swedish cohort. *Int. J. Cancer*, **67**, 327–332

Persson, I., Bergkvist, L., Lindgren, C. & Yuen, J. (1997a) Hormone replacement therapy and major risk factors for reproductive cancer, osteoporosis and cardiovascular diseases: Evidence of confounding by exposure characteristics. *J. clin. Epidemiol.*, **50**, 611–618

Persson, I., Thurfjell, E., Bergström, R. & Holmberg, L. (1997b) Hormone replacement therapy and the risk of breast cancer. Nested case–control study in a cohort of Swedish women attending mammography screening. *Int. J. Cancer*, **72**, 758–761

Persson, I., Bergström, R., Barlow, L. & Adami, H.-O. (1998) Recent trends in breast cancer incidence in Sweden. *Br. J. Cancer*, **77**, 167–169

Peters, R.K., Pike, M.C., Chang, W.W.L. & Mack, T.M. (1990) Reproductive factors and colon cancers. *Br. J. Cancer*, **61**, 741–748

Petitti, D.B., Perlman, J.A. & Sidney, S. (1987) Noncontraceptive estrogens and mortality: Long-term follow-up of women in the Walnut Creek Study. *Obstet. Gynecol.*, **70**, 289–293

Pike, M.C., Peters, R.K., Cozen, W., Probst-Hensch, N.M., Felix, J.C., Wan, P.C. & Mack, T.M. (1997) Estrogen–progestin replacement therapy and endometrial cancer. *J. natl Cancer Inst.*, **89**, 1110–1116

Polychronopoulou, A., Tzonou, A., Hsieh, C., Kaprinis, G., Rebelakos, A., Toupadaki, N. & Trichopoulos, D. (1993) Reproductive variables, tobacco, ethanol, coffee and somatometry as risk factors for ovarian cancer. *Int. J. Cancer*, **55**, 402–407

Porter, M., Penney, G.C., Russell, D., Russell, E. & Templeton, A. (1996) A population based survey of women's experience of the menopause. *Br. J. Obstet. Gynaecol.*, **103**, 1025–1028

Postmenopausal Estrogen/Progestin Interventions (PEPI) Trial (1996) Effects of hormone replacement therapy on endometrial histology in postmenopausal women. *J. Am. med. Assoc.*, **275**, 370–375

Potter, J.D. & McMichael, A.J. (1983) Large bowel cancer in women in relation to reproductive and hormonal factors: A case–control study. *J. natl Cancer Inst.*, **71**, 703–709

Potter, J.D., Bostick, R.M., Grandits, G.A., Fosdick, L., Elmer, P., Wood, J., Grambsch, P. & Louis, T.A. (1996) Hormone replacement therapy is associated with lower risk of adenomatous polyps of the large bowel: The Minnesota Cancer Prevention Research Unit Case–Control Study. *Cancer Epidemiol. Biomarkers Prev.*, **5**, 779–784

Price, T.M., Blauer, K.L., Hansen, M., Stanczyk, F., Lobo, R. & Bates, W.G. (1997) Single-dose pharmacokinetics of sublingual versus oral administration of micronized 17β-estradiol. *Obstet. Gynecol.*, **89**, 340–345

Purdie, D., Green, A., Bain, C., Siskind, V., Ward, B., Hacker, N., Quinn, M., Wright, G., Russell, P. & Susil, B. for the Survey of Women's Health Group (1995) Reproductive and other factors and risk of epithelial ovarian cancer: An Australian case–control study. *Int. J. Cancer*, **62**, 678–684

Ravnihar, B., Primic Zakeli, M., Kosmeli, K. & Stare, J. (1988) A case–control study of breast cancer in relation to oral contraceptive use in Slovenia. *Neoplasma*, **35**, 109–121

Reynolds, J.E.F., ed. (1998) *Martindale, The Extra Pharmacopoeia*, 13th Ed., London, The Pharmaceutical Press [MicroMedex CD-ROM]

Ringa, V., Ledésert, B., Gueguen, R., Schiele, F. & Breart, G. (1992) Determinants of hormonal replacement therapy in recently postmenopausal women. *Eur. J. Obstet. Gynecol. reprod. Biol.*, **45**, 193–200

Risch, H.A. (1996) Estrogen replacement therapy and risk of epithelial ovarian cancer. *Gynecol. Oncol.*, **63**, 254–257

Risch, H.A. & Howe, G.R. (1994) Menopausal hormone usage and breast cancer in Saskatchewan: A record-linkage cohort study. *Am. J. Epidemiol.*, **139**, 670–683

Risch, H.A. & Howe, G.R. (1995) Menopausal hormone use and colorectal cancer in Saskatchewan: A record linkage cohort study. *Cancer Epidemiol. Biomarkers Prev.*, **4**, 21–28

Risch, H.A., Marrett, L.D., Jain, M. & Howe, G.R. (1996) Differences in risk factors for epithelial ovarian cancer by histologic type. Results of a case–control study. *Am. J. Epidemiol., 144*, 363–372

Rodriguez, C., Calle, E.E., Coates, R.J., Miracle-McMahill, H.L., Thun, M.J. & Heath, C.W., Jr (1995) Estrogen replacement therapy and fatal ovarian cancer. *Am. J. Epidemiol., 141*, 828–835

Rohan, T.E. & McMichael, A.J. (1988) Non-contraceptive exogenous oestrogen therapy and breast cancer. *Med. J. Aust., 148*, 217–221

Ron, E., Kleinerman, R.A., Boice, J.D., Jr, LiVolsi, V.A., Flannery, J.T. & Fraumeni, J.F., Jr (1987) A population-based case–control study of thyroid cancer. *J. natl Cancer Inst., 79*, 1–12

Rookus, M.A., van Leeuwen, F.E., for the Netherlands Oral Contraceptives and Breast Cancer Study Group (1994) Oral contraceptives and risk of breast cancer in women aged 20–54 years. *Lancet, 344*, 844–851

Ross, R.K., Paganini-Hill, A., Gerkins, V.R., Mack, T.M., Pfeffer, R., Arthur, M. & Henderson, B.E. (1980) A case–control study of menopausal estrogen therapy and breast cancer. *J. Am. med. Assoc., 243*, 1635–1639

Ross, R.K., Paganini-Hill, A., Roy, S., Chao, A. & Henderson, B.E. (1988) Past and present preferred prescribing practices of hormone replacement therapy among Los Angeles gynecologists: Possible implications for public health. *Am. J. public Health, 78*, 516–519

Roy, D. & Thomas, R.D. (1994) Catalysis of the redox cycling reactions of estrogens by nuclear enzymes. *Arch. Biochem. Biophys., 315*, 310–316

Roy, D., Kalyanaraman, B. & Liehr, J.G. (1991) Superoxide radical mediated reduction of estrogen quinones to semiquinones and hydroquinones. *Biochem. Pharmacol., 42*, 1627–1631

Rozenbaum, H. (1996) Advantages and disadvantages of estrogen treatment by transdermal or oral administration. *Eur. J. Obstet. Gynecol. reprod. Biol., 65*, 33–37

Rubin, G.L., Peterson, H.B., Lee, N.C., Maes, E.F., Wingo, P.A. & Becker, S. (1990) Estrogen replacement therapy and the risk of endometrial cancer: Remaining controversies. *Am. J. Obstet. Gynecol., 162*, 148–154

Ruoff, W.L. & Dziuk, P.J. (1994a) Absorption and metabolism of estrogens from the stomach and duodenum of pigs. *Domest. Anim. Endocrinol., 11*, 197–208

Ruoff, W.L. & Dziuk, P.J. (1994b) Circulation of estrogens introduced into the rectum or duodenum in pigs. *Domest. Anim. Endocrinol., 11*, 383–391

Rutanen, E.-M. (1997) Biology of the endometrium. In: Wren, B.G., ed., *Progress in the Management of the Menopause*, New York, Parthenon Publishing Group, pp. 217–225

Ruzycky, A.L. (1996) Effects of 17β-estradiol and progesterone on mitogen-activated protein kinase expression and activity in rat uterine smooth muscle. *Eur. J. Pharmacol., 300*, 247–254

Ruzycky, A.L. & Kulick, A. (1996) Estrogen increases the expression of uterine protein kinase C isozymes in a tissue specific manner. *Eur. J. Pharmacol., 313*, 257–263

Sakamato, S., Kudo, H., Suzuki, S., Mitamura, T., Sassa, S., Kuwa, K., Chun, Z., Yoshimura, S., Maemura, M., Nakayama, T. & Shinoda, H. (1997) Additional effects of medroxyprogesterone acetate on mammary tumors in oophorectomized, estrogenized, DMBA-treated rats. *Anticancer Res., 17*, 4583–4588

Sakr, S.A., El-Mofty, M.M. & Mohamed, A.M. (1989) Enhancement of hepatic tumors induced by N-nitrosodimethylamine in female toads *Bufo regularis* by oestrone. *Arch. Geschwulstforsch.*, **59**, 7–10

Salamone, L.M., Pressman, A.R., Seeley, D.G. & Cauley, J.A. (1996) Estrogen replacement therapy: A survey of older women's attitudes. *Arch. intern. Med.*, **156**, 1293–1297

Salmi, T. (1980) Endometrial carcinoma risk factors, with special reference to the use of oestrogens. *Acta endocrinol.*, **Suppl. 233**, 37–43

Sandberg, A.A. & Slaunwhite, W.R. (1957) Studies on phenolic steroids in humans subjects. II. The metabolic fate and hepatobiliary–enteric circulation of ¹⁴C-estrone and ¹⁴C-estradiol in women. *J. clin. Invest.*, **36**, 1266–1278

Santner, S.J., Ohlsson-Wilhelm, B. & Santen, R.J. (1993) Estrone sulfate promotes human breast cancer cell replication and nuclear uptake of estradiol in MCF-7 cell cultures. *Int. J. Cancer*, **54**, 119–124

Sarabia, S.F., Zhu, B.T., Kurosawa, T., Tohma, M. & Liehr, J.G. (1997) Mechanism of cytochrome P450-catalyzed hydroxylation of estrogens. *Chem. Res. Toxicol.*, **10**, 767–771

Satoh, H., Kajimura, T., Chen, C.-J., Yamada, K., Furuhama, K. & Nomura, M. (1997) Invasive pituitary tumors in female F344 rats induced by estradiol dipropionate. *Toxicol. Pathol.*, **25**, 462–469

Schairer, C., Byrne, C., Keyl, P.M., Brinton, L.A., Sturgeon, S.R. & Hoover, R.N. (1994) Menopausal estrogen and estrogen–progestin replacement therapy and risk of breast cancer (United States). *Cancer Causes Control*, **5**, 491–500

Schairer, C., Adami, H.-O., Hoover, R. & Persson, I. (1997) Cause-specific mortality in women receiving hormone replacement therapy. *Epidemiology*, **8**, 59–65

Schiff, I., Wentworth, B., Koos, B., Ryan, K.J. & Tulchinsky, D. (1978) Effect of estriol administration on the hypogonadal woman. *Fertil. Steril.*, **30**, 278–282

Schleyer-Saunders, E. (1973) Hormone replacement therapy for menopausal symptoms (Letter to the Editor). *Lancet*, **ii**, 389

Schnitzler, R., Foth, J., Degen, G.H. & Metzler, M. (1994) Induction of micronuclei by stilbene-type and steroidal estrogens in Syrian hamster embryo and ovine seminal vesicle cells *in vitro*. *Mutat. Res.*, **311**, 85–93

Schoonen, W.G.E.J., Joosten, J.W.H. & Kloosterboer, H.J. (1995a) Effects of two classes of progestagens, pregnane and 19-nortestosterone derivatives, on cell growth of human breast tumor cells: I. MCF-7 cell lines. *J. Steroid Biochem. mol. Biol.*, **55**, 423–437

Schoonen, W.G.E.J., Joosten, J.W.H. & Kloosterboer, H.J. (1995b) Effects of two classes of progestagens, pregnane and 19-nortestosterone derivatives, on cell growth of human breast tumor cells: II. T47D cell lines. *J. Steroid Biochem. mol. Biol.*, **55**, 439–444

Schulte-Hermann, R., Ochs, H., Bursch, W. & Parzefall, W. (1988) Quantitative structure–activity studies on effects of sixteen different steroids on growth and monooxygenases of rat liver. *Cancer Res.*, **48**, 2462–2468

Schuppler, J., Damme, J. & Schulte-Hermann, R. (1983) Assay of some endogenous and synthetic sex steroids for tumor-initiating activity in rat liver using the Solt–Faber system. *Carcinogenesis*, **4**, 239–241

Schuurman, A.G., van den Brandt, P.A. & Goldbohm, R.A. (1995) Exogenous hormone use and the risk of postmenopausal breast cancer: Results from the Netherlands cohort study. *Cancer Causes Control*, **6**, 416–424

Schwartz, U., Volger, H., Schneller, E., Moltz, L. & Hammerstein, J. (1983) Effects of various replacement oestrogens on hepatic transcortin synthesis in climacteric women. *Acta endocrinol.*, **102**, 103–106

Setnikar, I., Rovati, L.C., Vens-Cappel, B. & Hilgenstock, C. (1996) Pharmacokinetics of estradiol and of estrone during repeated transdermal or oral administration of estradiol. *Arzneim.-Forsch./Drug Res.*, **46**, 766–773

Shapiro, S., Kaufman, D.W., Slone, D., Rosenberg, L., Miettinen, O.S., Stolley, P.D., Rosenshein, N.B., Watring, W.G., Leavitt, T. & Knapp, R.C. (1980) Recent and past use of conjugated estrogens in relation to adenocarcinoma of the endometrium. *New Engl. J. Med.*, **303**, 485–489

Shapiro, S., Kelly, J.P., Rosenberg, L., Kaufman, D.W., Helmrich, S.P., Rosenshein, N.B., Lewis, J.L., Knapp, R.C., Stolley, P.D. & Schottenfeld, D. (1985) Risk of localized and widespread endometrial cancer in relation to recent and discontinued use of conjugated estrogens. *New Engl. J. Med.*, **313**, 969–972

Sheehan, D.M., Frederik, C.B., Branham, W.S. & Heath, J.E. (1982) Evidence for estradiol promotion of neoplastic lesions in the rat vagina after initiation with *N*-methyl-*N*-nitrosourea. *Carcinogenesis*, **3**, 957–959

Shen, L., Pisha, E., Huang, Z., Pezzuto, J.M., Krol, E., Alam, Z. , van Breemen, R.B. & Bolton, J.L. (1997) Bioreductive activation of catechol estrogen-*ortho*-quinones: Aromatization of the B ring in 4-hydroxyequilenin markedly alters quinoid formation and reactivity. *Carcinogenesis*, **18**, 1093–1101

Shifren, J.L., Tseng, J.F., Zaloudek, C.J, Ryan, I.P., Meng, Y.G., Ferrara, N., Jaffe, R.B. & Taylor, R.N. (1996) Ovarian steroid regulation of vascular endothelial growth factor in the human endometrium: Implications for angiogenesis during the menstrual cycle and in the pathogenesis of endometriosis. *J. clin. Endocrinol. Metab.*, **81**, 3112–3118

Shull, J.D., Spady, T.J., Snyder, M.C., Johansson S.L. & Pennington, K.L. (1997) Ovary-intact, but not ovariectomized female ACI rats treated with 17β-estradiol rapidly develop mammary carcinoma. *Carcinogenesis*, **18**, 1595–1601

Siddle, N.C., Townsend, P.T., Young, O., Minardi, J., King, R.J.B. & Whitehead, M.I. (1982) Dose-dependent effects of synthetic progestins on the biochemistry of the estrogenized postmenopausal endometrium. *Acta. obstet. gynecol. scand.*, **Suppl. 106**, 17–22

Siegfried, S., Pekonen, F., Nyman, T. & Ämmälä, M. (1995) Expression of mRNA for keratinocyte growth factor and its receptor in human endometrium. *Acta obstet. gynecol. scand.*, **74**, 410–414

Siiteri, P.K. (1987) Adipose tissue as a source of hormones. *Am. J. clin. Nutr.*, **45**, 277–282

Sina, J.F., Bean, C.L., Dysart, G.R., Taylor, V.I. & Bradley, M.O. (1983) Evaluation of the alkaline elution/rat hepatocyte assay as a predictor of carcinogenic/mutagenic potential. *Mutat. Res.*, **113**, 357–391

Sinclair, H.K., Bond, C.M. & Taylor, R.J. (1993) Hormone replacement therapy: A study of women's knowledge and attitudes. *Br. J. gen. Prac.*, **43**, 365–370

Siskind, V., Schofield, F., Rice, D. & Bain, C. (1989) Breast cancer and breast feeding: Results from an Australian case–control study. *Am. J. Epidemiol.*, **130**, 229–236

Slikker, W., Hill, D.E. & Young, J.F. (1982) Comparison of the transplacental pharmacokinetics of 17β-estradiol and diethylstilbestrol in the subhuman primate. *J. Pharmacol. exp. Ther.*, **221**, 173–182

Smith, D.C., Prentice, R., Thompson, D.J. & Herrmann, W.L. (1975) Association of exogenous estrogen and endometrial carcinoma. *New Engl. J. Med.*, **293**, 1164–1167

Snedeker, S.M. & Diaugustine, R.P. (1996) Hormonal and environmental factors affecting cell proliferation and neoplasia in the mammary gland. In: Huff, J., Boyd, J. & Barrett, J.C., eds, *Cellular and Molecular Mechanisms of Hormonal Carcinogenesis: Environmental Influences*, New York, Wiley-Liss, pp. 211–253

Spector, T.D. (1989) Use of oestrogen replacement therapy in high risk groups in the United Kingdom. *Br. med. J.*, **299**, 1434–1435

Spengler, R.F., Clarke, E.A., Woolever, C.A., Newman, A.M. & Osborn, R.W. (1981) Exogenous estrogens and endometrial cancer: A case–control study and assessment of potential biases. *Am. J. Epidemiol.*, **114**, 497–506

Stadberg, E., Mattsson, L.Å. & Milsom, I. (1997) The prevalence and severity of climacteric symptoms and the use of different treatment regimens in a Swedish population. *Acta obstet. gynecol. scand.*, **76**, 442–448

Stadel, B.V. & Weiss, N. (1975) Characteristics of menopausal women: A survey of King and Pierce counties in Washington, 1973–1974. *Am. J. Epidemiol.*, **102**, 209–216

Standeven, M., Criqui, M.H., Klauber, M.R., Gabriel, S. & Barrett-Connor, E. (1986) Correlates of change in postmenopausal estrogen use in a population-based study. *Am. J. Epidemiol.*, **124**, 268–274

Stanford, J.L., Weiss, N.S., Voigt, L.F., Daling, J.R., Habel, L.A. & Rossing, M.A. (1995) Combined estrogen and progestin hormone replacement therapy in relation to risk of breast cancer in middle-aged women. *J. Am. med. Assoc.*, **274**, 137–142

Stavraky, K.M., Collins, J.A., Donner, A. & Wells, G.A. (1981) A comparison of estrogen use by women with endometrial cancer, gynecologic disorders, and other illnesses. *Am. J. Obstet. Gynecol.*, **141**, 547–555

Stenchever, M.A., Jarvis, J.A. & Kreger, N.K. (1969) Effect of selected estrogens and progestins on human chromosomes in vitro. *Obstet. Gynecol.*, **34**, 249–252

Stern, M.D. (1982) Pharmacology of conjugated oestrogens. *Maturitas*, **4**, 333–339

Studd, J.W.W. (1976) Hormone implants in the climacteric syndrome. In: Campbell, S., ed., *The Management of the Menopause and the Post-menopausal Years*, Lancaster, MTP Press Ltd, pp. 383–385

Stumpf, P.G. (1990) Pharmacokinetics of estrogen. *Obstet. Gynecol.*, **75**, 9S–14S

Sturgis, S.H. (1979) Estrogen use and endometrial cancer (Letter to the Editor). *New Engl. J. Med.*, **300**, 922

Sumi, C., Yokoro, K. & Matsushima, R. (1984) Effects of 17β-estradiol and diethylstilbestrol on concurrent development of hepatic, mammary, and pituitary tumors in WF rats: Evidence for differential effect on liver. *J. natl Cancer Inst.*, **73**, 1229–1234

Swenberg, J.A. (1981) Utilization of the alkaline elution assay as a short-term test for chemical carcinogens. In: Stich, H.F. & San, R.H.C., eds, *Short-term Tests for Chemical Carcinogens*, New York, Springer-Verlag, pp. 48–58

Takahashi, M., Iijima, T., Suzuki, K., Ando-Lu, J., Yoshida, M., Kitamura, T., Nishiyama, K., Miyajima, K. & Maekawa, A. (1996) Rapid and high yield induction of endometrial adeno-carcinomas in CD-1 mice by a single intrauterine administration of *N*-ethyl-*N*-nitrosourea combined with chronic 17β estradiol treatment. *Cancer Lett.*, **104**, 7–12

Talamini, R., La Vecchia, C., Franceschi, S., Colombo, F., DeCarli, A., Grattoni, E., Grigoletto, E. & Tognoni, G. (1985) Reproductive and hormonal factors and breast cancer in a northern Italian population. *Int. J. Epidemiol.*, **14**, 70–74

Talamini, R., Franceschi, S., Dal Maso, L., Negri, E., Conti, E., Filiberti, R., Montella, M., Nanni, O. & La Vecchia, C. (1998) The influence of reproductive and hormonal factors on the risk of colon and rectal cancer in women. *Eur. J. Cancer*, **34**, 1070–1076

Tang, M. & Subbiah, M.T.R. (1996) Estrogens protect against hydrogen peroxide and archidonic acid induced DNA damage. *Biochim. biophys. Acta*, **1299**, 155–159

Taton, G., Servais, P. & Galand, P. (1990) Modulation by estrogen of the incidence of diethyl-nitrosamine-induced gamma-glutamyltranspeptidase-positive foci in rat liver. *Cancer Lett.*, **55**, 45–51

Tavani, A., Negri, E. & La Vecchia, C. (1996) Menstrual and reproductive factors and biliary tract cancers. *Eur. J. Cancer Prev.*, **5**, 241–247

Tavani, A., Braga, C., La Vecchia, C., Negri, E. & Franceschi, S. (1997) Hormone replacement treatment and breast cancer risk: An age-specific analysis. *Cancer Epidemiol. Biomarkers Prev.*, **6**, 11–14

Telang, N.T., Suto, A., Wong, G.Y., Osborne, M.P. & Bradlow, H.L. (1992) Induction by estrogen metabolite 16α-hydroxyestrone of genotoxic damage and aberrant proliferation in mouse mammary epithelial cells. *J. natl Cancer Inst.*, **84**, 634–638

Thomas, D.B., Persing, J.P. & Hutchinson, W.B. (1982) Exogenous oestrogens and other risk factors for breast cancer in women with benign breast diseases. *J. natl Cancer Inst.*, **69**, 1017–1025

Topo, P., Køster, A., Holte, A., Collins, A., Landgren, B.-M., Hemminki, E. & Uutela, A. (1995) Trends in the use of climacteric and postclimacteric hormones in Nordic countries. *Maturitas*, **22**, 89–95

Townsend, J. (1998) Hormone replacement therapy: Assessment of present use, costs and trends. *Br. J. gen. Pract.*, **48**, 955–958

Troisi, R., Schairer, C., Chow, W.-H., Schatzkin, A., Brinton, L.A. & Fraumeni, J.F., Jr (1997) A prospective study of menopausal hormones and risk of colorectal cancer (United States). *Cancer Causes Control*, **8**, 130–138

Tsutsui, T., Suzuki, N., Fukuda, S., Sato, M., Maizumi, H., McLacklan, J.A. & Barrett, J.C. (1987) 17β-Estradiol-induced cell transformation and aneuploidy of Syrian hamster embryo cells in culture. *Carcinogenesis*, **8**, 1715–1719

Tsutsui, T., Suzuki, N., Maizumi, H. & Barrett, J.C. (1990) Aneuploidy induction in human fibro-blasts: Comparison with results in Syrian hamster fibroblasts. *Mutat. Res.*, **240**, 241–249

Tsutsui, T., Taguchi, S., Tanaka, Y. & Barrett, C. (1997) 17β-Estradiol, diethylstilbestrol, tamo-xifen, toremifene and ICI 164,384 induce morphological transformation and aneuploidy in cultured Syrian hamster embryo cells. *Int. J. Cancer*, **70**, 188–193

Tzonou, A., Day, N.E., Trichopoulos, D., Walker, A., Saliaraki, M., Papapostolou, M. & Poly-chronopoulou, A. (1984) The epidemiology of ovarian cancer in Greece: A case–control study. *Eur. J. Cancer clin. Oncol.*, **20**, 1045–1052

Ueda, M., Fujii, H., Yoshizawa, K., Abe, F. & Ueki, M. (1996) Effects of sex steroids and growth factors on migration and invasion of endometrial adenocarcinoma SNG-M cells *in vitro*. *Jpn. J. Cancer Res.*, **87**, 524–533

Ursin, G., Aragaki, C.C., Paganini-Hill, A., Siemiatycki, J., Thompson, W.D. & Haile, R.W. (1992) Oral contraceptives and premenopausal bilateral breast cancer: A case–control study. *Epidemiology*, **3**, 414–419

Vakil, D.V., Morgan, R.W. & Halliday, M. (1983) Exogenous estrogens and development of breast and endometrial cancer. *Cancer Detect. Prev.*, **6**, 415–424

Vessey, M., Baron, J., Doll, R., McPherson, K. & Yeates, D. (1983) Oral contraceptives and breast cancer: Final report of an epidemiogic study. *Br. J. Cancer*, **47**, 455–62

Vessey, M.P., McPherson, K., Villard-Mackintosh, L. & Yeates, D. (1989) Oral contraceptives and breast cancer: Latest findings in a large cohort study. *Br. J. Cancer*, **59**, 613–617

Voigt, L.F., Weiss, N.S., Chu, J., Daling, J.R., McKnight, B. & van Belle, G. (1991) Progestagen supplementation of exogenous oestrogens and risk of endometrial cancer. *Lancet*, **338**, 274–277

Wang, D.Y., De Stavola, B.L., Bulbrook, R.D., Allen, D.S., Kwa, H.G., Verstraeten, A.A., Moore, J.W., Fentiman, I.S., Chaudary, M., Hayward, J.L. & Gravelle, I.H. (1987) The relationship between blood prolactin levels and risk of breast cancer in premenopausal women. *Eur. J. Cancer clin. Oncol.*, **23**, 1541–1548

Weinstein, A.L., Mahoney, M.C., Nasca, P.C., Hanson, R.L., Leske, M.C. & Varma, A.O. (1993) Oestrogen replacement therapy and breast cancer risk: A case–control study. *Int. J. Epidemiol.*, **22**, 781–789

Weiss, N.S., Szekely, D.R., English, D.R. & Schweid, A.I. (1979) Endometrial cancer in relation to patterns of menopausal estrogen use. *J. Am. med. Assoc.*, **242**, 261–264

Weiss, N.S., Daling, J.R. & Chow, W.H. (1981) Incidence of cancer of the large bowel in women in relation to reproductive and hormonal factors. *J. natl Cancer Inst.*, **67**, 57–60

Weiss, N.S., Lyon, J.L., Krishnamurthy, S., Dietert, S.E., Liff, J.M. & Daling, J.R. (1982) Non-contraceptive estrogen use and the occurrence of ovarian cancer. *J. natl Cancer Inst.*, **68**, 95–98

Westerdahl, J., Olsson, H., Måsbäck, A., Ingvar, C. & Jonsson, N. (1996) Risk of malignant mela-noma in relation to drug intake, alcohol, smoking and hormonal factors. *Br. J. Cancer*, **73**, 1126–1131

Wheeler, W.J., Cherry, L.M., Downs, T. & Hsu, T.C. (1986) Mitotic inhibition and aneuploidy induction by naturally occurring and synthetic estrogens in Chinese hamster cells *in vitro*. *Mutat. Res.*, **171**, 31–41

White, E., Malone, K.E., Weiss, N.S. & Daling, J.R. (1994) Breast cancer among young US women in relation to oral contraceptive use. *J. natl Cancer Inst.*, **86**, 505–514

Whitehead, M.I., Townsend, P.T., Pryse-Davis, J., Ryder, T.A. & King, R.J.B. (1981) Effects of estrogens and progestins on the biochemistry and morphology of the postmenopausal endometrium. *New Engl. J. Med.*, **305**, 1599–1605

Whittaker, P.G., Morgan, M.R.A., Dean, P.D.G., Cameron, E.H.D. & Lind, T. (1980) Serum equilin, estrone, and oestradiol levels in postmenopausal women after conjugated equine administration. *Lancet*, **i**, 14–16

Whittemore, A.S., Harris, R., Itnyre, J. & the Collaborative Ovarian Cancer Group (1992) Characteristics relating to ovarian cancer risk: Collaborative analysis of 12 US case–control studies. II. Invasive epithelial ovarian cancers in white women. *Am. J. Epidemiol.*, **136**,1184–1203

WHO Collaborative Study of Neoplasia and Steroid Contraceptives (1990) Breast cancer and combined oral contraceptives: Results from a multinational study. *Br. J. Cancer*, **61**, 110–119

Wilcox, J.G., Stanczyk, F.Z., Morris, R.S., Gentzschein, E. & Lobo, R.A. (1996) Biologic effects of 17α-dihydroequilin sulfate. *Fertil. Steril.*, **66**, 748–752

Williams, C.L. & Stancel, G.M. (1996) Estrogens and progestogens. In: Wonsiewicz, M.J. & McCurdy, P., eds, *Goodman & Gilman's The Pharmacological Basis of Therapeutics*, 9th Ed., New York, McGraw-Hill, pp. 1411–1440

Willis, D.B., Calle, E.E., Miracle-McMahill, H.L. & Heath, C.W., Jr (1996) Estrogen replacement therapy and risk of fatal breast cancer in a prospective cohort of postmenopausal women in the United States. *Cancer Causes Control*, **7**, 449–457

Wingo, P.A., Layde, P.M., Lee, N.C., Rubin, G. & Ory, H.W. (1987) The risk of breast cancer in postmenopausal women who have used estrogen replacement therapy. *J. Am. med. Assoc.*, **257**, 209–215

Wotiz, H.H., Beebe, D.R. & Müller, E. (1984) Effect of estrogens on DMBA induced breast tumors. *J. Steroid Biochem.*, **20**, 1067–1075

Writing Group for the PEPI Trial (1995) Effects of estrogen or estrogen/progestin regimens on heart disease risk factors in postmenopausal women. The Postmenopausal Estrogen/Progestin Interventions (PEPI) Trial. *J. Am. med. Assoc.*, **273**, 199–208 (Published erratum in 1995. *J. Am. med. Assoc.*, **274**, 1676)

Wu, A.H., Paganini-Hill, A., Ross, R.K. & Henderson, B.E. (1987) Alcohol, physical activity and other risk factors for colorectal cancer: A prospective study. *Br. J. Cancer*, **55**, 687–694

Wu-Williams, A.H., Lee, M., Whittemore, A.S., Gallagher, R.P., Jiao, D., Zheng, S., Zhou, L., Wang, X., Chen, K., Jung, D., Teh, C.-Z., Ling, C., Xu, J.Y. & Paffenbarger, R.S., Jr (1991) Reproductive factors and colorectal cancer risk among Chinese females. *Cancer Res.*, **51**, 2307–2311

Wysowski, D.K., Golden, L. & Burke, L. (1995) Use of menopausal estrogens and medroxyprogesterone in the United States, 1982–1992. *Obstet. Gynecol.*, **85**, 6–10

Xu, L.H., Rinehart, C.A. & Kaufman, D.G. (1995) Estrogen-induced anchorage-independence in human endometrial stromal cells. *Int. J. Cancer*, **62**, 772–776

Yager, J.D. & Liehr, J.G. (1996) Molecular mechanisms of estrogen carcinogenesis. *Ann. Rev. Pharmacol. Toxicol.*, **36**, 203–32

Yager, J.D., Campbell, H.A., Longnecker, D.S., Roebuck, B.D. & Benoit, M.C. (1984) Enhancement of hepatocarcinogenesis in female rats by ethinyl estradiol and mestranol but not estradiol. *Cancer Res.*, **44**, 3862–3869

Yamafuji, K., Iiyama, S. & Shinohara, K. (1971) Mode of action of steroid hormones on deoxyribonucleic acid. *Enzymology*, **40**, 259–264

Yamamoto, T., Terada, N., Nishizawa, Y. & Petrow, V. (1994) Angiostatic activities of medroxyprogesterone acetate and its analogues. *Int. J. Cancer*, **56**, 393–399

Yang, C.P., Daling, J.R., Band, P.R., Gallagher, R.P., White, E. & Weiss, N.S. (1992) Noncontraceptive hormone use and risk of breast cancer. *Cancer Causes Control*, **3**, 475–479

Yood, S.M., Ulcickas Yood, M. & McCarthy, B. (1998) A case-control study of hormone replacement therapy and colorectal cancer (Abstract). *Ann. Epidemiol.*, **8**, 133

Yu, M.C., Tong, M.J., Govindarajan, S. & Henderson, B.E. (1991) Nonviral risk factors for hepatocellular carcinoma in a low-risk population, the non-Asians of Los Angeles County, California. *J. natl Cancer Inst.*, **83**, 1820–1826

Yuen, J., Persson, I., Bergkvist, L., Hoover, R., Schairer, C. & Adami, H.O. (1993) Hormone replacement therapy and breast cancer mortality in Swedish women: Results after adjustment for 'healthy drug-user' effect. *Cancer Causes Control*, **4**, 369–374

Zhu, B.T. & Conney, A.H. (1998) Functional role of estrogen metabolism in target cells: review and perspectives. *Carcinogenesis*, **19**, 1–27

Ziel, H.K. & Finkle, W.D. (1975) Increased risk of endometrial carcinoma among users of conjugated estrogens. *New Engl. J. Med.*, **293**, 1167–1170

POST-MENOPAUSAL OESTROGEN–PROGESTOGEN THERAPY

1. Exposure

Post-menopausal oestrogen–progestogen therapy involves administration of the oestrogens described in the monograph on 'Post-menopausal oestrogen therapy' accompanied by a progestogen or progesterone to women around the time of the menopause, primarily for the treatment of menopausal symptoms but also for the prevention of conditions that become more common after the menopause, such as osteoporosis and ischaemic heart disease. The progestogen can be administered orally or transdermally and either continuously or at various intervals. Intermittent progestogen administration causes withdrawal uterine bleeding, while continuous therapy generally does not. In 'peri-menopausal hormonal therapy', the components are not specified but are usually oestrogen with or without a progestogen. Annex 2 (Table 5) gives examples of brands of post-menopausal oestrogen–progestogen therapy. Progestogens that can be given in combination with the oestrogens are listed in Annex 1, with their constituents, doses, routes of administration and the names of some countries in which the brands are available; Annex 1 also gives the chemical formulae and some information on indications for use.

1.1 Historical overview

The earliest forms of hormones used for the treatment of ovarian failure or after oophorectomy were natural extracts of ovarian tissue, placenta and urine from pregnant women and thus contained both oestrogen and progestogen, as well as other substances. Crystalline progesterone was first identified in 1934, and shortly afterwards experimental treatment of women with injected oestrogen and progesterone began (Hirvonen, 1996). In the decades that followed, however, menopausal symptoms were treated mainly with oestrogen alone rather than with combined oestrogen–progestogen therapy.

Oral progesterone equivalents did not become readily available until the 1940s, when Russell Marker synthesized diosgenin from extracts of the Mexican yam. Further experimentation yielded the synthesis of norethisterone (norethindrone) by Carl Djerassi in 1950 and norethynodrel by Frank B. Colton in 1952. These compounds were named progestogens (or progestins) owing to their progesterone-like actions (Kleinman, 1990). They were ultimately used in combined oral contraceptives (see section 1 of the monograph on 'Oral contraceptives, combined' for details), developed in the late 1950s.

During the 1960s and early 1970s, most hormonal therapy was used in the United States (particularly in California) and took the form of post-menopausal oestrogen therapy, without progestogen. At that time, some clinicians, especially those in Europe, prescribed oestrogen–progestogen therapy, primarily for better control of uterine bleeding during treatment, as post-menopausal oestrogen therapy sometimes causes irregular bleeding in women with a uterus (Maddison, 1973; Studd, 1976; Bush & Barrett-Connor, 1985). Figure 1 of the monograph on 'Post-menopausal oestrogen therapy' shows the estimated numbers of prescriptions of non-contraceptive progestogens and medroxyprogesterone acetate in the United States between 1966 and 1992.

Studies linking post-menopausal oestrogen therapy with increased rates of endometrial cancer were first published in 1975 (Ziel & Finkle, 1975). These led to a rapid decrease in prescription of such therapy in the United States and the recommendation by many clinicians and researchers that progestogen be added to oestrogen when treating post-menopausal women with an intact uterus, as this had been shown to attenuate the risk of endometrial cancer associated with the use of oestrogen alone (Bush & Barrett-Connor, 1985; Kennedy et al., 1985). In Europe, when post-menopausal hormonal therapy was indicated for women with an intact uterus, it became accepted practice to administer combined oestrogen–progestogen therapy; post-menopausal oestrogen therapy was still given to hysterectomized women. In the United States, some clinicians continued to prescribe post-menopausal oestrogen therapy to women with a uterus, following guidelines to monitor the endometrium (American College of Physicians, 1992), although increasing prescription of progestogens was noted after 1975 (see Figure 1 in the monograph on 'Post-menopausal oestrogen therapy'). In the United States in 1980, approximately 5% of the Premarin®, the commonest oestrogen sold, was accompanied by oral Provera®, the commonest progestogen, while in 1983 this figure had risen to 12% (Kennedy et al., 1985). In the United Kingdom, prescription of oestrogen–progestogen therapy increased throughout the late 1970s and early 1980s, until in 1984 almost equal amounts of oestrogen alone and oestrogen–progestogen therapy were used (Townsend, 1998).

The Women's Health Initiative trial of post-menopausal hormonal therapy was begun in the United States in 1992. In this trial, women with a uterus could be randomized to post-menopausal oestrogen therapy with monitoring of the endometrium, reflecting a proportion of clinical practice at the time (Finnegan et al., 1995). In 1995, the results of the Postmenopausal Estrogen/Progestin Interventions (PEPI) trial showed adenomatous or atypical endometrial hyperplasia in 34% of women receiving 0.625 mg unopposed conjugated equine oestrogens daily (Writing Group for the PEPI Trial, 1995). The protocol of the Women's Health Initiative trial was therefore amended so that women with a uterus could be randomized to receive only combined oestrogen–progestogen therapy or placebo (Finnegan et al., 1995). No figures on the prevalence of post-menopausal oestrogen–progestogen therapy after this publication are available, but it is expected that use will increase relative to that of post-menopausal oestrogen therapy.

1.2   Post-menopausal oestrogen–progestogen therapy preparations

The oestrogens used in post-menopausal oestrogen–progestogen therapy are described in the monograph on 'Post-menopausal oestrogen therapy' and in Annex 1; the progestogens used in oestrogen–progestogen therapy are derived from 17α-hydroxyprogesterone and 19-nortestosterone, although progesterone itself is sometimes used. Tibolone is a centrally acting compound with both oestrogenic and progestogenic actions. Of the 17α-hydroxyprogesterone derivatives, medroxyprogesterone acetate is the most widely used; dydrogesterone is also available. Of the 19-nortestosterone derivatives, norethisterone, norethisterone acetate, norgestrel and levonorgestrel are used in post-menopausal oestrogen–progestogen therapy. Progesterone is now administered orally in a micronized form but was given by injection in the past (British Medical Association, 1997).

In the commonest treatment regimen, the oestrogen component is taken daily orally or transdermally, usually at a constant dose, with a progestogen given for 10–14 days per month, causing withdrawal bleeding. A typical dose of progestogen is 5–10 mg medroxyprogesterone acetate orally, daily for 10–14 days. Preparations are also available in which the progestogen is given every three months, causing quarterly bleeding. Another widely used regimen is a constant dose of oestrogen taken daily continuously, accompanied by continuous progestogen. A typical continuous progestogen dose would be about 2.5 mg medroxyprogesterone acetate orally per day (British Medical Association, 1997). The continuous progestogen can also be given transdermally as 0.25 mg norethisterone acetate per 24 h; this regimen usually does not result in withdrawal bleeding (Cameron *et al.*, 1997). Tibolone is given orally, continuously and does not usually result in bleeding, except if treatment is started within 12 months of the woman's last menstrual period (British Medical Association, 1997).

In some countries, primarily in Europe, a progestogen is sometimes given alone for the treatment of menopausal symptoms. A progestogen can also be given in the form of a levonorgestrel-releasing intrauterine device, accompanying oral or transdermal oestrogen, to deliver the progestogen directly to the endometrium (British Medical Association, 1997). This system is not widely licensed for use as post-menopausal oestrogen–progestogen therapy.

1.2.1   Patterns of use

Like post-menopausal oestrogen therapy, combined oestrogen–progestogen therapy is started around the time of the menopause and can be used for both short- and long-term treatment. Table 1 in the monograph on 'Post-menopausal oestrogen therapy' shows the prevalence of current and any use of post-menopausal hormonal therapy in selected studies internationally, with post-menopausal oestrogen therapy and oestrogen–progestogen therapy use shown in the studies in which they were reported separately; very few studies mentioned use of post-menopausal oestrogen–progestogen therapy. In the United States, post-menopausal oestrogen–progestogen therapy was being used currently by 1–5% of women aged 45–64 and had ever been used by 14% of a nationally representative sample of post-menopausal women aged 25–76 in the late 1980s. In Denmark, 12% of 40–59-year-old and 17% of 51-year-old women had ever used post-menopausal oestrogen–progestogen therapy in 1983 and 1987, respectively. In Sweden, combined oestradiol–progestogen use (usually with levonorgestrel or norethisterone acetate) became popular in the early 1970s and is now standard practice. Thus, the increase in the sales of replacement hormones in Sweden since the early 1990s almost entirely entails progestogen-combined regimens. In England, prescription data showed that an estimated 1% of women aged 40–64 used post-menopausal oestrogen–progestogen therapy in 1989, compared with an estimated 11% of women in 1994. About 1% of women in this age group were using tibolone in 1994 (Townsend, 1998).

In a study of general medical practices in the United Kingdom in 1993, 96% of women with a hysterectomy who were taking post-menopausal hormonal therapy were taking oestrogen alone, and 96% of women who had not undergone hysterectomy were taking combinations of oestrogen and progestogen (Lancaster *et al.*, 1995).

2.   Studies of Cancer in Humans

2.1   Breast cancer

The progesterone present during natural cycles and the progestogens added in hormonal therapy may be important in cancer etiology (Stanford & Thomas, 1993). Some epidemiological data suggest that short menstrual cycles or having many regular cycles during a life-time, reflecting exposure to progesterone, may have an adverse effect on the risk for breast cancer (Kelsey *et al.*, 1993). Several studies (Anderson *et al.*, 1982; Longacre & Bartow, 1986; Going *et al.*, 1988; Potten *et al.*, 1988; Anderson *et al.*, 1989), but not all (Vogel *et al.*, 1981), indicate that progesterone in natural cycles and exogenous progestogens in the cycles of users of combined oral contraceptives augment proliferative activity in breast epithelial cells (Key & Pike, 1988). Furthermore, progesterone probably down-regulates oestrogen receptors but maintains the numbers of progesterone receptors in natural cycles (Söderqvist *et al.*, 1993). As increased proliferation may cause neoplastic cell transformation (Preston-Martin *et al.*, 1990), progestogens in treatment regimens may further enhance the risk for breast cancer.

The use of added progestogens to control menstrual bleeding and to prevent development of hyper- and neoplasia of the endometrium in women with an intact uterus has increased markedly since the 1970s, when reports of an increased risk for endometrial cancer after unopposed oestrogen therapy were first published. Both use and the number of progestogen compounds (progesterone- or testosterone-derived) and treatment schedules (cyclical, sequential, long cycle and continuous) have surged. For these reasons, the effects of progestogen combinations on the risk for breast cancer is an important topic in epidemiological research; however, epidemiological data on the effects of oestrogen plus progestogen treatment are rather scarce, especially for long-term use. Some data on the risks associated with combined use are available in nine cohort studies and five case–control studies. The Collaborative Group on Hormonal Factors in Breast Cancer (1997) pooled and re-analysed individual data on such use from some of these and other studies (see section 2.1.3).

2.1.1   *Cohort studies*

The cohort studies on use of post-menopausal oestrogen–progestogen therapy and breast cancer are summarized in Table 1.

Hunt *et al.* (1987) reported the results of the surveillance of a cohort of 4544 women recruited at 21 menopause clinics in Great Britain, all of whom had been placed on hormones and 43% with a variety of combined progestogens for an average of 67 months. The incidence of breast cancer was ascertained through several sources, including mailed questionnaires, morbidity registers and hospital notes. On the basis of about 20 000 person–years of observation and 50 observed cases, a standardized incidence ratio (SIR) of 1.6 (95% confidence interval [CI], 1.2–2.1) was calculated for any use. Analyses of use of oestrogens only or oestrogens plus progestogens, by classifying the different regimens, did not produce any interpretable results. A trend of increasing risk with increasing time since first use (SIR, 3.1; 95% CI, 1.5–5.6 after 10 years or longer) was found for all types of treatment.

In the cohort study of Bergkvist *et al.* (1989), over 23 000 women were recruited by analysing registered prescriptions for various types of hormonal treatment dispensed in six counties in central Sweden. These women were followed-up by record-linkage with the National Cancer Registry. Individual data on exposure and risk factors were obtained from the accumulated prescriptions and from questionnaires sent to a sample of the cohort and all 253 women with newly diagnosed cases of breast cancer. In cohort and nested case–control analyses, exposure to oestrogens alone for nine years or longer was associated with a relative risk of 1.8 (95% CI, 1.0–3.1); for exposure to oestradiol combined with levonorgestrel, the relative risk was 4.4 (based on 10 cases only) after use for more than six years. In women with mixed intakes of oestrogens only and oestrogens plus progestogens exceeding six years, the relative risk estimates varied between 1.2 and 7.2 (not significant).

This cohort was also followed-up for death from breast cancer by linkage to a population-based mortality registry (Yuen *et al.*, 1993). On the basis of prescription data collected during 1977–80 and corrected external mortality rates (calculated from newly diagnosed cases of breast cancer only), an overall standardized mortality ratio (SMR) of 0.8 (95% CI, 0.2–1.1) emerged. When only those women to whom an oestradiol–levonorgestrel combination had been prescribed were included, the SMR was similarly close to baseline, 0.8 (95% CI, 0.4–1.3). In the same study, Persson *et al.* (1996) conducted a 13-year record-linkage follow-up, yielding 634 new cases of breast cancer. Any use of an oestradiol–levonorgestrel combination conferred a slightly increased relative risk (1.3; 95% CI, 1.1–1.4), whereas women receiving oestradiol or conjugated oestrogens only had no alteration of their risk (RR, 0.9; 95% CI, 0.8–1.1).

The results of the Nurses' Health Study were reported on at least two occasions by Colditz *et al.* (1992, 1995). Data on exposure and risk factors were obtained from a baseline questionnaire in 1976 which was administered every two years for up-dates and ascertainment of breast cancer outcome. In the latest report (1995), the cohort of over 121 000 women had been followed-up for 16 years, resulting in over 700 000 person–years of observation and 1935 cases of breast cancer. The results were similar to those reported

Table 1. Summary of cohort studies on post-menopausal oestrogen–progestogen therapy and breast cancer

Reference	Study base	Design: cohort, follow-up, data	Risk relationships: relative risk (RR) and 95% confidence intervals (95% CI)	Comments
Hunt et al. (1987)	Menopause clinics in the UK, 1978–82; women given counsel for menopausal symptoms	Cohort of 4 544 women who used hormones ≥ 1 year; 17 830 person–years; follow-up through contact letters and medical record data; exposure data through baseline interview	**Incidence**: 50 cases Any use of hormones: incidence: SIR, 1.6 (95% CI, 1.2–2.1) Time since first intake: trend for incidence ≥ 10 years: SIR, 3.1 (95% CI, 1.5–5.6) 43% of all treatment episodes combined with progestogens, analyses by subcategories not feasible	Possible selection bias in study of mortality Heterogeneous exposure regimens with regard to progestogens
Bergkvist et al. (1989)	Six counties in Sweden, 1977–83; women given hormonal therapy; age, ≥ 35 years	Population-based cohort; 23 244 women; 133 375 person–years; follow-up through record linkage with National Cancer Registry; exposure data from prescriptions; questionnaire data in a random sample; cohort, case–cohort and case–control analyses	**Incidence**: 253 cases Regimens, duration ≥ 9 years: oestrogens alone: RR, 1.8 (95% CI, 1.0–3.1) oestrogen and progestogens > 6 years: RR, 4.4 (95% CI, 0.9–22)	Low power to examine long-term progestogen combined regimens
Colditz et al. (1992)	Nurses' Health Cohort, USA, 1976–88, 30–55 years at entry	Cohort, 118 300 nurses at post-menopausal ages; 480 665 person–years; individual follow-up through questionnaires, 95% complete for incidence and 98% for deaths; internal comparisons; baseline questionnaire, 1976; up-dated questionnaires every 2 years	**Incidence**: 12 years' follow-up, 1 050 cases Post-menopausal hormones: any use: RR,1.1 (95% CI, 1.0–1.2) current use: RR, 1.3 (1.1–1.5) Oestrogen and progestogen, current intake: RR, 1.5 (95% CI, 1.0–2.4)	Main relationship with current intake
Yuen et al. (1993)	Uppsala health care region, Sweden, 1977–80; women given hormonal therapy	See Bergkvist et al. above; follow-up through record linkage with Causes of Death Registry; comparison with external, *corrected* mortality rates; exposure data from prescriptions	**Mortality**, 12 years' follow-up, 73 deaths Any use: oestradiol and progestogen: SMR, 0.8 (95% CI, 0.4–1.3)	Exposure only from prescription data (population rates corrected for prevalent cases)

Table 1 (contd)

Reference	Study base	Design: cohort, follow-up, data	Risk relationships: relative risk (RR) and 95% confidence intervals (95% CI)	Comments
Schairer et al. (1994)	Populations in 27 cities, USA, breast cancer screening, 1980–89	Cohort of 49 017 participants; 313 902 person–years; follow-up through interviews and questionnaires; information on exposure and risk factors from questionnaires	**Incidence**, both in-situ and invasive tumours, 1 185 cases Conjugated oestrogens, combinations with progestogens All tumours: any use: oestrogens and progestogens: RR, 1.2 (95% CI, 1.0–1.6) In-situ tumours: oestrogens and progestogens: any use: RR, 2.3 (95% CI, 1.3–3.9) current use: RR, 2.4 (95% CI, 1.2–4.7) past use: RR, 2.3 (95% CI, 1.0–5.4)	Risk relationship limited to in-situ tumours Low power to assess long-term duration of oestrogen and progestogen regimens
Risch & Howe (1994)	Inhabitants of Saskatchewan, Canada, 43–49 years of age, 1976–91	Registry-based cohort; 33 003 women followed-up through linkage to cancer registry; 448 716 person–years; exposure data from prescription roster	**Incidence**: 15 years' follow-up, 742 cases Conjugated oestrogens, added progestogens Oestrogens and progestogens: no significant risk increase	Limited power to study long-term oestrogen–progestogen combined treatment
Colditz et al. (1995)	Nurses' Health Cohort, see Colditz et al. (1992) above	Cohort of 121 700 nurses; 725 550 person–years; baseline questionnaire in 1976, questionnaires every two years, up-dates on exposure and outcome (follow-up)	**Incidence**: 16 years' follow-up, 1 935 cases Conjugated oestrogens and added progestogens Current intake: conjugated oestrogen: RR, 1.3 (95% CI, 1.1–1.5) Any use: oestrogen and progestogen: RR, 1.4 (95% CI, 1.2–1.7)	No relationship with past use Detection bias unlikely First study to show an increased risk for death with hormonal therapy
Persson et al. (1996)	See Yuen et al. (1993) above, Swedish cohort	22 597 women with registered hormone prescriptions; record linkage follow-up of incidence and mortality; risk factor data in questionnaire survey	**Incidence**: 13 years' follow-up, 634 cases Prescriptions for various regimens any use: oestradiol/levonorgestrel: RR, 1.3 (95% CI, 1.1–1.4)	No data on duration

Table 1 (contd)

Reference	Study base	Design: cohort, follow-up, data	Risk relationships: relative risk (RR) and 95% confidence intervals (95% CI)	Comments
Persson *et al.* (1997)	Participants in mammography screening, Uppsala, Sweden, 1990–92, 40–74 years	Cohort of 30 982 women participating in two screening rounds; follow-up through screening and in diagnostic registry of pathology department; questionnaires at visits; nested case–control approach.	Follow-up through June 1995: 435 cases (87% invasive), 1 740 controls any use: all compounds: odds ratio, 1.1 (95% CI, 0.8–1.4) Duration ≥ 11 years: Oestradiol and progestogen: odds ratio, 2.4 (95% CI, 0.7–8.6) Oestradiol–conjugated oestrogen alone: odds ratio, 1.3 (95% CI, 0.5–3.7)	Low power in regimen subgroups

SIR, standardized incidence ratio; SMR, standardized mortality ratio

earlier, showing increased risks for current intake of conjugated oestrogens alone (relative risk, 1.3; 95% CI, 1.1–1.5) and for combinations with progestogens (chiefly medroxy-progesterone acetate; relative risk, 1.4; 95% CI, 1.2–1.7). Owing to the low statistical power, no data were presented on the risk for use of combinations with progestogens by categories of duration.

Schairer *et al.* (1994) followed a cohort of some 49 000 women participating in a breast cancer screening programme in several cities in the United States. To ascertain data on their exposure, risk factors and occurrence of breast cancer, the women were sent questionnaires or were interviewed. After a mean follow-up of 7.2 years, 1185 cases of in-situ or invasive breast cancer had occurred. For both types of tumour together, any use of oestrogens plus progestogens yielded a relative risk of 1.2 (95% CI, 1.0–1.6); for in-situ tumours only, a significant excess risk was noted (2.3; 95% CI, 1.3–3.9). The risk estimates were 2.4 (95% CI, 1.2–4.7) for current use and 2.3 (95% CI, 1.0–5.4) for past use.

Risch and Howe (1994) used a prescription database to establish a cohort of some 33 000 women in the province of Saskatchewan, Canada, who had received hormonal treatment. Through linkage with the population-based cancer registry, 742 newly dia-gnosed cases of breast cancer were ascertained during 15 years of follow-up. Use of oestro-gens plus progestogens was not associated with a significant change in the risk for breast cancer. In this study, the power to show any effects of combined use was low, with only three exposed cases.

Persson *et al.* (1997) investigated breast cancer incidence in relation to hormonal treatment in a cohort of some 31 000 women who had participated in mammography scree-ning on two regular visits. Data on their exposure to hormones and reproductive factors were collected through interviews at the visits. In all, 435 new cases of breast cancer were ascertained during five years of follow-up, chiefly through mammography screening but also through linkage to a local pathology register; 87% of the cases were invasive. In a nested case–control study, use of oestradiol plus a progestogen (usually norethisterone acetate) for 11 years or longer was associated with a relative risk of 2.4 (95% CI, 0.7–8.6), whereas use of oestradiol alone was associated with a relative risk of 1.3 (95% CI, 0.5–3.7). The risk for combined long-term use seemed to be greater than for other use, but the diffe-rence in risk estimates between the two treatment types was not statistically significant.

2.1.2   *Case–control studies*

The results of case–control studies on use of post-menopausal oestrogen–proges-togen therapy and breast cancer are shown in Table 2.

In a case–control study in Denmark of 1486 cases and 1336 controls, Ewertz (1988) had the opportunity to examine the effects of various treatment regimens. Data were collected through mailed questionnaires, filled in by 88% of the cases and 78% of the controls, with details on reproductive factors and hormone use. Women who had ever used oestradiol–progestogen combined treatments had a non-significantly increased relative risk of 1.4 (95% CI, 0.9–2.1) compared with a relative risk of 1.0 (95% CI, 0.8–1.3) for use of oestrogen only. Analyses by duration were not possible owing to the small numbers.

Table 2. Summary of case–control studies of post-menopausal oestrogen-progestogen therapy and breast cancer

Reference	Study base	Design: number of cases and controls, data	Risk relationships: relative risk (RR) and 95% confidence intervals (95% CI)	Comments
Ewertz (1988)	Denmark, 1983–84, > 70 years	Population-based, national. 1 486 cases/1 336 controls (random); self-administered, mailed questionnaire	Oestradiol and oestradiol–progestogen combinations: Combination oestradiol–progestogens any use: RR, 1.4 (95% CI, 0.9–2.1)	First study to show similar risk with combined treatments
Kaufman et al. (1991)	Metropolitan areas, primarily eastern USA, 1980–86, post-menopausal women, 40–69 years	Hospital-based; 1 686 cases/2 077 controls; interviews	Oestrogens and progestogens, any use: RR, 1.7 (95% CI, 0.9–3.6)	Low power for long-term treatment with oestrogen-progestogen combinations
Yang et al. (1992)	British Columbia, Canada, 1988–89, post-menopausal women, < 75 years	Population-based; 699 cases/685 controls (random); mailed questionnaire	Mainly conjugated oestrogens: any use: oestrogens and progestogens: RR, 1.2 (95% CI, 0.6–2.2)	Low power in analyses of use of oestrogen plus progestogen
Stanford et al. (1995)	13 counties, Washington State, USA, 1998–90, cancer survey system, white women, 50–64 years	Population-based; 537 cases/492 controls (random-digit dialling); personal interviews	Conjugated oestrogens, added progestogens: Combined, any use: odds ratio, 0.9 (95% CI, 0.7–1.3) Duration ≥ 8 years: odds ratio, 0.4 (95% CI, 0.2–1.0)	Low power for long-term use
Newcomb et al. (1995)	Four states in northern/eastern USA, tumour registries, 1988–91, age < 75	Population-based; 3 130 cases/3 698 controls (from rosters); personal interviews	'Non-contraceptive hormones, oestrogens and progestogen combinations': any use of progestogen in combination: RR, 1.0 (95% CI, 0.8–1.3) Duration ≥ 15 years: RR, 1.1 (95% CI, 0.5–2.3) No trend with timing	Limited power for long-duration categories No effects in sub-groups

In a study by Kaufman *et al.* (1991), 1686 case and 2077 hospital-based control women were interviewed. Only 1% of the controls had used oestrogen–progestogen combinations. Women who had ever used such combined treatments showed an elevated relative risk, but with wide confidence limits (relative risk, 1.7; 95% CI, 0.9–3.6). Use of oestrogen only, at any time or for several years, was not associated with an excess risk.

Yang *et al.* (1992) examined the effects of conjugated oestrogens and combinations with progestogens in a population-based study of 699 cases and 685 controls. Data on exposure and risk factors were acquired from mailed questionnaires. Use of oestrogens plus progestogens, reported by 3% of the controls, was linked to a risk near the baseline (1.2; 95% CI, 0.6–2.2).

Stanford *et al.* (1995) conducted a population-based study on 537 cases of breast cancer and 492 controls in Washington State, United States, using random-digit dialling to recruit controls. Data from personal interviews revealed that 21% of the controls had used combined treatments. The relative risk was 0.9 (95% CI, 0.7–1.3) for any use and 0.4 (95% CI, 0.2–1.0) for use for eight years and more.

Newcomb *et al.* (1995) presented data on combined use from the largest population-based study of breast cancer hitherto reported, 3130 cases and 3628 controls, from four states in northern and eastern United States. Data obtained at interview showed that about 4% of the healthy controls had used combined progestogen treatment, but few of these women had had long-term treatment. Any use of progestogen combinations was associated with a baseline risk (1.0; 95% CI, 0.8–1.3), whereas use for 15 years or longer (based on 15 cases and 15 controls) gave a relative risk of 1.1 (95% CI, 0.5–2.3). There was no indication of a trend with categories of duration of intake.

2.1.3 *Pooled analysis of individual data*

The Collaborative Group on Hormonal Factors in Breast Cancer (1997) compiled and re-analysed the original data from 51 studies, of which 22 provided data on the hormonal constituents of the preparations. Of the eligible women in the re-analysis, such data were available for 4640, 12% of whom had received combinations of oestrogens and progestogens. Current use or last use 1–4 years before diagnosis, with a duration of less than five years, was associated with a relative risk of 1.2 (95% CI, 0.8–1.5), and a duration of five years or longer with a relative risk of 1.5 (95% CI, 0.9–2.2). These estimates were not statistically different from those for the corresponding categories of oestrogen-only use (RR, 1.3).

These limited data do not provide a basis for firm conclusions on the effects of oestrogen–progestogen use on the risk for breast cancer. One major limitation is the small amount of information available on use for many years. Overall, there is little evidence to suggest that added progestogens confer a risk different from that associated with oestrogens alone.

2.2   Endometrial cancer

Women who use oestrogen–progestogen regimens have a lower occurrence of endo-metrial hyperplasia than those who use oestrogen-only therapy, especially when the progestogen is used for 10 or more days per month or continuously with oestrogen (Sturdee *et al.*, 1978; Thom *et al.*, 1979; Paterson *et al.*, 1980; Postmenopausal Estrogen/ Progestin Interventions Trial, 1996; Speroff *et al.*, 1996). Depending on the type, dose and duration of progestogen supplementation, it may be given for 10–14 days once every three months as well, in a so-called 'long cycle' regimen. In two studies in which women were followed-up for one to two years while receiving a 14-day supplementation with 10 or 20 mg medroxyprogesterone acetate, less than 2% developed hyperplasia (Ettinger *et al.*, 1994; Hirvonen *et al.*, 1995). In contrast, in a Scandinavian randomized controlled trial, a higher occurrence of hyperplasia was found in women who received a 10-day supplemen-tation of 1 mg norethisterone (6%) than in women who received monthly progestogen supplementation (< 1%) (Cerin *et al.*, 1996). Although information is available on endo-metrial hyperplasia, there is much less information on combined oestrogen–progestogen therapy and the risk for endometrial cancer.

2.2.1   *Randomized trial*

In a very small randomized trial in which 168 institutionalized women were rando-mized to receive post-menopausal oestrogen–progestogen therapy or placebo, no case of endometrial cancer occurred in the treated group and one occurred in those receiving placebo (Nachtigall *et al.*, 1979).

2.2.2   *Cohort studies*

Only three cohort studies have provided information on the risk for endometrial cancer among women who used combined therapy relative to women who did not use any post-menopausal hormonal therapy.

Hammond *et al.* (1979) (see Table 5 of the monograph on 'Post-menopausal oestrogen therapy') followed-up approximately 600 hyperoestrogenic women, roughly half of whom used either oestrogen-only or oestrogen–progestogen preparations and half of whom did not use hormones. No cases of endometrial cancer were observed among the 72 women who received oestrogen–progestogen therapy, whereas three cases were observed among the non-users.

In the cohort study of Gambrell (1986) (summarized in Table 5 of the monograph on 'Post-menopausal oestrogen therapy'), the incidence of endometrial cancer among women who used combined hormonal therapy (eight cases/16 327 woman–years) was lower than that among women who did not use any hormonal therapy (nine cases/4480 woman–years) [no age-adjusted results were reported].

A Swedish cohort study (Persson *et al.*, 1989) (see Table 5 of the monograph on 'Post-menopausal oestrogen therapy') of endometrial cancer occurrence among women using combination therapy identified through pharmacy records in comparison with the popu-lation rates in the Uppsala health care region, showed that women using oestrogen-only therapy (predominantly oestradiol) had an increased risk (48 cases observed versus 34.3 expected; relative risk, 1.4; 95% CI, 1.1–1.9), whereas no increase in risk was found in women using combination therapy (seven cases observed versus 7.6 expected; relative risk, 0.9; 95% CI, 0.4–2.0).

2.2.3   Case–control studies

The case–control studies on post-menopausal oestrogen–progestogen therapy and endometrial cancer risk are summarized in Table 3.

Jick *et al.* (1993) studied women who were members of a large health maintenance organization in western Washington State, United States. Women with endometrial cancer were identified from the tumour registry of the organization, and the control women were other members; both groups included only those women who used the pharmacies of the organization, and who had previously completed a questionnaire sent to all female members for a study of mammography. Use of post-menopausal hormonal therapy was ascertained from the pharmacy database. Relative to women who had never or briefly (≤ six months) used menopausal hormones, those who had used any oestrogen–progestogen therapy within the previous year had a slightly increased risk (odds ratio, 1.9; 95% CI, 0.9–3.8), after adjustment for age, calendar year, age at menopause, body mass index and history of oral contraceptive use, although those with a longer duration of use (≥ three years) did not. Former users (last use ≥ one year earlier) had no increase in risk (odds ratio, 0.9; 95% CI, 0.3–3.4). Women with recent (within the past year) oestrogen-only use (32 cases and 26 controls) had a strongly elevated risk for endometrial cancer (odds ratio, 6.5; 95% CI, 3.1–13), but no increased risk was seen for past users of oestrogen alone (odds ratio, 1.0; 95% CI, 0.5–2.0).

A multicentre study was conducted with 300 menopausal women with endometrial cancer diagnosed at seven hospitals, in Chicago, Illinois; Hershey, Pennsylvania; Irvine and Long Beach, California; Minneapolis, Minnesota; and Winston-Salem, North Carolina, United States, and 207 age-, race- and residence-matched control women from the general population (Brinton *et al.*, 1993). Any oestrogen–progestogen therapy for three months or longer was reported by 4% of the case women and 5% of the control women (odds ratio, 1.8; 95% CI, 0.3–0.7), after adjustment for age, parity, weight and years of oral contraceptive use. Use of oestrogens only was associated with a relative risk of 3.4 (95% CI, 1.8–6.3).

Pike *et al.* (1997) identified 833 women with endometrial cancer from a population-based cancer registry in Los Angeles County, United States, and matched them to control women of similar age and race (white) who lived in the same neighbourhood block as the matched case or to 791 randomly identifed women on the United States Health Care Financing Administration computer tapes. The risk for endometrial cancer was investigated among women who had used unopposed oestrogens, oestrogen–progestogen with progestogen added for fewer than 10 days per cycle, oestrogen–progestogen with progestogen added for 10 or more days per cycle and continuous combined therapy. An elevated risk was noted for women with longer use of oestrogen–progestogen if the

Table 3. Summary of case–control studies of post-menopausal oestrogen–progestogen therapy and endometrial cancer risk, by number of days progestogen was added per cycle and duration, when available

Reference	Location; period	Age (years)	Source of controls	Participation (%)		Type/measure of combined therapy	No. of subjects		Adjusted odds ratio (95% CI)
				Cases	Controls		Cases	Controls	
Jick et al. (1993)	Washington; USA; 1979–89	50–64	Members of health maintenance organization	NR	NR	No use, ≤ 6 months' use	97	606	Referent
						Any use within past year[a]	18	83	1.9 (0.9–3.8)
						Duration (years)			
						< 3	NR	NR	2.2 (0.7–7.3)
						≥ 3	NR	NR	1.3 (0.5–3.4)
						Any use ≥ 1 year previously	6	64	0.9 (0.3–3.4)
Brinton et al. (1993)	Five US areas; 1987–90	20–74	General population	86	66	No use	222	176	Referent
						Any use for ≥ 3 months[a]	11	9	1.8 (0.6–4.9)
Pike et al. (1997)	California, USA; 1987–93	50–74	General population (neighbours)	57	NR	*Any use, progestogen < 10 days/cycle*[b]			
						Duration (months)			
						0	759	744	Referent
						1–24	35	22	1.4 (NR)
						25–60	12	12	1.5 (NR)
						> 60	27	13	3.5 (NR)
						Any use, progestogen ≥ 10 days/cycle			
						Duration (months)			
						0	754	703	Referent
						1–24	37	30	1.0 (NR)
						25–60	19	25	0.7 (NR)
						> 60	23	33	1.1 (NR)
						Any use, progestogen all days/cycle			
						Duration (months)			
						0	739	710	Referent
						1–24	45	41	1.1 (NR)
						25–60	25	15	1.4 (NR)
						> 60	24	25	1.3 (NR)

Table 3 (contd)

Reference	Location; period	Age (years)	Source of controls	Participation (%) Cases	Participation (%) Controls	Type/measure of combined therapy	No. of subjects Cases	No. of subjects Controls	Adjusted odds ratio (95% CI)
Beresford et al. (1997)	Washington, USA; 1985–91	45–74	General population	72	73	No use, ≤ 6 months' use	337	685	Referent
						Any use[c]	67	134	1.4 (1.0–1.9)
						Progestogen ≤ 10 days/cycle			
						Duration (months)			
						6–35	12	14	2.1 (0.9–4.7)
						36–59	3	7	1.4 (0.3–5.4)
						≥ 60	15	12	3.7 (1.7–8.2)
						Progestogen > 10 days/cycle			
						Duration (months)			
						6–35	10	31	0.8 (0.4–1.8)
						36–59	5	23	0.6 (0.2–1.6)
						≥ 60	12	16	2.5 (1.1–5.5)
						Current use only			
						Progestogen ≤ 10 days/cycle			
						Duration (months)			
						6–59	11	13	2.2 (0.9–5.2)
						≥ 60	14	9	4.8 (2.0–11)
						Progestogen > 10 days/cycle			
						Duration (months)			
						6–59	12	48	0.7 (0.4–1.4)
						≥ 60	12	15	2.7 (1.2–6.0)

CI, confidence interval; NR, not reported

[a] Women with unopposed oestrogen use included

[b] Use of unopposed oestrogen and other combined therapy adjusted for in the analysis

[c] Women with unopposed oestrogen use excluded

progestogen was added for fewer than 10 days per cycle, but not if it was added for 10 or more days per cycle; the odds ratio was 1.9 (95% CI, 1.3–2.7) for each additional five years of use and 1.1 (95% CI, 0.8–1.4) after adjustment for age at menarche, time to regular cycles, parity, duration of incomplete pregnancies, weight, duration of breast-feeding, amenorrhoea, smoking, duration of oral contraceptive use, age at menopause and the other hormonal treatments. No increase in risk was noted for women who had had continuous combined therapy; the odds ratio for each additional five years of use was 1.1 (95% CI, 0.8–1.4). Each additional five years of unopposed oestrogen use was associated with a roughly twofold elevation in risk, with an odds ratio of 2.1 for each five-year period (95% CI, 1.9–2.5).

Beresford *et al.* (1997) expanded the study population originally investigated by Voigt *et al.* (1991) and evaluated the risk for endometrial cancer among women who had used only oestrogen–progestogen therapy. Women with endometrial cancer were identified from a population-based cancer registry and compared with control women from the general population in western Washington State, United States. After some exclusions, 394 cases and 788 controls were available for the analysis. Relative to women who had never or briefly (≤ six months) used menopausal hormones, women who had used only oestrogen–progestogen therapy had a slightly increased risk (odds ratio, 1.4; 95% CI, 1.0–1.9), after adjustment for age, body mass and county of residence. An elevated risk was noted among women with five or more years of exclusive oestrogen–progestogen use, regardless of the number of days a progestogen had been used. For women using oestrogen–progestogen therapy for ≤ 10 days/cycle, the odds ratio was 3.7 (95% CI, 1.7–8.2); the risk was similar for use on more than 10 days/cycle (odds ratio, 2.5; 95% CI, 1.1–5.5), and similar results were found when the analysis was restricted to current oestrogen–progestogen users. The small numbers of women (eight cases and 11 controls) who had used only oestrogen–progestogen therapy for five or more years, with the highest dose of medroxyprogesterone acetate (10 mg) added for more than 10 days/cycle, still had a significant increase in risk (odds ratio, 2.7; 95% CI, 1.0–6.8). Unopposed oestrogen therapy taken for at least six months was associated with a relative risk for endometrial cancer of 4.0 (95% CI, 3.1–5.1).

In summary, most of the small number of epidemiological studies conducted to date have shown no effect or a modest increase in the risk for endometrial cancer among women using combined hormonal therapy relative to women who had not used menopausal hormones. In all of the studies summarized above, a lower risk for endometrial cancer was associated with use of combined hormonal therapy than with oestrogen-only therapy. The two studies that were large enough to evaluate cyclic use of progestogen reported two- to fourfold increases in risk associated with use of oestrogen–progestogen if the progestogen was added for approximately 10 days or less per cycle (Beresford *et al.*, 1997; Pike *et al.*, 1997), but only one found an elevated risk if the progestogen was added for 10 days or more per cycle (Beresford *et al.*, 1997). It is not clear whether the few cancers appearing in women taking oestrogens and progestogens represent failure of the progestogen to protect the endometrium or failure of the women to take the prescribed progestogen.

2.3   Ovarian cancer

2.3.1   *Cohort study*

In the cohort study of Hunt *et al.* (1987) described in section 2.1.1, six cases of ovarian cancer were observed up to 1986 among users of post-menopausal hormonal therapy versus 6.92 expected, corresponding to a nonsignificant SIR of 0.9 (95% CI, 0.3–1.9). In a follow-up until 1988 on mortality only (Hunt *et al.*, 1990), four more deaths from ovarian cancer were observed versus 6.33 expected (SMR, 0.63; 95% CI, 0.0–1.4).

2.3.2   *Case–control study*

In a multicentre case–control study of 377 cases of ovarian cancer and 2030 controls conducted between 1976 and 1985 in various areas of Canada, Israel and the United States (Kaufman *et al.*, 1989), only 1–2% of cases and controls had ever used combination post-menopausal therapy. The multivariate relative risk was 0.7 (95% CI, 0.2–1.8).

2.4   Liver cancer

Persson *et al.* (1996) studied cancer risks after post-menopausal hormonal therapy in a population-based cohort of 22 579 women aged 35 or more living in the Uppsala health care region in Sweden. Women who had ever received a prescription for post-menopausal hormonal therapy between 1977 and 1980 were identified and followed until 1991; information on hormone use was obtained from pharmacy records. The expected numbers of cases were calculated from national incidence rates. There was no information on smoking or alcohol consumption. The SIR for all cancers was 1.0 (95% CI, 0.9–1.0). There were 43 cancers of the hepatobiliary tract, comprising 14 hepatocellular carcinomas, five cholangiocarcinomas, 23 gall-bladder cancers and one unclassified. The expected number was 73.2, giving an SIR of 0.6 (95% CI, 0.4–0.8) for any type of post-menopausal hormonal therapy. The SIRs for treatment with oestradiol combined with levonorgestrel were 0.6 (95% CI, 0.1–2.3) for hepatocellular carcinoma and 0.7 (95% CI, 0.0–3.8) for cholangiocarcinoma. There was no information on infection with hepatitis viruses.

2.5   Colorectal cancer

In most of the studies on the influence of post-menopausal hormonal therapy on the risk for colorectal cancer, it was not possible to distinguish formulations. Only a few investigations provided separate information on combinations of oestrogens and progestogens, but in all instances the use of opposed hormonal therapy was very limited and was generally restricted to recent use. The available studies are summarized in Table 4.

2.5.1   *Cohort studies*

In a Canadian record linkage study described in detail in the monograph on 'Post-menopausal oestrogen therapy' (Risch & Howe, 1995), no case of colon or rectal cancer occurred in women who had used both oestrogens and progestogens and not oestrogens only; however, the number of such women (171) was small. One case of colon cancer

Table 4. Studies on use of post-menopausal oestrogen–progestogen therapy and colorectal cancer

Reference	Country	Population (follow-up) or cases/controls	Relative risk (RR) (95% confidence interval [CI]) (any versus no use)		Adjustment/comments
			Colon	Rectum	
Cohort					
Risch & Howe (1995)	Canada	33 003 (14 years) 230 cancers	–	–	Age No case of colorectal cancer among 171 hormone users
Persson *et al.* (1996)	Sweden	23 244 (13 years) 233 cancers, 62 deaths	0.6 (0.4–1.0)	0.8 (0.4–1.3)	Age No effect among 5 573 hormone users Refers to a fixed combined brand. RR for colon cancer mortality, 0.6 (95% CI, 0.2–1.1)
Troisi *et al.* (1997)	USA	33 779 (7.7 years) 313	1.4 (0.7–2.5)		Age (but unaltered by education, body mass index, parity or use of combined oral contraceptives)
Case–control					
Newcomb & Storer (1995)	Wisconsin, USA	694/1 622	Recent use: 0.54 (0.28–1.0)	1.1 (0.51–2.5)	Age, alcohol, body mass index, family history of cancer and sigmoidoscopy Combined post-menopausal hormonal therapy was used by 18% of users

occurred among 648 women who had used both oestrogen and progestogen and also oestrogens alone. [No estimates for relative risks were provided in the paper.]

In the Swedish cohort followed by Persson *et al.* (1996) (see section 2.4), 5573 women (i.e. about 25% of the total cohort) had received prescriptions for combined post-menopausal hormonal therapy consisting of 2 mg oestradiol and 250 mg levonorgestrol for 10–21 days. They had an age-adjusted relative risk of 0.6 (95% CI, 0.4–1.0) for colon cancer and 0.8 (95% CI, 0.4–1.3) for rectal cancer. The rate of mortality from colorectal cancer was marginally decreased (relative risk, 0.6; 95% CI, 0.2–1.1).

In the North American cohort described in detail in the monograph on 'Post-menopausal oestrogen therapy' (Troisi *et al.*, 1997), the age-adjusted relative risk associated with use of combined oestrogen and progestogen therapy (i.e. 16% of woman–years of hormone therapy use) for colon cancer was 1.4 (95% CI, 0.7–2.5); there were insufficient numbers of exposed cases to evaluate the risk for rectal cancer or for cancers of the colon at sub-sites.

2.5.2 *Case–control study*

Only one case–control investigation (Newcomb & Storer, 1995), described in detail in the monograph on 'Post-menopausal oestrogen therapy', included detailed information on the influence of recent use of post-menopausal hormonal therapy on the risk for colon cancer. The relative risk, adjusted for age, alcohol, body mass index, family history of cancer and sigmoidoscopy, was 0.54 (95% CI, 0.28–1.0; 11 cases) and that for rectal cancer was 1.1 (95% CI, 0.51–2.5; 8 cases). Use of this formulation had been reported by 18% of hormone users, and the risk estimates were close to those for use of post-menopausal oestrogen therapy of any type.

2.6 Cutaneous malignant melanoma

2.6.1 *Cohort study*

In the study of Persson *et al.* (1996) (see section 2.4), an age-adjusted relative risk of 0.6 (95% CI, 0.3–1.1) was found for cutaneous malignant melanoma, with nine cases.

2.6.2 *Case–control study*

Østerlind *et al.* (1988) (see Table 11 of the monograph on 'Post-menopausal oestrogen therapy') reported a multivariate relative risk adjusted for age, naevi and sunbathing for any use of oestrogens and opposed progestogens of 1.5 (95% CI, 0.8–2.8), on the basis of 28 users among cases and 45 among controls.

3. Studies of Cancer in Experimental Animals

Oestrogen plus progestogen hormonal therapy is usually given in the form of conjugated oestrogens (Premarin®; for oestrogen composition, see the monograph on 'Post-menopausal oestrogen therapy', Table 2) plus medroxyprogesterone acetate or cyproterone acetate. Studies of the carcinogenicity of conjugated oestrogens in experimental animals are described in the monograph on 'Post-menopausal oestrogen therapy', those on medroxyprogesterone acetate and implanted levonorgestrel are described in the monograph on 'Hormonal contraceptives, progestogens only', and those on cyproterone acetate and the 19-nortestosterone derivatives norethisterone, norethisterone acetate and lynoestrenol are summarized in the monograph on 'Oral contraceptives, combined'. No studies on micronized progesterone were available. For studies on progesterone, see IARC (1979).

Female Sprague-Dawley rats, 48 days of age, were given a single intravenous injection of 5 mg 7,12-dimethylbenz[a]anthracene (DMBA), separated into four groups of seven rats per group and given DMBA only, DMBA plus oophorectomy, DMBA plus oophorectomy plus Premarin® at a concentration of 1.875 mg/kg of diet or DMBA plus oophorectomy plus Premarin® plus medroxyprogesterone acetate at a concentration of 7.5 mg/kg of diet. The animals were observed for 285 days, at which time body and organ weights, tumour incidence, the plasma concentrations of prolactin, oestradiol and progesterone and bone density were determined in all rats. In two rats per group, the numbers of S-phase cells in mammary tumours were assessed by immunohistochemistry, after injection with bromodeoxyuridine (BdUr) 6 h before killing. Mammary tumours were found in 6/7 rats given DMBA, 0/7 given DMBA plus oophorectomy, 5/7 given DMBA plus oophorectomy plus Premarin® and 5/7 given the preceding treatment plus medroxyprogesterone acetate. The percentages of cells in S phase were (mean ± standard error) 7 ± 0.5 in tumours from rats given DMBA, 5.5 ± 0.8 in those from oophorectomized rats given DMBA plus Premarin® and 3.1 ± 0.5 in those from oophorectomized rats given DMBA, Premarin® and medroxyprogesterone acetate, the last value being significantly different from the percentage with DMBA alone ($p < 0.01$). Thus, oophorectomy completely inhibited mammary tumour development, and medroxyprogesterone acetate significantly decreased the percentage of S-phase cells in the tumours [number of tumours/rat not specified] (Sakamoto et al., 1997).

4. Other Data Relevant to an Evaluation of Carcinogenicity and its Mechanisms

4.1 Absorption, distribution, metabolism and excretion

4.1.1 Humans

The pharmacokinetics of the newer progestogens, desogestrel, norgestimate and gestodene, has been reviewed (Fotherby, 1996). There are only a few reports of studies on the disposition of these progestogens, mostly in combination with ethinyloestradiol, and these are discussed in detail in the monograph on 'Oral contraceptives, combined'.

After oral administration of crystalline progesterone, the progestogen undergoes a first-pass effect due to extensive metabolism in the gut and liver; it thus has minimal systemic bioavailability. Micronized progesterone is rapidly absorbed and provides an adequate concentration in the blood (Whitehead *et al.*, 1980; Ottoson *et al.*, 1984; Kuhl, 1990; Simon *et al.*, 1993). After oral intake of 100 or 200 mg micronized progesterone, maximal serum levels of 10–15 and 20 ng/mL, respectively, are achieved within 1–4 h; these decrease thereafter (Whitehead *et al.*, 1980; Morville *et al.*, 1982; Maxson & Hargrove, 1985). After oral intake, absorption is enhanced about twofold by the presence of food, but the bioavailability appears to be low, the integrated area under the curve of concentration versus time (area under the curve) after intramuscular injection of progesterone being about 10 times larger than after oral intake (Simon *et al.*, 1993).

Both single and multiple treatments with progesterone or with most modified progesterone derivatives result in rapid absorption and maximum blood level within 1–2 h. Accumulation occurs in blood after multiple treatments as a result of binding to sex hormone-binding globulin until a steady-state concentration is reached. These progestogens are largely stored in fat tissues (Kuhl, 1990; Fotherby, 1996).

Gestodene, levonorgestrel, cyproterone acetate and chlormadinone acetate taken orally in combination with ethinyloestradiol do not undergo first-pass metabolism and consequently have a bioavailability of almost 100%, whereas norethisterone, desogestrel and norgestimate in combination with ethinyloestradiol are rapidly and extensively metabolized in the gastrointestinal tract, with a bioavailability of 50–75% (Kuhl, 1990; Fotherby, 1996). Specific examples of the disposition of some progestogens are given below. There are large interindividual variations in the pharmacokinetic parameters.

When gestodene is taken alone, a high serum concentration is found; the mean absorption time is 0.8–1.9 h. Subjects vary widely in the area under the curve for gestodene. When combined with ethinyloestradiol, daily treatment with gestodene or 3-keto-desogestrel results in accumulation of these progestogens in serum. Poor elimination as a result of binding to sex hormone-binding globulin and inactivation of metabolizing enzymes are considered to be a likely explanation for this effect (Fotherby, 1994).

Cyproterone acetate at 5 mg taken orally with 50 µg ethinyloestradiol is rapidly absorbed, and its bioavailability is 100%. The maximum serum concentration is reached within 1–2 h after both single and multiple doses. It is largely stored in fat tissue. An increase from 11 ng/mL after a single intake to 17 ng/mL within a week of multiple intakes suggests that long-term intake leads to accumulation. After multiple oral doses, the elimination half-life remains unchanged at 2.5 days (Schleusener *et al.*, 1980; Kuhl, 1990).

In most of the pharmacokinetic studies of orally administered medroxyprogesterone acetate, high doses have been used. Absorption of orally administered compound is rapid, and the time to reach the maximum serum concentration is 1–3 h (Pannuti *et al.*, 1982; Johansson *et al.*, 1986).

Norethisterone is rapidly absorbed, and peak serum concentrations occur within 2–4 h. The bioavailability is about 60%, because of first-pass metabolism. Micronized norethisterone is quickly absorbed and results in a higher serum concentration within a shorter time (Shi *et al.*, 1987; Kuhl, 1990; Fotherby, 1996).

4.1.2   *Experimental systems*

Most of the experimental data relate to the disposition of progesterone; very limited information is available on oestrogen and progestogen combinations.

In ovariectomized rats, the distribution and elimination half-lives of progesterone after a single intravenous administration of 500 μg/kg bw were 0.13 and 1.21 h, respectively. Progesterone was eliminated rapidly, with a total clearance of 2.75 L/h per kg bw (Gangrade *et al.*, 1992).

Intravenous administration of ^{3}H-progesterone to cynomolgus monkeys (*Macaca fascicularis*) resulted in the total disappearance of the hormone from the circulation within 3 h; 0.5–1.75 h later, about 5% of the initial maximal concentration of the hormone reappeared, perhaps as a result of delayed release from tissue stores (Kowalski *et al.*, 1996). In female cynomolgus monkeys (*Macaca fascicularis*), progesterone has a volume of distribution of 1.75 L/kg bw and a plasma clearance of 0.06 L/kg bw per min. In comparison with humans, plasma progesterone binding is greater and progesterone clearance is slower in cynomolgus monkeys (Braasch *et al.*, 1988). In baboons (*Papio anubis*), the bioavailability of chlormadinone acetate was 100%, and the peak serum concentration was reached within 1–2 h (Honjo *et al.*, 1976).

4.2   Receptor-mediated effects

4.2.1   *Humans*

A group of 14 post-menopausal women was given ethinyloestradiol for one month at a daily dose of 50 μg, followed by a dose escalation of 50 μg per day over four days to a final dose of 200 μg; half of the women received 5 mg per day chlormadinone acetate during the four-day period. Endometrial biopsy samples were taken at the end of the first month and at the end of the four-day dose escalation period. The addition of chlormadinone decreased the twofold increase in uterine progesterone receptor concentration induced by the ethinyloestradiol dose escalation to that observed after the first month of ethinyloestradiol treatment (approximately 2150 fmol/mg DNA). The uterine oestrogen receptor concentration was not affected by the chlormadinone treatment (Kreitmann *et al.*, 1979).

Post-menopausal women continuously receiving either 2 mg/day oestradiol valerate, 1.5 mg/day oestropipate, 0.625 or 1.25 mg/day conjugated equine oestrogens (Premarin®), 50 mg oestradiol implants or 5 g/day of a skin cream which contained 3 mg oestradiol received an oral progestogen during the last 7–10 days of each month. In endometrial biopsy samples, the soluble progesterone receptor content was found to be elevated by approximately 40% as compared with proliferative-phase endometrium from 12 unexposed women; this increase occurred only in the nine women receiving oestradiol implants and the seven women receiving oestrone sulfate. The nuclear content of oestrogen receptor was increased (by about 30%) only in the endometrial samples from the 12–15 women who had received the high dose of Premarin® before progestogen as compared with proliferative-phase endometrium from 16 unexposed women. Progestogen treatment reduced the oestrogen receptor concentration to that found in secretory-phase endometrium within six days, regardless of the type of progestogen or dose. The percentage of endometrial glandular cells from five women receiving 1.25 mg/day Premarin® that incorporated tritiated thymidine *in vitro* was similar to that of proliferative-phase endometrium of 12 unexposed women. After the start of progestogen treatment, the labelling index decreased to the very low levels found in secretory-phase endometrium within six days. This effect of progestogens was also found with norethisterone at doses of 1, 2.5 and 5 mg/day and with norgestrel at doses of 150 and 500 µg/day. At a dose of 10 mg/day, norethisterone showed less inhibition of cell proliferation than at lower doses (Whitehead *et al.*, 1981). Similar effects of norgestrel and norethisterone were observed in a separate study of the same design, confirming the absence of a dose–response relationship at the doses tested. Medroxyprogesterone (at 2.5, 5 and 10 mg/day), dydrogesterone (5, 10 and 20 mg/day) and progesterone (at 100, 200 and 300 µg/day) also inhibited the oestrogen-induced increase in labelling index, but these effects were dose-related, reaching a maximal effect at doses of 10 mg, 20 mg and 200 µg, respectively. All of these progestogens decreased the nuclear oestrogen receptor content and had clear progestational effects on endometrial morphology (King & Whitehead, 1986).

In groups of four to six post-menopausal women given Premarin® alone at 1.25 mg/day or Premarin® and norgestrel at a dose of 150 or 500 µg/day or norethisterone at a dose of 1, 2.5, 5 or 10 mg/day for three months, the progestogens reduced the high tritiated thymidine labelling index found in the epithelial cells (approximately 9%) and stromal cells (approximately 13%) in endometrial biopsy samples from Premarin®-treated women to values found in secretory-phase endometrium from unexposed women. The highest dose of norethisterone (10 mg/day) was less effective than the lower doses; the nuclear oestrogen receptor content of the endometrium was also reduced by more than 65% (Siddle *et al.*, 1982). Identical findings were reported from a study in groups of 6–12 post-menopausal women given dydrogesterone as the progestogen. Reduction of the endometrial labelling index and oestrogen receptor content was maximal at a dose of 10 mg/day of progestogen. With dydrogesterone at a dose of 20 mg/day, the labelling index was suppressed to a lesser extent than at 10 mg/day. An apparently positive relation was observed between the dose of Premarin® and induction of the endometrial enzymes oestradiol and isocitrate dehydrogenase (Lane *et al.*, 1986).

Oestradiol was given transdermally at a dose of 50 µg/day throughout the cycle and norethisterone acetate at a transdermal dose of 170 or 350 µg/day either for the last 14 days of each cycle or continuously. A reference group received the same transdermal dose of oestrogen, but norethisterone acetate (1 mg/day) or dydrogesterone (20 mg/day) was given orally for the last 14 days of each cycle. Each group consisted of at least 150 women who were followed for at least one year. Atrophy, presumably induced by the progestogens, was more frequent in the group receiving the progestogen transdermally in a continuous regimen (66 and 84% for high and low dose, respectively) than in the group given the progestogen orally or transdermally in a sequential regimen (32–38%). No hyperplastic changes occurred in women in any group (Johannison *et al.*, 1997).

Post-menopausal women received norethisterone at 5 mg/day, ethinyloestradiol at 50 µg/day or their combination orally, each for one month. Cervical biopsy samples were taken at baseline and at the end of each treatment period. Multivariate analysis indicated that the oestrogen increased the percentage of cells in S-phase (by flow cytometry) and the endometrial content of both oestrogen and progesterone receptors. There were no significant effects of progestogen, and there was no interaction between the progestogen and oestrogen treatment on these three parameters (Bhattacharya *et al.*, 1997).

Dydrogesterone was given at 10 mg/day in combination with conjugated equine oestrogens at 0.625 mg/day orally to 12 post-menopausal women. The serum concentrations of sex hormone-binding globulin more than doubled, whereas the circulating concentrations of insulin-like growth factor-I decreased by approximately 20%. When the therapy of the women was changed after six months to an oral regimen of norethisterone at 6 mg/day and the oestrogens for three months, the increase in sex hormone-binding globulin was largely abolished and the decrease in insulin-like growth factor-I disappeared. In another six women given oestradiol at 0.05 mg/day transdermally, the combination with dydrogesterone and norethisterone did not alter these parameters, except for a small decrease in sex hormone-binding globulin concentration (Campagnoli *et al.*, 1994).

Six post-menopausal women were given 20 μg/day ethinyloestradiol, 1.25 mg/day conjugated equine oestrogens (Premarin®) or 2 mg/day oestradiol valerate for subsequent periods of four weeks; during the last 12 days of each treatment cycle, the women also received 10 mg/day medroxyprogesterone acetate. The serum concentrations of insulin-like growth factor-I were decreased by approximately 15–25% with all three treatments when compared with the pretreatment period, while the serum concentrations of growth hormone and growth hormone-binding protein were increased by two- to threefold when compared with the pretreatment period (Kelly *et al.*, 1993).

Women receiving transdermal oestradiol developed histological signs of progestational endometrial effects when given levonorgestrel in an intrauterine device releasing 20 μg/day of the progestogen; such effects were not seen in women receiving progesterone orally at 100 mg/day or vaginally at 100–200 mg/day (Suvanto-Luukkonen *et al.*, 1995). Insulin-like growth factor binding protein-I was also induced by intrauterine exposure to levonorgestrel but not by the other routes of exposure. The observations for the binding protein-I were confirmed in a similar comparison of intrauterine and subcutaneous treatment with levonorgestrel (Suhonen *et al.*, 1996).

In the Postmenopausal Estrogen/Progestin Interventions Trial (1996) 875 post-menopausal women were assigned randomly to placebo, conjugated equine oestrogens (0.625 mg/day), conjugated equine oestrogens plus cyclic medroxyprogesterone acetate (10 mg/day for 12 days per month) or conjugated equine oestrogens plus cyclic micronized progestogen (200 mg/day for 12 days per month). During the three-year study, the women assigned to oestrogen were more likely to develop simple (cystic), complex, adenomatous or atypical hyperplasia than those given placebo (27.7 versus 0.8%, 22.7 versus 0.8% and 11.8 versus 0%, respectively). The rates of hyperplasia were similar in all groups, and the occurrence of hyperplasia was distributed across the three-year trial.

4.2.2   *Experimental systems*

The relevant effects in experimental systems of combinations of progestogens and oestrogens used in post-menopausal hormonal therapy are summarized in detail in the monographs on 'Oral contraceptives, combined', section 4.2, and 'Hormonal contraceptives, oestrogens only', section 4.2. These effects are briefly mentioned for each of the progestogens covered in this monograph, but the effects of oestrogen–progestogen combinations *in vivo* at doses similar to those used for humans are described in detail.

In some but not all of the studies, cyproterone acetate inhibited the stimulatory effects of oestradiol on human breast cancer cells in culture; it was not oestrogenic. Desogestrel, gestodene, norethisterone and levonorgestrel have oestrogenic properties but also inhibited the stimulatory effects of oestradiol on human breast cancer cells in culture. In some but not all of the studies, medroxyprogesterone acetate inhibited the stimulatory effects of oestradiol on human breast cancer cells in culture; it was not oestrogenic.

Medroxyprogesterone acetate at 2 µg/rat per day decreased the hyperplastic effects of conjugated equine oestrogens at 50 µg/rat per day on the endometrium of ovariectomized rats, whereas dydrogesterone and cyproterone acetate at the same dose appeared to enhance these oestrogen-induced hyperplastic effects slightly (Kumasaka *et al.*, 1994).

Subcutaneous administration of medroxyprogesterone acetate at 1–1.5 mg/rat twice daily over 18 days inhibited stimulation by oestrone (1 µg/rat, subcutaneously twice daily) of the growth of mammary gland carcinomas induced by DMBA in female Sprague-Dawley rats which were ovariectomized after tumours had developed. The reductive activity of 17β-hydroxysteroid oxidoreductase [dehydrogenase] on mammary tumour tissue was altered by medroxyprogesterone acetate in such a way that the formation of oestradiol in tumours of these oestrone-treated animals was reduced by more than 50%. In the uterus, however, medroxyprogesterone acetate decreased the activity of this enzyme by less than 20% (Luo *et al.*, 1997).

The effects of a combination of dietary administration of conjugated equine oestrogens (Premarin®) and medroxyprogesterone acetate on the mammary glands of 25 adult female cynomolgus monkeys (*Macaca fascicularis*) were studied in comparison with 22 monkeys receiving control diet; all of the animals had been ovariectomized before the experiment. The daily dose of Premarin® was approximately 7.2 µg per animal for the first eight months of the experiment and 166 µg per animal for the subsequent duration of the 30-month study. The latter dose was stated by the authors to be equivalent to a human dose of 0.625 mg/day. The dose of medroxyprogesterone acetate was 650 µg/day throughout the experiment; this dose was stated by the authors to be equivalent to a human dose of 2.5 mg/day. The combined oestrogen–progestogen treatment increased the concentration of circulating oestradiol from 5 to 161 pg/mL; the concentration of medroxyprogesterone acetate in the blood was 116 pg/mL. Exposure to the hormones increased the thickness of the mammary tissue by 70% and significantly enlarged the estimated surface areas of lobular tissue and epithelial tissue; it also induced mammary gland hyperplasia in 18/21 animals, as compared with 41% of animals given Premarin® alone and none in the control group. The mean percentage of epithelial breast cells that stained for Ki-67 MIB-1 antibody (a marker of cell proliferation) was increased from 2.5 to 8.0% in alveoli, from 0.6 to 1.9% in terminal ducts and from 1.2 to 5.5% in major mammary ducts. These effects on labelling were not different from those in monkeys given Premarin® alone (see the monograph on 'Post-menopausal oestrogen therapy', section 4.2). The mean percentage of epithelial breast cells that stained for progesterone receptor was not changed in these mammary structures, but the percentage of cells that stained for oestrogen receptor was decreased by approximately 65% in alveoli, by 40% in terminal ducts and by more than 90% in major mammary ducts (Cline et al., 1996).

4.3   Genetic and related effects

4.3.1   *Humans*

No data were available to the Working Group.

4.3.2   *Experimental systems*

Relevant data are contained in section 4.3.2 of the monographs on 'Oral contraceptives, combined' and 'Post-menopausal oestrogen therapy'.

5.   Summary of Data Reported and Evaluation

5.1   Exposure

Use of regimens in which a progestogen is added to post-menopausal oestrogen therapy has been increasing in order to reduce the increased risk for endometrial cancer observed with oestrogens alone. Regimens vary with respect to dose and timing of oestrogen and progestogen administration and in the number of days on which the progestogen is given per month. Several routes of administration are used, including oral (as tablets), injection, implantation, percutaneous application and intrauterine administration. The frequency and type of hormonal supplementation used vary widely within and between countries.

5.2   Human carcinogenicity

Breast cancer

Separate information on the effects of use of post-menopausal oestrogen–progestogen therapy was provided in only a minority of the studies on the risk for breast cancer. The results of nine cohort and five case–control studies that did include such information and the findings of a pooled analysis of the original data from these and other studies indicate that the increased relative risk observed with long-term use of post-menopausal oestrogen–progestogen therapy is not materially different from that for long-term use of oestrogens alone. The available information on long-term use of the combination is, however, limited. The data are insufficient to assess the effects of past use and of different progestogen compounds, doses and treatment schedules.

Endometrial cancer

The relationship between use of post-menopausal oestrogen–progestogen therapy and the risk for endometrial cancer was addressed in four follow-up and four case–control studies. In comparison with women who did not use hormonal therapy, the risk of women who did was no different or modestly increased, but the increase was smaller than that for women who used oestrogens alone. In the two studies that were recent and large enough to evaluate different durations of progestogen supplementation during each cycle, an increase in risk was found relative to non-users when the progestogen was added to the cycle for 10 days or fewer. The risk for endometrial cancer associated with different monthly durations of progestogen supplementation per cycle and different doses of progestogen supplementation remains unclear.

Ovarian cancer

One cohort and one case–control study are available on the possible relationship between use of post-menopausal oestrogen–progestogen therapy and the risk for ovarian cancer. The limited data suggest no association.

Liver cancer

One cohort study suggested that there is no association between use of post-menopausal oestrogen–progestogen therapy and the risk for liver cancer.

Other cancers

Very few studies were available of the risks for colorectal cancer, cutaneous malignant melanoma or thyroid cancer that allowed a distinction between use of post-menopausal oestrogen–progestogen and oestrogen therapy. They do not suggest an increased risk, but all included few exposed subjects.

5.3   Carcinogenicity in experimental animals

Only one study was available on combined oestrogen and progestogen therapy, in which conjugated equine oestrogens were tested with medroxyprogesterone acetate. Oral administration of this combination or of the conjugated oestrogens alone in the diet of ovariectomized female rats which had been given 7,12-dimethylbenz[*a*]anthracene, a known mammary carcinogen, increased the incidence of mammary tumours to a level equal to that in non-ovariectomized controls treated with the carcinogen.

5.4   Other relevant data

Combinations of oestrogens and progestogens are absorbed rapidly and reach maximal serum concentrations quickly. The proportion of absorbed hormones that becomes biologically available depends on the extent of enterohepatic circulation and metabolic transformation of pro-drugs. Oestrogens and progestogens may affect each other's disposition. Many progestogens have oestrogenic activity and can modify the effects of oestrogens. The addition of progestogens to therapy may decrease cell proliferation in human endometrium over that with oestrogen alone. The extent of the cell proliferation response depends on the doses of oestrogen and progestogen, increasing with higher doses of oestrogen and decreasing with more progestogen, as compared with oestrogen alone.

In ovariectomized cynomolgus monkeys, the conjugated oestrogen–progestogen combination caused a higher incidence of mammary gland hyperplasia than did conjugated equine oestrogens alone. No information was available on whether the effect of oestrogen–progestogen combinations on the mammary gland is modified by sequential exposure to progestogens, by body weight or by the recency or duration of exposure in experimental animals. Similarly, no information was available on the possible relationship between exposure to oestrogen–progestogen combinations and the degree of malignancy of breast tumours.

No information was available on the genotoxic effects of formulations similar to those used in post-menopausal oestrogen–progestogen therapy.

5.5   Evaluation

There is *limited evidence* in humans for the carcinogenicity of post-menopausal oestrogen–progestogen therapy.

There is *inadequate evidence* in experimental animals for the carcinogenicity of conjugated equine oestrogens plus progestogen.

Overall evaluation

Post-menopausal oestrogen–progestogen therapy is *possibly carcinogenic to humans (Group 2B)*.

6.   References

American College of Physicians (1992) Guidelines for counselling postmenopausal women about preventive hormone therapy. *Ann. intern. Med.*, **117**, 1038–1041

Anderson, T.J., Ferguson, D.J. & Raab, G.M. (1982) Cell turnover in the 'resting' human breast: Influence of parity, contraceptive pill, age and laterality. *Br. J. Cancer*, **46**, 376–382

Anderson, T.J., Battersby, S., King, R.J.B., McPherson, K. & Going, J.J. (1989) Oral contraceptive use influences resting breast proliferation. *Hum. Pathol.*, **20**, 1139–1144

Beresford, S.A.A., Weiss, N.S., Voigt, L.F. & McKnight, B. (1997) Risk of endometrial cancer in relation to use of oestrogen combined with cyclic progestagen therapy in postmenopausal women. *Lancet*, **349**, 458–461

Bergkvist, L., Adami, H.O., Persson, I., Hoover, R. & Schairer, C. (1989) The risk of breast cancer after estrogen and estrogen–progestin replacement. *New Engl. J. Med.*, **321**, 293–297

Bhattacharya, D., Redkar, A., Mittra, I., Sutaria, U. & MacRae, K.D. (1997) Oestrogen increases S-phase fraction and oestrogen and progesterone receptors in human cervical cancer *in vivo*. *Br. J. Cancer*, **75**, 554–558

Braasch, H.V., Frederiksen, M.C. & Chaterton, R.T. (1988) Metabolism and pharmacokinetics of progesterone in the cynomolgus monkey (*Macaca fascicularis*). *Steroids*, **52**, 279–294

Brinton, L.A., Hoover, R.N. & the Endometrial Cancer Collaborative Group (1993) Estrogen replacement therapy and endometrial cancer risk: Unresolved issues. *Obstet. Gynecol.*, **81**, 265–271

British Medical Association (1997) Female sex hormones. In: *British National Formulary*, Vol. 34, London, Royal Pharmaceutical Society of Great Britain, pp. 313–321

Bush, T.L. & Barrett-Connor, E. (1985) Non contraceptive estrogen use and cardiovascular disease. *Epidemiol. Rev*, **7**, 80–104

Cameron, S.T., Critchley, H.O., Glasier, A.F., Williams, A.R. & Baird, D.T. (1997) Continuous transdermal oestrogen and interrupted progestogen as a novel bleed-free regimen of hormone replacement therapy for postmenopausal women. *Br. J. Obstet. Gynaecol.*, **104**, 1184–1190

Campagnoli, C., Biglia, N., Lanza, M.G., Lesca, L., Peris, C. & Sismondi, P. (1994) Androgenic progestogens oppose the decrease of insulin-like growth factor I serum level induced by conjugated oestrogens in postmenopausal women. Preliminary report. *Maturitas*, **19**, 25–31

Cerin, A., Heldaas, K. & Moeller, B. (1996) Adverse endometrial effects of long-cycle estrogen and progestogen replacement therapy. The Scandinavian Long Cycle Study Group (Letter to the Editor). *New Engl. J. Med.*, **334**, 668–669

Cline, J.M., Soderqvist, G., von Schoultz, E., Skoog, L. & von Schoutlz, B. (1996) Effects of hormone replacement therapy on the mammary gland of surgically postmenopausal cyno-molgus macaques. *Am. J. Obstet. Gynecol.*, **174**, 93–100

Colditz, G.A., Stampfer, M.J., Willett, W.C., Hunter, D.J., Manson, J.E., Hennekens, C.H., Rosner, B.A. & Speizer, F.E. (1992) Type of postmenopausal hormone use and risk of breast cancer: 12-year follow-up from the Nurses' Health Study. *Cancer Causes Control*, **3**, 433–439

Colditz, G.A., Hankinson, S.E., Hunter, D.J., Willett, W.C., Manson, J.E., Stampfer, M.J., Hennekens, C. & Rosner, B. (1995) The use of estrogens and progestins and the risk of breast cancer in postmenopausal women. *New Engl. J. Med.*, **332**, 1589–1593

Collaborative Group on Hormonal Factors in Breast Cancer (1997) Breast cancer and hormone replacement therapy: Collaborative reanalysis of data from 51 epidemiological studies of 52 705 women with breast cancer and 108 411 women without breast cancer. *Lancet*, **350**, 1047–1059

Ettinger, B., Selby, J., Citron, J.T., Bangessel, A., Ettinger, V.M. & Hendrickson, M.R. (1994) Cyclic hormone replacement therapy using quarterly progestin. *Obstet. Gynecol.*, **83**, 693–700

Ewertz, M. (1988) Influence of non-contraceptive exogenous and endogenous sex hormones on breast cancer risk in Denmark. *Int. J. Cancer*, **42**, 832–838

Finnegan, L.P., Rossouw, J. & Harlan, W.R. (1995) A peppy response to PEPI results. *Nature Med.*, **1**, 205–206

Fotherby, K. (1994) Pharmacokinetics and metabolism of progestins in humans. In: Goldzieher, J.W. & Fotherby, K., eds, *Pharmacology of the Contraceptive Steroids*, New York, Raven Press, pp. 99–126

Fotherby, K. (1996) Bioavailability of orally administered sex steroids used in oral contraception and hormone replacement therapy. *Contraception*, **54**, 59–69

Gambrell, R.D. (1986) Prevention of endometrial cancer with progestogens. *Maturitas*, **8**, 159–168

Gangrade, N.K., Boudinot, F.D. & Price, J.C. (1992) Pharmacokinetics of progesterone in ovariectomized rat after single dose intravenous administration. *Biopharm. Drug Disposition*, **13**, 703–709

Going, J.J., Anderson, T.J., Battersby, S. & MacIntyre, C.C. (1988) Proliferative and secretory activity in human breast during natural and artificial menstrual cycles. *Am. J. Pathol.*, **130**, 193–204

Hammond, C.B., Jelovsek, F.R., Lee, K.L., Creasman, W.T. & Parker, R.T. (1979) Effects of long-term estrogen replacement therapy. II. Neoplasia. *Am. J. Obstet. Gynecol.*, **133**, 537–547

Hirvonen, E. (1996) Progestins. *Maturitas*, **23** (Suppl.), S13–S18

Hirvonen, E., Allonen, H., Anttila, M., Kulmala, Y., Ranta, T., Rautiainen, H., Sipila, P. & Ylostalo, P. (1995) Oral contraceptive containing natural estradiol for premenopausal women. *Maturitas*, **21**, 27–32

Honjo, H., Ishihara, M., Osawa, Y., Kirdani, R.Y. & Sandberg, A.A. (1976) The metabolic fate of chlormadinone acetate in the baboon. *Steroids*, **27**, 79–98

Hunt, K., Vessey, M., McPherson, K. & Coleman, M. (1987) Long-term surveillance of mortality and cancer incidence in women receiving hormone replacement therapy. *Br. J. Obstet. Gynaecol.*, **94**, 620–635

Hunt, K., Vessey, M. & McPherson, K. (1990) Mortality in a cohort of long-term users of hormone replacement therapy: An updated analysis. *Br. J. Obstet. Gynaecol.*, **97**, 1080–1086

IARC (1979) *IARC Monographs on the Evaluation of the Carcinogenic Risk of Chemicals to Humans*, Vol. 21, *Sex Hormones (II)*, Lyon

Jick, S.S., Walker, A.M. & Jick, H. (1993) Oral contraceptives and endometrial cancer. *Obstet. Gynecol.*, **82**, 931–935

Johanisson, E., Holinka, C.F. & Arrenbrecht, S. (1997) Transdermal sequential and continuous hormone replacement regimens with estradiol and norethisterone acetate in postmenopausal women: Effects on the endometrium. *Int. J. Fertil.*, **42** (Suppl. 2), 388–398

Johansson, E.D.B., Johansson, P.B. & Rasmussen, S.N.A. (1986) MPA pharmacokinetics after oral administration. *Acta pharmacol. toxicol.*, **58**, 311–317

Kaufman, D.W., Kelly, J.P., Welch, W.R., Rosenberg, L., Stolley, P.D., Warshauer, M.E., Lewis, J., Woodruff, J. & Shapiro, S. (1989) Noncontraceptive estrogen use and epithelial ovarian cancer. *Am. J. Epidemiol.*, **130**, 1142–1151

Kaufman, D.W., Palmer, J.R., de Mouzon, J., Rosenberg, L., Stolley, P.D., Warshauer, M.E., Zauber, A.G. & Shapiro, S. (1991) Estrogen replacement therapy and the risk of breast cancer: Results from the case–control surveillance study. *Am. J. Epidemiol.*, **134**, 1375–1385

Kelly, J.J., Rajkovic, I.A., O'Sullivan, A.J., Sernia, C. & Ho, K.K.Y. (1993) Effects of different oral oestrogen formulations on insulin-like growth factor-I, growth hormone and growth hormone binding protein in post-menopausal women. *Clin. Endocrinol.*, **39**, 561–567

Kelsey, J.L., Gammon, M.D. & John, E.M. (1993) Reproductive factors and breast cancer. *Epidemiol. Rev.*, **15**, 36–47

Kennedy, D.L., Baum, C. & Forbes, M.B. (1985) Noncontraceptive estrogens and progestins: Use patterns over time. *Obstet. Gynecol.*, **65**, 441–446

Key, T.J. & Pike, M.C. (1988) The role of oestrogens and progestagens in the epidemiology and prevention of breast cancer. *Eur. J. Cancer clin. Oncol.*, **24**, 29–43

King, R.J.B. & Whitehead, M.I. (1986) Assessment of the potency of orally administered progestins in women. *Fertil. Steril.*, **46**, 1062–1066

Kleinman, R.L. (1990) *Hormonal Contraception*, London, IPPF Medical Publications

Kowalski, W.B., Chatterton, R.T., Kazer, R.R. & Severini, T.A. (1996) Disappearance and unexpected reappearance of progesterone in the circulation of the monkey: Novel hormone kinetics. *J. Physiol.*, **493**, 877–884

Kreitmann, B., Bugat, R. & Bayard, F. (1979) Estrogen and progestin regulation of the progesterone receptor concentration in human endometrium. *J. clin. Endocrinol. Metab.*, **49**, 926–929

Kuhl, H. (1990) Pharmacokinetics of oestrogens and progestogens. *Maturitas*, **12**, 171–197

Kumasaka, T., Itoh, E., Watanabe, H., Hoshino, K., Yoshinaka, A. & Masawa, N. (1994) Effects of various forms of progestin on the endometrium of the estrogen-primed, ovariectomized rat. *Endocrine J.*, **41**, 161–169

Lancaster, T., Surman, G., Lawrence, M., Mant, D., Vessey, M., Thorogood, M., Yudkin, P. & Daly, E. (1995) Hormone replacement therapy: Characteristics of users and non-users in a British general practice cohort identified through computerised prescribing records. *J. Epidemiol. Community Health*, **49**, 389–394

Lane, G., Siddle, N.C., Ryder, T.A., Pryse-Davies, J., King, R.J.B. & Whitehead, M.I. (1986) Effects of dydrogesterone on the oestrogenized postmenopausal endometrium. *Br. J. Obstet. Gynaecol.*, **93**, 55–62

Li, J.J., Li, S.A., Oberley, T.D. & Parsons, J.A. (1995) Carcinogenic activities of various steroidal and nonsteroidal estrogens in the hamster kidney: Relation to hormonal activity and cell proliferation. *Cancer Res.*, **55**, 4347–4351

Longacre, T.A. & Bartow, S.A. (1986) A correlative morphologic study of human breast and endometrium in the menstrual cycle. *Am. J. Surg. Pathol.*, **10**, 382-393

Luo, S., Stojanovic, M., Labrie, C. & Labrie, F. (1997) Inhibitory effect of the novel anti-estrogen EM-800 and medroxyprogesterone acetate on estrone-stimulated growth of dimethylbenz[a]-anthracene-induced mammary carcinoma in rats. *Int. J. Cancer*, **73**, 580–586

Maddison, J. (1973) Hormone replacement therapy for menopausal symptoms (Letter to the Editor). *Lancet*, **i**, 1507

Maxson, W.S. & Hargrove, J.T. (1985) Bioavailability of oral micronized progesterone. *Fertil. Steril.*, **44**, 622–626

Morville, R., Dray, F., Reynier, J. & Barrat, J. (1982) The bioavailability of natural progesterone given by mouth. Measurement of steroid concentrations in plasma, endometrium and breast tissue. *J. Gynécol. Obstét. Biol. Reprod. (Paris)*, **11**, 355–363 (in French)

Nachtigall, L.E., Nachtigall, R.H., Nachtigall, R.D. & Beckman, E.M. (1979) Estrogen replacement therapy. I. A 10-year prospective study in the relationship to osteoporosis. *Obstet. Gynecol.*, **53**, 277–281

Newcomb, P.A. & Storer, B.E. (1995) Postmenopausal hormone use and risk of large-bowel cancer. *J. natl Cancer Inst.*, **87**, 1067–1071

Newcomb, P.A., Longnecker, M.P., Storer, B.E., Mittendorf, R., Baron, J., Clapp, R.W., Bogdan, G. & Willett, W.C. (1995) Long-term hormone replacement therapy and risk of breast cancer in postmenopausal women. *Am. J. Epidemiol.*, **142**, 788–795

Østerlind, A., Tucker, M.A., Stone, B.J. & Jensen, O.M. (1988) The Danish case–control study of cutaneous malignant melanoma. III. Hormonal and reproductive factors in women. *Int. J. Cancer*, **42**, 821–824

Ottoson, U.B., Carlstrom, K., Damber, J.E. & von Schoultz, B. (1984) Serum levels of progesterone and some of its metabolites including deoxycorticosterone after oral and parenteral administration. *Br. J. Obstet. Gynaecol.*, **91**, 1111–1119

Pannuti, F., Camaggi, C.M., Strocchi, E., Giovannini, M., DiMarco, A.R. & Costanti, B. (1982) MPA relative availability after single high dose administration. *Cancer Treat. Rep.*, **66**, 2043–2049

Paterson, M.E.L., Wade-Evans, T., Sturdee, D.W., Thom, M.H. & Studd, J.W.W. (1980) Endometrial disease after treatment with oestrogens and progestogens in the climacteric. *Br. med. J.*, **i**, 822–824

Persson, I., Adami, H.-O., Bergkvist, L., Lindgren, A., Pettersson, B., Hoover, R. & Schairer, C. (1989) Risk of endometrial cancer after treatment with oestrogens alone or in conjunction with progestogens: Results of a prospective study. *Br. med. J.*, **298**, 147–151

Persson, I., Yuen, J., Bergkvist, L. & Schairer, C. (1996) Cancer incidence and mortality in women receiving estrogen and estrogen-progestin replacement therapy—Long-term follow-up of a Swedish cohort. *Int. J. Cancer*, **67**, 327–332

Persson, I., Bergkvist, L., Lindgren, C. & Yuen, J. (1997) Hormone replacement therapy and major risk factors for reproductive cancers, osteoporosis, and cardiovascular diseases: Evidence of confounding by exposure characteristics. *J. clin. Epidemiol.*, **50**, 611–618

Pike, M.C., Peters, R.K., Cozen, W., Probst-Hensch, N.M., Felix, J.C., Wan, P.C. & Mack, T.M. (1997) Estrogen–progestin replacement therapy and endometrial cancer. *J. natl Cancer Inst.*, **89**, 1110–1116

Postmenopausal Estrogen/Progestin Interventions Trial (PEPI) (1996) Effects of hormone replacement therapy on endometrial histology in postmenopausal women. *J. Am. med. Assoc.*, **275**, 370–375

Potten, C.S., Watson, R.J., Williams, G.T., Tickle, S., Roberts, S.A., Harris, M. & Howell, A. (1988) The effect of age and menstrual cycle upon proliferative activity of the normal human breast. *Br. J. Cancer*, **58**, 163–170

Preston-Martin, S., Pike, M.C., Ross, R.K., Jones, P.A. & Henderson, B.E. (1990) Increased cell division as a cause of human cancer. *Cancer Res.*, **50**, 7415–7421

Risch, H.A. & Howe, G.R. (1994) Menopausal hormone usage and breast cancer in Saskatchewan: A record-linkage cohort study. *Am. J. Epidemiol.*, **139**, 670–683

Risch, H.A. & Howe, G.R. (1995) Menopausal hormone use and colorectal cancer in Saskatchewan: A record linkage cohort study. *Cancer Epidemiol. Biomarkers Prev.*, **4**, 21–28

Sakamoto, S., Kudo, H., Suzuki, S., Mitamura, T., Sassa, S., Kuwa, K., Chun, Z., Yoshimura, S., Maemura, M., Nakayama, T. & Shinoda, H. (1997) Additional effects of medroxyprogesterone acetate on mammary tumors in oophorectomized, estrogenized, DMBA-treated rats. *Anticancer Res.*, **17**, 4583–4588

Schairer, C., Byrne, C., Keyl, P.M., Brinton, L.A., Sturgeon, S.R. & Hoover, R.N. (1994) Menopausal estrogen and estrogen–progestin replacement therapy and risk of breast cancer (United States). *Cancer Causes Control*, 5, 491–500

Schleusener, A., Nishino, Y., Albring, M., Neumann, F. & Beier S. (1980) Endocrine profile of cyproterone acetate metabolite and its potential clinical use. *Acta endocrinol.*, 234S, 94–106

Shi, Y.E., He, C.H., Gu, J. & Fotherby, K. (1987) Pharmacokinetics of norethisterone in humans. *Contraception*, 35, 465–475

Siddle, N.C., Townsend, P.T., Young, O., Minardi, J., King, R.J.B. & Whitehead, M.I. (1982) Dose-dependent effects of synthetic progestins on the biochemistry of the estrogenized post-menopausal endometrium. *Acta obstet. gynecol. scand.*, **Suppl. 106**, 17–22

Simon, J.A., Robinson, D.E., Andrews, M.C., Hildebrand, J.R., Rocci, M.L., Jr, Blake, R.E. & Hodgen, G.D. (1993) The absorption of oral micronized progesterone: The effect of food dose proportionality, and comparison with intramuscular progesterone. *Fertil. Steril.*, 60, 26–33

Söderqvist, G., von Schoultz, B., Tani, E. & Skoog, L. (1993) Estrogen and progesterone receptor content in breast epithelial cells from healthy women during the menstrual cycle. *Am. J. Obstet. Gynecol.*, 168, 874–879

Speroff, L., Rowan, J., Symons, J., Genant, H. & Wilborn, W. for the CHART Study Group (1996) The comparative effect on bone density, endometrium, and lipids of continuous hormones as replacement therapy (CHART Study). A randomized controlled trial. *J. Am. med. Assoc.*, 276, 1397–1403

Stanford, J.L. & Thomas, D.B. (1993) Exogenous progestins and breast cancer. *Epidemiol. Rev.*, 15, 98–107

Stanford, J.L., Weiss, N.S., Voigt, L.F., Daling, J.R., Habel, L.A. & Rossing, M.A. (1995) Combined estrogen and progestin hormone replacement therapy in relation to risk of breast cancer in middle-aged women. *J. Am. med. Assoc.*, 274, 137–142

Studd, J.W.W. (1976) Hormone implants in the climacteric syndrome. In: Campbel, S., ed., *The Management of the Menopause and the Post-menopausal Years*, Lancaster, MTP Press Ltd, pp. 383–385

Sturdee, D.W., Wade-Evans, T., Paterson, M.E., Thom, M. & Studd, J.W. (1978) Relations between bleeding pattern, endometrial histology, and oestrogen treatment in menopausal women. *Br. med. J.*, i, 1575–1577

Suhonen, S., Haukkamaa, M., Holmström, T., Lähteenmäki, P. & Rutanen, E.-M. (1996) Endometrial response to hormone replacement therapy as assessed by expression of insulin-like growth factor-binding protein-1 in the endometrium. *Fertil. Steril.*, 65, 776–782

Suvanto-Luukkonen, E., Sundström, H., Penttinen, J., Kauppila, A. & Rutanen, E.-M. (1995) Insulin-like growth factor-binding protein-1: A biochemical marker of endometrial response to progestin during hormone replacement therapy. *Maturitas*, 22, 255–262

Thom, M.H., White, P.J., Williams, R.M., Sturdee, D.W., Paterson, M.E., Wade-Evans, T. & Studd, J.W. (1979) Prevention and treatment of endometrial disease in climacteric women receiving oestrogen therapy. *Lancet*, ii, 455–457

Townsend, J. (1998) Hormone replacement therapy: Assessment of present use, costs and trends. *Br. J. gen. Pract.*, 48, 955–958

Troisi, R., Schairer, C., Chow, W.-H., Schatzkin, A., Brinton, L.A. & Fraumeni, J.F., Jr (1997) A prospective study of menopausal hormones and risk of colorectal cancer (United States). *Cancer Causes Control*, **8**, 130–138

Vogel, P.M., Georgiade, N.G., Fetter, B.F., Vogel, F.S. & McCarty, K.S., Jr (1981) The correlation of histologic changes in the human breast with the menstrual cycle. *Am. J. Pathol.*, **104**, 23–34

Voigt, L.F., Weiss, N.S., Chu, J., Daling, J.R., McKnight, B. & van Belle, G. (1991) Progestogen supplementation of exogenous oestrogens and risk of endometrial cancer. *Lancet*, **338**, 274–277

Whitehead, M.I., Townsend, P.T., Gill, D.K., Collins, W.P. & Campbell, S. (1980) Absorption and metabolism of oral progesterone. *Br. med J.*, **i**, 825–827

Whitehead, M.I., Townsend, P.T., Pryse-Davies, J., Ryder, T.A. & King, R.J.B. (1981) Effects of estrogens and progestins on the biochemistry and morphology of the postmenopausal endometrium. *New Engl. J. Med.*, **305**, 1599–1605

Writing Group for the PEPI Trial (1995) Effects of estrogen or estrogen/progestin regimens on heart disease risk factors in postmenopausal women. The Postmenopausal Estrogen/Progestin Interventions (PEPI) Trial. *J. Am. med. Assoc.*, **273**, 199–208

Yang, C.P., Daling, J.R., Band, P.R., Gallagher, R.P., White, E. & Weiss, N.S. (1992) Noncontraceptive hormone use and risk of breast cancer. *Cancer Causes Control*, **3**, 475–479

Yuen, J., Persson, I., Bergkvist, L., Hoover, R., Schairer, C. & Adami, H.O. (1993) Hormone replacement therapy and breast cancer mortality in Swedish women: Results after adjustment for 'healthy drug-user' effect. *Cancer Causes Control*, **4**, 369–374

Ziel, H.K. & Finkle, W.D. (1975) Increased risk of endometrial carcinoma among users of conjugated estrogens. *New Engl. J. Med.*, **293**, 1167–1170

SUMMARY OF FINAL EVALUATIONS

Agent	Degree of evidence of carcinogenicity		Overall evaluation of carcinogenicity to humans
	Human	Animal	
Oral contraceptives, combined	S[a]		1
Hormonal contraceptives, progestogen-only	I		2B
Post-menopausal oestrogen therapy	S		1
Post-menopausal oestrogen–progestogen therapy	L		2B
Oestrogens			
Conjugated equine oestrogens		L	
d-Equilenin		I	
Equilin		L	
Ethinyloestradiol		S	
Mestranol		S	
Oestradiol		S	
Oestriol		L	
Oestrone		S	
Progestogens			
Chlormadinone acetate		L	
Cyproterone acetate		L	
Ethynodiol diacetate		L	
Levonorgestrel		I	
Lynoestrenol		S	
Medroxyprogesterone acetate		S	
Megestrol acetate		L	
Norethisterone		L	
Norethisterone acetate		L	
Norethynodrel		S	
Norgestrel		I	
Combinations			
Conjugated equine oestrogens (O) + progestogen (P)		I	
Ethinyloestradiol (O) + chlormadinone acetate (P)		L	
Ethinyloestradiol (O) + ethynodiol diacetate (P)		S	
Ethinyloestradiol (O) + megestrol acetate (P)		L	
Ethinyloestradiol (O) + norethisterone (P)		L	
Ethinyloestradiol (O) + norgestrel (P)		L	
Mestranol (O) + chlormadinone acetate (P)		L	
Mestranol (O) + ethynodiol diacetate (P)		L	
Mestranol (O) + lynoestrenol (P)		L	
Mestranol (O) + norethisterone (P)		L	
Mestranol (O) + norethynodrel (P)		S	

S, sufficient evidence; I, inadequate evidence; L, limited evidence; group 1, carcinogenic to humans; group 2B, possibly carcinogenic to humans; for definitions of criteria for degrees of evidence and groups, see preamble, pp. 23–27.

O, oestrogen; P, progestogen

[a] Hepatocellular carcinomas, high-dose preparations

ANNEXES

Annex 1.
Chemical and physical data and information on production and use for oestrogens and progestogens used in oral contraceptives, progestogen-only contraceptives and post-menopausal hormonal therapy

Trade names for these compounds alone and in combination with other hormonal drugs are given in Annex 2.

1. Oestrogens

1.1 Conjugated oestrogens

The term 'conjugated oestrogens' refers to mixtures of at least eight compounds, including sodium oestrone sulfate and sodium equilin sulfate, derived wholly or in part from equine urine or synthetically from oestrone and equilin. Conjugated oestrogens contain as concomitant components the sodium sulfate conjugates of 17α-dihydroequilin, 17β-dihydroequilin and 17α-oestradiol (United States Pharmacopeial Convention, 1995).

1.1.1   *Nomenclature*
Sodium oestrone sulfate
    Chem. Abstr. Serv. Reg. No.: 438-67-5
    Chem. Abstr. Name: 3-(Sulfooxy)-estra-1,3,5(10)-trien-17-one, sodium salt
    IUPAC Systematic Name: Estrone, hydrogen sulfate sodium salt
    Synonyms: Estrone sodium sulfate; estrone sulfate sodium; estrone sulfate sodium salt; oestrone sodium sulfate; oestrone sulfate sodium; oestrone sulfate sodium salt; sodium estrone sulfate; sodium estrone-3-sulfate; sodium oestrone-3-sulfate

Sodium equilin sulfate
    Chem. Abstr. Serv. Reg. No.: 16680-47-0
    Chem. Abstr. Name: 3-(Sulfooxy)-estra-1,3,5(10),7-tetraen-17-one, sodium salt
    IUPAC Systematic Name: 3-Hydroxy-estra-1,3,5(10),7-tetraen-17-one, hydrogen sulfate, sodium salt
    Synonyms: Equilin, sulfate, sodium salt; equilin sodium sulfate; sodium equilin 3-monosulfate

1.1.2   *Structural and molecular formulae and relative molecular mass*
Sodium oestrone sulfate

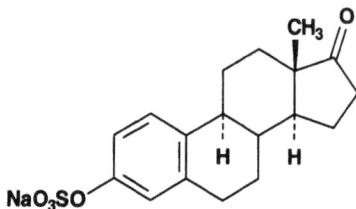

$C_{18}H_{21}O_5S.Na$ Relative molecular mass: 372.4

Sodium equilin sulfate

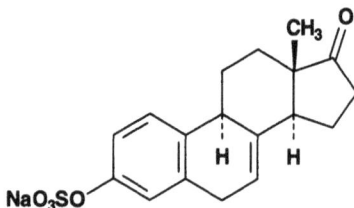

$C_{18}H_{19}O_5S.Na$ Relative molecular mass: 370.4

1.1.3   *Chemical and physical properties*
From Gennaro (1995)
  (*a*)   *Description*: Buff-coloured, odourless powder
  (*b*)   *Solubility*: Soluble in water

1.1.4   *Technical products and impurities*
Conjugated oestrogens contain not less than 52.5% and not more than 61.5% sodium oestrone sulfate and not less than 22.5% and not more than 30.5% sodium equilin sulfate, and the total of sodium oestrone sulfate and sodium equilin sulfate is not less than 79.5% and not more than 88.0% of the labelled content of conjugated oestrogens. Conjugated oestrogens contain as concomitant components (as sodium sulfate conjugates) not less than 13.5% and not more than 19.5% 17α-dihydroequilin, not less than 0.5% and not more than 4.0% 17β-dihydroequilin and not less than 2.5% and not more than 9.5% 17α-oestradiol, of the labelled content of conjugated oestrogens (United States Pharmacopeial Convention, 1995).

Conjugated oestrogens are available as tablets for oral administration, as an injection for parenteral administration and as a 0.0625% vaginal cream (American Hospital Formulary Service, 1997).

Conjugated oestrogens are also used in combination with several other pharmaceutical preparations, including medrogestone, medroxyprogesterone acetate and methyltestosterone (American Hospital Formulary Service, 1997; Reynolds, 1998).

Information available in 1995 indicated that conjugated oestrogens were manu-factured or formulated in Argentina, Belgium, Brazil, Canada, France, India, Mexico, the Netherlands, Portugal, Switzerland and the United States (CIS Information Services, 1995).

1.1.5   *Analysis*

Gas chromatography with flame ionization detection is used for identification and for establishing the purity of conjugated oestrogens, their components and impurities (United States Pharmacopeial Convention, 1995).

1.2   **Ethinyloestradiol**

1.2.1   *Nomenclature*

Chem. Abstr. Serv. Reg. No.: 57-63-6

Deleted CAS Reg. No.: 77538-56-8

Chem. Abstr. Name: (17α)-19-Norpregna-1,3,5(10)-trien-20-yne-3,17-diol

IUPAC Systematic Name: 19-Nor-17α-pregna-1,3,5(10)-trien-20-yne-3,17-diol

Synonyms: 17-Ethinyl-3,17-estradiol; 17-ethinylestradiol; 17α-ethinyl-17β-estradiol; 17α-ethynylestradiol; ethinylestradiol; 17-ethynylestradiol; ethynylestradiol; 17α-ethynylestradiol; ethynyloestradiol

1.2.2   *Structural and molecular formulae and relative molecular mass*

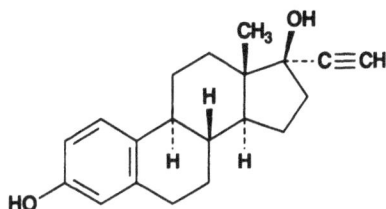

$C_{20}H_{24}O_2$ Relative molecular mass: 296.4

1.2.3   *Chemical and physical properties of the pure substance*

From Budavari (1996) and Reynolds (1998), unless otherwise specified

  (*a*) *Description:* White to creamy- or slightly yellowish-white, odourless, crystalline powder

  (*b*) *Melting-point:* 182–184°C

  (*c*) *Solubility:* Practically insoluble in water; soluble in acetone (1 part in 5), ethanol (1 part in 6), chloroform (1 part in 20), dioxane (1 part in 4), diethyl ether (1 part in 4) and vegetable oils

  (*d*) *Optical rotation:* $[\alpha]_D^{20}$, less than –27° to –30° (Council of Europe, 1997)

1.2.4   *Technical products and impurities*

Ethinyloestradiol is commercially available as tablets alone and in combination with progestogens, as described in the monograph on 'Oral contraceptives, combined'.

1.2.5   *Analysis*

Several international pharmacopoeias specify infra-red and ultra-violet absorption spectrophotometry and thin-layer chromatography as methods for identifying ethinyl-oestradiol; thin-layer chromatography, liquid chromatography, ultra-violet absorption spectrophotometry and potentiometric titration are used to assay the purity of ethinyl-oestradiol and to determine its content in pharmaceutical preparations (British Pharmaco-poeial Commission, 1993; Secretaria de Salud, 1994, 1995; United States Pharmacopeial Convention, 1995; Schweizerischen Bundesrat, 1996; Council of Europe, 1997).

1.3   Mestranol

1.3.1   *Nomenclature*

Chem. Abstr. Serv. Reg. No.: 72-33-3

Deleted CAS Reg. No.: 43085-54-7; 53445-46-8

Chem. Abstr. Name: (17α)-3-Methoxy-19-norpregna-1,3,5(10)-trien-20-yn-17-ol

IUPAC Systematic Name: 3-Methoxy-19-nor-17α-pregna-1,3,5(10)-trien-20-yn-17-ol

Synonyms: Ethinylestradiol 3-methyl ether; 17α-ethinylestradiol 3-methyl ether; ethi-nyloestradiol 3-methyl ether; 17α-ethinyloestradiol 3-methyl ether; ethynylestradiol methyl ether; ethynylestradiol 3-methyl ether; 17-ethynylestradiol 3-methyl ether; 17α-ethynylestradiol 3-methyl ether; 17α-ethynylestradiol methyl ether; ethynyl-oestradiol methyl ether; ethynyloestradiol 3-methyl ether; 17-ethynyloestradiol 3-methyl ether; 17α-ethynyloestradiol 3-methyl ether; 17α-ethynyloestradiol methyl ether; 3-methoxy-17α-ethinylestradiol; 3-methoxy-17α-ethinyloestradiol; 3-methoxy-17α-ethynylestradiol; 3-methoxyethynylestradiol; 3-methoxy-17α-ethynyloestradiol; 3-methoxyethynyloestradiol; 3-methylethynylestradiol; 3-*O*-methylethynylestradiol; 3-methylethynyloestradiol; 3-*O*-methylethynyloestradiol; Δ-MVE

1.3.2   *Structural and molecular formulae and relative molecular mass*

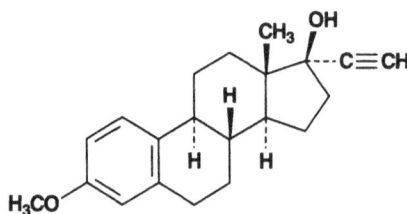

C$_{21}$H$_{26}$O$_2$ Relative molecular mass: 310.4

1.3.3   *Chemical and physical properties of the pure substance*

From Budavari (1996) and Reynolds (1998)

(a)   *Description*: White to creamy-white, odourless, crystalline powder

(b)   *Melting-point*: 150–151°C

(c)   *Solubility*: Practically insoluble in water; sparingly soluble in ethanol; slightly soluble in methanol; soluble in acetone, dioxane and diethyl ether; freely soluble in chloroform

1.3.4   *Technical products and impurities*

Mestranol is commercially available as a component of combination tablets with norethisterone, chlormadinone acetate, norethisterone, ethynodiol diacetate, lynoestrenol or norethynodrel (Reynolds, 1998; see the monograph on 'Oral contraceptives, combined' and Annex 2).

1.3.5   *Analysis*

Several international pharmacopoeias specify infra-red and ultra-violet absorption spectrophotometry with comparison to standards as methods for identifying mestranol; ultra-violet absorption spectrophotometry and potentiometric titration with sodium hydroxide are used to assay its purity. Mestranol is identified in pharmaceutical preparations by thin-layer chromatography; liquid chromatography is used to assay for mestranol content (British Pharmacopoeial Commission, 1988; Secretaria de Salud, 1994; United States Pharmacopeial Convention, 1995; Schweizerischen Bundesrat, 1996; Society of Japanese Pharmacopoeia, 1996; Council of Europe, 1997).

1.4   Oestradiol

1.4.1   *Nomenclature*

Chem. Abstr. Serv. Reg. No.: 50-28-2

Chem. Abstr. Name: (17β)-Estra-1,3,5(10)-triene-3,17-diol

IUPAC Systematic Name: Estra-1,3,5(10)-triene-3,17β-diol

Synonyms: Dihydrofollicular hormone; dihydrofolliculin; dihydromenformon; dihydrotheelin; dihydroxyestrin; 3,17β-dihydroxyestra-1,3,5(10)-triene; 3,17-epi-dihydroxyestratriene; β-estradiol; 17β-estradiol; 3,17β-estradiol; (d)-3,17β-estradiol; oestradiol-17β; 17β-oestradiol

1.4.2   *Structural and molecular formulae and relative molecular mass*

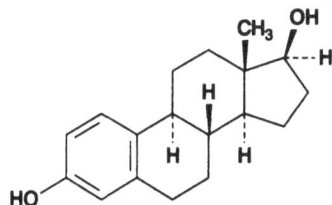

$C_{18}H_{24}O_2$ Relative molecular mass: 272.4

1.4.3   *Chemical and physical properties of the pure substance*

From Budavari (1996) and Reynolds (1998)

(*a*) *Description*: White or creamy-white, odourless, crystalline powder

(*b*) *Melting-point*: 173–179°C

(*c*) *Solubility*: Practically insoluble in water; soluble in ethanol (1 part in 28), chloroform (1 part in 435), diethyl ether (1 part in 150), acetone and dioxane

(*d*) *Optical rotation*: $[\alpha]_D^{25}$, +76° to +83°

Oestradiol hemihydrate is a white crystalline powder: it is practically insoluble in water, soluble in ethanol and acetone and slightly soluble in dichloromethane and diethyl ether. Approximately 1.03 g of oestradiol hemihydrate are equivalent to 1 g of the anhydrous substance (Reynolds, 1998).

1.4.4   *Technical products and impurities*

Oestradiol is commercially available as micronized tablets, as topical transdermal patches, as a vaginal cream and as an extended-release vaginal insert (ring) (United States Food & Drug Administration, 1996; American Hospital Formulary Service, 1997).

1.5   Oestradiol benzoate

1.5.1   *Nomenclature*

Chem. Abstr. Serv. Reg. No.: 50-50-0

Chem. Abstr. Name: (17β)-Estra-1,3,5(10)-triene-3,17-diol, 3-benzoate

IUPAC Systematic Name: Estradiol, 3-benzoate

Synonyms: Estradiol benzoate; β-estradiol benzoate; β-estradiol 3-benzoate; 17β-estradiol benzoate; 17β-estradiol 3-benzoate; estradiol monobenzoate; 1,3,5(10)-estratriene-3,17β-diol 3-benzoate; β-oestradiol benzoate; β-oestradiol 3 benzoate; 17β-oestradiol benzoate; 17β-oestradiol 3-benzoate; oestradiol monobenzoate; 1,3,5(10)-oestratriene-3,17β-diol 3-benzoate

1.5.2   *Structural and molecular formulae and relative molecular mass*

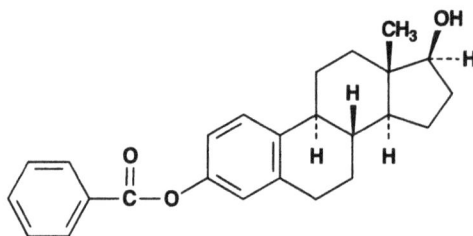

$C_{25}H_{28}O_3$ Relative molecular mass: 376.5

1.5.3   *Chemical and physical properties of the pure substance*

From Budavari (1996) and Reynolds (1996)

- (*a*)   *Description*: White crystalline powder
- (*b*)   *Melting-point*: 191–196°C
- (*c*)   *Solubility*: Practically insoluble in water; slightly soluble in ethanol and diethyl ether; and sparingly soluble in acetone and vegetable oils
- (*d*)   *Optical rotation*: $[\alpha]_D^{25}$, +58° to +63°

1.5.4   *Technical products and impurities*

Oestradiol benzoate is commercially available as an injection (oily or aqueous suspension) and as implants (British Pharmacopoeial Commission, 1993; Society of Japanese Pharmacopoeia, 1996).

1.6   Oestradiol cypionate

1.6.1   *Nomenclature*

Chem. Abstr. Serv. Reg. No.: 313-06-4

Chem. Abstr. Name: (17β)-Estra-1,3,5(10)-triene-3,17-diol, 17-cyclopentanepropanoate

IUPAC Systematic Name: Oestradiol, 17-cyclopentanepropionate

Synonyms: Cyclopentanepropionic acid, 17-ester with oestradiol; cyclopentanepropionic acid, 3-hydroxyestra-1,3,5(10)-trien-17β-yl ester; depo-estradiol cyclopentylpropionate; depoestradiol cypionate; estradiol 17β-cyclopentanepropionate; estradiol cyclopentylpropionate; estradiol 17-cyclopentylpropionate; estradiol 17β-cyclopentylpropionate; 17β-estradiol 17-cyclopentylpropionate; estradiol cypionate; estradiol 17-cypionate; estradiol 17β-cypionate

1.6.2   *Structural and molecular formulae and relative molecular mass*

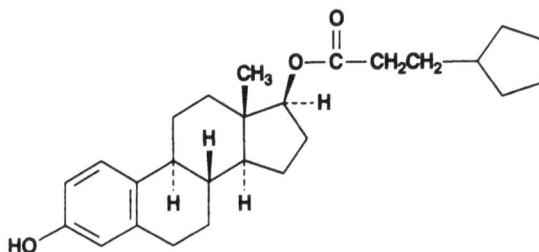

$C_{26}H_{36}O_3$ Relative molecular mass: 396.6

1.6.3   *Chemical and physical properties of the pure substance*

From Budavari (1996) and Reynolds (1996)

(a)   *Description*: White, odourless crystalline powder

(b)   *Melting-point*: 151–152°C

(c)   *Solubility*: Practically insoluble in water; soluble in ethanol (1 part in 40), chloroform (1 in 7), diethyl ether (1 in 2800), acetone and dioxane

(d)   *Optical rotation*: $[\alpha]_D^{25}$, +45°

1.6.4   *Technical products and impurities*

Oestradiol cypionate is commercially available as injectable suspensions in oil for parenteral administration (United States Food & Drug Administration, 1996; American Hospital Formulary Service, 1997).

1.7   Oestradiol valerate

1.7.1   Nomenclature

Chem. Abstr. Serv. Reg. No.: 979-32-8

Deleted CAS Nos.: 907-12-0; 69557-95-5

Chem. Abstr. Name: (17β)-Estra-1,3,5(10)-triene-3,17-diol, 17-pentanoate

IUPAC Systematic Name: Estradiol 17-valerate

Synonyms: Oestradiol valerate; estradiol 17β-valerate; estradiol valerianate; estra-1,3,5(10)-triene-3,17β-diol 17-valerate; 3-hydroxy-17β-valeroyloxyestra-1,3,5(10)-triene

1.7.2   *Structural and molecular formulae and relative molecular mass*

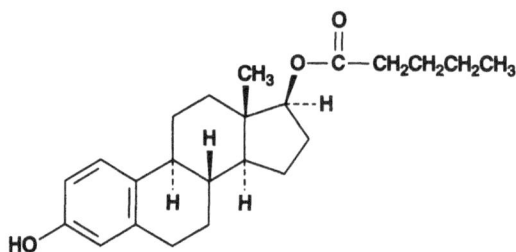

$C_{23}H_{32}O_3$ Relative molecular mass: 356.5

1.7.3   *Chemical and physical properties of the pure substance*

From Budavari (1996) and Reynolds (1996)

(*a*)   *Description*: White, crystalline, odourless powder

(*b*)   *Melting-point*: 144–145°C

(*c*)   *Solubility*: Practically insoluble in water; soluble in benzyl benzoate, dioxane, methanol and castor oil; sparingly soluble in arachis oil and sesame oil

1.7.4   *Technical products and impurities*

Oestradiol valerate is commercially available as injectable suspensions in oil for parenteral administration; it is also commercially available as tablets alone or in combination with progestogens (Reynolds, 1996; United States Food & Drug Administration, 1996; American Hospital Formulary Service, 1997; Editions du Vidal, 1997).

Other esters of oestradiol that have been reported and that may have been used as pharmaceuticals include oestradiol 17β-acetate 3-benzoate, oestradiol 3,17β-dipropionate, oestradiol 3,17β-diundecylenate, oestradiol 17β-oenanthate, oestradiol 17β-hexahydro-benzoate, oestradiol 17β-phenylpropionate, oestradiol 17β-stearate, oestradiol 17β-un-decylate and polyoestradiol phosphate.

1.7.5   *Analysis*

Several international pharmacopoeias specify infra-red and ultra-violet absorption spectrophotometry with comparison to standards and thin-layer chromatography as methods for identifying oestradiol and its hemihydrate; ultra-violet absorption and liquid chromatography are used to assay its purity. Oestradiol in vaginal creams and tablets is identified by thin-layer chromatography; liquid chromatography is used to assay the oestradiol content of these preparations. Oestradiol in pellets and sterile suspensions is identified by infra-red spectroscopy with comparison to standards; ultra-violet absorption spectrophotometry is used to assay the oestradiol content. Methods for identifying oestradiol benzoate include infra-red absorption spectrophotometry with comparison to standards, fluorescence and thin-layer chromatography. Ultra-violet absorption spectrophotometry, thin-layer chromatography and liquid chromatography are used to assay its purity. Methods for identifying oestradiol cypionate include infra-red and ultra-violet absorption spectroscopy with comparison to standards; high-pressure liquid chromatography is used to assay its purity. Oestradiol valerate is identified in pharmaceutical preparations by infra-red absorption spectroscopy with comparison to standards, and liquid chromatography is used to assay the oestradiol valerate content (British Pharmacopoeial Commission, 1988, 1993; United States Pharmacopeial Convention, 1995; Society of the Japanese Pharmacopoeia, 1996; Council of Europe, 1997).

1.8   Oestriol

1.8.1   *Nomenclature*

    Chem. Abstr. Serv. Reg. No.: 50-27-1

    Chem. Abstr. Name: (16α,17β)-Estra-1,3,5(10)-triene-3,16,17-triol

    IUPAC Systematic Name: Estriol

    Synonyms: Estra-1,3,5(10)-triene-3,16α,17β-triol; estratriol; 16α-estriol; 16α,17β-estriol; 3,16α,17β-estriol; follicular hormone hydrate; 16α-hydroxyestradiol; 3,16α,17β-trihydroxyestra-1,3,5(10)-triene; trihydroxyestrin

1.8.2   *Structural and molecular formulae and relative molecular mass*

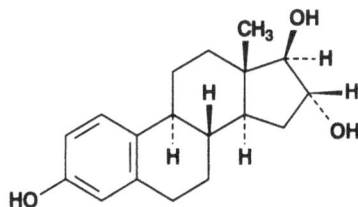

$C_{18}H_{24}O_3$ Relative molecular mass: 288.4

1.8.3   *Chemical and physical properties of the pure substance*

From Budavari (1996) and Reynolds (1998)

    (*a*) *Description*: White, odourless, crystalline powder

    (*b*) *Melting-point*: 282°C

    (*c*) *Solubility*: Practically insoluble in water; sparingly soluble in ethanol; soluble in acetone, chloroform, dioxane, diethyl ether and vegetable oils

(d)   *Specific rotation*: $[\alpha]_D^{25}$, +58°

1.8.4   *Technical products and impurities*

Oestriol is commercially available as tablets and as a cream. Sodium succinate and succinate salts of oestriol are also available (Morant & Ruppanner, 1991; Thomas, 1997).

1.8.5   *Analysis*

The Japanese and United States pharmacopoeias specify infra-red and ultra-violet absorption spectrophotometry with comparison to standards as methods for identifying oestriol; ultra-violet absorption spectrophotometry, thin-layer chromatography and liquid chromatography are used to assay its purity (United States Pharmacopeial Convention, 1995; Society of Japanese Pharmacopoeia, 1996).

1.9   Oestrone

1.9.1   *Nomenclature*

Chem. Abstr. Serv. Reg. No.: 53-16-7
Deleted CAS Reg. No.: 37242-41-4
Chem. Abstr. Name: 3-Hydroxyestra-1,3,5(10)-trien-17-one
IUPAC Systematic Name: 3-Hydroxyestra-1,2,5(10)-triene-17-one
Synonyms: d-Estrone; d-oestrone

1.9.2   *Structural and molecular formulae and relative molecular mass*

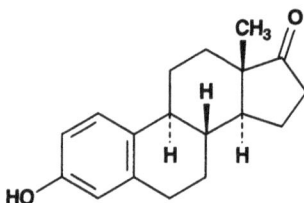

$C_{18}H_{22}O_2$ Relative molecular mass: 270.4

1.9.3   *Chemical and physical properties of the pure substance*

From Budavari (1996) and Reynolds (1998)

(a)   *Description*: White to creamy-white, crystalline powder
(b)   *Melting-point*: 254.5–256°C
(c)   *Solubility*: Practically insoluble in water (0.003 g/100 mL at 25°C); soluble in ethanol (1 in 250), chloroform (1 in 110 at 15°C), acetone (1 in 50 at 50°C), dioxane and vegetable oils; slightly soluble in diethyl ether and solutions of alkali hydroxides
(d)   *Specific rotation*: $[\alpha]_D^{22}$, +152°

1.9.4 *Technical products and impurities*

Oestrone is commercially available as pessaries and as a sterile suspension in water or 0.9% sodium chloride for injection. Oestrone benzoate and oestrone sodium sulfate are also available (Thomas, 1991; Gennaro, 1995; American Hospital Formulary Service, 1997).

1.9.5 *Analysis*

The United States Pharmacopeia specifies infra-red and ultra-violet absorption spectrophotometry with comparison to standards and thin-layer chromatography as methods for identifying oestrone; liquid chromatography is used to assay the purity of oestrone and to determine its content in pharmaceutical preparations (United States Pharmacopeial Convention, 1995).

1.10 Oestropipate

1.10.1 *Nomenclature*

Chem. Abstr. Serv. Reg. No.: 7280-37-7

Deleted CAS No.: 29080-16-8

Chem. Abstr. Name: 3-(Sulfooxy)-estra-1,3,5(10)-trien-17-one, compd. with piperazine (1:1)

IUPAC Systematic Name: Estrone, hydrogen sulfate, compd. with piperazine (1:1)

Synonyms: Piperazine estrone sulfate; piperazine oestrone sulfate; 3-sulfatoxyestra-1,3,5(10)-trien-17-one piperazine salt; 3-sulfatoxyoestra-1,3,5(10)-trien-17-one piperazine salt

1.10.2 *Structural and molecular formulae and relative molecular mass*

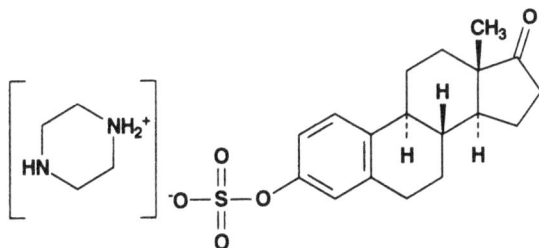

$C_{22}H_{32}N_2O_5S$ Relative molecular mass: 436.6

1.10.3 *Chemical and physical properties of the pure substance*

From Budavari (1996) and Reynolds (1998)

(*a*) *Description*: White to yellowish-white, odourless, fine crystalline powder

(*b*) *Melting-point*: 190°C; solidifies on further heating and decomposes at 245°C

(*c*) *Solubility*: Very slightly soluble in water, ethanol, chloroform and diethyl ether; soluble in warm water and warm ethanol (1 part in 500)

(*d*) *Optical rotation*: $[\alpha]_D^{25}$, +87.8°

1.10.4   *Technical products and impurities*

Oestropipate is available as tablets and as a vaginal cream (Gennaro, 1995; American Hospital Formulary Service, 1997). Information available in 1996 indicated that it was manufactured or formulated in the United Kingdom and the United States (Reynolds, 1996).

1.10.5   *Analysis*

Methods for the identification of oestropipate include infra-red absorption with comparison to standards and thin-layer chromatography; liquid chromatography and high-pressure liquid chromatography are used to assay its purity (United States Pharmacopeial Convention, 1995).

1.11   Production and use

1.11.1   *Production*

Oestrogens are either isolated from the urine of pregnant mares (conjugated and esterified oestrogens) or synthesized. The synthesis of ethinyloestradiol was first reported in 1938 by treatment of oestrone with potassium acetylide in liquid ammonia. It is believed to be produced commercially by the same method (Sittig, 1988). It was produced in the United States between 1945 and 1955 (United States Tariff Commission, 1947, 1956). Information available in 1995 indicated that ethinyloestradiol was manufactured or formulated in Argentina, Australia, Austria, Belgium, Brazil, Canada, Denmark, Finland, France, Germany, India, Italy, Japan, Mexico, the Netherlands, Norway, Poland, Portugal, South Africa, Spain, Switzerland, the United Kingdom and the United States (CIS Information Services, 1995).

The first synthesis of mestranol was reported in 1954 (Sittig, 1988). Commercial production in the United Kingdom was first reported in 1955. It was first marketed in Japan in 1960 (IARC, 1979). Mestranol is prepared by converting oestrone to its 3-methoxy analogue by reaction with methyl sulfate. The ethinyl group may then be introduced at position 17, either by reaction with sodium acetylide in liquid ammonia followed by hydrolysis or through a Grignard reaction with ethynyl bromide (Sittig, 1988; Gennaro, 1995). Information available in 1995 indicated that mestranol was manufactured or formulated in Argentina, Australia, Belgium, Brazil, Canada, Denmark, Germany, India, Japan, Mexico, New Zealand, South Africa, Spain, Switzerland, the United Kingdom and the United States (CIS Information Services, 1995).

The countries in which oestrogens used in oestrogen replacement therapy are manufactured and/or formulated are listed in Table 1.

1.11.2   *Use*

Conjugated oestrogens, oestradiol and its semisynthetic esters, especially oestradiol valerate, are used mainly in the treatment of menopausal disorders and for the prevention and treatment of osteoporosis; they have been proposed for use in the prevention of cardiovascular diseases (Sullivan & Fowlkes, 1996) and of Alzheimer disease (Paganini-Hill & Henderson, 1994). Conjugated oestrogens are usually administered orally in a dose of

Table 1. Countries in which oestrogens used in oestrogen replacement therapy are manufactured or formulated

Country	Oestradiol	Oestradiol benzoate	Oestradiol valerate	Oestradiol oenanthate	Oestrone	Oestrone sulfate	Oestriol
Argentina	X	X	X	X			X
Australia	X	X	X		X	X	X
Austria	X		X				X
Belgium	X	X	X				X
Brazil	X	X	X	X		X	X
Canada	X	X	X	X	X		
Denmark	X	X	X				X
Finland	X		X			X	X
France	X	X	X		X		X
Germany	X	X	X		X	X	X
India	X	X					
Italy	X	X					
Japan	X	X	X				X
Mexico	X	X	X	X			X
Netherlands	X	X	X				X
New Zealand	X	X	X				
Poland		X					
Portugal	X	X		X	X		X
South Africa	X	X	X		X		X
Spain	X	X	X	X		X	X
Sweden	X	X					X
Switzerland	X	X	X		X		X
United Kingdom	X	X	X		X		X
United States	X	X	X				X

From CIS Information Services (1995)

0.3–1.25 mg/day and have been used extensively in the United Kingdom and the United States for the treatment of climacteric symptoms. In Europe, micronized oestradiol and oestradiol valerate are the most popular preparations used in post-menopausal oestrogen therapy. Oestropipate at a dose of 0.75–3 mg per day has also been used (Ellerington *et al.*, 1992; American Hospital Formulary Service, 1997; British Medical Association, 1997).

Oestradiol is the main naturally occurring oestrogen. It is given in the form of oestradiol or one of its semisynthetic esters in cases of oestrogen deficiency, such as primary and secondary amenorrhoea, and in the menopause (Reynolds, 1996).

Oestradiol can be administered via a percutaneous patch in which the dose of hormone absorbed can be regulated by the surface area of the patch (Corson, 1993; Birkhäuser & Haenggi, 1994; Judd, 1994; Gordon, 1995). Patches are available that deliver oestradiol at a dose of 25, 37.7, 50, 75 or 100 µg daily. The patches should be changed once or twice weekly. Oestradiol can also be administered in the form of a gel applied directly to the skin (American Hospital Formulary Service, 1997; British Medical Association, 1997).

The metabolic products of oestradiol, oestrone and oestriol, are also used in clinical practice. Oestrone is a less potent oestrogen, but it is metabolized back to oestradiol (Williams & Stancel, 1996). It is administered orally, mainly as the sulfate. Oestriol is a weak oestrogen, with mainly local effects. It is used in vaginal creams and vaginal suppositories at a daily dose of 0.5–1 mg in the treatment of urogenital symptoms in women in whom systemic effects should be avoided (Reynolds, 1996; American Hospital Formulary Service, 1997; Editions du Vidal, 1997).

Ethinyloestradiol is used most extensively in oral contraceptives in combination with a progestogen. Other indications include peri-menopausal symptoms, hormonal therapy for hypogonadal women, treatment of post-partum breast engorgement and dysfunctional uterine bleeding and therapy for carcinoma of the breast and prostate. It is also used in conjunction with progestogens for the treatment of post-menopausal symptoms. Ethinyloestradiol is also used in conjunction with a progestogen as a post-coital contraceptive (Gennaro, 1995; Reynolds, 1996; Hatcher *et al.*, 1997).

Mestranol is an effective oestrogen for the typical uses of oestrogens, but it is marketed only in combination regimens typically containing 0.05 mg mestranol (Reynolds, 1996). Other indications for use of mestranol combined with a progestogen are in the treatment of dysmenorrhoea and menorrhagia, to produce cyclic withdrawal bleeding, in the treatment of pre-menstrual tension, amenorrhoea and idiopathic infertility, for emergency control of dysfunctional uterine bleeding, for endometriosis or to delay menstruation (Gennaro, 1995). Mestranol is also used with a progestogen to treat menopausal symptoms and for the prevention and treatment of osteoporosis (British Medical Association, 1997).

1.12 Regulations and guidelines

The only guidelines that could be found for use of oestrogens are those in national and international pharmacopoeias (Secretaria de Salud, 1994, 1995; United States Pharmacopeial Convention, 1995; Reynolds, 1996; Society of Japanese Pharmacopoeia, 1996; Council of Europe, 1997; Reynolds, 1998; Swiss Pharmaceutical Society, 1998).

2. Progestogens

2.1 Chlormadinone acetate

2.1.1 *Nomenclature*

Chem. Abstr. Serv. Reg. No.: 302-22-7
Chem. Abstr. Name: 17-(Acetyloxy)-6-chloropregna-4,6-diene-3,20-dione
IUPAC Systematic Name: 6-Chloro-17-hydroxypregna-4,6-diene-3,20-dione, acetate
Synonyms: 17α-Acetoxy-6-chloro-4,6-pregnadiene-3,20-dione; 6-chloro-Δ⁶-17-acetoxyprogesterone; 6-chloro-Δ⁶-[17α]acetoxyprogesterone

2.1.2 *Structural and molecular formulae and relative molecular mass*

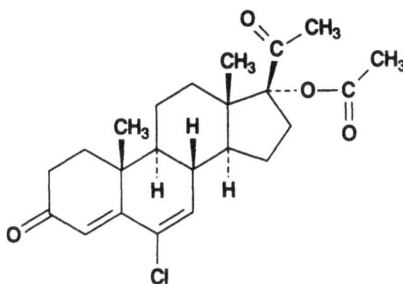

$C_{23}H_{29}ClO_4$ Relative molecular mass: 404.9

2.1.3 *Chemical and physical properties of the pure substance*

From Budavari (1996) and Society of Japanese Pharmacopoeia (1996)

(a) *Description*: White to light-yellow, odourless crystals
(b) *Melting-point*: 212–214°C
(c) *Solubility*: Practically insoluble in water; very soluble in chloroform; soluble in acetonitrile; slightly soluble in ethanol and diethyl ether
(d) *Optical rotation*: $[\alpha]_D^{20}$, –10.0° to –14.0°

2.1.4 *Technical products and impurities*

Trade names for pharmaceutical preparations of chlormadinone acetate include Gestafortin and Luteran (Reynolds, 1996).

2.1.5 *Analysis*

Several international pharmacopoeias specify infra-red and ultra-violet absorption spectrophotometry with comparison to standards and liquid chromatography as methods for identifying chlormadinone acetate; liquid chromatography and ultra-violet absorption spectrophotometry are used to assay its purity (Secretaria de Salud, 1994, 1995; Society of Japanese Pharmacopoeia, 1996).

2.1.6   *Production and use*

Chlormadinone acetate does not occur naturally. Its synthesis was first reported in 1960, by the treatment of 17α-acetoxyprogesterone with ethyl orthoformate in the presence of an acid catalyst to produce the 3-enol ether of the corresponding 3,5-dione; conversion of this enol ether to 6-chloro-17α-acetoxyprogesterone with *N*-chlorosuccinimide is followed by dehydrogenation with chloranil (Brückner *et al.*, 1961).

Information available in 1995 indicated that chlormadinone acetate was manufactured or formulated in Argentina, Austria, France, Germany, Japan, Mexico and Switzerland (CIS Information Services, 1995).

Chlormadinone acetate has not been used in the United States since 1970, when the only product (an oral contraceptive) was removed from the market. Its use in the United Kingdom was suspended in the same year. Before suspension, chlormadinone acetate was used in oral contraceptives either together with mestranol as a 'sequential' contraceptive or as a 'progestogen only' oral contraceptive (IARC, 1979). Chlormadinone acetate has been used (frequently in combination with mestranol) for treatment of threatened abortion (Notter & Durand, 1969) and dysmenorrhoea (Roland *et al.*, 1966).

2.2   Cyproterone acetate

2.2.1   *Nomenclature*

Chem. Abstr. Serv. Reg. No.: 427-51-0

Chem. Abstr. Name: (1β,2β)-17-(Acetyloxy)-6-chloro-1,2-dihydro-3′H-cyclopropa-[1,2]pregna-1,4,6-triene-3,20-dione

IUPAC Systematic Name: 6-Chloro-1β,2β-dihydro-17-hydroxy-3′H-cyclopropa[1,2]-pregna-1,4,6-triene-3,20-dione acetate

Synonyms: Cyproterone 17-*O*-acetate; cyproterone 17α-acetate; 1,2α-methylene-6-chloro-17α-acetoxy-4,6-pregnadiene-3,20-dione; 1,2α-methylene-6-chloro-Δ^{4,6}-pre-gnadien-17α-ol-3,20-dione acetate; 1,2α-methylene-6-chloro-pregna-4,6-diene-3,20-dione 17α-acetate; methylene-6-chloro-17-hydroxy-1α,2α-pregna-4,6-diene-3,20-dione acetate

2.2.2   *Structural and molecular formulae and relative molecular mass*

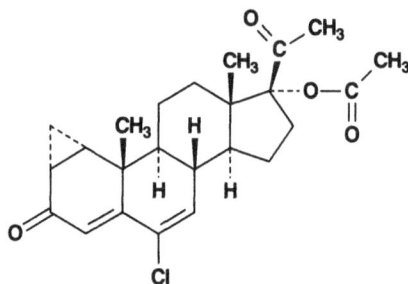

$C_{24}H_{29}ClO_4$ Relative molecular mass: 416.9

2.2.3 *Chemical and physical properties of the pure substance*
From Budavari (1996) and Council of Europe (1997)
(a) *Description:* White crystalline powder
(b) *Melting-point:* 200–201°C
(c) *Solubility:* Practically insoluble in water; very soluble in dichloromethane and acetone; soluble in methanol; sparingly soluble in ethanol
(d) *Specific rotation:* $[\alpha]_D^{20}$, +152° to +157°

2.2.4 *Technical products and impurities*
Cyproterone acetate is commercially available as tablets and as an injectable solution (Organizzazione Editoriale Medico Farmaceutica, 1995; British Medical Association, 1997).

2.2.5 *Analysis*
The European Pharmacopoeia specifies infra-red absorption spectrophotometry and thin-layer chromatography as methods for identifying cyproterone acetate; liquid chromatography and ultra-violet absorption spectrophotometry are used to assay its purity (Council of Europe, 1997).

2.2.6 *Production and use*
Cyproterone acetate does not occur naturally. No information was available on its synthesis. Information available in 1995 indicated that its was manufactured or formulated in Argentina, Australia, Austria, Belgium, Brazil, Canada, Finland, France, Germany, Japan, Mexico, New Zealand, South Africa, Spain, Switzerland and the United Kingdom (CIS Information Services, 1995).

Cyproterone acetate has a strong gonadotrophin-inhibiting effect and has clinical use as an anti-androgen for the treatment of hyperandrogenic disorders such as hirsutism, acne and seborrhoea in women. It is used as an oral contraceptive in combination with ethinyl-oestradiol. It is given in combination with oestradiol valerate to women over 35 up to the climacteric because its effects on the coagulation system are minimal (Hirvonen *et al.*, 1988; Reynolds, 1996). Cyproterone acetate is also used in the treatment of prostate cancer and hypersexuality disorders (Cooper, 1986; Neumann & Topert, 1986; Namer, 1988) and is being investigated as a means of oral contraception in men (Moltz *et al.*, 1980; Wang & Yeung, 1980; Meriggiola *et al.*, 1996). In some European countries, cyproterone acetate is used in sequential preparations with oestradiol valerate in the treatment of climacteric complaints (Editions du Vidal, 1997).

2.3 Desogestrel
2.3.1 *Nomenclature*
Chem. Abstr. Serv. Reg. No.: 54024-22-5
Chem. Abstr. Name: (17α)-13-Ethyl-11-methylene-18,19-dinorpregn-4-en-20-yn-17-ol

IUPAC Systematic Name: 13-Ethyl-11-methylene-18,19-dinor-17α-pregn-4-en-20-yn-17-ol

Synonyms: 13-Ethyl-11-methylene-18,19-dinor-17α-4-pregnen-20-yn-17-ol; 17α-ethynyl-18-methyl-11-methylene-Δ⁴-oestren-17β-ol

2.3.2   *Structural and molecular formulae and relative molecular mass*

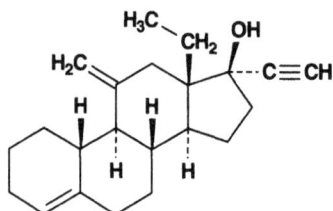

C$_{22}$H$_{30}$O   Relative molecular mass: 310.5

2.3.3   *Chemical and physical properties of the pure substance*
From Budavari (1996) and British Pharmacopoeial Commission (1997)

(*a*)   *Description*: White crystalline powder

(*b*)   *Melting-point*: 109–110°C

(*c*)   *Solubility*: Practically insoluble in water; slightly soluble in ethanol and ethyl acetate; sparingly soluble in *n*-hexane

(*d*)   *Optical rotation*: $[\alpha]_D^{20}$, +53° to +57°

2.3.4   *Technical products and impurities*
Desogestrel is commercially available only in combination with ethinyloestradiol (Reynolds, 1996; American Hospital Formulary Service, 1997; British Medical Association, 1997; Editions du Vidal, 1997; LINFO Läkemedelsinformation AB, 1997; Reynolds, 1998).

2.3.5   *Analysis*
The British Pharmacopoeia specifies infra-red absorption spectrophotometry and thin-layer chromatography as methods for identifying desogestrel; liquid chromatography is used to assay its purity (British Pharmacopoeial Commission, 1997).

2.3.6   *Production and use*
Desogestrel does not occur naturally. It is produced by adding a solution of 11,11-methylene-18-methyl-Δ⁴-oestren-17-one in tetrahydrofuran to potassium acetylide solution in tetrahydrofuran and acidified (Sittig, 1988).

Information available in 1995 indicated that desogestrel was manufactured or formulated in Argentina, Australia, Belgium, Brazil, Canada, France, Germany, India, Mexico, the Netherlands, South Africa, Spain, Switzerland, the United Kingdom and the United States (CIS Information Services, 1995).

Desogestrel is a synthetic progestogen structurally related to levonorgestrel, with actions and uses similar to those of progestogens in general. It is reported to have potent progestogenic activity and little or no androgenic activity. It is used as the progestogenic component of combined mono- and multiphasic oral contraceptive preparations and as a subdermal implantable 'progestogen-only' contraceptive. A typical daily dose in combined oral contraceptives is 150 μg (Reynolds, 1997) with 30 μg ethinyloestradiol (Williams & Stancel, 1996; Editions du Vidal, 1997).

2.4 Dydrogesterone

2.4.1 *Nomenclature*
Chem. Abstr. Serv. Reg. No.: 152-62-5
Chem. Abstr. Name: (9β,10α)-Pregna-4,6-diene-3,20-dione
IUPAC Systematic Name: 10α-Pregna-4,6-diene-3,20-dione
Synonyms: 10α-Isopregnenone; dehydro-retroprogesterone; dehydroprogesterone

2.4.2 *Structural and molecular formulae and relative molecular mass*

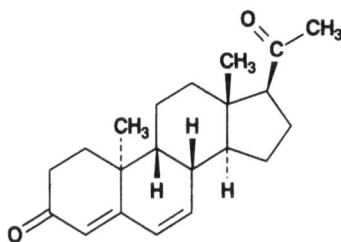

$C_{21}H_{28}O_2$ Relative molecular mass: 312.5

2.4.3 *Chemical and physical properties of the pure substance*
From Budavari (1996) and Reynolds (1996)
(*a*) *Description*: White to off-white, odourless, crystalline powder
(*b*) *Melting-point*: 169–170°C
(*c*) *Solubility*: Practically insoluble in water; soluble in acetone, chloroform (1 in 2), ethanol (1 in 40) and diethyl ether (1 in 200); slightly soluble in fixed oils; sparingly soluble in methanol
(*d*) *Specific rotation*: $[\alpha]_D^{25}$, −484.5° (in chloroform)

2.4.4 *Technical products and impurities*
Trade names for pharmaceutical preparations containing dydrogesterone are listed in Annex 2 (Table 5).

2.4.5 *Analysis*
Several international pharmacopoeias specify infra-red and ultra-violet absorption spectrophotometry with comparison to standards as methods for identifying dydroges-

terone; ultra-violet absorption spectrophotometry and liquid chromatography are used to assay its purity. Dydrogesterone is identified in pharmaceutical preparations by infra-red and ultra-violet absorption spectrophotometry; ultra-violet absorption spectrophotometry and liquid chromatography are used to assay for dydrogesterone content (British Pharmacopoeial Commission,1988; United States Pharmacopeial Convention, 1990).

2.4.6   Production and use

Dydrogesterone does not occur naturally. It is believed to be prepared commercially from lumisterol (9β,10α-ergosta-5,7,22-trien-3β-ol derived from ultra-violet-irradiated ergosterol) via a multistep synthesis involving oxidation, isomerization, lithium reduction, ozonolysis of the side-chain and a final zinc reduction (Budavari, 1996).

In hormonal therapy, dydrogesterone is used at doses of 10–20 mg per day for 10–14 days per cycle. Together with cyclic or continuous oestrogen, it gives effective cycle control and good protection of the endometrium. It does not inhibit secretion of follicle-stimulating hormone and does not increase basal body temperature (Reynolds, 1996; British Medical Association, 1997; Crook *et al.*, 1997).

2.5   Ethynodiol diacetate

2.5.1   Nomenclature

Chem. Abstr. Serv. Reg. No.: 297-76-7
Chem. Abstr. Name: (3β,17α)-19-Norpregn-4-en-20-yne-3,17-diol, diacetate
IUPAC Systematic Name: 19-Nor-17α-pregn-4-en-20-yne-3β,17β-diol, diacetate
Synonyms: Ethinodiol diacetate; ethynodiol acetate; β-ethynodiol diacetate

2.5.2   Structural and molecular formulae and relative molecular mass

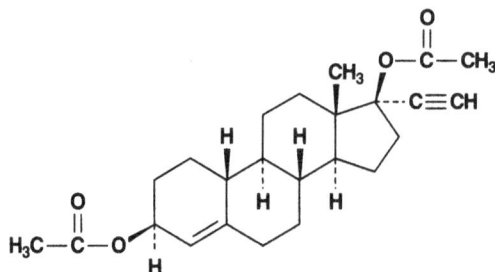

$C_{24}H_{32}O_4$ Relative molecular mass: 384.5

2.5.3   Chemical and physical properties of the pure substance

(a) *Description:* White, odourless, crystalline powder (Reynolds, 1998)
(b) *Melting-point:* ~126–127°C (Budavari, 1996)
(c) *Solubility:* Very slightly soluble to practically insoluble in water; soluble in ethanol; freely to very soluble in chloroform; freely soluble in diethyl ether (Reynolds, 1998)

(*d*) *Optical rotation*: $[\alpha]_D^{20}$, −70° to −76° (British Pharmacopoeial Commission, 1993)

2.5.4   *Technical products and impurities*

Ethynodiol diacetate is commercially available alone or as a component of a combination tablet containing ethynodiol diacetate plus ethinyloestradiol or mestranol (Thomas, 1991; Kleinman, 1996; Medical Economics, 1996; US Food & Drug Administration, 1996; American Hospital Formulary Service, 1997; British Medical Association, 1997; Reynolds, 1998).

2.5.5   *Analysis*

The British and United States pharmacopoeias specify infra-red and ultra-violet absorption spectrophotometry with comparison to standards as methods for identifying ethynodiol diacetate; potentiometric titration with sodium hydroxide and liquid chromatography are used to assay its purity. Thin-layer chromatography is specified to identify ethynodiol diacetate in combination formulations; liquid chromatography is used to assay the quantity of ethynodiol diacetate in combination tablets (British Pharmacopoeial Commission, 1993; United States Pharmacopeial Convention, 1995).

2.5.6   *Production and use*

Ethynodiol diacetate does not occur naturally. A method for its synthesis was first patented in the United States in 1965. Ethindrone is reduced to ethynodiol, which is acetylated with acetic anhydride in pyridine to produce ethynodiol diacetate. Ethynodiol diacetate can also be prepared from ethynodiol or from norethisterone by reducing the keto group to the carbinol and acetylating the 3- and 17-hydroxyls (Sittig, 1988; Gennaro, 1995). It is not known which process is used for commercial production.

Ethynodiol diacetate was introduced in France in 1965, in the United States in 1966, in Italy in 1971 and in the United Kingdom in 1973 (Sittig, 1988).

Information available in 1995 indicated that ethynodiol diacetate was manufactured or formulated in Argentina, Australia, Brazil, Canada, France, India, the Netherlands, New Zealand, South Africa, Switzerland, the United Kingdom and the United States (CIS Information Services, 1995).

Ethynodiol diacetate is a progestogen with actions and uses similar to those of norethisterone; however, because it has a hydroxyl rather than a keto group at the 3-position of the A ring, it has stronger oestrogenic activity and is essentially devoid of androgenic activity. For use as an oral contraceptive, it has been combined with an oestrogen at a typical dose of 1 mg ethynodiol diacetate and either 35 or 50 µg ethinyloestradiol or 0.1 mg mestranol (Gennaro, 1995). It is also used as a 'progestogen-only' contraceptive (British Medical Association, 1997).

2.6   Gestodene

2.6.1   *Nomenclature*

    Chem. Abstr. Serv. Reg. No.: 60282-87-3

    Deleted CAS Reg. No.: 110541-55-4

    Chem. Abstr. Name: (17α)-13-Ethyl-17-hydroxy-18,19-dinorpregna-4,15-dien-20-yn-3-one

    IUPAC Systematic Name: 13-Ethyl-17-hydroxy-18,19-dinor-17α-pregna-4,15-dien-20-yn-3-one

2.6.2   *Structural and molecular formulae and relative molecular mass*

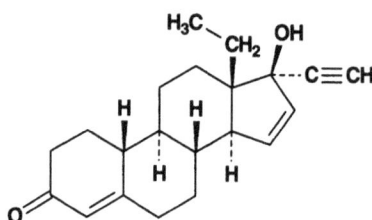

$C_{21}H_{26}O_2$ Relative molecular mass: 310.4

2.6.3   *Chemical and physical properties of the pure substance*

    From Budavari (1996)

    (*a*)   *Description*: Crystals

    (*b*)   *Melting-point*: 197.9°C

2.6.4   *Technical products and impurities*

    Gestodene is commercially available as a component of combination tablets with ethinyloestradiol (Morant & Ruppanner, 1991; British Medical Association, 1997; Editions du Vidal, 1997; Thomas, 1997).

2.6.5   *Analysis*

    No information was available to the Working Group.

2.6.6   *Production and use*

    Gestodene does not occur naturally. It can be prepared from the 17-keto steroid [18-methyloestrone methyl ether] in a multistep synthesis involving palladium-catalysed conversion of its enol ether to an enone, reduction to the corresponding allylic alcohol, partial reduction of the aromatic ring, regeneration of the enone and ethinylation (Bohlman *et al.*, 1989).

    Information available in 1995 indicated that gestodene was manufactured or formulated in Argentina, Austria, Belgium, Brazil, Finland, France, Germany, Mexico, the Netherlands, New Zealand, Portugal, South Africa, Spain, Switzerland and the United Kingdom (CIS Information Services, 1995).

Gestodene is used only in combination with ethinyloestradiol as an oral contraceptive, at a dose of 0.075 mg gestodene and 20 or 30 µg ethinyloestradiol, and in a triphasic regimen at 0.05, 0.07 and 0.1 mg gestodene and 30, 40 and 30 µg ethinyloestradiol (Kleinman, 1996).

2.7 Levonorgestrel

2.7.1 *Nomenclature*

Chem. Abstr. Serv. Reg. No.: 797-63-7
Deleted CAS Reg. No.: 797-62-6; 4222-79-1; 121714-72-5
Chem. Abstr. Name: (17α)-13-Ethyl-17-hydroxy-18,19-dinorpregn-4-en-20-yn-3-one
IUPAC Systematic Name: 13-Ethyl-17-hydroxy-18,19-dinor-17α-pregn-4-en-20-yn-3-one
Synonyms: 13-Ethyl-17-ethynyl-17β-hydroxy-4-gonen-3-one; 13-ethyl-17α-ethynyl-17-hydroxygon-4-en-3-one; 13-ethyl-17α-ethynylgon-4-en-17β-ol-3-one; 13β-ethyl-17α-ethynyl-17β-hydroxygon-4-en-3-one; 13-ethyl-17-hydroxy-18,19-dinor-17α-pregn-4-en-20-yn-3-one; 17-ethynyl-18-methyl-19-nortestosterone; 18-methylnorethindrone; l-norgestrel; D-l-norgestrel; D-norgestrel

2.7.2 *Structural and molecular formulae and relative molecular mass*

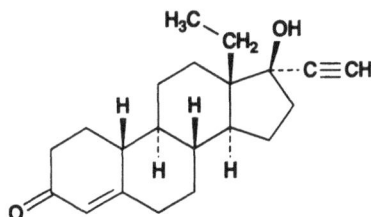

$C_{21}H_{28}O_2$ Relative molecular mass: 312.5

2.7.3 *Chemical and physical properties of the pure substance*

From Budavari (1996) and Reynolds (1998)

(a) *Description*: White, odourless, crystalline powder
(b) *Melting-point*: 235–237°C
(c) *Solubility:* Practically insoluble in water; slightly soluble in ethanol, acetone and diethyl ether; sparingly soluble in dichloromethane; soluble in chloroform
(d) *Specific rotation:* $[\alpha]_D^{20}$, –32.4°

2.7.4 *Technical products and impurities*

Levonorgestrel is commercially available as a single-ingredient tablet (Kleinman, 1996; Editions du Vidal, 1997); it is also available as an interuterine system and as a flexible, closed-capsule implant made of silicone rubber tubing (Medical Economics, 1996; LINFO Läkemedelsinformation AB, 1997). Levonorgestrel is also used in combination with ethinyloestradiol for contraception (Kleinman, 1996; Medical Economics, 1996; Editions du Vidal, 1997) and in combination with several other pharmaceutical preparations including oestradiol, oestradiol valerate, oestriol and ethinyloestradiol for hormonal replacement therapy (British Medical Association, 1997; Reynolds, 1998).

2.7.5   *Analysis*

Several international pharmacopoeias specify infra-red and ultra-violet visible absorption spectrophotometry and optical rotation with comparison to standards as methods for identifying levonorgestrel; potentiometric titration and ultra-violet absorption spectrophotometry are used to assay its purity. Levonorgestrel is identified in pharmaceutical preparations by ultra-violet absorption visible spectrophotometry and thin-layer chromatography (British Pharmacopoeial Commission, 1993; United States Pharmacopeial Convention, 1995; Council of Europe, 1997).

2.7.6   *Production and use*

Levonorgestrel does not occur naturally. Several methods for the synthesis of norgestrel were reported in the early 1960s (Sittig, 1988; Budavari, 1996).

The activity of norgestrel is found in the levorotatory form D-l-norgestrel or levonorgestrel. Synthesis of the levorotatory form involves *meta*-cresol methyl ether, dimethyl malonate and *trans*-1,4-dibromo-2-butene as starting materials. The steroid skeleton was constructed by using an intramolecular Diels-Alder reaction of an *ortho*-quinodimethane derivative, preceded by photo-enolization of an appropriate methyl-substituted acetophenone derivative. Chirality was introduced at an early stage during a nucleophilic substitution reaction (Baier *et al.*, 1985). It is not known if this synthesis is used commercially.

Information available in 1995 indicated that levonorgestrel was manufactured or formulated in Argentina, Australia, Austria, Belgium, Brazil, Canada, Finland, France, Germany, India, Mexico, the Netherlands, New Zealand, Portugal, South Africa, Spain, Switzerland, the United Kingdom and the United States (CIS Information Services, 1995).

Levonorgestrel is used as a combined oral contraceptive with ethinyloestradiol in monophasic, biphasic and triphasic regimens. It is also used as a 'progestogen-only' contraceptive pill and subdermal implant (Kleinman, 1996).

2.8   Lynoestrenol

2.8.1   *Nomenclature*

Chem. Abstr. Serv. Reg. No.: 52-76-6

Deleted CAS Reg. No.: 60416-16-2

Chem. Abstr. Name: (17α)-19-Norpregn-4-en-20-yn-17-ol

IUPAC Systematic Name: 19-Nor-17α-pregn-4-en-20-yn-17-ol

Synonyms: 3-Desoxynorlutin; Δ⁴-17α-ethinylestren-17β-ol; Δ⁴-17α-ethinyloestren-17β-ol; ethynylestrenol; ethynyloestrenol; 17α-ethynylestrenol; 17α-ethynyloestrenol; 17α-ethynyl-17β-hydroxy-Δ⁴-estrene; 17α-ethynyl-17β-hydroxy-Δ⁴-oestrene

2.8.2   *Structural and molecular formulae and relative molecular mass*

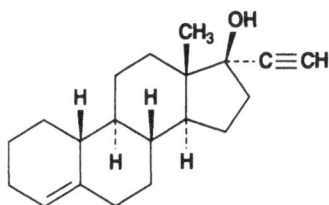

$C_{20}H_{28}O$ Relative molecular mass: 284.4

2.8.3   *Chemical and physical properties of the pure substance*
From Budavari (1996) and Reynolds (1998)
(*a*)   *Description*: White crystalline powder
(*b*)   *Melting-point*: 158–160°C
(*c*)   *Solubility*: Practically insoluble in water; freely soluble in chloroform; soluble in ethanol, acetone and diethyl ether
(*d*)   *Specific rotation*: $[\alpha]_D^{25}$, –13° (chloroform)

2.8.4   *Technical products and impurities*
Lynoestrenol is commercially available as a single-ingredient tablet and as a component of combination tablets containing ethinyloestradiol or mestranol (Kleinman, 1996; Editions du Vidal, 1997; Reynolds, 1998).

2.8.5   *Analysis*
Several international pharmacopoeias specify infra-red absorption spectrophotometry with comparison to standards as the method for identifying lynoestrenol; potentiometric titration with sodium hydroxide is used to assay its purity (British Pharmacopoeial Commission, 1993; Schweizerischen Bundesrat, 1996; Council of Europe, 1997).

2.8.6   *Production and use*
Lynoestrenol does not occur naturally. Synthesis of lynoestrenol was first reported in 1959 (de Winter *et al.*, 1959), by treatment of 19-nortestosterone with ethane-1,2-dithiol and boron trifluoride to give the 3-thioketal; treatment with sodium in liquid ammonia gives 17β-hydroxyoestr-4-ene, which by oxidation with chromic acid gives oestr-4-en-17-one. This can be converted to lynoestrenol by treatment with lithium acetylide or Grignard reagent. Whether this is the method used for commercial production is not known.

Information available in 1995 indicated that lynestrenol was manufactured or formulated in Argentina, Austria, Belgium, Brazil, France, Germany, Mexico, the Netherlands, South Africa, Spain and Switzerland (CIS Information Services, 1995).

Lynoestrenol is used primarily as a component of contraceptive tablets at a dose of 0.75–2.5 mg in conjunction with ethinyloestradiol. It is also used as a 'progestogen-only'

contraceptive. It can be used in the treatment of dysfunctional uterine bleeding and endometriosis (Kleinman, 1996; Reynolds, 1996).

2.9   Medroxyprogesterone acetate

2.9.1   *Nomenclature*

   Chem. Abstr. Serv. Reg. No.: 71-58-9

   Chem. Abstr. Name: (6α)-17-(Acetyloxy)-6-methylpregn-4-ene-3,20-dione

   IUPAC Systematic Name: 17-Hydroxy-6α-methylpregn-4-ene-3,20-dione, acetate

   Synonyms: 17α-Acetoxy-6α-methylprogesterone; depomedroxyprogesterone acetate;
   depo-progestin; depot-medroxyprogesterone acetate; DMPA; 17-hydroxy-6α-methyl-
   progesterone, acetate; 17α-hydroxy-6α-methylprogesterone acetate; MAP; medroxyprogesterone 17-acetate; 6α-methyl-17-acetoxyprogesterone; 6α-methyl-17α-
   hydroxyprogesterone acetate

2.9.2   *Structural and molecular formulae and relative molecular mass*

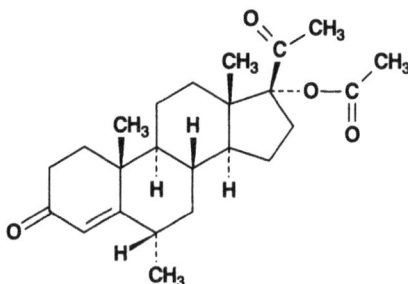

$C_{24}H_{34}O_4$ Relative molecular mass: 386.5

2.9.3   *Chemical and physical properties of the pure substance*

   From Budavari (1996) and Reynolds (1998)

   (*a*)   *Description*: White to off-white, odourless, crystalline powder

   (*b*)   *Melting-point*: 207–209.5°C

   (*c*)   *Solubility*: Practically insoluble in water; slightly soluble in diethyl ether;
            sparingly soluble in ethanol and methanol; soluble in acetone and dioxane;
            freely soluble in chloroform

   (*d*)   *Specific rotation*: $[\alpha]_D^{25}$, +61° (in chloroform)

2.9.4   *Technical products and impurities*

   Medroxyprogesterone acetate is commercially available as a single-ingredient tablet
and as combination tablets with conjugated oestrogens, oestradiol or oestradiol valerate,
and as sterile suspensions (Gennaro, 1995; Medical Economics, 1996; American Hospital
Formulary Service, 1997; British Medical Association, 1997; Editions du Vidal, 1997).

2.9.5 *Analysis*

Several international pharmacopoeias specify infra-red and ultra-violet absorption spectrophotometry with comparison to standards and thin-layer chromatography as methods for identifying medroxyprogesterone acetate; ultra-violet absorption spectrophotometry and liquid chromatography are used to assay its purity. Medroxyprogesterone acetate is identified in pharmaceutical preparations by infra-red absorption spectrophotometry and liquid chromatography; ultra-violet absorption spectrophotometry and liquid chromatography are used to assay for its content in these preparations (British Pharmacopoeial Commission, 1993; Secretaria de Salud, 1994; United States Pharmacopeial Convention, 1995; Council of Europe, 1997).

2.9.6 *Production and use*

Medroxyprogesterone acetate does not occur naturally. Its synthesis was first reported in 1958. The bisethylene acetal of 17α-hydroxyprogesterone was treated with peracetic acid to give a mixture of 5α,6α-epoxy-17α-hydroxypregnane-3,20-dione bisethylene acetal and the corresponding 5β,6β-epoxide. The 5α,6α-epoxide was refluxed with methylmagnesium bromide in tetrahydrofuran to afford the bisethylene acetal of 5α,17α-dihydroxy-6β-methylpregnane-3,20-dione. Dehydration by dilute sodium hydroxide in pyridine produced 6β-methyl-17α-hydroxyprogesterone which was epimerized in chloroform saturated with gaseous hydrogen chloride to 6α-methyl-17α-hydroxyprogesterone. Alternatively, dehydration and epimerization of 5α,17β-dihydroxy-6β-methylpregnane-3,20-dione bisethylene acetal could be effected directly with chloroform or hydrogen chloride. Acylation with acetic anhydride, acetic acid and *para*-toluenesulfonic acid produced medroxyprogesterone acetate (Babcock *et al.*, 1958)

Information available in 1995 indicated that medroxyprogesterone acetate is manufactured or formulated in Argentina, Australia, Belgium, Brazil, Canada, Denmark, Finland, France, Germany, Japan, Italy, Mexico, the Netherlands, New Zealand, Portugal, South Africa, Spain, Sweden, Switzerland, the United Kingdom and the United States (CIS Information Services, 1995).

For contraception, medroxyprogesterone acetate is given intramuscularly at a dose of 150 mg once every three months (depot medroxyprogesterone acetate). It is usually given within the first five days of the menstrual cycle (Reynolds, 1996).

Medroxyprogesterone acetate is used for post-menopausal hormonal therapy, for the treatment of dysfunctional uterine bleeding, secondary amenorrhoea and mild to moderate endometriosis. It is also used in the palliative treatment of some hormone-dependent malignant neoplasms, including breast, endometrial, renal and prostatic carcinoma (Reynolds, 1996).

Medroxyprogesterone acetate is also being explored as a means of oral contraception in men, given in combination with testosterone (Melo & Coutinho, 1977; Soufir *et al.*, 1983).

2.10   Megestrol acetate

2.10.1   *Nomenclature*

Chem. Abstr. Serv. Reg. No.: 595-33-5
Chem. Abstr. Name: 17-(Acetyloxy)-6-methylpregna-4,6-diene-3,20-dione
IUPAC Systematic Name: 17-Hydroxy-6-methylpregna-4,6-diene-3,20-dione, acetate
Synonyms: DMAP; megestryl acetate; MGA

2.10.2   *Structural and molecular formulae and relative molecular mass*

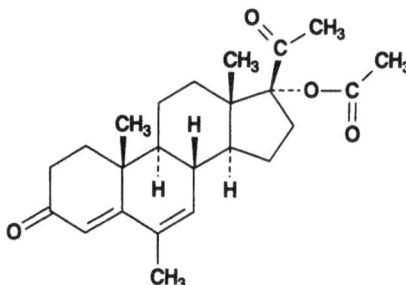

$C_{24}H_{32}O_4$ Relative molecular mass: 384.5

2.10.3   *Chemical and physical properties of the pure substance*

From Budavari (1996) and Reynolds (1998)

(a)   *Description*: White to creamy-white, odourless, crystalline powder
(b)   *Melting-point*: 214–216°C
(c)   *Solubility*: Practically insoluble in water (2 μg/mL at 37°C); very soluble in chloroform; soluble in acetone; slightly soluble in diethyl ether and fixed oils; sparingly soluble in ethanol
(d)   *Specific rotation*: $[\alpha]_D^{24}$, +5° (in chloroform)

2.10.4   *Technical products and impurities*

Megestrol acetate is commercially available as tablets and as an oral suspension (Medical Economics, 1996; Editions du Vidal, 1997; LINFO Läkemedelsinformation AB, 1997).

2.10.5   *Analysis*

The British and United States pharmacopoeias specify ultra-violet and infra-red absorption spectrophotometry with comparison to standards as methods for identifying megestrol acetate alone and in pharmaceutical preparations; ultra-violet absorption spectrophotometry and liquid chromatography are used to assay its purity (British Phar-macopoeial Commission, 1993; United States Pharmacopeial Convention, 1995).

2.10.6 *Production and use*

Megestrol acetate does not occur naturally. It was first synthesized in 1959 and is now prepared by oxidation of 17α-acetoxy-3β-hydroxy-6-methylpregn-5-en-20-one with aluminium *tert*-butoxide and *para*-quinone in dry benzene (Sittig, 1988).

Commercial production of megestrol acetate in the United States was first reported in 1976 (United States International Trade Commission, 1977). Information available in 1995 indicated that megestrol acetate was manufactured or formulated in Argentina, Australia, Belgium, Canada, Finland, France, Germany, Italy, the Netherlands, New Zealand, South Africa, Spain, Switzerland, the United Kingdom and the United States (CIS Information Services, 1995).

Megestrol acetate is used in a few countries as an oral contraceptive, usually in combination with ethinyloestradiol. It is not used as an oral contraceptive in the United States, and such usage was discontinued in the United Kingdom in 1975 (IARC, 1979). It is used for palliative treatment of carcinoma of the breast or endometrium, in the treatment of acne, hirsutism and sexual infantilism in females and in the treatment of anorexia and cachexia in patients with AIDS or cancer (IARC, 1979; Gennaro, 1995; Reynolds, 1996).

2.11   Norethisterone

2.11.1 *Nomenclature*

Chem. Abstr. Serv. Reg. No.: 68-22-4

Chem. Abstr. Name: (17α)-17-Hydroxy-19-norpregn-4-en-20-yn-3-one

IUPAC Systematic Name: 17-Hydroxy-19-nor-17α-pregn-4-en-20-yn-3-one

Synonyms: Ethinylnortestosterone; 17α-ethinyl-19-nortestosterone; ethynylnortestosterone; 17-ethynyl-19-nortestosterone; 17α-ethynyl-19-nortestosterone; norethindrone; norethisteron; norethynodrone; 19-nor-17α-ethynyltestosterone; norpregneninolone

2.11.2 *Structural and molecular formulae and relative molecular mass*

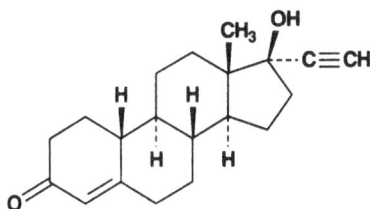

$C_{20}H_{26}O_2$ Relative molecular mass: 298.4

2.11.3 *Chemical and physical properties of the pure substance*

From Budavari (1996) and Reynolds (1998)

(*a*) *Description*: White or yellowish-white, odourless, crystalline powder

(*b*) *Melting-point*: 203–204°C

(c) *Solubility*: Practically insoluble in water; slightly to sparingly soluble in ethanol; slightly soluble in diethyl ether; soluble in chloroform and dioxane

(d) *Specific rotation*: $[\alpha]_D^{20}$, $-31.7°$

2.11.4 *Technical products and impurities*

Norethisterone is commercially available as single-ingredient tablets or as a component of combination tablets with ethinyloestradiol or mestranol (Morant & Ruppanner, 1991; Kleinman, 1996; Medical Economics, 1996; British Medical Association, 1997; Editions du Vidal, 1997).

2.11.5 *Analysis*

Several international pharmacopoeias specify infra-red and ultra-violet absorption spectrophotometry with comparison to standards and thin-layer chromatography as methods for identifying norethisterone; potentiometric titration, ultra-violet absorption spectrophotometry and thin-layer chromatography are used to assay its purity. Norethisterone is identified in pharmaceutical preparations by infra-red absorption spectrophotometry, thin-layer and liquid chromatography; potentiometric titration, ultra-violet absorption spectrophotometry and liquid chromatography are used to assay for norethisterone content (British Pharmacopoeial Commission, 1993; Secretaria de Salud, 1994, 1995; United States Pharmacopeial Convention, 1995; Schweizerischen Bundesrat, 1996; Society of the Japanese Pharmacopoeia, 1996; Council of Europe, 1997).

2.11.6 *Production and use*

Norethisterone does not occur naturally. A method for synthesizing norethisterone was first reported in 1954 (Djerassi *et al.*, 1954). It is prepared by reacting the methyl ester of oestrone with lithium metal in liquid ammonia to reduce ring A to the 4-ene state; the reduced product is oxidized with chromic acid in aqueous acetic acid to form oestr-4-ene-3,17-dione. In order to prevent the 3-keto group from participating in the ensuing ethynylation reaction, oestr-4-ene-3,17-dione is reacted with ethyl orthoformate in the presence of pyridine hydrochloride to form the 3-ethoxy-3,5-diene compound. Acetylene is passed into a solution of this compound in toluene, previously admixed with a solution of sodium in *tert*-amyl alcohol, to form the 17-ethynyl-17-hydroxy compound. Hydrolysis at the 3-ethoxy linkage by heating with dilute hydrochloric acid is accompanied by rearrangement of the 3-hydroxy-3,5-diene compound to the 3-oxo-4-ene compound.

Information available in 1995 indicated that norethisterone was manufactured or formulated in Australia, Brazil, Canada, France, Germany, India, Italy, Japan, Mexico, New Zealand, South Africa, Switzerland, the United Kingdom and the United States (CIS Information Services, 1995).

Norethisterone is used as an oral contraceptive alone or combined with mestranol or ethinyloestradiol in monophasic, biphasic and triphasic regimens (Kleinman, 1996).

It is also used to delay menstruation and in the treatment of amenorrhoea, dysfunctional uterine bleeding, premenstrual tension, dysmenorrhoea and endometriosis (Gennaro, 1995; Taitel & Kafrisse, 1995; Reynolds, 1996).

2.12 Norethisterone acetate

2.12.1 *Nomenclature*

Chem. Abstr. Serv. Reg. No.: 51-98-9

Chem. Abstr. Name: (17α)-17-(Acetyloxy)-19-norpregn-4-en-20-yn-3-one

IUPAC Systematic Name: 17-Hydroxy-19-nor-17α-pregn-4-en-20-yn-3-one, acetate

Synonyms: 17α-Ethinyl-19-nortestosterone 17β-acetate; 17α-ethinyl-19-nortestosterone acetate; 17α-ethynyl-19-nortestosterone acetate; norethindrone acetate; norethindrone 17-acetate; norethisteron acetate; norethisterone 17-acetate; 19-norethisterone acetate; norethynyltestosterone acetate; 19-norethynyltestosterone acetate; norethysterone acetate

2.12.2 *Structural and molecular formulae and relative molecular mass*

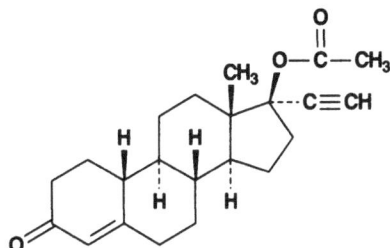

$C_{22}H_{28}O_3$ Relative molecular mass: 340.5

2.12.3 *Chemical and physical properties of the pure substance*

(*a*) *Description*: White or creamy-white, odourless, crystalline powder (Reynolds, 1998)

(*b*) *Melting-point*: 161–162°C (Budavari, 1996)

(*c*) *Solubility*: Practically insoluble in water (1 g in > 10 L); soluble in ethanol (1 g in 10 mL), chloroform (1 g in < 1 mL), dioxane (1 g in 2 mL) and diethyl ether (1 g in 18 mL) (Gennaro, 1995; Reynolds, 1998)

(*d*) *Specific rotation*: $[\alpha]_D^{25}$, –32° to –38° (United States Pharmacopeial Convention, 1995)

2.12.4 *Technical products and impurities*

Norethisterone acetate is commercially available as single-ingredient tablets or as a component of combination tablets with ethinyloestradiol. For post-menopausal hormonal therapy, norethisterone acetate is used in combination with oestradiol, oestradiol hemihydrate or oestriol. It is also available as a percutaneous patch with oestradiol (Morant &

Ruppanner, 1991; Kleinman, 1996; Medical Economics, 1996; British Medical Association, 1997; Editions du Vidal, 1997).

2.12.5 *Analysis*

Several international pharmacopoeias specify infra-red absorption spectrophotometry with comparison to standards and thin-layer chromatography as methods for identifying norethisterone acetate; potentiometric titration and ultra-violet absorption spectrophotometry are used to assay its purity. Norethisterone acetate is identified in pharmaceutical preparations by infra-red absorption spectrophotometry and thin-layer chromatography; ultra-violet absorption spectrophotometry is used to assay for norethisterone acetate content (British Pharmacopoeial Commission, 1993; United States Pharmacopeial Convention, 1995; Council of Europe, 1997).

2.12.6 *Production and use*

Norethisterone acetate does not occur naturally. In a method for synthesizing norethisterone acetate, first patented in 1957, it is acetylated with acetic anhydride in pyridine (IARC, 1979).

Information available in 1995 indicated that norethisterone acetate was manufactured or formulated in Argentina, Australia, Austria, Belgium, Brazil, Canada, Denmark, France, Germany, India, Mexico, New Zealand, Poland, Portugal, South Africa, Spain, Switzerland, the United Kingdom and the United States (CIS Information Services, 1995).

Norethisterone acetate is used in combination with ethinyloestradiol for oral contraception at doses of 0.5–2.5 mg norethisterone acetate and 20–50 µg ethinyloestradiol (Gennaro, 1995; Kleinman, 1996; Editions du Vidal, 1997). It is also used as a 'progestogen-only' contraceptive (Kleinman, 1996; Editions du Vidal, 1997) and in post-menopausal hormonal therapy, both as tablets and percutaneously by a patch (British Medical Association, 1997).

Norethisterone acetate is used in the treatment of primary and secondary amenorrhoea, dysfunctional uterine bleeding, endometriosis and inoperable malignant neoplasms of the breast (Reynolds, 1996; British Medical Association, 1997).

2.13   Norethisterone oenanthate

2.13.1 *Nomenclature*

Chem. Abstr. Serv. Reg. No.: 3836-23-5

Chem. Abstr. Name: (17α)-17-(Heptanoyl)-19-norpregn-4-en-20-yn-3-one

IUPAC Systematic Name: 17-Hydroxy-19-nor-17α-pregn-4-en-20-yn-3-one, heptanoate

Synonyms: Norethindrone enanthate; norethindrone oenanthate; norethisterone enanthate; norethisterone heptanoate; 17β-hydroxy-19-nor-17α-pregn-4-en-20-yn-3-one heptanoate

2.13.2   *Structural and molecular formulae and relative molecular mass*

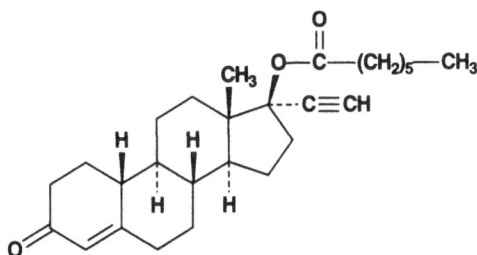

$C_{27}H_{38}O_3$ Relative molecular mass: 410.6

2.13.3   *Chemical and physical properties of the pure substance*
No information was available to the Working Group.

2.13.4   *Technical products and impurities*
Norethisterone oenanthate is available commercially in an oily solution for depot injection (Kleinman, 1996; Editions du Vidal, 1997).

2.13.5   *Analysis*
Norethisterone oenanthate is identified by thin-layer and liquid chromatography; liquid chromatography is used to assay its content (Secretaria de Salud, 1994).

2.13.6   *Production and use*
Norethisterone oenanthate does not occur naturally. It is probably synthesized by esterification with heptanoic acid.

Norethisterone oenanthate is used as a 'progestogen-only' contraceptive, mainly given intramuscularly at a dose of 200 mg once every two months, usually within the first five days of the menstrual cycle (Reynolds, 1996).

2.14   Norethynodrel
2.14.1   *Nomenclature*
Chem. Abstr. Serv. Reg. No.: 68-23-5
Chem. Abstr. Name: (17α)-17-Hydroxy-19-norpregn-5(10)-en-20-yn-3-one
IUPAC Systematic Name: 17-Hydroxy-19-nor-17α-pregn-5(10)-en-20-yn-3-one
Synonyms: Enidrel; noretynodrel

2.14.2   *Structural and molecular formulae and relative molecular mass*

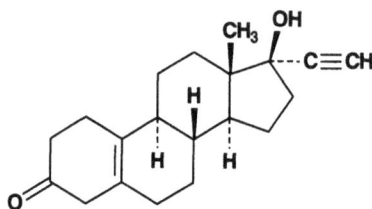

$C_{20}H_{26}O_2$ Relative molecular mass: 298.4

2.14.3   *Chemical and physical properties of the pure substance*
From Budavari (1996) and Reynolds (1998)
(a)   *Description*: White, odourless, crystalline powder
(b)   *Melting-point*: 169–170°C
(c)   *Solubility*: Very slightly soluble in water; freely soluble in chloroform; soluble in acetone; sparingly soluble in ethanol
(d)   *Optical rotation*: $[\alpha]_D^{25}$, +108° (in 1% chloroform)

2.14.4   *Technical products and impurities*
Norethynodrel was commercially available as a component of a combination tablet with mestranol (United States Food & Drug Administration, 1996).

2.14.5   *Analysis*
Several international pharmacopoeias specify infra-red absorption spectrophotometry with comparison to standards as the method for identifying norethynodrel; ultra-violet absorption spectrophotometry and potentiometric titration are used to assay its purity (British Pharmacopoeial Commission, 1980; United States Pharmacopeial Convention, 1995).

2.14.6   *Production and use*
Norethynodrel does not occur naturally. Synthesis of norethynodrel was first reported in 1954, in which oestradiol 3-methyl ether was reduced with lithium in liquid ammonia and the intermediate oxidized; ethynolation produced the 3-methyl ether of norethynodrel; treatment of this ether with acetic acid in methanol gave norethynodrel (Colton, 1954, 1955). Norethynodrel is now prepared by simultaneously saponifying and oxidizing dehydroepiandrosterone acetate by a series of reactions to 19-hydroxyandrost-6(6)-ene-3,17-dione. The hydroxymethyl group at the 10-position is then oxidized to carboxyl. The resulting acid is decarboxylated with simultaneous shifting of the double bond to give oestr-5(10)-ene-3,17-dione. Selective addition of acetylene at the expense of the 17-keto group yields norethynodrel (Gennaro, 1995).

Commercial production of norethynodrel was first begun in the United Kingdom in 1957 and in Japan and the United States in 1962. In 1960, the United States Food and Drug Administration licensed the first combined oral contraceptive pill, Enovid (norethynodrel and mestranol), which contained much higher doses of hormones than are now routinely used (Drill, 1966; McLaughlin, 1982). It was introduced in the United Kingdom two years later (Thorogood & Villard-Mackintosh, 1993). Enovid was voluntarily withdrawn from the United States market in July 1992.

Norethynodrel is also used in the treatment of dysfunctional bleeding and endometriosis (Reynolds, 1996).

2.15   Norgestimate

2.15.1   *Nomenclature*

Chem. Abstr. Serv. Reg. No.: 35189-28-7
Chem. Abstr. Name: (17α)-17-(Acetyloxy)-13-ethyl-18,19-dinorpregn-4-en-20-yn-3-one, 3-oxime
IUPAC Systematic Name: 13-Ethyl-17-hydroxy-18,19-dinor-17α-pregn-4-en-20-yn-3-one oxime acetate (ester)
Synonyms: 17α-Acetoxy-13-ethyl-17-ethynylgon-4-en-3-one oxime; dexnorgestrel acetime

2.15.2   *Structural and molecular formulae and relative molecular mass*

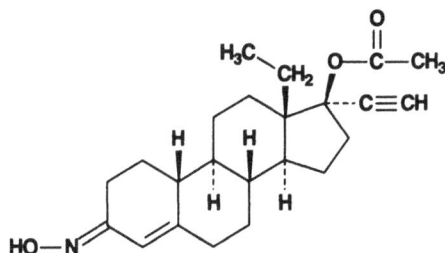

$C_{23}H_{31}NO_3$ Relative molecular mass: 369.5

2.15.3   *Chemical and physical properties of the pure substance*

From Budavari (1996)

(*a*)   *Description*: Crystals
(*b*)   *Melting-point*: 214–218°C
(*c*)   *Specific rotation*: $[\alpha]_D^{25}$, +110°

2.15.4   *Technical products and impurities*

Norgestimate is commercially available as a component of a combination tablet with ethinyloestradiol (Morant & Ruppanner, 1991; Kleinman, 1996; Medical Economics, 1996; British Medical Association, 1997; Editions du Vidal, 1997).

2.15.5   *Analysis*

Norgestimate can be separated and quantified in pharmaceutical preparations by high-performance liquid chromatography (Lane *et al.*, 1987).

2.15.6   *Production and use*

Norgestimate does not occur naturally. It can be prepared by pyrrolidine cyclo-condensation of the appropriate secoestranedione followed by conversion to the 3-oxime with hydroxylamine (Roussel-UCLAF, 1979).

Information available in 1995 indicated that norgestimate was produced in Canada, Germany, Mexico, Switzerland, the United Kingdom and the United States (CIS Information Services, 1995).

Norgestimate is a synthetic progestogen structurally related to levonorgestrel, with actions and uses similar to those described for the progestogens in general. It is used as the progestogenic component of combined oral contraceptives in tablets containing 0.18, 0.215 and 0.25 mg norgestimate plus 35 μg ethinyloestradiol for a triphasic regimen (Kleinman, 1996; Reynolds, 1998).

2.16   Norgestrel

2.16.1   *Nomenclature*

Chem. Abstr. Serv. Reg. No.: 6533-00-2

Chem. Abstr. Name: (17α)-dl-13-Ethyl-17-hydroxy-18,19-dinorpregn-4-en-20-yn-3-one

IUPAC Systematic Name: dl-13-Ethyl-17-hydroxy-18,19-dinor-17α-pregn-4-en-20-yn-3-one

Synonyms: (17α)-13-Ethyl-17-hydroxy-18,19-dinorpregn-4-en-20-yn-3-one; methyl-norethindrone; α-norgestrel; dl-norgestrel; DL-norgestrel

2.16.2   *Structural and molecular formulae and relative molecular mass*

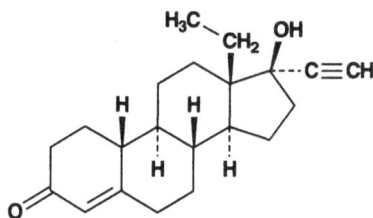

$C_{21}H_{28}O_2$ Relative molecular mass: 312.5

2.16.3   *Chemical and physical properties of the pure substance*

From Budavari (1996) and Reynolds (1998), unless otherwise specified

  (*a*)   *Description*: White, practically odourless crystalline powder

  (*b*)   *Boiling-point*: 205–207°C

  (*c*)   *Solubility*: Practically insoluble in water; slightly to sparingly soluble in ethanol; sparingly soluble in dichloromethane; freely soluble in chloroform

  (*d*)   *Optical rotation*: $[\alpha]_D^{25}$, –0.1° to +0.1° (United States Pharmacopeial Convention, 1995)

2.16.4   *Technical products and impurities*

Norgestrel is commercially available as a single-ingredient tablet and as a component of combination tablets with ethinyloestradiol, oestradiol valerate or conjugated oestrogens (Morant & Ruppanner, 1991; Kleinman, 1996; Medical Economics, 1996; British Medical Association, 1997; Editions du Vidal, 1997).

2.16.5   *Analysis*

Several international pharmacopoeias specify infra-red and ultra-violet absorption spectrophotometry with comparison to standards as methods for identifying norgestrel; potentiometric titration and ultra-violet absorption spectrophotometry are used to assay its purity. Norgestrel is identified in pharmaceutical preparations by ultra-violet absorption spectrophotometry and thin-layer chromatography; potentiometric titration and liquid chromatography are used to assay for norgestrel content in these preparations (United States Pharmacopeial Convention, 1995; Society of Japanese Pharmacopoeia, 1996; Council of Europe, 1997).

2.16.6   *Production and use*

Norgestrel does not occur naturally. It was first synthesized in 1963 (Smith *et al.*, 1963) and was first isolated as a racemic mixture of dl-13β-ethyl-17β-hydroxygon-4-en-3-one, which contains 50% of dextro- and levorotatory enantiomers (Edgren, 1963).

The activity of norgestrel is found in the levorotatory form of D-l-norgestrel or levo-norgestrel. In a representative chemical synthesis, 6-methoxy-α-tetralone is reacted with vinylmagnesium bromide, and the resulting 1,2,3,4-tetrahydro-6-methoxy-1-vinyl-1-naphthol is condensed with 2-ethyl-1,3-cyclopentanedione to form initially a tricyclic intermediate (secosteroid) containing all of the gonane skeleton carbon atoms. Cyclization of the secosteroid via dehydration yields a 13-ethylgona-1,3,5(10)-8,14-pentaene structure which is then successively reduced and ethynylated (Klimstra, 1969).

Information available in 1995 indicated that norgestrel was manufactured or formulated in Argentina, Austria, Belgium, Brazil, France, Germany, India, Japan, Mexico, the Netherlands, New Zealand, Portugal, South Africa, Spain, Swizerland, the United Kingdom and the United States (CIS Information Services, 1995).

Norgestrel is marketed as an oral contraceptive, both as a single entity and in combination with ethinyloestradiol. As a combination oral contraceptive, the dose is 0.25, 0.3 or 0.5 mg norgestrel plus 30 or 50 µg ethinyloestradiol per day (Kleinman, 1996). It is also marketed as a sequential preparation for post-menopausal hormonal therapy and has been used in combination with ethinyloestradiol to control menstrual disorders and endometriosis (Reynolds, 1996; British Medical Association, 1997).

2.17   Progesterone

2.17.1   *Nomenclature*

Chem. Abst. Services Reg. No.: 57-83-0

Chem. Abstr. Name: Pregn-4-ene-3,20-dione

Synonyms: Corpus luteum hormone; luteal hormone; luteine; luteohormone; Δ^4-pregnene-3,20-dione

2.17.2   *Structural and molecular formulae and relative molecular mass*

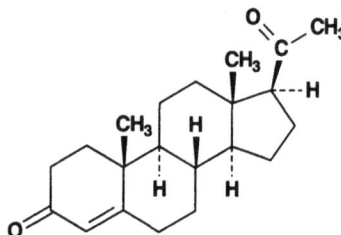

$C_{21}H_{30}O_2$ Relative molecular mass: 314.5

2.17.3   *Chemical and physical properties*

From Weast (1977) and Windholz (1976), unless otherwise specified

(a) *Description*: Exists in two readily interconvertible crystalline forms: the α form, in white orthorhombic prisms, and the β form, in white orthorhombic needles

(b) *Melting-point*: α form, 128.5–131°C; β form, 121–122°C

(c) *Optical rotation*: $[\alpha]_D^{20}$, α form, +192°; β form, +172° to +182° (in 2% w/v dioxane)

(d) *Solubility*: Practically insoluble in water; soluble in ethanol (1 in 8), arachis oil (1 in 60), chloroform (1 in < 1), diethyl ether (1 in 16), ethyl oleate (1 in 60) and light petroleum (1 in 100) (Wade, 1977); soluble in acetone, dioxane and concentrated sulfuric acid; sparingly soluble in vegetable oils

2.17.4   *Technical products and impurities*

Progesterone is available in an oily solution for injection, as pessaries or suppositories and as an intrauterine device (Reynolds, 1996; British Medical Association, 1997; Editions du Vidal, 1997).

2.17.5   *Analysis*

Several international pharmacopoeias specify infra-red absorption spectrophotometry with comparison to standards and thin-layer chromatography as methods for identifying progesterone; thin-layer chromatography is used to assay its purity. Ultra-violet absorption spectrophotometry and high-pressure liquid chromatography are used to assay the progesterone content in pharmaceutical preparations (British Pharmacopoeial Commission, 1988; United States Pharmacopeial Convention, 1990; Society of Japanese Pharmacopeia, 1996).

2.17.6   *Production and use*

Progesterone is a naturally occurring steroidal hormone found in a wide variety of tissues and biological fluids, including cow's milk. It has also been found in certain plant species (IARC, 1979).

Progesterone was isolated in 1929 from the corpora lutea of sows by Corner and Allen and was first synthesized by Butenandt and Schmidt in 1934 by heating 4β-bromo-5β-pregnane-3,20-dione with pyridine (IARC, 1979). Progesterone is produced commercially by (1) the degradation of diosgenin (obtained from the Mexican yam, *Dioscorea mexicana*) to pregnenolone, which is converted to progesterone by Oppenauer oxidation; or (2) the oxidation of stigmasterol (obtained from soya bean oil) to stigmastadienone, which undergoes further modifications to progesterone. Progesterone can also be produced from cholesterol as a starting material (Dorfman, 1966; Harvey, 1975).

Commercial production of progesterone in the United States was first reported in 1939, and that in the United Kingdom was first reported in 1950. Progesterone was first marketed commercially in Japan in 1954–55 (IARC, 1979).

Progesterone is used in human medicine for the treatment of secondary amenorrhoea and dysfunctional uterine bleeding, although progestational agents which are active orally are generally preferred to progesterone. Dosage regimens for the administration of progesterone as an intramuscular injection vary, depending on whether it is administered as an aqueous suspension or as an oily solution. Micronized progesterone can be given orally in a dose of 100–300 mg per day; however, it causes progestogenic side-effects, of which drowsiness is the most common (Reynolds, 1996).

Progesterone-delivering intrauterine devices are used for contraception. Like those containing levonorgestrel, they are also suitable for post-menopausal hormone therapy, but the fact that they must be changed each year may diminish compliance (Treiman *et al.*, 1995; Reynolds, 1996).

2.18   Regulations and guidelines

Concern about an enhanced risk for thrombosis related to use of desogestrel and gestodene in comparison with other oral contraceptives resulted in various responses from national authorities in Europe and New Zealand, although no action has been taken in some other countries (Griffin, 1996).

Chlormadinone acetate was removed from the market in the United Kingdom and the United States in 1970 (IARC, 1979). Ethynodiol diacetate is also no longer used in the United States (United States Food & Drug Administration, 1996). Megestrol has not been used as an oral contraceptive in the United Kingdom since 1975 and is not used in the United States (Wade, 1977). Norethynodrel as part of an oral contraceptive with mestranol (Enovid) was withdrawn from the United States market in July 1992.

The only guidelines that could be found for use of progestogens are those in national and international pharmacopoeias (Secretariat de Salud, 1994, 1995; United States Pharmacopeial Convention, 1995; Reynolds, 1996; Society of Japanese Pharmacopoeia, 1996; Council of Europe, 1997; Reynolds, 1998; Swiss Pharmaceutical Society, 1998).

3. References

American Hospital Formulary Service (1997) *AHFS Drug Information® 97*, Bethesda, MD, American Society of Health-System Pharmacists, pp. 2389, 2390, 2401–2408, 2472–2473

Babcock, J.C., Gutsell, E.S., Herr, M.E., Hogg, J.A., Stucki, J.C., Barnes, L.E. & Dulin, W.E. (1958) 6α-Methyl-17α-hydroxy-progesterone 17-acylates; a new class of potent progestins. *J. Am. chem. Soc.*, **80**, 2904–2905

Baier, H., Durner, G. & Quinkert, G. (1985) [Total synthesis of (–)-norgestrel.] *Helvet. chim. Acta*, **68**, 1054–1068 (in German)

Birkhaüser, M.H. & Haenggi, W. (1994) Benefits of different routes of administration. *Int. J. Fertil.*, **39** (Suppl. 1), 11–19

Bohlmann, R., Laurent, H., Hofmeister, H. & Weichert, R. (1989) *Preparation of Gestodene by a Novel Method*, German Patent issued to Schering AG, German Patent No. DE 3710728-1A

British Medical Association (1997) *British National Formulary*, No. 34, London, British Medical Association & The Pharmaceutical Press, pp. 313–353

British Pharmacopoeial Commission (1980) *British Pharmacopoeia 1980*, Vol. I, London, Her Majesty's Stationery Office, p. 310

British Pharmacopoeial Commission (1988) *British Pharmacopoeia 1988*, Vol. I, London, Her Majesty's Stationery Office, pp. 214, 361, 399–400, 468, 587

British Pharmacopoeial Commission (1993) *British Pharmacopoeia 1993*, Vol. I, London, Her Majesty's Stationery Office, pp. 263, 270, 382, 393, 406–408, 456–457, 1032–1033

British Pharmacopoeial Commission (1997) *British Pharmacopoeia 1993, Addendum 1997*, London, Her Majesty's Stationery Office, pp. 1971–1972

Brückner, K., Hampel, B. & Johnsen, U. (1961) [Synthesis and properties of monohalogenated 3-keto-$\Delta^{4,6}$-diene-steroids.] *Ber. Dtsch. chem. Ges.*, **94**, 1225–1240 (in German)

Budavari, S., ed. (1996) *The Merck Index*, 12th Ed., Whitehouse Station, NJ, Merck & Co., pp. 350–351, 469, 495, 587, 630–632, 637–638, 654, 749, 962, 988–990, 1010, 1149–1151

CIS Information Services (1995) *International Directory of Pharmaceutical Ingredients 1995/96 Edition*, Dallas, TX, pp. 204, 277, 283, 348–349, 376–378, 422, 546–547, 557, 605, 677–678, 746

Colton, F.B. (1954) Estradienes. *US Patent*, 2,691,028, 5 Oct. to G.D. Searle & Co. [*Chem. Abstr.*, **49**, 11729i]

Colton, F.B. (1955) 13-Methyl-17-ethynyl-17-hydroxy-1,2,3,4,6,7,8,9,11,12,13,14,16,17-tetradecahydro-15*H*-cyclopentaphenanthren-3-one. *US Patent*, 2,725,389, 29 Nov. to G.D. Searle & Co. [*Chem. Abstr.*, **50**, 9454f]

Cooper, A.J. (1986) Progestogens in the treatment of male sex offenders: A review. *Can. J. Psychiatr.*, **31**, 73–79

Corson, S.L. (1993) Clinical experiment with Systen, a new transdermal form of hormone replacement therapy. *Int. J. Fertil.*, **38** (Suppl. 1), 36–44

Council of Europe (1997) *European Pharmacopoeia*, 3rd Ed., Strasbourg, pp. 700–701, 815–817, 821–822, 1094–1095, 1112–1113, 1153–1154, 1162–1163, 1245–1249

Crook, D., Godsland, I.F., Hull, J. & Stevenson, J.C. (1997) Hormone replacement therapy with dydrogesterone and 17β-oestradiol: Effects on serum lipoproteins and glucose tolerance during 24 month follow up. *Br. J. Obstet. Gynaecol.*, **104**, 298–304

Djerassi, C., Miramontes, L., Rosenkranz, G. & Sondheimer, F. (1954) Steroids. LIV. Synthesis of 19-nor-17α-ethynyltestosterone and 19-nor-17α-methyltestosterone. *J. Am. chem. Soc.*, **76**, 4092–4094

Dorfman, R.I. (1966) Hormones (sex). In: Kirk, R.E. & Othmer, D.F., eds, *Encyclopedia of Chemical Technology*, 2nd Ed., Vol. II, New York, Wiley & Sons, pp. 122–124

Drill, V.A. (1966). *Oral Contraceptives*, New York, McGraw-Hill, pp. 6–7

Edgren, R.A., Smith, H., Hughes, G.A., Smith, L.L. & Greenspan, G. (1963) Biological effects of racemic and resolved 13-ethyl-4-gonen-3-ones. *Steroids*, **2**, 731–737

Editions du Vidal (1997) *Vidal*, 73rd Ed., Paris, OVP, pp. 359–361, 412–413, 452–453, 474–475, 509, 561–562, 758–759, 903–904, 983, 1014, 1016–1017, 1023, 1036, 1042–1043, 1045–1046, 1051–1052, 1071–1072, 1125–1126, 1166, 1214, 1290–1291, 1335, 1346–1347, 1352–1353, 1356–1357, 1558, 1695–1696, 1699–1700, 1747–1748

Ellerington, M.C., Whitcroft, S.I. & Whitehead, M.I. (1992) HRT: Developments in therapy. *Br. med. Bull.*, **48**, 401–425

Gennaro, A.R. (1995) *The Science and Practice of Pharmacy*, 19th Ed., Vol. II, Easton, PA, Mack Publishing Co., pp. 1089–1093, 1095–1097, 1099

Gordon, S.F. (1995) Clinical experience with a seven-day estradiol transdermal system for estrogen replacement therapy. *Am. J. Obstet. Gynecol.*, **173**, 998–1004

Griffin, J.P. (1996) Editorial—Third generation oral contraceptives containing desogestrel and gestodene and the risk of thrombosis. *Adverse Drug React. Toxicol. Rev.*, **15**, 5–7

Harvey, S.C. (1975) Hormones. In: Osol, A. et al., eds, *Remington's Pharmaceutical Sciences*, 15th Ed., Easton, PA, Mack, pp. 924–925

Hatcher, R.A., Rinckart, W., Blackburn, R. & Geller, J.S. (1997) *The Essentials of Contraceptive Technolology*, Baltimore, Population Information Program, Center for Communication Programs, The Johns Hopkins School of Public Health, pp. 5–23

Hirvonen, E., Stenman, U.H., Malkonen, M., Rasi, V., Vartiainen, E. & Ylostalo, P. (1988) New natural oestradiol/cyproterone acetate oral contraceptive for pre-menopausal women. *Maturitas*, **10**, 201–213

IARC (1979) *IARC Monographs on the Evaluation of the Carcinogenic Risk of Chemicals to Humans*, Vol. 21, *Sex Hormones (II)*, Lyon, pp. 257–278, 365–375, 431–439, 441–460, 491–515

Judd, H.L. (1994) Transdermal estradiol—A potentially improved method of hormone replacement. *J. reprod. Med.*, **39**, 343–352

Kleinman, R.L. (1996) *Directory of Hormonal Contraceptives*, London, IPPF Medical Publications

Klimstra, P.D. (1969) The role of progestin and estrogen in fertility control and maintenance. In: Chinn, L.J., Klimstra, P.D., Baran, J.S. & Pappo, R., eds, *The Chemistry and Biochemistry of Steroids*, Los Altos, CA, Geron-X, pp. 65–66

Lane, P.A., Mayberry, D.O. & Young, R.W. (1987) Determination of norgestimate and ethinyl estradiol in tablets by high-performance liquid chromatography. *J. pharm. Sci.*, **76**, 44–47

LINFO Läkemedelsinformation AB (1997) *FASS 1997 Läkemedel I Sverige*, Stockholm, pp. 336–338, 672, 721, 723–725, 827

McLaughlin, L. (1982) *The Pill, John Rock and the Church*, Toronto, Little, Brown & Co., pp. 138–145

Medical Economics (1996) *PDR®: Physicians' Desk Reference*, 50th Ed., Montvale, NJ, Medical Economics Data Production Co., pp. 699–702, 974–976, 1858–1865, 1872–1880, 2087–2093, 2428, 2602–2607, 2636–2637, 2746–2764, 2770–2772, 2787–2807

Melo, J.F. & Coutinho, E.M. (1977) Inhibition of spermatogenesis in men with monthly injections of medroxyprogesterone acetate and testosterone enanthate. *Contraception*, 15, 627–634

Meriggiola, M.C., Bremner, W.J., Paulsen, C.A., Valdiserri, A., Incorvaia, L., Motta, R., Pavani, A., Capelli, M. & Flamigni, C. (1996) A combined regimen of cyproterone acetate and testosterone enanthate as a potentially highly effective male contraceptive. *J. clin. Endocrinol. Metab.*, 81, 3018–3023

Moltz, L., Römmler, A., Post, K., Schwartz, U. & Hammerstein, J. (1980) Medium dose cyproterone acetate (CPA): Effects on hormone secretion and on spermatogenesis in men. *Contraception*, 21, 393–413

Morant, J. & Ruppanner, H., eds (1991) *Compendium Suisse des Medicaments* 1991, 12th Ed., Basel, Documed, pp. 38, 418–419, 521–523, 804, 985, 988–989, 1207–1208, 1439–1440, 1457–1458, 1711–1712, 1725–1726, 1901–1906, 2262–2263, 2452, 2462–2463

Namer, M. (1988) Clinical applications of antiandrogens. *J. Steroid Biochem.*, 31, 719–729

Neumann, F. & Topert, M. (1986) Pharmacology of antiandrogens. *J. Steroid Biochem.*, 25, 885–895

Notter, A. & Durand, P.M. (1969) Advantage of chlormadinone in threatened abortion. *Lyon méd.*, 221, 659–666 (in French)

Organizzazione Editoriale Medico Farmaceutica (1995) *L'Informatore Farmaceutico* (Part I), 55th Ed., Milan, OEMF, p. 46

Paganini-Hill, A. & Henderson, V.W. (1994) Estrogen deficiency and risk of Alzheimer's disease in women. *Am. J. Epidemiol.*, 140, 256–261

Reynolds, J.E.F., ed. (1996) *Martindale: The Extra Pharmacopoeia*, 31st Ed., London, The Pharmaceutical Press, pp. 1470–1510

Reynolds, J.E.F., ed. (1998) *Martindale, The Extra Pharmacopoeia* [Micromedex database CD-ROM]

Roland, M., Clyman, M., Decker, A. & Ober, W.B. (1966) Significance of dysmenorrhea in infertility. *Pac. med. Surg.*, 74, 135–138

Roussel-UCLAF (1979) Steroid oximes. *Japanese Patent issued to Roussel-UCLAF, France*, Patent No. JP54048750

Schweizerischen Bundesrat (1996) *Pharmacopea Helvetica*, 7th Ed., Bern, Eidgenössicher Departement des Innern

Secretaria de Salud (1994) *Farmacopea de los Estados Unidos Mexicanos (Pharmacopoeia of the Mexican United States)*, 6th Ed., Mexico City, Comision Permanente de la Farmacopea de los Estados Unidos Mexicanos, pp. 538–540, 543–544, 634–635, 640–641, 1006–1007, 1308–1312

Secretaria de Salud (1995) *Farmacopea de los Estados Unidos Mexicanos (Pharmacopoeia of the Mexican United States)*, 6th Ed., Suppl. 1, Mexico City, Comision Permanente de la Farmacopea de los Estados Unidos Mexicanos, pp. 1774–1775, 1896–1900

Sittig, M. (1988) *Pharmaceutical Manufacturing Encyclopedia*, 2nd Ed., Vols 1 and 2, Park Ridge, NJ, Noyes Publications, pp. 445, 588–589, 598–599, 922, 954–955, 1100–1101

Smith, H., Hughes, G.A., Douglas, G.H., Hartley, D., McLoughlin, B.J., Siddall, J.B., Wendt, G.R., Buzby, G.C., Jr, Herbst, D.R., Ledig, K.W., McMenamin, J.R., Pattison, T.W., Suida, J., Tokolics, J., Edgren, R.A., Jansen, A.B.A., Gadsby, B., Watson, D.H.R. & Phillips, P.C. (1963) Totally synthetic (+)-13-alkyl-3-hydroxy and methoxy-gona-1,3,5(10)-trien-17-ones and related compounds. *Experientia*, **19**, 394–396

Society of Japanese Pharmacopoeia (1996) *JP XIII The Japanese Pharmacopoeia*, 13th Ed., Tokyo, pp. 281, 371–375, 500, 536—539, 593–594

Soufir, J.-C., Jouannet, P., Marson, J. & Soumah, A. (1983) Reversible inhibition of sperm production and gonadotrophin secretion in men following combined oral medroxyprogesterone acetate and percutaneous testosterone treatment. *Acta endocrinol.*, **102**, 625–632

Sullivan, J.M. & Fowlkes, L.P. (1996) The clinical aspects of estrogen and the cardiovascular system. *Obstet. Gynecol.*, **87**, 36S–43S

Swiss Pharmaceutical Society, ed. (1998) *Index Nominum, International Drug Directory*, 16th Ed., Stuttgart, Medpharm Scientific Publishers [MicroMedex CD-ROM]

Taitel, H.F. & Kafrissen, M.E. (1995) Norethindrone—A review of therapeutic applications. *Int. J. Fertil. menopausal Stud.*, **40**, 207–223

Thomas, J., ed. (1991) *Prescription Products Guide*, 20th Ed., Vol. 1, Victoria, Australian Pharmaceutical Publishing Co. Ltd, pp. 719, 968–969, 1249, 1285

Thomas, J., ed. (1997) *Australian Prescription Products Guide*, 26th Ed., Vol. 1, Victoria, Australian Pharmaceutical Publishing Co. Ltd, pp. 1177, 1890–1891

Thorogood, M. & Villard-Mackintosh, L. (1993) Combined oral contraceptives: Risks and benefits. *Br. med. Bull.*, **49**, 124–139

Treiman, K., Liskin, L., Kols, A. & Ward, R. (1995) IUDs—An update. *Popul. Rep.*, **23**, 1–35

United States Food & Drug Administration (1996) *Approved Drug Products with Therapeutic Equivalence Evaluations*, 16th Ed., Washington DC, United States Department of Health and Human Services, pp. 3-124–3-125, 3-127, 3-378, 3-424

United States International Trade Commission (1977) *Synthetic Organic Chemicals, US Production and Sales, 1976* (USITC Publication 833), Washington DC, United States Government Printing Office, p. 149

United States Pharmacopeial Convention (1990) *The United States Pharmacopeia*, 22nd rev./*The National Formulary*, 17th rev., Rockville, MD, pp. 486–487, 1154–1156

United States Pharmacopeial Convention (1995) *The 1995 US Pharmacopeia*, 23rd rev./*The National Formulary*, 18th rev., Rockville, MD, pp. 622–633, 638, 880–882, 941–945, 963, 1098–1103, 1105–1106

United States Tariff Commission (1947) *Synthetic Organic Chemicals, US Production and Sales, 1945* (TC Publication 157), Second Series, Washington DC, United States Government Printing Office, p. 141

United States Tariff Commission (1956) *Synthetic Organic Chemicals, US Production and Sales, 1955* (TC Publication 198), Second Series, Washington DC, United States Government Printing Office, p. 112

Wade, A., ed. (1977) *Martindale, The Extra Pharmacopoeia*, 27th Ed., London, Pharmaceutical Press, pp. 1422–1424

Wang, C. & Yeung, K.K. (1980) Use of low-dosage oral cyproterone acetate as a male contraceptive. *Contraception*, **21**, 245–272

Weast, R.C., ed. (1977) *CRC Handbook of Chemistry and Physics*, 58th Ed., Cleveland, OH, Chemical Rubber Co., p. C-444

Williams, C.L. & Stancel, G.M. (1996) Estrogens and progestins. In: Wonsiewicz, M.J. & McCurdy, P., eds, *Goodman & Gilman's The Pharmacological Basis of Therapeutics*, 9th Ed., New York, McGraw-Hill, pp. 1411–1440

Windholz, M., ed. (1976) *The Merck Index*, 9th Ed., Rahway, NJ, Merck & Co., p. 1007

de Winter, M.S., Siegmann, C.M. & Szpilfogel, S.A. (1959) 17-Alkylated 3-deoxo-19-nortestosterones. *Chem. Ind.*, **11 July**, 905

Annex 2.
Preparations of oestrogens, progestogens and combinations of oestrogens and progestogens that are or have been used as hormonal contraceptives and for post-menopausal hormonal therapy, with known trade names

Table 1. Some combinations of oestrogens and progestogens used in oral contraceptives, with known trade names

Combination		Progestogen	Dose (mg)	Trade names
Oestrogen	Dose (µg)			
Ethinyloestradiol				
Biphasic	50	Chlormadinone acetate	1/2	Neo-Eunomin
Monophasic	35	Cyproterone acetate	2	Diane, Diane-35, Diane-Mite, Diane Nova, Dianette, Gynofen 35
Monophasic	20	Desogestrel	0.15	Cycléane-20, Lovelle, Marvelon 20, Mercilon, Microdosis, Myralon, Securgin, Segurin
Monophasic	30	Desogestrel	0.15	Cycléane-30, Desogen, Desolett, Frilavon, Marvelon, Marvelon 30, Marviol, Microdiol, Novelon, Ortho-Cept, Planum, Practil, Prevenon, Varnoline
Biphasic	40/30	Desogestrel	0.025/0.125	Gracial
Biphasic	50	Desogestrel	0/0.125	Ovidol, Oviol
Triphasic	35/30	Desogestrel	0.05/0.1/0.15	Trimiron
Monophasic	30	Dienogest	2	Valette
Monophasic	20	Gestodene	0.075	Harmonet, Meliane
Monophasic	30	Gestodene	0.075	Ciclomex, Evacin, Femodeen, Femoden, Femodene, Femovan, Ginera, Ginoden, Gynera, Gynovin, Minulet, Minulette, Moneva, Myvlar
Triphasic	30/40/30	Gestodene	0.05/0.07/0.1	Milvane, Phaeva, Triadene, Tricilomex, Tri-Femoden, Trigynera, Tri-Gynera, Trigynovin, Triminulet, Trioden, Triodeen, Triodena, Triodene
Monophasic	20	Levonorgestrel	0.1	Miranova
Monophasic	30	Levonorgestrel	0.125	Minisiston, Monostep

Table 1 (contd)

Combination			Trade names
Oestrogen	Dose (µg)	Progestogen	Dose (mg)	

Ethinyloestradiol (contd)

Combination	Dose (µg)	Progestogen	Dose (mg)	Trade names
Monophasic	30	Levonorgestrel	0.15	Ciclo, Ciclon, Combination 3, Contraceptive L.D., Duofem[a], Egogyn 30, Femigoa, Femranette mikro, Follimin, Gynatrol, Levlen, Levonorgestrel Pill, Levora, Lo-Femenal[a], Lo-Gentrol[a], Lo-Ovral[a], Lo/Ovral[a], Lo-Rondal[a], Lorsax, Mala D, Microgest, Microginon 30, Mycrogyn, Microgyn 30, Microgynon, Microgynon 30, Microgynon-30, Microvlar, Minibora, Minidril, Minigynon, Minigynon 30, Minivlar, MinOvral[a], Mithuri, Neo-Gentrol 150/30, Neomonovar, Neovletta, Nordet, Nordette, Nordette 150/30, Norgestrel Pill[a], Norgylene, Norvetal, Ologyn-micro, Ovoplex 30/150, Ovral L[a], Ovranet, Ovranette, Riget, Rigevidon, Sexcon, Stediril-30, Stediril-d 150/30, Stediril-M, Suginor
Monophasic	30	Levonorgestrel	0.25	Combination 5, Eugynon 30, Eugynon-30, Neogynon 30 MCG, Nordiol 30, Ovran 30, Primovlar-30
Monophasic	50	Levonorgestrel	0.125	Ediwal, Gravistat 125, Microgynon, Microgynon-50, Minigynon 50, Neo-Gentrol 125/50, Neostediril, Neo-Stediril, Nordette 50, Regunon, Stediril-50

Table 1 (contd)

Combination				
Oestrogen	Dose (µg)	Progestogen	Dose (mg)	Trade names
Ethinyloestradiol (contd)				
Monophasic	50	Levonorgestrel	0.25	Anfertil[a], Anulette[a], Anulit[a], Contraceptive H.D., Daphiron[a], Denoval, Denoval-Wyeth, D-Norginor, Duoluton, Duoluton L, Duotone, Dystrol, Eugynon[a], Eugynon-50[a], Eugynon 250, Evanor, Evanor-d, Follinett, Gentrol[a], Gravistat, Gravistat 250, Monovar, Neogentrol, Neo-Gentrol, Neo-Gentrol 250/50, Neogynon, Neogynona, Neo-Primovlar, Neovlar, Noral, Nordiol, Norginor, Normanor, Novogyn 21, Novogynon, Ologyn, Ovidon, Ovlar, Ovoplex, Ovral[a], Ovral 0.25, Ovran, Planovar[a], Primovlar[a], Primovlar-50, Stediril[a], Stediril-d
Biphasic	30/40	Levonorgestrel	0.15/0.2	Adepal, Adépal
Biphasic	50	Levonorgestrel	0.05/0.125	Anteovin, Binordiol, Biphasil, Bivlar, Duophasal, Normovlar, Perikursal, Prolorfin, Sekvilar, Sequilar, Sequilarum
Triphasic	30/40/30	Levonorgestrel	0.05/0.075/0.125	Fironetta, Levordiol, Logynon, Modutrol, Triagynon, Triciclor, Triette, Trigoa, Trigynon, Trikvilar, Tri-Levlen, Trinordiol, Trionetta, Triovlar, Triphasil, Triquilar, Tri-Regol, Trisiston, Tri-Stediril, Trolit
Triphasic	30/50/40	Levonorgestrel	0.05/0.05/0.125	Tristep
Monophasic	37.5	Lynoestrenol	0.75	Ginotex, Mini Pregnon, Ministat, Ovamezzo, Ovoresta M, Ovostat Micro, Restovar
Monophasic	40	Lynoestrenol	2	Ermonil, Yermonil
Monophasic	50	Lynoestrenol	1	Anacyclin, Lyndiol 1, Lyndiolett, Miniol, Noracyclin, Novostat, Ovoresta, Ovostat, Pregnon

Table 1 (contd)

Ethinyloestradiol (contd)

| Combination | | | | Trade names |
Oestrogen	Dose (µg)	Progestogen	Dose (mg)	
Monophasic	50	Lynoestrenol	2.5	Lindiol, Lindiol 2.5, Lyndiol, Lyndiol 2.5, Lyn-ratiopharm, Minilyn, Neo-Lyndiol, Ovariostat, Sukhi
Biphasic	50	Lynoestrenol	0/1.0	Fysioquens, Normofasico, Normophasic, Physiostat
Biphasic		Lynoestrenol	0/2.5	Lyn-radiopharm Sequenz, Ovanon
Monophasic	35	Megestrol acetate	1	No 2 Oral Pill
Monophasic	30	Norethisterone	0.5	Conceplan M, Sinovula mikro
Monophasic	35	Norethisterone	0.4	Micropil, Norquen, Ovcon 35, Oviprem
Monophasic	35	Norethisterone	0.5	Brevicon, Brevinor, Genora 0.5/35, Gynex 0.5/35 E, Intercon 5/35, Mikro Plan, Modicon, Nelova 0.5/35 E, Nilocan, Norminest, Orthonett Novum, Ovacon, Ovysmen 0.5/35, Perle LD
Monophasic		Norethisterone	0.6	No 1 Oral Pill
Monophasic		Norethisterone	1	Brevicon 1, Brevinor-1, Genora 1/35, Gynex 1/35 E, Intercon 1/35, Kanchan, Nelova 1+35 E, Neocon, Norcept-E 1/35, Norimin, Norimin-1, Norinyl 1/35, Norquest, Ortho Novum 1/35, Ovysmen 1/35, Secure
Monophasic	50	Norethisterone	1	Anovulatorio MK, Apranax, Arona, Non-Ovlon, Norlesterire, Ovcon 50, Syntracept
Biphasic	35	Norethisterone	0.5/1	Binovum, Jenest, Nelova 10/11, Ortho Novum 10/11
Triphasic	35	Norethisterone	0.5/0.75/1.0	Ortho Novum 7/7/7, Triella, Trinovum
Triphasic		Norethisterone	0.5/1.0/0.5	Improvil, Synfase, Synphase, Tri-Norinyl
Monophasic	35	Norethisterone + megestrol acetate	0.3 + 0.5	No 0 Oral Pill
Monophasic	20	Norethisterone acetate	1	Loestrin, Loestrin 1/20, Loestrin 20, Minestril-20, Minestrin 1/20

Table 1 (contd)

Combination				Trade names
Oestrogen	Dose (μg)	Progestogen	Dose (mg)	
Ethinyloestradiol (contd)				
Monophasic	30	Norethisterone acetate	0.6	Neorlest
Monophasic	30	Norethisterone acetate	1	Econ 30, Econ Mite, Loestrin 30, Mala N, Trentovlane
Monophasic	30	Norethisterone acetate	1.5	Loestrin 1.5/30, Minestril-30
Monophasic	50	Norethisterone acetate	0.5	Loveston
Monophasic	50	Norethisterone acetate	1	Anovlar 1 mg, Anovlar-1 mg, Anovulatorio, Milli-Anovlar, Nodiol, Nonovlon, Non-Ovlon, Orlest, Prolestrin
Monophasic	50	Norethisterone acetate	2	Econ, Gynovlane
Monophasic	50	Norethisterone acetate	2.5	Norlestrin
Monophasic	50	Norethisterone acetate	3	Anovlar-3 mg, Gynovlar
Biphasic	30/40	Norethisterone acetate	1/2	Miniphase
Biphasic	50	Norethisterone acetate	0/5	Sequostat
			1/2	Gynophase, Sinovula
Monophasic	35	Norgestimate	0.25	Cilest, Effiprev, Effiprev 35, Ortho-Cyclen
Triphasic	35	Norgestimate	0.18/0.215/0.25	Ortho Tri-Cyclen, Pramino, Tricilest
Monophasic	50	Norgestrienone	2	Planor
Monophasic	50	Quingestanol acetate	0.5	Piloval

Table 1 (contd)

Combination				Trade names
Oestrogen	Dose (μg)	Progestogen	Dose (mg)	
Ethinyloestradiol sulfonate				
Biphasic	1/0 (mg)	Norethisterone acetate	0/5	Deposiston (weekly)
Mestranol				
Monophasic	50	Chlormadinone acetate	2	Femigen, Gestamestrol N, Lutestral
Monophasic	50	Ethynodiol diacetate	1	Angravid, Neo-Ovulen, Ovulen 50
Triphasic	30/40/30	Levonorgestrel	0.05/0.075/0.125	Tridestan
Monophasic	50	Norethisterone	1	Combiginor, Conceplan, Conlumin, Genora 1+50, Gulaf, Nelova 1/50 M, Norimin, Norinyl, Norinyl-1, Norinyl 1/50, Norit, Orthonett 1/50, Ortho Novin 1/50, Ortho Novum 1/50, Perle, Plan mite, Ultranovulance
Biphasic	50	Norethisterone	1/2	Norbiogest

From Kleinman (1996)

a Product containing norgestrel (levonorgestrel + dextronorgestrel)

Table 2. Some oral 'progestogen-only' contraceptives

Composition	Drug name	Dose (mg)	Countries in which available (not comprehensive)
Ethynodiol diacetate	Femulen	0.5	Australia, Ethiopia, Israel, South Africa, United Kingdom
Levonorgestrel	Follistrel	0.03	Sweden
	Microval	0.03	Australia, Belgium, Denmark, Ethiopia, Finland, France, Morocco, Romania, South Africa, Sudan, United Kingdom, Venezuela
	Microlut	0.03	Algeria, Australia, Belgium, Ethiopia, Germany, Ireland, Italy, Kenya, Mexico, Sudan, Switzerland, Tanzania, Thailand
	Microluton	0.03	Denmark, Finland, Norway
	Mikro-30 Wyeth	0.03	Germany
	Neogest[a]	0.0375	Czech Republic, Slovakia, United Kingdom
	Norgeal[a]	0.0375	Argentina
	Norgeston	0.03	United Kingdom
	Nortrel	0.03	Brazil
	Ovrette[a]	0.0375	Democratic Republic of Congo (Kinshasa), Nigeria, Russian Federation, United States
Lynoestrenol	Exlutena	0.5	Germany, Sweden, Switzerland
	Exluton	0.5	Algeria, Argentina, Belgium, Democratic Republic of Congo (Kinshasa), Ethiopia, Finland, France, Indonesia, Iran, Mexico, Netherlands, Nigeria, Portugal, Romania, Peru, South Africa, Thailand, Venezuela
	Exlutona	0.5	Denmark, Iceland, Norway
Norethisterone	Conludag	0.3	Norway
	Dianor	0.35	Mexico
	Gesta Plan	0.3	Denmark
	Locilan	0.35	Australia
	Micronor	0.35	Australia, Austria, Brazil, Canada, Germany, Ireland, Russian Federation, South Africa, Sudan, Switzerland, United Kingdom, United States
	Mini-Pe	0.3	Denmark, Sweden

Table 2 (contd)

Composition	Drug name	Dose (mg)	Countries in which available (not comprehensive)
Norethisterone (contd)	Mini-Pill	0.3	Finland
	Monogest	0.3	Czech Republic, Slovakia
	Noriday	0.35	Australia, Ireland, United Kingdom
	Nor-QD	0.35	United States
Norgestrienone	Ogyline	0.35	France

From Kleinman (1996)

[a] Product containing norgestrel (levonorgestrel and dextronorgestrel)

Table 3. Post-menopausal oestrogen-only hormonal therapy

Drug name	Route	Composition	Dose (mg)	Countries or regions in which available (not comprehensive)
Climaval	Oral	Oestradiol valerate	1 2	United Kingdom
Climara	Patch	Oestradiol	0.05[a] 0.1	Canada, much of Europe, New Zealand, Republic of Korea, South Africa, United States
Delestrogen	Injectable	Oestradiol valerate	10–40	Canada, United States
Estinyl	Oral	Ethinyloestradiol	0.02 0.05	Canada, United States
Estrace	Oral	Oestradiol	0.5 1.0 2.0	Brazil, Canada, United States
Estraderm Estraderm matrix Estraderm mx Estraderm TTS	Patch	Oestradiol	0.025[a] 0.05 0.1	Much of Asia, Australia, Canada, most of Europe, most of Latin America, Middle East, New Zealand, Scandinavia, South Africa, United States
Estratab	Oral	Esterified oestrogens	0.3 0.625 1.25 2.5	United States
Estrofem Estrofem Forte	Oral	Oestradiol (± oestriol)	2 (1) 4 (2)	Argentina, Austria, Belgium, Central America, Ecuador, Finland, France, Indonesia, Ireland, much of the Middle East, Netherlands, Philippines, Portugal, Poland, South Africa, Switzerland
Evex	Oral	Esterified oestrogens	0.625 1.25 2.5	United States
Evorel	Patch	Oestradiol	0.025[a] 0.05 0.075 0.1	Argentina, Germany, Ireland, Peru, Scandinavia, South Africa, United Kingdom

Table 3 (contd)

Drug name	Route	Composition	Dose (mg)	Countries or regions in which available (not comprehensive)
Fem 7/seven	Patch	Oestradiol	0.05[a]	Austria, Finland, Germany, Netherlands, Sweden, Switzerland, United Kingdom
Femogen	Oral	Esterified oestrogens	0.625 1.25 2.5	United States
FemPatch	Patch	Oestradiol	0.025[a]	Puerto Rico, United States
Harmogen	Oral	Oestrone	0.93	Ecuador, Netherlands, United Kingdom
Hormonin	Oral	Oestriol Oestrone Oestradiol	0.135/0.27 0.7/1.4 0.3/0.6	Canada, United Kingdom, United States
Menest	Oral	Esterified oestrogens	0.3 0.625 1.25 2.5	Canada, United States
Menorest	Patch	Oestradiol	0.037 0.05 0.075	Australia, Chile, Colombia, most of Europe, Singapore, Venezuela
Oestrogel	Gel	Oestradiol	0.75	Belgium, Egypt, Ireland, Israel, Malaysia, Singapore, Switzerland, Thailand, United Kingdom
Ogen	Oral	Oestropipate	0.75 1.5 3 6	Australia, Canada, Mexico, Venezuela, United States
Orthoest	Oral	Oestropipate	0.625 1.25	South Africa, United States
Østradiol-øestriol	Oral	Oestradiol Oestriol	1/2/4 0.5/1/2	Denmark
Ovestin	Oral	Oestriol	0.5 1 2	Denmark, Hong Kong (China), Malaysia, New Zealand, United Kingdom, United States

Table 3 (contd)

Drug name	Route	Composition	Dose (mg)	Countries or regions in which available (not comprehensive)
Premarin	Oral	Conjugated oestrogens	0.3 0.625 0.9 1.25 2.5	Australia, Canada, most of Europe, Japan, Latvia, South Africa, most of South America, United States
Progynova	Oral	Oestradiol valerate	1 2	Australia, most of Europe, Hong Kong (China), Israel, Malaysia, Philippines, Poland, Russian Federation, Singapore, South Africa
SK Estrogens	Oral	Esterified oestrogens	0.3 0.625 1.25 2.5	United States
Triovex	Oral	Oestriol	1	Sweden
Vallestril	Oral	Methallenestril	3 20	Canada, United States
Vivelle	Patch	Oestradiol	0.0375[a] 0.05 0.075 0.1	Canada, Puerto Rico, United States
Zeste	Oral	Esterified oestrogens	0.625 1.25 2.5	United States
Zumenon	Oral	Oestradiol	1 2	Austria, Belgium, Netherlands, United Kingdom

[a] Approximate dose per 24 h of use

Table 4. Combined oestrogen–androgen therapy

Drug name	Route	Oestrogen	Dose (mg)	Androgen	Dose (mg)	Countries or regions in which available (not comprehensive)
Climatone	Oral	Ethinyloestradiol	0.01	Methyltestosterone	5	United Kingdom
Estratest	Oral	Esterified oestrogens	0.625	Methyltestosterone	1.25	United States
			1.25		2.5	
Formatrix	Oral	Conjugated oestrogens	1.25	Methyltestosterone	10	United States
Gynetone	Oral	Ethinyloestradiol	0.02	Methyltestosterone	1.25	Canada, United States
			0.04		2.5	
Mixogen	Oral	Ethinyloestradiol	0.04	Methyltestosterone	3.6	Australia, South Africa, United Kingdom

Table 5. Post-menopausal oestrogen–progestogen therapy

Drug name	Route	Composition	Dose (mg)	Countries or regions in which available (not comprehensive)
Climagest	Oral	Oestradiol valerate (O)	1	United Kingdom
		Norethisterone (P)	2	
Cyclo-progynova	Oral	Oestradiol valerate (O)	1	Germany, Ireland, Netherlands, United Kingdom
		Levonorgestrel (P)	0.25	
		Oestradiol valerate (O)	2	
		Norgestrel (P)	0.5	
Divina	Oral	Oestradiol valerate (O)	2	Australia, Denmark, Finland, France, Greece, Morocco, Netherlands, New Zealand, Paraguay, Poland, Republic of Korea, South Africa, Sweden, Turkey
		Medroxyprogesterone acetate (P)	10	
Estracombi, Estracomb	Patch + oral	Oestradiol (O)	0.05[a]	Most of Europe, Hong Kong (China), Indonesia, Latin America, Malaysia, New Zealand, Philippines, Republic of Korea, Scandinavia, South Africa
		Norethisterone acetate (2 weeks) (P)	0.25[a]	
Estrapak	Patch + oral	Oestradiol (O)	0.05[a]	Australia, Ecuador, Ireland, Mexico, New Zealand, United Kingdom
		Norethisterone acetate (P)	0.1	
Femapak	Patch	Oestradiol (O)	0.04[a]	United Kingdom
			0.08[a]	
	Oral	Dydrogesterone (2 weeks) (P)	10	
Femoston	Oral	Oestradiol (O)	1	United Kingdom
			2	
		Dydrogesterone (P)	10	
Kliogest, Kliofem	Oral	Oestradiol (or oestriol) (O)	2 (1)	Australia, most of Europe, much of Latin America, Mexico, Morocco, New Zealand, Pakistan, South Africa, Taiwan, United States
		Norethisterone acetate (P)	1	
Livial	Oral	Tibolone[b]	2.5	Denmark, Italy, Netherlands, South Africa, United Kingdom

Table 5 (contd)

Drug name	Route	Composition	Dose (mg)	Countries or regions in which available (not comprehensive)
Menophase	Oral	Mestranol (O) Norethisterone (P)	0.0125–0.05 0.75–1.5	United Kingdom
Novafac	Oral	Conjugated oestrogens (O) Medroxyprogesterone acetate (P)	0.625 1.25 5 10	Much of Latin America
Nuvelle	Oral	Oestradiol valerate (O) Levonorgestrel (12 days) (P)	2 0.075	Denmark, Ireland, Italy, New Zealand, Portugal, Spain, United Kingdom
Premique	Oral	Conjugated oestrogens (O) Medroxyprogesterone acetate (P)	0.625 5	Ireland, United Kingdom
Prempak-C/Prempak	Oral	Conjugated oestrogens (O) Norgestrel/medrogestone (P)	0.625 1.25 0.15/0.5	Most of Europe, Egypt, Kuwait, Malaysia, Singapore, South Africa, United Arab Emirates
Premphase	Oral	Conjugated oestrogens (O) Medroxyprogesterone acetate (P)	0.625 5	Puerto Rico, United States
Prempro	Oral	Conjugated oestrogens (O) Medroxyprogesterone acetate (P)	0.625 2.5	Puerto Rico, United States
Tridestra	Oral	Oestradiol valerate (O) Medroxyprogesterone acetate (P)	2 20	United Kingdom
Trisequens, Triskevens	Oral	Oestradiol (O) Norethisterone acetate (P)	2/1 1	Australia, most of Europe, Indonesia, much of Latin America, Middle East, New Zealand, Pakistan, Philippines, Taiwan, United Kingdom
Trisequens Forte	Oral	Oestradiol (O) Norethisterone acetate (P)	4/1 1	Australia, Netherlands, United Kingdom

O, oestrogen; P, progestogen

[a] Approximate dose per 24 h of use

[b] Tibolone has both oestrogenic and progestogenic properties.

CUMULATIVE CROSS INDEX TO *IARC MONOGRAPHS ON THE EVALUATION OF CARCINOGENIC RISKS TO HUMANS*

The volume, page and year of publication are given. References to corrigenda are given in parentheses.

A

A-α-C	*40*, 245 (1986); *Suppl. 7*, 56 (1987)
Acetaldehyde	*36*, 101 (1985) (*corr. 42*, 263); *Suppl. 7*, 77 (1987); *71*, 319 (1999)
Acetaldehyde formylmethylhydrazone (*see* Gyromitrin)	
Acetamide	*7*, 197 (1974); *Suppl. 7*, 389 (1987); *71*, 1211 (1999)
Acetaminophen (*see* Paracetamol)	
Acridine orange	*16*, 145 (1978); *Suppl. 7*, 56 (1987)
Acriflavinium chloride	*13*, 31 (1977); *Suppl. 7*, 56 (1987)
Acrolein	*19*, 479 (1979); *36*, 133 (1985); *Suppl. 7*, 78 (1987); *63*, 337 (1995) (*corr. 65*, 549)
Acrylamide	*39*, 41 (1986); *Suppl. 7*, 56 (1987); *60*, 389 (1994)
Acrylic acid	*19*, 47 (1979); *Suppl. 7*, 56 (1987); *71*, 1223 (1999)
Acrylic fibres	*19*, 86 (1979); *Suppl. 7*, 56 (1987)
Acrylonitrile	*19*, 73 (1979); *Suppl. 7*, 79 (1987); *71*, 43 (1999)
Acrylonitrile-butadiene-styrene copolymers	*19*, 91 (1979); *Suppl. 7*, 56 (1987)
Actinolite (*see* Asbestos)	
Actinomycin D (*see also* Actinomycins)	*Suppl. 7*, 80 (1987)
Actinomycins	*10*, 29 (1976) (*corr. 42*, 255)
Adriamycin	*10*, 43 (1976); *Suppl. 7*, 82 (1987)
AF-2	*31*, 47 (1983); *Suppl. 7*, 56 (1987)
Aflatoxins	*1*, 145 (1972) (*corr. 42*, 251); *10*, 51 (1976); *Suppl. 7*, 83 (1987); *56*, 245 (1993)
Aflatoxin B₁ (*see* Aflatoxins)	
Aflatoxin B₂ (*see* Aflatoxins)	
Aflatoxin G₁ (*see* Aflatoxins)	
Aflatoxin G₂ (*see* Aflatoxins)	
Aflatoxin M₁ (*see* Aflatoxins)	
Agaritine	*31*, 63 (1983); *Suppl. 7*, 56 (1987)
Alcohol drinking	*44* (1988)
Aldicarb	*53*, 93 (1991)
Aldrin	*5*, 25 (1974); *Suppl. 7*, 88 (1987)
Allyl chloride	*36*, 39 (1985); *Suppl. 7*, 56 (1987); *71*, 1231 (1999)

Allyl isothiocyanate	*36*, 55 (1985); *Suppl. 7*, 56 (1987)
Allyl isovalerate	*36*, 69 (1985); *Suppl. 7*, 56 (1987); *71*, 1241 (1999)
Aluminium production	*34*, 37 (1984); *Suppl. 7*, 89 (1987)
Amaranth	*8*, 41 (1975); *Suppl. 7*, 56 (1987)
5-Aminoacenaphthene	*16*, 243 (1978); *Suppl. 7*, 56 (1987)
2-Aminoanthraquinone	*27*, 191 (1982); *Suppl. 7*, 56 (1987)
para-Aminoazobenzene	*8*, 53 (1975); *Suppl. 7*, 390 (1987)
ortho-Aminoazotoluene	*8*, 61 (1975) (*corr. 42*, 254); *Suppl. 7*, 56 (1987)
para-Aminobenzoic acid	*16*, 249 (1978); *Suppl. 7*, 56 (1987)
4-Aminobiphenyl	*1*, 74 (1972) (*corr. 42*, 251); *Suppl. 7*, 91 (1987)
2-Amino-3,4-dimethylimidazo[4,5-*f*]quinoline (*see* MeIQ)	
2-Amino-3,8-dimethylimidazo[4,5-*f*]quinoxaline (*see* MeIQx)	
3-Amino-1,4-dimethyl-5*H*-pyrido[4,3-*b*]indole (*see* Trp-P-1)	
2-Aminodipyrido[1,2-*a*:3′,2′-*d*]imidazole (*see* Glu-P-2)	
1-Amino-2-methylanthraquinone	*27*, 199 (1982); *Suppl. 7*, 57 (1987)
2-Amino-3-methylimidazo[4,5-*f*]quinoline (*see* IQ)	
2-Amino-6-methyldipyrido[1,2-*a*:3′,2′-*d*]imidazole (*see* Glu-P-1)	
2-Amino-1-methyl-6-phenylimidazo[4,5-*b*]pyridine (*see* PhIP)	
2-Amino-3-methyl-9*H*-pyrido[2,3-*b*]indole (*see* MeA-α-C)	
3-Amino-1-methyl-5*H*-pyrido[4,3-*b*]indole (*see* Trp-P-2)	
2-Amino-5-(5-nitro-2-furyl)-1,3,4-thiadiazole	*7*, 143 (1974); *Suppl. 7*, 57 (1987)
2-Amino-4-nitrophenol	*57*, 167 (1993)
2-Amino-5-nitrophenol	*57*, 177 (1993)
4-Amino-2-nitrophenol	*16*, 43 (1978); *Suppl. 7*, 57 (1987)
2-Amino-5-nitrothiazole	*31*, 71 (1983); *Suppl. 7*, 57 (1987)
2-Amino-9*H*-pyrido[2,3-*b*]indole (*see* A-α-C)	
11-Aminoundecanoic acid	*39*, 239 (1986); *Suppl. 7*, 57 (1987)
Amitrole	*7*, 31 (1974); *41*, 293 (1986) (*corr. 52*, 513; *Suppl. 7*, 92 (1987)
Ammonium potassium selenide (*see* Selenium and selenium compounds)	
Amorphous silica (*see also* Silica)	*42*, 39 (1987); *Suppl. 7*, 341 (1987); *68*, 41 (1997)
Amosite (*see* Asbestos)	
Ampicillin	*50*, 153 (1990)
Anabolic steroids (*see* Androgenic (anabolic) steroids)	
Anaesthetics, volatile	*11*, 285 (1976); *Suppl. 7*, 93 (1987)
Analgesic mixtures containing phenacetin (*see also* Phenacetin)	*Suppl. 7*, 310 (1987)
Androgenic (anabolic) steroids	*Suppl. 7*, 96 (1987)
Angelicin and some synthetic derivatives (*see also* Angelicins)	*40*, 291 (1986)
Angelicin plus ultraviolet radiation (*see also* Angelicin and some synthetic derivatives)	*Suppl. 7*, 57 (1987)
Angelicins	*Suppl. 7*, 57 (1987)
Aniline	*4*, 27 (1974) (*corr. 42*, 252); *27*, 39 (1982); *Suppl. 7*, 99 (1987)
ortho-Anisidine	*27*, 63 (1982); *Suppl. 7*, 57 (1987)
para-Anisidine	*27*, 65 (1982); *Suppl. 7*, 57 (1987)
Anthanthrene	*32*, 95 (1983); *Suppl. 7*, 57 (1987)
Anthophyllite (*see* Asbestos)	
Anthracene	*32*, 105 (1983); *Suppl. 7*, 57 (1987)
Anthranilic acid	*16*, 265 (1978); *Suppl. 7*, 57 (1987)
Antimony trioxide	*47*, 291 (1989)

B

Benzo[*b*]fluoranthene	*3*, 69 (1973); *32*, 147 (1983); *Suppl. 7*, 58 (1987)
Benzo[*j*]fluoranthene	*3*, 82 (1973); *32*, 155 (1983); *Suppl. 7*, 58 (1987)
Benzo[*k*]fluoranthene	*32*, 163 (1983); *Suppl. 7*, 58 (1987)
Benzo[*ghi*]fluoranthene	*32*, 171 (1983); *Suppl. 7*, 58 (1987)
Benzo[*a*]fluorene	*32*, 177 (1983); *Suppl. 7*, 58 (1987)
Benzo[*b*]fluorene	*32*, 183 (1983); *Suppl. 7*, 58 (1987)
Benzo[*c*]fluorene	*32*, 189 (1983); *Suppl. 7*, 58 (1987)
Benzofuran	*63*, 431 (1995)
Benzo[*ghi*]perylene	*32*, 195 (1983); *Suppl. 7*, 58 (1987)
Benzo[*c*]phenanthrene	*32*, 205 (1983); *Suppl. 7*, 58 (1987)
Benzo[*a*]pyrene	*3*, 91 (1973); *32*, 211 (1983) (*corr. 68*, 477); *Suppl. 7*, 58 (1987)
Benzo[*e*]pyrene	*3*, 137 (1973); *32*, 225 (1983); *Suppl. 7*, 58 (1987)
1,4-Benzoquinone (see *para*-Quinone)	
1,4-Benzoquinone dioxime	*29*, 185 (1982); *Suppl. 7*, 58 (1987); *71*, 1251 (1999)
Benzotrichloride (*see also* α-Chlorinated toluenes and benzoyl chloride)	*29*, 73 (1982); *Suppl. 7*, 148 (1987); *71*, 453 (1999)
Benzoyl chloride (*see also* α-Chlorinated toluenes and benzoyl chloride)	*29*, 83 (1982) (*corr. 42*, 261); *Suppl. 7*, 126 (1987); *71*, 453 (1999)
Benzoyl peroxide	*36*, 267 (1985); *Suppl. 7*, 58 (1987); *71*, 345 (1999)
Benzyl acetate	*40*, 109 (1986); *Suppl. 7*, 58 (1987); *71*, 1255 (1999)
Benzyl chloride (*see also* α-Chlorinated toluenes and benzoyl chloride)	*11*, 217 (1976) (*corr. 42*, 256); *29*, 49 (1982); *Suppl. 7*, 148 (1987); *71*, 453 (1999)
Benzyl violet 4B	*16*, 153 (1978); *Suppl. 7*, 58 (1987)
Bertrandite (*see* Beryllium and beryllium compounds)	
Beryllium and beryllium compounds	*1*, 17 (1972); *23*, 143 (1980) (*corr. 42*, 260); *Suppl. 7*, 127 (1987); *58*, 41 (1993)
Beryllium acetate (*see* Beryllium and beryllium compounds)	
Beryllium acetate, basic (*see* Beryllium and beryllium compounds)	
Beryllium-aluminium alloy (*see* Beryllium and beryllium compounds)	
Beryllium carbonate (*see* Beryllium and beryllium compounds)	
Beryllium chloride (*see* Beryllium and beryllium compounds)	
Beryllium-copper alloy (*see* Beryllium and beryllium compounds)	
Beryllium-copper-cobalt alloy (*see* Beryllium and beryllium compounds)	
Beryllium fluoride (*see* Beryllium and beryllium compounds)	
Beryllium hydroxide (*see* Beryllium and beryllium compounds)	
Beryllium-nickel alloy (*see* Beryllium and beryllium compounds)	
Beryllium oxide (*see* Beryllium and beryllium compounds)	
Beryllium phosphate (*see* Beryllium and beryllium compounds)	
Beryllium silicate (*see* Beryllium and beryllium compounds)	
Beryllium sulfate (*see* Beryllium and beryllium compounds)	
Beryl ore (*see* Beryllium and beryllium compounds)	
Betel quid	*37*, 141 (1985); *Suppl. 7*, 128 (1987)
Betel-quid chewing (*see* Betel quid)	
BHA (*see* Butylated hydroxyanisole)	
BHT (*see* Butylated hydroxytoluene)	

C

Cadmium oxide (*see* Cadmium and cadmium compounds)
Cadmium sulfate (*see* Cadmium and cadmium compounds)
Cadmium sulfide (*see* Cadmium and cadmium compounds)
Caffeic acid   *56*, 115 (1993)
Caffeine   *51*, 291 (1991)
Calcium arsenate (*see* Arsenic and arsenic compounds)
Calcium chromate (see Chromium and chromium compounds)
Calcium cyclamate (*see* Cyclamates)
Calcium saccharin (*see* Saccharin)
Cantharidin   *10*, 79 (1976); *Suppl. 7*, 59 (1987)
Caprolactam   *19*, 115 (1979) (*corr. 42*, 258);
                                                               39, 247 (1986) (*corr. 42*, 264);
                                                               Suppl. 7, 390 (1987); *71*, 383
                                                               (1999)
Captafol   *53*, 353 (1991)
Captan   *30*, 295 (1983); *Suppl. 7*, 59 (1987)
Carbaryl   *12*, 37 (1976); *Suppl. 7*, 59 (1987)
Carbazole   *32*, 239 (1983); *Suppl. 7*, 59
                                                               (1987); *71*, 1319 (1999)
3-Carbethoxypsoralen   *40*, 317 (1986); *Suppl. 7*, 59 (1987)
Carbon black   *3*, 22 (1973); *33*, 35 (1984);
                                                               Suppl. 7, 142 (1987); *65*, 149
                                                               (1996)
Carbon tetrachloride   *1*, 53 (1972); *20*, 371 (1979);
                                                               Suppl. 7, 143 (1987); *71*, 401
                                                               (1999)
Carmoisine   *8*, 83 (1975); *Suppl. 7*, 59 (1987)
Carpentry and joinery   *25*, 139 (1981); *Suppl. 7*, 378
                                                               (1987)
Carrageenan   *10*, 181 (1976) (*corr. 42*, 255); *31*,
                                                               79 (1983); *Suppl. 7*, 59 (1987)
Catechol   *15*, 155 (1977); *Suppl. 7*, 59
                                                               (1987); *71*, 433 (1999)
CCNU (*see* 1-(2-Chloroethyl)-3-cyclohexyl-1-nitrosourea)
Ceramic fibres (see Man-made mineral fibres)
Chemotherapy, combined, including alkylating agents (*see* MOPP and
    other combined chemotherapy including alkylating agents)
Chloral   *63*, 245 (1995)
Chloral hydrate   *63*, 245 (1995)
Chlorambucil   *9*, 125 (1975); *26*, 115 (1981);
                                                               Suppl. 7, 144 (1987)
Chloramphenicol   *10*, 85 (1976); *Suppl. 7*, 145
                                                               (1987); *50*, 169 (1990)
Chlordane (*see also* Chlordane/Heptachlor)   *20*, 45 (1979) (*corr. 42*, 258)
Chlordane/Heptachlor   *Suppl. 7*, 146 (1987); *53*, 115
                                                               (1991)
Chlordecone   *20*, 67 (1979); *Suppl. 7*, 59 (1987)
Chlordimeform   *30*, 61 (1983); *Suppl. 7*, 59 (1987)
Chlorendic acid   *48*, 45 (1990)
Chlorinated dibenzodioxins (other than TCDD) (*see also*
    Polychlorinated dibenzo-*para*-dioxins)   *15*, 41 (1977); *Suppl. 7*, 59 (1987)
Chlorinated drinking-water   *52*, 45 (1991)
Chlorinated paraffins   *48*, 55 (1990)

Ferbam   *12*, 121 (1976) (*corr. 42*, 256);
                                                               Suppl. 7, 63 (1987)
Ferric oxide   *1*, 29 (1972); *Suppl. 7*, 216 (1987)
Ferrochromium (*see* Chromium and chromium compounds)
Fluometuron   *30*, 245 (1983); *Suppl. 7*, 63 (1987)
Fluoranthene   *32*, 355 (1983); *Suppl. 7*, 63 (1987)
Fluorene   *32*, 365 (1983); *Suppl. 7*, 63 (1987)
Fluorescent lighting (exposure to) (*see* Ultraviolet radiation)
Fluorides (inorganic, used in drinking-water)   *27*, 237 (1982); *Suppl. 7*, 208
                                                               (1987)
5-Fluorouracil   *26*, 217 (1981); *Suppl. 7*, 210
                                                               (1987)
Fluorspar (*see* Fluorides)
Fluosilicic acid (*see* Fluorides)
Fluroxene (*see* Anaesthetics, volatile)
Formaldehyde   *29*, 345 (1982); *Suppl. 7*, 211
                                                               (1987); *62*, 217 (1995) (*corr. 65*,
                                                               549; *corr. 66*, 485)
2-(2-Formylhydrazino)-4-(5-nitro-2-furyl)thiazole   *7*, 151 (1974) (*corr. 42*, 253);
                                                               Suppl. 7, 63 (1987)
Frusemide (*see* Furosemide)
Fuel oils (heating oils)   *45*, 239 (1989) (*corr. 47*, 505)
Fumonisin B₁ (*see* Toxins derived from *Fusarium moniliforme*)
Fumonisin B₂ (*see* Toxins derived from *Fusarium moniliforme*)
Furan   *63*, 393 (1995)
Furazolidone   *31*, 141 (1983); *Suppl. 7*, 63 (1987)
Furfural   *63*, 409 (1995)
Furniture and cabinet-making   *25*, 99 (1981); *Suppl. 7*, 380 (1987)
Furosemide   *50*, 277 (1990)
2-(2-Furyl)-3-(5-nitro-2-furyl)acrylamide (*see* AF-2)
Fusarenon-X (*see* Toxins derived from *Fusarium graminearum*,
        F. culmorum and *F. crookwellense*)
Fusarenone-X (*see* Toxins derived from *Fusarium graminearum*,
        F. culmorum and *F. crookwellense*)
Fusarin C (*see* Toxins derived from *Fusarium moniliforme*)

G

Gasoline   *45*, 159 (1989) (*corr. 47*, 505)
Gasoline engine exhaust (*see* Diesel and gasoline engine exhausts)
Gemfibrozil   *66*, 427 (1996)
Glass fibres (*see* Man-made mineral fibres)
Glass manufacturing industry, occupational exposures in   *58*, 347 (1993)
Glasswool (*see* Man-made mineral fibres)
Glass filaments (*see* Man-made mineral fibres)
Glu-P-1   *40*, 223 (1986); *Suppl. 7*, 64 (1987)
Glu-P-2   *40*, 235 (1986); *Suppl. 7*, 64 (1987)
L-Glutamic acid, 5-[2-(4-hydroxymethyl)phenylhydrazide]
        (*see* Agaritine)
Glycidaldehyde   *11*, 175 (1976); *Suppl. 7*, 64
                                                               (1987); *71*, 1459 (1999)
Glycidyl ethers   *47*, 237 (1989); *71*, 1285, 1417,
                                                               1525, 1539 (1999)

Hydrochlorothiazide	*50*, 293 (1990)
Hydrogen peroxide	*36*, 285 (1985); *Suppl. 7*, 64 (1987); *71*, 671 (1999)
Hydroquinone	*15*, 155 (1977); *Suppl. 7*, 64 (1987); *71*, 691 (1999)
4-Hydroxyazobenzene	*8*, 157 (1975); *Suppl. 7*, 64 (1987)
17α-Hydroxyprogesterone caproate (*see also* Progestins)	*21*, 399 (1979) (*corr. 42*, 259)
8-Hydroxyquinoline	*13*, 101 (1977); *Suppl. 7*, 64 (1987)
8-Hydroxysenkirkine	*10*, 265 (1976); *Suppl. 7*, 64 (1987)
Hypochlorite salts	*52*, 159 (1991)

I

Indeno[1,2,3-*cd*]pyrene	*3*, 229 (1973); *32*, 373 (1983); *Suppl. 7*, 64 (1987)
Inorganic acids (*see* Sulfuric acid and other strong inorganic acids, occupational exposures to mists and vapours from)	
Insecticides, occupational exposures in spraying and application of	*53*, 45 (1991)
IQ	*40*, 261 (1986); *Suppl. 7*, 64 (1987); *56*, 165 (1993)
Iron and steel founding	*34*, 133 (1984); *Suppl. 7*, 224 (1987)
Iron-dextran complex	*2*, 161 (1973); *Suppl. 7*, 226 (1987)
Iron-dextrin complex	*2*, 161 (1973) (*corr. 42*, 252); *Suppl. 7*, 64 (1987)
Iron oxide (*see* Ferric oxide)	
Iron oxide, saccharated (*see* Saccharated iron oxide)	
Iron sorbitol-citric acid complex	*2*, 161 (1973); *Suppl. 7*, 64 (1987)
Isatidine	*10*, 269 (1976); *Suppl. 7*, 65 (1987)
Isoflurane (*see* Anaesthetics, volatile)	
Isoniazid (*see* Isonicotinic acid hydrazide)	
Isonicotinic acid hydrazide	*4*, 159 (1974); *Suppl. 7*, 227 (1987)
Isophosphamide	*26*, 237 (1981); *Suppl. 7*, 65 (1987)
Isoprene	*60*, 215 (1994); *71*, 1015 (1999)
Isopropanol	*15*, 223 (1977); *Suppl. 7*, 229 (1987); *71*, 1027 (1999)
Isopropanol manufacture (strong-acid process) (*see also* Isopropanol; Sulfuric acid and other strong inorganic acids, occupational exposures to mists and vapours from)	*Suppl. 7*, 229 (1987)
Isopropyl oils	*15*, 223 (1977); *Suppl. 7*, 229 (1987); *71*, 1483 (1999)
Isosafrole	*1*, 169 (1972); *10*, 232 (1976); *Suppl. 7*, 65 (1987)

J

Jacobine	*10*, 275 (1976); *Suppl. 7*, 65 (1987)
Jet fuel	*45*, 203 (1989)
Joinery (*see* Carpentry and joinery)	

Malathion	*30*, 103 (1983); *Suppl. 7*, 65 (1987)
Maleic hydrazide	*4*, 173 (1974) (*corr. 42*, 253);
	Suppl. 7, 65 (1987)
Malonaldehyde	*36*, 163 (1985); *Suppl. 7*, 65
	(1987); *71*, 1037 (1999)
Malondialdehyde (*see* Malonaldehyde)	
Maneb	*12*, 137 (1976); *Suppl. 7*, 65 (1987)
Man-made mineral fibres	*43*, 39 (1988)
Mannomustine	*9*, 157 (1975); *Suppl. 7*, 65 (1987)
Mate	*51*, 273 (1991)
MCPA (*see also* Chlorophenoxy herbicides; Chlorophenoxy	*30*, 255 (1983)
herbicides, occupational exposures to)	
MeA-α-C	*40*, 253 (1986); *Suppl. 7*, 65 (1987)
Medphalan	*9*, 168 (1975); *Suppl. 7*, 65 (1987)
Medroxyprogesterone acetate	*6*, 157 (1974); *21*, 417 (1979)
	(*corr. 42*, 259); *Suppl. 7*, 289
	(1987); *72*, 339 (1999)
Megestrol acetate	*Suppl. 7*, 293 (1987); *72*, 49 (1999)
MeIQ	*40*, 275 (1986); *Suppl. 7*, 65
	(1987); *56*, 197 (1993)
MeIQx	*40*, 283 (1986); *Suppl. 7*, 65 (1987)
	56, 211 (1993)
Melamine	*39*, 333 (1986); *Suppl. 7*, 65 (1987)
Melphalan	*9*, 167 (1975); *Suppl. 7*, 239 (1987)
6-Mercaptopurine	*26*, 249 (1981); *Suppl. 7*, 240
	(1987)
Mercuric chloride (*see* Mercury and mercury compounds)	
Mercury and mercury compounds	*58*, 239 (1993)
Merphalan	*9*, 169 (1975); *Suppl. 7*, 65 (1987)
Mestranol	*6*, 87 (1974); *21*, 257 (1979)
	(*corr. 42*, 259); *Suppl. 7*, 288
	(1987); *72*, 49 (1999)
Metabisulfites (*see* Sulfur dioxide and some sulfites, bisulfites	
and metabisulfites)	
Metallic mercury (*see* Mercury and mercury compounds)	
Methanearsonic acid, disodium salt (*see* Arsenic and arsenic compounds)	
Methanearsonic acid, monosodium salt (*see* Arsenic and arsenic	
compounds	
Methotrexate	*26*, 267 (1981); *Suppl. 7*, 241
	(1987)
Methoxsalen (*see* 8-Methoxypsoralen)	
Methoxychlor	*5*, 193 (1974); *20*, 259 (1979);
	Suppl. 7, 66 (1987)
Methoxyflurane (*see* Anaesthetics, volatile)	
5-Methoxypsoralen	*40*, 327 (1986); *Suppl. 7*, 242
	(1987)
8-Methoxypsoralen (*see also* 8-Methoxypsoralen plus ultraviolet	*24*, 101 (1980)
radiation)	
8-Methoxypsoralen plus ultraviolet radiation	*Suppl. 7*, 243 (1987)
Methyl acrylate	*19*, 52 (1979); *39*, 99 (1986);
	Suppl. 7, 66 (1987); *71*, 1489
	(1999)
5-Methylangelicin plus ultraviolet radiation (*see also* Angelicin	
and some synthetic derivatives)	*Suppl. 7*, 57 (1987)

Methyl selenac (*see also* Selenium and selenium compounds)   *12*, 161 (1976); *Suppl. 7*, 66 (1987)
Methylthiouracil   *7*, 53 (1974); *Suppl. 7*, 66 (1987)
Metronidazole   *13*, 113 (1977); *Suppl. 7*, 250
                                                                (1987)
Mineral oils   *3*, 30 (1973); *33*, 87 (1984)
                                                                (*corr. 42*, 262); *Suppl. 7*, 252
                                                                (1987)
Mirex   *5*, 203 (1974); *20*, 283 (1979)
                                                                (*corr. 42*, 258); *Suppl. 7*, 66 (1987)
Mists and vapours from sulfuric acid and other strong inorganic acids   *54*, 41 (1992)
Mitomycin C   *10*, 171 (1976); *Suppl. 7*, 67 (1987)
MNNG (*see N*-Methyl-*N′*-nitro-*N*-nitrosoguanidine)
MOCA (*see* 4,4′-Methylene bis(2-chloroaniline))
Modacrylic fibres   *19*, 86 (1979); *Suppl. 7*, 67 (1987)
Monocrotaline   *10*, 291 (1976); *Suppl. 7*, 67 (1987)
Monuron   *12*, 167 (1976); *Suppl. 7*, 67
                                                              (1987); *53*, 467 (1991)
MOPP and other combined chemotherapy including   *Suppl. 7*, 254 (1987)
    alkylating agents
Mordanite (*see* Zeolites)
Morpholine   *47*, 199 (1989); *71*, 1511 (1999)
5-(Morpholinomethyl)-3-[(5-nitrofurfurylidene)amino]-2-   *7*, 161 (1974); *Suppl. 7*, 67 (1987)
    oxazolidinone
Musk ambrette   *65*, 477 (1996)
Musk xylene   *65*, 477 (1996)
Mustard gas   *9*, 181 (1975) (*corr. 42*, 254);
                                                             Suppl. 7, 259 (1987)
Myleran (*see* 1,4-Butanediol dimethanesulfonate)

N

Nafenopin   *24*, 125 (1980); *Suppl. 7*, 67 (1987)
1,5-Naphthalenediamine   *27*, 127 (1982); *Suppl. 7*, 67 (1987)
1,5-Naphthalene diisocyanate   *19*, 311 (1979); *Suppl. 7*, 67
                                                             (1987); *71*, 1515 (1999)
1-Naphthylamine   *4*, 87 (1974) (*corr. 42*, 253);
                                                             Suppl. 7, 260 (1987)
2-Naphthylamine   *4*, 97 (1974); *Suppl. 7*, 261 (1987)
1-Naphthylthiourea   *30*, 347 (1983); *Suppl. 7*, 263
                                                             (1987)
Nickel acetate (*see* Nickel and nickel compounds)
Nickel ammonium sulfate (*see* Nickel and nickel compounds)
Nickel and nickel compounds   *2*, 126 (1973) (*corr. 42*, 252); *11*,
                                                             75 (1976); *Suppl. 7*, 264 (1987)
                                                             (*corr. 45*, 283); *49*, 257 (1990)
                                                             (*corr. 67*, 395)
Nickel carbonate (*see* Nickel and nickel compounds)
Nickel carbonyl (*see* Nickel and nickel compounds)
Nickel chloride (*see* Nickel and nickel compounds)
Nickel-gallium alloy (*see* Nickel and nickel compounds)
Nickel hydroxide (*see* Nickel and nickel compounds)
Nickelocene (*see* Nickel and nickel compounds)
Nickel oxide (*see* Nickel and nickel compounds)

N-Nitrosodi-*n*-propylamine	*17*, 177 (1978); *Suppl. 7*, 68 (1987)
N-Nitroso-*N*-ethylurea (*see N*-Ethyl-*N*-nitrosourea)	
N-Nitrosofolic acid	*17*, 217 (1978); *Suppl. 7*, 68 (1987)
N-Nitrosoguvacine	*37*, 263 (1985); *Suppl. 7*, 68 (1987)
N-Nitrosoguvacoline	*37*, 263 (1985); *Suppl. 7*, 68 (1987)
N-Nitrosohydroxyproline	*17*, 304 (1978); *Suppl. 7*, 68 (1987)
3-(*N*-Nitrosomethylamino)propionaldehyde	*37*, 263 (1985); *Suppl. 7*, 68 (1987)
3-(*N*-Nitrosomethylamino)propionitrile	*37*, 263 (1985); *Suppl. 7*, 68 (1987)
4-(*N*-Nitrosomethylamino)-4-(3-pyridyl)-1-butanal	*37*, 205 (1985); *Suppl. 7*, 68 (1987)
4-(*N*-Nitrosomethylamino)-1-(3-pyridyl)-1-butanone	*37*, 209 (1985); *Suppl. 7*, 68 (1987)
N-Nitrosomethylethylamine	*17*, 221 (1978); *Suppl. 7*, 68 (1987)
N-Nitroso-*N*-methylurea (*see N*-Methyl-*N*-nitrosourea)	
N-Nitroso-*N*-methylurethane (*see N*-Methyl-*N*-nitrosourethane)	
N-Nitrosomethylvinylamine	*17*, 257 (1978); *Suppl. 7*, 68 (1987)
N-Nitrosomorpholine	*17*, 263 (1978); *Suppl. 7*, 68 (1987)
N'-Nitrosonornicotine	*17*, 281 (1978); *37*, 241 (1985); *Suppl. 7*, 68 (1987)
N-Nitrosopiperidine	*17*, 287 (1978); *Suppl. 7*, 68 (1987)
N-Nitrosoproline	*17*, 303 (1978); *Suppl. 7*, 68 (1987)
N-Nitrosopyrrolidine	*17*, 313 (1978); *Suppl. 7*, 68 (1987)
N-Nitrososarcosine	*17*, 327 (1978); *Suppl. 7*, 68 (1987)
Nitrosoureas, chloroethyl (*see* Chloroethyl nitrosoureas)	
5-Nitro-*ortho*-toluidine	*48*, 169 (1990)
2-Nitrotoluene	*65*, 409 (1996)
3-Nitrotoluene	*65*, 409 (1996)
4-Nitrotoluene	*65*, 409 (1996)
Nitrous oxide (*see* Anaesthetics, volatile)	
Nitrovin	*31*, 185 (1983); *Suppl. 7*, 68 (1987)
Nivalenol (*see* Toxins derived from *Fusarium graminearum*, *F. culmorum* and *F. crookwellense*)	
NNA (*see* 4-(*N*-Nitrosomethylamino)-4-(3-pyridyl)-1-butanal)	
NNK (*see* 4-(*N*-Nitrosomethylamino)-1-(3-pyridyl)-1-butanone)	
Nonsteroidal oestrogens	*Suppl. 7*, 273 (1987)
Norethisterone	*6*, 179 (1974); *21*, 461 (1979); *Suppl. 7*, 294 (1987); *72*, 49 (1999)
Norethisterone acetate	*72*, 49 (1999)
Norethynodrel	*6*, 191 (1974); *21*, 461 (1979) (*corr. 42*, 259); *Suppl. 7*, 295 (1987); *72*, 49 (1999)
Norgestrel	*6*, 201 (1974); *21*, 479 (1979); *Suppl. 7*, 295 (1987); *72*, 49 (1999)
Nylon 6	*19*, 120 (1979); *Suppl. 7*, 68 (1987)

O

Ochratoxin A	*10*, 191 (1976); *31*, 191 (1983) (*corr. 42*, 262); *Suppl. 7*, 271 (1987); *56*, 489 (1993)
Oestradiol	*6*, 99 (1974); *21*, 279 (1979); *Suppl. 7*, 284 (1987); *72*, 399 (1999)
Oestradiol-17β (*see* Oestradiol)	

Propylene	*19*, 213 (1979); *Suppl. 7*, 71 (1987); *60*, 161 (1994)
Propyleneimine (*see* 2-Methylaziridine)	
Propylene oxide	*11*, 191 (1976); *36*, 227 (1985) (*corr. 42*, 263); *Suppl. 7*, 328 (1987); *60*, 181 (1994)
Propylthiouracil	*7*, 67 (1974); *Suppl. 7*, 329 (1987)
Ptaquiloside (*see also* Bracken fern)	*40*, 55 (1986); *Suppl. 7*, 71 (1987)
Pulp and paper manufacture	*25*, 157 (1981); *Suppl. 7*, 385 (1987)
Pyrene	*32*, 431 (1983); *Suppl. 7*, 71 (1987)
Pyrido[3,4-*c*]psoralen	*40*, 349 (1986); *Suppl. 7*, 71 (1987)
Pyrimethamine	*13*, 233 (1977); *Suppl. 7*, 71 (1987)
Pyrrolizidine alkaloids (*see* Hydroxysenkirkine; Isatidine; Jacobine; Lasiocarpine; Monocrotaline; Retrorsine; Riddelliine; Seneciphylline; Senkirkine)	

Q

Quartz (*see* Crystalline silica)	
Quercetin (*see also* Bracken fern)	*31*, 213 (1983); *Suppl. 7*, 71 (1987)
para-Quinone	*15*, 255 (1977); *Suppl. 7*, 71 (1987); *71*, 1245 (1999)
Quintozene	*5*, 211 (1974); *Suppl. 7*, 71 (1987)

R

Radon	*43*, 173 (1988) (*corr. 45*, 283)
Reserpine	*10*, 217 (1976); *24*, 211 (1980) (*corr. 42*, 260); *Suppl. 7*, 330 (1987)
Resorcinol	*15*, 155 (1977); *Suppl. 7*, 71 (1987); *71*, 1119 (1990)
Retrorsine	*10*, 303 (1976); *Suppl. 7*, 71 (1987)
Rhodamine B	*16*, 221 (1978); *Suppl. 7*, 71 (1987)
Rhodamine 6G	*16*, 233 (1978); *Suppl. 7*, 71 (1987)
Riddelliine	*10*, 313 (1976); *Suppl. 7*, 71 (1987)
Rifampicin	*24*, 243 (1980); *Suppl. 7*, 71 (1987)
Ripazepam	*66*, 157 (1996)
Rockwool (*see* Man-made mineral fibres)	
Rubber industry	*28* (1982) (*corr. 42*, 261); *Suppl. 7*, 332 (1987)
Rugulosin	*40*, 99 (1986); *Suppl. 7*, 71 (1987)

S

Saccharated iron oxide	*2*, 161 (1973); *Suppl. 7*, 71 (1987)
Saccharin	*22*, 111 (1980) (*corr. 42*, 259); *Suppl. 7*, 334 (1987)
Safrole	*1*, 169 (1972); *10*, 231 (1976); *Suppl. 7*, 71 (1987)

Stannous fluoride (*see* Fluorides)
Steel founding (*see* Iron and steel founding)
Sterigmatocystin   *1*, 175 (1972); *10*, 245 (1976);
                                                        Suppl. 7, 72 (1987)
Steroidal oestrogens   *Suppl. 7*, 280 (1987)
Streptozotocin   *4*, 221 (1974); *17*, 337 (1978);
                                                        Suppl. 7, 72 (1987)
Strobane® (*see* Terpene polychlorinates)
Strong-inorganic-acid mists containing sulfuric acid (*see* Mists and
        vapours from sulfuric acid and other strong inorganic acids)
Strontium chromate (*see* Chromium and chromium compounds)
Styrene   *19*, 231 (1979) (*corr. 42*, 258);
                                                        Suppl. 7, 345 (1987); *60*, 233
                                                        (1994) (*corr. 65*, 549)
Styrene-acrylonitrile-copolymers   *19*, 97 (1979); *Suppl. 7*, 72 (1987)
Styrene-butadiene copolymers   *19*, 252 (1979); *Suppl. 7*, 72 (1987)
Styrene-7,8-oxide   *11*, 201 (1976); *19*, 275 (1979);
                                                        36, 245 (1985); *Suppl. 7*, 72
                                                        (1987); *60*, 321 (1994)
Succinic anhydride   *15*, 265 (1977); *Suppl. 7*, 72 (1987)
Sudan I   *8*, 225 (1975); *Suppl. 7*, 72 (1987)
Sudan II   *8*, 233 (1975); *Suppl. 7*, 72 (1987)
Sudan III   *8*, 241 (1975); *Suppl. 7*, 72 (1987)
Sudan Brown RR   *8*, 249 (1975); *Suppl. 7*, 72 (1987)
Sudan Red 7B   *8*, 253 (1975); *Suppl. 7*, 72 (1987)
Sulfafurazole   *24*, 275 (1980); *Suppl. 7*, 347
                                                        (1987)
Sulfallate   *30*, 283 (1983); *Suppl. 7*, 72 (1987)
Sulfamethoxazole   *24*, 285 (1980); *Suppl. 7*, 348
                                                        (1987)
Sulfites (*see* Sulfur dioxide and some sulfites, bisulfites and metabisulfites)
Sulfur dioxide and some sulfites, bisulfites and metabisulfites   *54*, 131 (1992)
Sulfur mustard (*see* Mustard gas)
Sulfuric acid and other strong inorganic acids, occupational exposures   *54*, 41 (1992)
        to mists and vapours from
Sulfur trioxide   *54*, 121 (1992)
Sulphisoxazole (*see* Sulfafurazole)
Sunset Yellow FCF   *8*, 257 (1975); *Suppl. 7*, 72 (1987)
Symphytine   *31*, 239 (1983); *Suppl. 7*, 72 (1987)

T

2,4,5-T (*see also* Chlorophenoxy herbicides; Chlorophenoxy   *15*, 273 (1977)
        herbicides, occupational exposures to)
Talc   *42*, 185 (1987); *Suppl. 7*, 349
                                                        (1987)
Tamoxifen   *66*, 253 (1996)
Tannic acid   *10*, 253 (1976) (*corr. 42*, 255);
                                                        Suppl. 7, 72 (1987)
Tannins (*see* also Tannic acid)   *10*, 254 (1976); *Suppl. 7*, 72 (1987)
TCDD (*see* 2,3,7,8-Tetrachlorodibenzo-*para*-dioxin)
TDE (*see* DDT)
Tea   *51*, 207 (1991)

ortho-Toluidine	*16*, 349 (1978); *27*, 155 (1982) (*corr. 68*, 477); *Suppl. 7*, 362 (1987)
Toremifene	*66*, 367 (1996)
Toxaphene	*20*, 327 (1979); *Suppl. 7*, 72 (1987)
T-2 Toxin (*see* Toxins derived from *Fusarium sporotrichioides*)	
Toxins derived from *Fusarium graminearum, F. culmorum* and F. crookwellense	*11*, 169 (1976); *31*, 153, 279 (1983); *Suppl. 7*, 64, 74 (1987); *56*, 397 (1993)
Toxins derived from *Fusarium moniliforme*	*56*, 445 (1993)
Toxins derived from *Fusarium sporotrichioides*	*31*, 265 (1983); *Suppl. 7*, 73 (1987); *56*, 467 (1993)
Tremolite (*see* Asbestos)	
Treosulfan	*26*, 341 (1981); *Suppl. 7*, 363 (1987)
Triaziquone (*see* Tris(aziridinyl)-*para*-benzoquinone)	
Trichlorfon	*30*, 207 (1983); *Suppl. 7*, 73 (1987)
Trichlormethine	*9*, 229 (1975); *Suppl. 7*, 73 (1987); *50*, 143 (1990)
Trichloroacetic acid	*63*, 291 (1995) (*corr. 65*, 549)
Trichloroacetonitrile (*see also* Halogenated acetonitriles)	*71*, 1533 (1999)
1,1,1-Trichloroethane	*20*, 515 (1979); *Suppl. 7*, 73 (1987); *71*, 881 (1999)
1,1,2-Trichloroethane	*20*, 533 (1979); *Suppl. 7*, 73 (1987); *52*, 337 (1991); *71*, 1153 (1999)
Trichloroethylene	*11*, 263 (1976); *20*, 545 (1979); *Suppl. 7*, 364 (1987); *63*, 75 (1995) (*corr. 65*, 549)
2,4,5-Trichlorophenol (*see also* Chlorophenols; Chlorophenols occupational exposures to; Polychlorophenols and their sodium salts)	*20*, 349 (1979)
2,4,6-Trichlorophenol (*see also* Chlorophenols; Chlorophenols, occupational exposures to; Polychlorophenols and their sodium salts)	*20*, 349 (1979)
(2,4,5-Trichlorophenoxy)acetic acid (*see* 2,4,5-T)	
1,2,3-Trichloropropane	*63*, 223 (1995)
Trichlorotriethylamine-hydrochloride (*see* Trichlormethine)	
T₂-Trichothecene (*see* Toxins derived from *Fusarium sporotrichioides*)	
Tridymite (*see* Crystalline silica)	
Triethylene glycol diglycidyl ether	*11*, 209 (1976); *Suppl. 7*, 73 (1987); *71*, 1539 (1999)
Trifluralin	*53*, 515 (1991)
4,4′,6-Trimethylangelicin plus ultraviolet radiation (*see also* Angelicin and some synthetic derivatives)	*Suppl. 7*, 57 (1987)
2,4,5-Trimethylaniline	*27*, 177 (1982); *Suppl. 7*, 73 (1987)
2,4,6-Trimethylaniline	*27*, 178 (1982); *Suppl. 7*, 73 (1987)
4,5′,8-Trimethylpsoralen	*40*, 357 (1986); *Suppl. 7*, 366 (1987)
Trimustine hydrochloride (*see* Trichlormethine)	
2,4,6-Trinitrotoluene	*65*, 449 (1996)
Triphenylene	*32*, 447 (1983); *Suppl. 7*, 73 (1987)
Tris(aziridinyl)-*para*-benzoquinone	*9*, 67 (1975); *Suppl. 7*, 367 (1987)
Tris(1-aziridinyl)phosphine-oxide	*9*, 75 (1975); *Suppl. 7*, 73 (1987)
Tris(1-aziridinyl)phosphine-sulphide (*see* Thiotepa)	
2,4,6-Tris(1-aziridinyl)-*s*-triazine	*9*, 95 (1975); *Suppl. 7*, 73 (1987)

U

V

W

Welding	*49*, 447 (1990) (*corr. 52*, 513)
Wollastonite	*42*, 145 (1987); *Suppl. 7*, 377 (1987); *68*, 283 (1997)
Wood dust	*62*, 35 (1995)
Wood industries	*25* (1981); *Suppl. 7*, 378 (1987)

X

Xylenes	*47*, 125 (1989); *71*, 1189 (1999)
2,4-Xylidine	*16*, 367 (1978); *Suppl. 7*, 74 (1987)
2,5-Xylidine	*16*, 377 (1978); *Suppl. 7*, 74 (1987)
2,6-Xylidine (*see* 2,6-Dimethylaniline)	

Y

Yellow AB	*8*, 279 (1975); *Suppl. 7*, 74 (1987)
Yellow OB	*8*, 287 (1975); *Suppl. 7*, 74 (1987)

Z

Zearalenone (*see* Toxins derived from *Fusarium graminearum*, *F. culmorum* and *F. crookwellense*)	
Zectran	*12*, 237 (1976); *Suppl. 7*, 74 (1987)
Zeolites other than erionite	*68*, 307 (1997)
Zinc beryllium silicate (*see* Beryllium and beryllium compounds)	
Zinc chromate (*see* Chromium and chromium compounds)	
Zinc chromate hydroxide (*see* Chromium and chromium compounds)	
Zinc potassium chromate (*see* Chromium and chromium compounds)	
Zinc yellow (*see* Chromium and chromium compounds)	
Zineb	*12*, 245 (1976); *Suppl. 7*, 74 (1987)
Ziram	*12*, 259 (1976); *Suppl. 7*, 74 (1987); *53, 423* (1991)

List of IARC Monographs on the Evaluation of Carcinogenic Risks to Humans*

Volume 1
Some Inorganic Substances, Chlorinated Hydrocarbons, Aromatic Amines, N-Nitroso Compounds, and Natural Products
1972; 184 pages (out-of-print)

Volume 2
Some Inorganic and Organo-metallic Compounds
1973; 181 pages (out-of-print)

Volume 3
Certain Polycyclic Aromatic Hydrocarbons and Heterocyclic Compounds
1973; 271 pages (out-of-print)

Volume 4
Some Aromatic Amines, Hydra-zine and Related Substances, N-Nitroso Compounds and Miscellaneous Alkylating Agents
1974; 286 pages (out-of-print)

Volume 5
Some Organochlorine Pesticides
1974; 241 pages (out-of-print)

Volume 6
Sex Hormones
1974; 243 pages (out-of-print)

Volume 7
Some Anti-Thyroid and Related Substances, Nitrofurans and Industrial Chemicals
1974; 326 pages (out-of-print)

Volume 8
Some Aromatic Azo Compounds
1975; 357 pages

Volume 9
Some Aziridines, N-, S- and O-Mustards and Selenium
1975; 268 pages

Volume 10
Some Naturally Occurring Substances
1976; 353 pages (out-of-print)

Volume 11
Cadmium, Nickel, Some Epoxides, Miscellaneous Industrial Chemicals and General Considerations on Volatile Anaesthetics
1976; 306 pages (out-of-print)

Volume 12
Some Carbamates, Thio-carbamates and Carbazides
1976; 282 pages (out-of-print)

Volume 13
Some Miscellaneous Pharmaceutical Substances
1977; 255 pages

Volume 14
Asbestos
1977; 106 pages (out-of-print)

Volume 15
Some Fumigants, the Herbicides 2,4-D and 2,4,5-T, Chlorinated Dibenzodioxins and Miscella-neous Industrial Chemicals
1977; 354 pages (out-of-print)

Volume 16
Some Aromatic Amines and Related Nitro Compounds—Hair Dyes, Colouring Agents and Miscellaneous Industrial Chemicals
1978; 400 pages

Volume 17
Some N-Nitroso Compounds
1978; 365 pages

Volume 18
Polychlorinated Biphenyls and Polybrominated Biphenyls
1978; 140 pages (out-of-print)

Volume 19
Some Monomers, Plastics and Synthetic Elastomers, and Acrolein
1979; 513 pages (out-of-print)

Volume 20
Some Halogenated Hydrocarbons
1979; 609 pages (out-of-print)

Volume 21
Sex Hormones (II)
1979; 583 pages

Volume 22
Some Non-Nutritive Sweetening Agents
1980; 208 pages

Volume 23
Some Metals and Metallic Compounds
1980; 438 pages (out-of-print)

Volume 24
Some Pharmaceutical Drugs
1980; 337 pages

Volume 25
Wood, Leather and Some Associated Industries
1981; 412 pages

Volume 26
Some Antineoplastic and Immunosuppressive Agents
1981; 411 pages

Volume 27
Some Aromatic Amines, Anthraquinones and Nitroso Compounds, and Inorganic Fluorides Used in Drinking-water and Dental Preparations
1982; 341 pages

Volume 28
The Rubber Industry
1982; 486 pages

Volume 29
Some Industrial Chemicals and Dyestuffs
1982; 416 pages

Volume 30
Miscellaneous Pesticides
1983; 424 pages

---

*Certain older volumes, marked out-of-print, are still available directly from IARCPress. Further, high-quality photo-copies of all out-of-print volumes may be purchased from University Microfilms International, 300 North Zeeb Road, Ann Arbor, MI 48106-1346, USA (Tel.: 313-761-4700, 800-521-0600).

All IARC publications are available directly from
IARCPress, 150 Cours Albert Thomas, F-69372 Lyon cedex 08, France
(Fax: +33 4 72 73 83 02; E-mail: press@iarc.fr).

IARC Monographs and Technical Reports are also available from the
World Health Organization Distribution and Sales, CH-1211 Geneva 27 (Fax: +41 22 791 4857)
and from WHO Sales Agents worldwide.

IARC Scientific Publications, IARC Handbooks and IARC CancerBases are also available from
Oxford University Press, Walton Street, Oxford, UK OX2 6DP (Fax: +44 1865 267782).

www.ingramcontent.com/pod-product-compliance
Lightning Source LLC
Chambersburg PA
CBHW081755200326
41597CB00023B/4031